INTRODUCTION TO CLINICAL NEUROSCIENCE

Second Edition

SIR JOHN WALTON

TD, MD, DSc, MA, FRCP, Dr de l'Univ (Hon) (Aix-Marseille),
Hon MD (Sheff), Hon DSc (Leeds and Leic), Hon FACP,
Hon FRCP (Edin), Hon FRCP (Canada),
Warden, Green College, Oxford
former Professor of Neurology, University of Newcastle upon Tyne
and Consultant Neurologist, Newcastle District Hospitals

Baillière Tindall
LONDON PHILADELPHIA TORONTO
SYDNEY TOKYO HONG KONG

Baillière Tindall:	24–28 Oval Road,
W. B. Saunders	Camden Town, London NW1

West Washington Square
Philadelphia, PA 19105, USA

1 Goldthorne Avenue
Toronto, Ontario M8Z 5T9, Canada

ABP Australia Ltd, 44 Waterloo Road
North Ryde, NSW 2064, Australia

Ichibancho Central Building, 22-1 Ichibancho
Chiyoda-ku, Tokyo 102, Japan

10/fl, Inter-Continental Plaza, 94 Granville Rd
Tsim Sha Tsui East, Kowloon, Hong Kong

© 1987 Baillière Tindall. All rights reserved. No part of this publication may be reproduced, stored in a retrieval system or transmitted, in any form or by any means, electronic, mechanical, photocopying or otherwise, without the prior permission of Baillière Tindall, 33 The Avenue, Eastbourne, East Sussex BN21 3UN, England

First published 1983
Second edition 1987

Typeset and printed in Great Britain by
Butler & Tanner Ltd, Frome and London

British Library Cataloguing in Publication Data

Walton, *Sir* John, *1922–*
   Introduction to clinical neuroscience.
   —2nd ed.
   1. Neurology
   I. Title
   616.8   RC346

ISBN 0 7020 1201 7

PREFACE TO THE FIRST EDITION

These chapters, intended to introduce the reader to clinical neuroscience, originally constituted the section on neurology (pages 1265–1565 inclusive) of *Pathophysiology: The Biological Principles of Disease* edited by Lloyd H. Smith Jr and Samuel O. Thier and published in 1981 by WB Saunders Company as Volume I of the International Textbook of Medicine.

One of the primary concepts underlying the planning of that volume was that the authors chosen would be clinicians who both teach and utilize pathophysiology in medical practice. The objective of each section was to describe the simpler scientific facts and principles relating to the structure and function of each of the bodily systems covered in order to introduce the reader to the ways in which such structure and function is often modified by disease. Now that a second edition of the International Textbook of Medicine is in the planning stage, its editors have concluded that the section on the pathophysiology of the nervous system in Volume I should be more closely integrated with, and should be prepared under the same authorship as, the section on clinical neurology which is to appear in Volume III. I am most grateful, therefore, to the volume editors and to the directors and staff of WB Saunders and of Baillière Tindall in the United Kingdom for their suggestion that the chapters which I prepared for the first edition of the International Textbook (dealing with the pathophysiology of the nervous system) should be re-published without modification in this format as a clinical introduction to neuroscience.

The content of the book is thus intended to be no more and no less than the title implies. It is neither a textbook of neuroanatomy nor one of neurophysiology, nor is it a comprehensive commentary upon neurobiology. The primary aim of these chapters is simply to provide for the medical student or practising doctor who already has some understanding of neurobiology a simple commentary upon nervous structure and function and upon the ways in which its dysfunction may be made manifest by the production of clinical symptoms and signs. Inevitably there are omissions, and equally inevitably some of the scientific concepts included are oversimplified. Nevertheless, I hope that this short volume will be found useful by many readers, not only within the medical profession, but also by those in the allied health care professions who have an interest in the nervous system and its diseases.

As I acknowledged in *Pathophysiology*, I drew extensively in preparing these chapters upon textual and illustrative material previously used by myself in *Essentials of Neurology*, 4th edition (Pitman Medical, 1975) and in *Brain's Diseases of the Nervous System*, 8th edition (Oxford University Press, 1977). I am particularly grateful to Mr Stephen Neal of Pitman Medical Publishing Company and to Mr Richard Charkin of Oxford University Press for permission to reproduce this material in these chapters. Some of it, with modification, has appeared in the 5th edition of *Essentials of Neurology* and other material also included in these chapters will appear in the 9th edition of *Brain's Diseases of the Nervous System*, which was published in 1985.

When I selected illustrations for these chapters, I also drew extensively upon *An Introduction to Basic Neurology* by Patton, Sundsten, Crill and Swanson, and *Fundamentals of Neurology* by Gardner (6th edition), both published by WB Saunders. I am especially pleased and grateful to acknowledge the willingness with which the authors of these books and the publishers agreed that I should be allowed complete freedom to reproduce any of the illustrations which had appeared. Several had been published in previous papers and monographs and the sources of these are quoted in the captions to the individual figures. Here again I wish to express my appreciation to the authors and publishers concerned for their permission to reproduce the material so identified.

Other illustrations have been derived from *Atlas of Neuropathology*, 2nd edition, by Blackwood, Dodds and Sommerville (Churchill Livingstone, 1964); *The Essentials of Neuroanatomy*, 2nd edition, by Mitchell (Churchill Livingstone, 1971); *The Anatomy of the Nervous System: Its Development and Function* by Ranson and Clark (WB Saunders, 1959); *Disorders of Peripheral Nerves* by Bradley (Blackwell Scientific, 1974); *A Physiological Approach to Clinical Neurology*, 2nd edition, by Lance and McLeod (Butterworth, 1975); *Gray's Anatomy*, 35th British edition, chapter by Warwick and Williams (Longman, 1973); *Textbook of Medical Physiology*, 5th edition, by Guyton (WB Saunders, 1976); *The Biochemical Basis of Neuropharmacology*, 2nd edition, by Cooper, Bloom and Roth (Oxford University Press, 1974); *Aids to the Examination of the Peripheral Nervous System* by the Medical Research Council (HMSO, 1976); *Scientific Approaches to Clinical Neurology*, edited by Goldensohn and Appel (Lea & Febiger, 1977); and *Scientific Foundations of Neurology*, edited by Critchley, O'Leary and Jennett (Heinemann, 1972). Here again, the authors and publishers of these works willingly gave permission for the reproduction of specific illustrations, and their kind agreement is acknowledged in the captions to the figures concerned. Similarly, wherever tables have been reproduced from original articles published in scientific journals, the original sources are indicated by footnotes, and the agreement of the authors, editors and publishers was obtained before this material was published in the International Textbook.

It will be noted that the US style of English as distinct from the British style has been adopted throughout this volume, as it was in the original publication from which these chapters are derived.

To all of those concerned, to Dr Barend ter Haar of Baillière Tindall and staff, and to my secretary, Rosemary Allan, who willingly shouldered the task of typing the original manuscript, I would like to express my gratitude.

JOHN WALTON

Newcastle upon Tyne
June 1983

PREFACE TO THE SECOND EDITION

Since this book first appeared, there have been so many exciting developments in neurobiology and in clinical neurology and their related disciplines that extensive revision has been needed. I am particularly grateful to those who reviewed the first edition, and especially for the very helpful comments made by Professor M. J. T. FitzGerald, author of *Neuroanatomy: Basic and Applied* published by Baillière Tindall, and Dr M. FitzGerald, who drew my attention to many important points relating to the presentation of anatomical and neurobiological material. And when I had provisionally completed my revision, my publishers helpfully obtained two further opinions from independent authorities working in neurophysiology whose comments also proved to be invaluable. In the light of all this advice and published reviews, the book has been completely updated and much new information has been included. This applies particularly to the sections on the physiology of the neuron, the structure and behaviour of biological membranes and excitable structures (including commentaries on sodium, potassium and calcium channels, and the patch and voltage clamp techniques of investigation), and receptors and neurotransmitters, to name but a few of the areas in neurobiology where there have been major developments. These advances have necessitated extensive additions and much rewriting. Similarly, major changes have been made in the chapters on the special senses in the light of new knowledge. And in those chapters with a greater clinical orientation, equally radical updating has been needed, not least in Chapters 10 and 11 where, respectively, new knowledge derived from neurochemical research on the one hand and the revolution in neuroimaging techniques resulting from computed tomography and nuclear magnetic resonance on the other has made substantial changes in emphasis obligatory. I hope therefore that, in consequence, this volume will be even more useful, as many reviewers of the first edition suggested, either for introducing the embryo clinician with a grounding in neurobiology to those pathophysiological principles so necessary to a full understanding of clinical neuroscience, or alternatively as a vehicle through which the busy physician, neurologist or neurosurgeon can update his knowledge of neurobiology by being presented with such information in that clinical context with which he is more familiar.

Not only am I most grateful to the reviewers, both known and anonymous, mentioned above, but also to Sir Roger Bannister and Mr John Manger of Oxford University Press for permission to reproduce seven CT scans and five NMR scans from the 6th edition of *Brain's Clinical Neurology*; to Professor M. J. T. FitzGerald for permission to include, again with acknowledgement indicated in the respective captions, a number of line drawings from *Neuroanatomy: Basic and Applied*; to Dr J. K. Aronson, clinical pharmacologist and Fellow of Green College, for his very helpful advice on Table 2; to Professor R. Fishman for permission to reproduce Table 15; to Dr R. D. Adams and Dr G. Lyon for their agreement to the reproduction of Table 12; to Drs D. O'Brian and S. Goodman for Table 13, and to Drs H. H. White and J. H. Menkes for Table 14. The last five items had been previously used by myself, with full permission and acknowledgement, in the 9th edition of *Brain's Diseases of the Nervous System* (Oxford University Press). Yet again, as in the first edition of this book, I have drawn upon some overlapping material previously published in that volume and in my *Essentials of Neurology*, 5th edition (Pitman Medical, now Churchill Livingstone); here again I wish to express my appreciation for permission to do so.

Whereas the first edition maintained American spelling and usage (see Preface to the First Edition, p. vi), for this extensively revised edition, British spelling and usage have been followed.

Finally, I also wish to thank my indefatigable secretary, Miss Rosemary Allan, whose unfailing help and support has been such that without her this revision would have been impossible, as well as Mr Nicholas Dunton and his staff at Baillière Tindall for the effective and efficient manner in which they have steered this second edition through the press.

JOHN WALTON
Oxford
November 1986

CONTENTS

Preface to the second edition   iii
Preface to the first edition   iv

1 Structure and Function of the Nervous System   1

Part 1: Units of structure and their functional characteristics: Introduction, 1; The neuron and its structure, 1; The neuroglia, 5; The neuron and its function, 6; Some neuropharmacological principles, 12; *Part 2: General morphology and organization:* Introduction, 19; The skull, spine and meninges, 20; Development and growth of the nervous system, 22; The blood supply of the brain and spinal cord, 26; The cerebrum, 33; The cerebellum, 38; The brain stem, 41; The spinal cord and ganglia, 46

2 Some General Principles of Value in Interpreting the Pathophysiology of the Nervous System   53

Introduction, 53; Some important pathophysiological influences, 53; Some pathophysiological foundations of neurological diagnosis, 54; Degeneration and regeneration in the nervous system, 55; Pathological reactions in the nervous system, 57; Constitution and heredity, 61; The approach to the patient, 62; The nosology of nervous system dysfunction, 62

3 Human Verbal Communication and Conceptual Aspects of Movement and Sensory Perception   72

Introduction, 72; The organization of speech, 72; Aphasia, 73; Dysarthria, 76; Palilia and echolalia, 77; Mutism, 77; Aphonia, 77; Speech disorders in childhood, 77; Apraxia, 78; Agnosia, 79; The body image, 79; Developmental apraxia and agnosia, 80; Disconnection syndromes, 80; Conclusions, 80

4 Consciousness and its Disorders   82

Introduction, 82; Sleep, 83; Stupor, 86; Coma, 86; Delirium and confusion, 90; Transient disorders of consciousness, 91

5 Behaviour, Memory, Intellect, Personality and their Disorders   99

Introduction, 99; The function of the diencephalon, 99; The limbic system: behavioural functions, 101; The limbic system and emotion, 101; Memory, 102; The functions of the frontal lobe, 104; Brain, mind and intellect, 104; Hallucinations and allied disorders of perception, 105; Abnormalities of memory, mood, intellect and personality, 106

6	**The Autonomic Nervous System and Hypothalamus**	112
	Introduction, 112; Anatomy and physiology, 112; Some common disorders of the autonomic nervous system, 121; Conclusions, 124	
7	**The Special Senses**	125
	Introduction, 125; Smell, 125; Taste, 126; Vision, 127; Hearing, 144; The vestibular system, 152	
8	**The Motor System**	158
	Introduction, 158; The organization of movement, 158; Weakness and paralysis, 172; Muscle 'tone' and its disorders, 174; Ataxia and incoordination, 178; The reflexes, 179; The clinical features of upper and lower motor neuron lesions, 180; Involuntary movements, 182; The pathophysiology of neuromuscular disease, 184; Conclusions, 192	
9	**The Sensory System**	194
	Introduction, 194; The anatomical and physiological organization of somatic sensation, 194; The pathophysiology and clinical significance of sensory abnormalities, 203; Pain, 205	
10	**Cerebral Metabolism and its Disorders**	213
	Introduction, 213; Some general principles, 213; The pathological substrate of cerebral metabolic disorders, 214; The biochemical substrate of cerebral metabolic disorders, 214; Other important disorders of cerebral metabolism, 224	
11	**The Cerebrospinal Fluid, Raised Intracranial Pressure, Brain Oedema, Craniocerebral and Spinal Trauma, Spinal Cord Compression and Relevant Investigations—Some Pathophysiological Principles**	238
	Introduction, 238; The cerebrospinal fluid (CSF), 238; Raised intracranial pressure—pathophysiology, 243; Craniocerebral trauma—pathophysiology, 248; The spinal cord—the pathophysiology of injury and compression, 252; Investigations in neurology—some general principles, 253	
	Index	273

1

STRUCTURE AND FUNCTION OF THE NERVOUS SYSTEM

Part 1: Units of structure and their functional characteristics

INTRODUCTION

The interpretation of the clinical manifestations of disease or dysfunction in the central or peripheral nervous system or in the voluntary muscles must be based upon a thorough understanding of their structure and function. The study of pathophysiological mechanisms is thus dependent upon a knowledge of anatomy, physiology, biochemistry and pharmacology, disciplines which when applied to the nervous system are generally grouped together as the basic neurosciences or neurobiology. The aim of the first two chapters in this book is to describe first the principal units of structure of the nervous system and some principles which govern their function, and then the general organization of the nervous system and of one of its principal effector organs, namely voluntary or skeletal muscle. An understanding of the structure and function of cells is a prerequisite to reading this chapter. The discussion here will therefore be confined to the highly specialized aspects of structure and function characteristic of the central nervous and neuromuscular systems.

THE NEURON AND ITS STRUCTURE

General morphology

The nerve cell or neuron is one of the few cells in the human body which, with the exception of the olfactory bipolar neurons, cannot be replaced once destroyed. No other neurons can divide or regenerate after the first few weeks of extrauterine life. Each neuron is a separate cell which consists of (a) a cell body or soma, (b) dendrites, which are processes extending only a short distance from the cell, and (c) an axon varying in length from a few millimetres to more than a metre. By means of nerve endings, axons make contact with dendrites or cell bodies of other neurons or with effector cells, such as muscle. Each embryonic neuron forms a single adult nerve cell. When axons and dendrites meet, there is a synaptic junction with structural discontinuity so that protoplasm never passes from one cell to another (even though *electrical* continuity does exist at some synapses). It follows that a process of degeneration in one nerve cell and its processes does not necessarily spread to other cells with which it is in synaptic contact. Nerve processes always arise by direct growth from parent cells and never by differentiation from intercellular material, a fact readily demonstrable in tissue culture.

The cell body or soma (Fig. 1.1) contains a nucleus of variable size which in turn contains a nucleolus. The cytoplasm of the soma is called the perikaryon. Neuronal mitochondria are especially concentrated in synaptic regions. Aggregates of ribosomes with rough endoplasmic reticulum form granules of so-called Nissl substance, which stains intensely with basic dyes and which may extend for a short distance into the dendrites but never into the axon hillock (from which the axon originates) or into the axon itself. Channels and cisternae of endoplasmic reticulum without attached ribosomes are also present

Figure 1.1 A, A multipolar neuron, as seen under the light microscope. B, A synapse. C, The neuron soma, as shown by light microscopy. [Reproduced from Patton et al (1976) *Introduction to Basic Neurology*, by kind permission of the authors and publisher.]

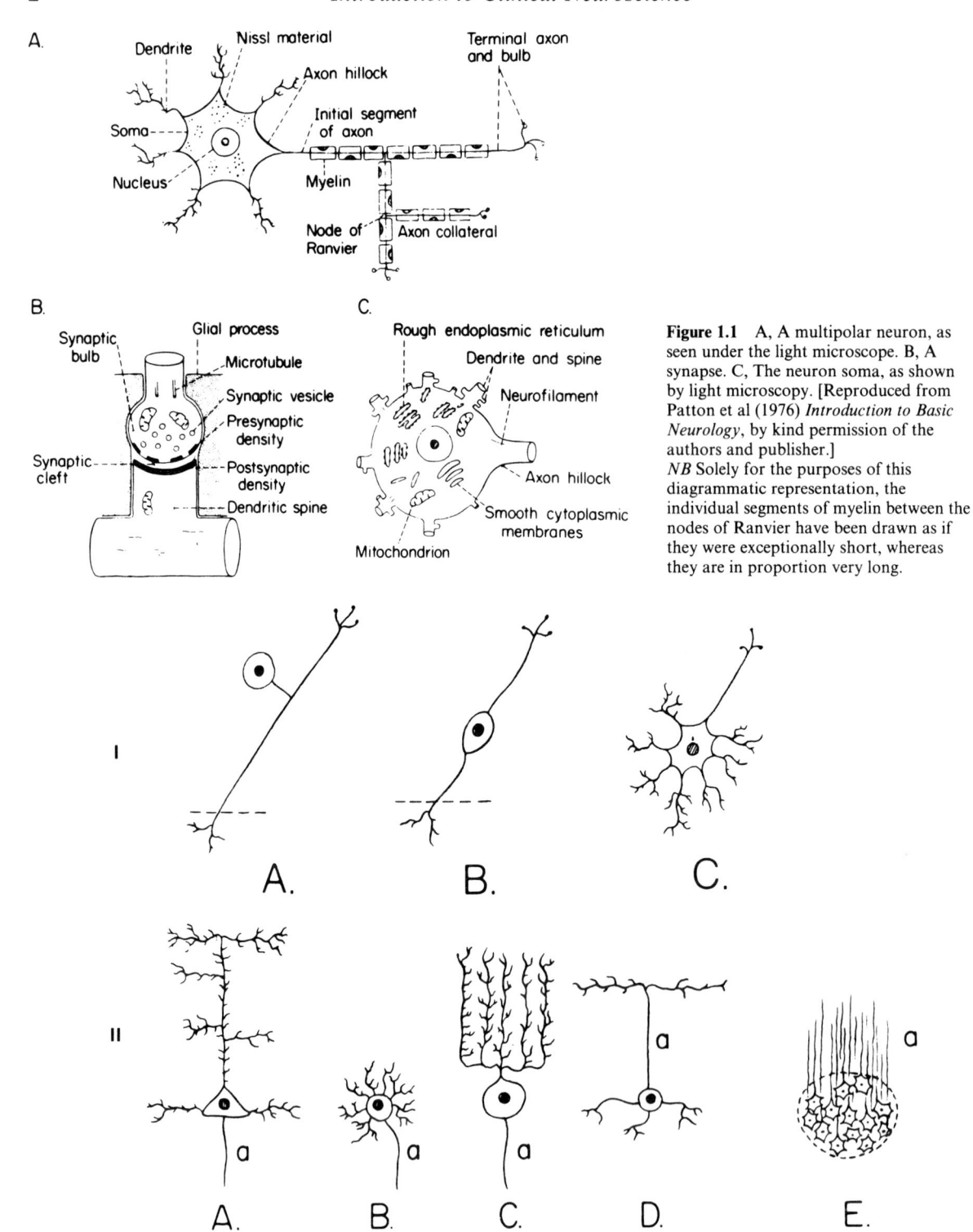

NB Solely for the purposes of this diagrammatic representation, the individual segments of myelin between the nodes of Ranvier have been drawn as if they were exceptionally short, whereas they are in proportion very long.

Figure 1.2 I, Morphological types of neurons. The unipolar (pseudobipolar) neuron (A) is typical of all dorsal root ganglia and general sensory ganglia associated with cranial nerves. The bipolar neuron (B) occurs in the cranial nerves for special senses. The multipolar neurons differ widely in shape; the motoneuron type is shown here (C).

II, Various representative configurations of multipolar neurons. A, pyramidal cell. B, stellate cell. C, Purkinje cell. D, granule cell. E, a nucleus of multipolar cells (dendrites have been omitted for clarity). The small letter a indicates axon. [Reproduced from Patton et al (1976) *Introduction to Basic Neurology* by kind permission of the authors and publisher.]

and often connect to form the so-called Golgi apparatus.

Even smaller microtubules are present and are believed to provide a rapid transport system to distant parts of the cell, while protein threads or neurofilaments, present in the soma, become arranged in a parallel and longitudinal manner in the axons and dendrites. Special classes of proteins, polypeptides, amines, or enzymes may be synthesized within the cytoplasm of selected nerve cells and are transported along the axons either to enter the bloodstream through end-feet upon capillaries or to stimulate effector organs or other neurons at synaptic junctions. Some of these form secretory granules or pigment inclusions. Transport from soma to nerve ending is called orthograde; transport in the reverse direction is called retrograde.

There are many millions of neurons within the central nervous system, and they vary greatly in size, shape, and functional characteristics (Fig. 1.2). Unipolar and bipolar neurons are primarily afferent and convey sensory information from receptor endings into the central nervous system. They are largely confined to the spinal dorsal root ganglia and the cranial nerves. The unipolar neuron has a single process which divides into two parts, one entering the spinal cord, the other extending to the peripheral sensory receptor (as in the skin). Bipolar neurons have an axon which enters the nervous system, and a dendrite extending peripherally; these relatively primitive neurons are virtually confined to the sense organs concerned with olfaction, vision, hearing and equilibrium. The great majority of the neurons in the central nervous system are of the more complex multipolar type (Fig. 1.2), with a single axon (though this always branches) and multiple branching dendrites. The point of origin of the axon is called the axon hillock. Often these cells are grouped together into conglomerates of uniform function called nuclei (e.g. the motor nucleus of a cranial nerve). Within the nervous system there are some neurons, such as the anterior horn cells of the spinal cord, which have very large cell bodies (50–100 μm diameter) with long axons, and these are often classified as Golgi type I. But very many more cells in both brain and cord are small (with a soma of 5–10 μm diameter) and are called Golgi type II. Alternative classifications are projector neurons (with long axons), interneurons (which play a linking role between other neurons), and motor (effector) or sensory (afferent) neurons. Close to their terminations, axons usually divide into a number of fine terminal twigs or telodendria, which enter a peripheral end-organ or make synaptic contact with cell bodies or dendrites of other neurons.

DENDRITES AND AXONS

Dendrites are usually short and invariably branched, sometimes forming a dendritic tree (Fig. 1.2). They contain endoplasmic reticulum, microtubules and neurofilaments, but in contrast to axons they are never myelinated. They are usually irregular in outline because of the presence of spines (Fig. 1.3) which are devoid of organelles. The dendrites of unipolar and bipolar neurons end in sensory receptors which are sometimes highly specialized (e.g. the rods and cones of the retina and the hair cells of the cochlea and labyrinth).

The axon, sometimes called the axis cylinder or nerve fibre, is smooth in outline, usually of constant diameter, and surrounded by a plasma membrane called the axolemma. Its cytoplasm, termed the axoplasm, contains mitochondria, smooth endoplasmic reticulum and many neurofilaments, but few microtubules. Proteins, enzymes and hormones, and indeed the transmitters which mediate transmission at the synapses in which the axons terminate, are synthesized in the soma but travel distally along the axoplasm in the process known as axoplasmic flow. The orthograde flow of proteins and polypeptides is usually slow (0.3–4 mm a day), whereas that of transmitter substances and of the hormones produced by some specialized neurons is usually fast (200–400 mm a day or more). There is also evidence of retrograde flow in many neurons. Smooth endoplasmic reticulum is involved in fast orthograde transport and contributes to renewal of axolemma and to the formation of synaptic vesicles. Degraded plasma membrane and mitochondria are involved in retrograde transport to the soma to be engulfed by lysosomes. Molecules are also acquired by pinocytosis at points of synaptic contact with target cells and are eventually incorporated into Golgi complexes in the perikaryon. This mechanism of pinocytosis of target cell markers is probably important during development for the recognition of target cells.

THE CELLULAR AND MYELIN SHEATHS

In the peripheral nervous system all dendrites and axons are surrounded by specialized cellular sheaths. Peripheral axons of more than 1–2 μm in diameter are ensheathed by neurilemmal cells (Schwann cells) whose cytoplasmic processes form and enclose a complex lipoprotein called myelin, containing sphingomyelin, cerebrosides and cholesterol. Unmyelinated axons are also surrounded by neurilemmal cells (Remak cells), one of which may enclose several axons. At regular intervals short gaps in myelin sheaths occur, known as the nodes of Ranvier; across

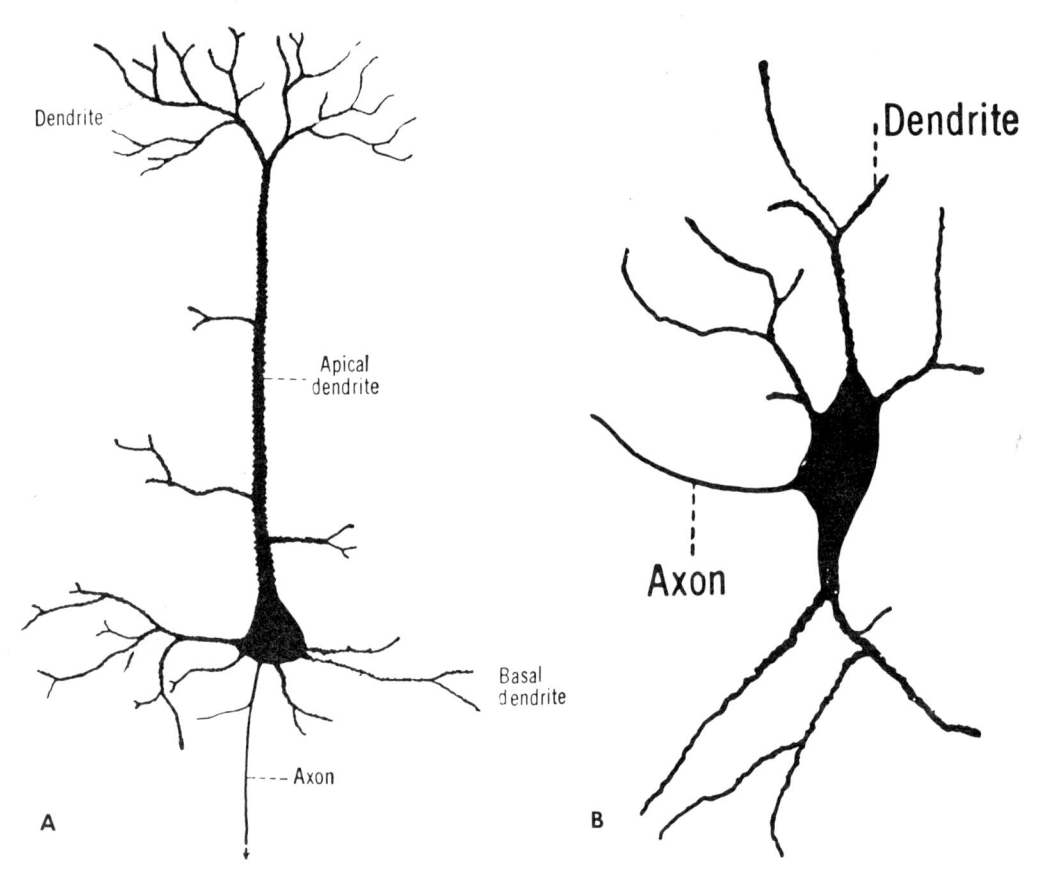

Figure 1.3 A, Drawing of a pyramidal cell from rabbit cortex. This is a Golgi type I neuron. Note the surface irregularities of the dendrites (dendritic spines). The axon of this type of cell in man may be a metre in length. Magnification about × 100. B, A spindle-shaped neuron from rabbit cortex, about 10 μm in diameter. This is a Golgi type II neuron. Only the first part of the axon is shown. Magnification about × 500. [Reproduced from Gardner (1975) *Fundamentals of Neurology*, 6th edn, by kind permission of the author and publisher.]

these nodes so-called saltatory conduction of the neuronal impulse takes place (see p. 8). Outside the Schwann cells are the basal lamina (a layer of protein and polysaccharide) and the collagen and reticulin of the endoneurium. The individual axons and their sheaths are bound together into nerves by connective tissue (see p. 49). In the central nervous system, in contrast to the peripheral nerves, dendrites have no sheaths, but axons may be myelinated or unmyelinated. The oligodendrocyte rather than the Schwann cell controls the myelin between the nodes of Ranvier, and unmyelinated fibres (which are invested by Remak cells) may also lie within indentations in the membrane of such cells. The speed of conduction in myelinated fibres is much faster than in unmyelinated axons, and is indeed faster the greater the diameter of the myelin sheath. The longer the internodal distances, the thicker the myelin sheath.

SYNAPSES AND NEUROEFFECTOR JUNCTIONS

Axons of multipolar neurons make contact with other neurons in synapses or in an effector organ (e.g. muscle or a secretory gland), or terminate on a blood vessel wall in order to release some substance into the circulation. These sites of axonal contact are highly specialized and of obvious functional importance. The terminal twigs (telodendria) of an axon are always unmyelinated. In both the central and autonomic nervous systems the axons may make contact with a dendrite (axodendritic synapse), with a cell body (axosomatic synapse), or with another axon (axonal synapse). Less commonly, dendrodendritic, dendrosomatic and somatosomatic synapses may occur. At most synapses transmission of the nervous impulse is chemically mediated and results from the release of a specific transmitter substance which is stored in synaptic vesicles in the

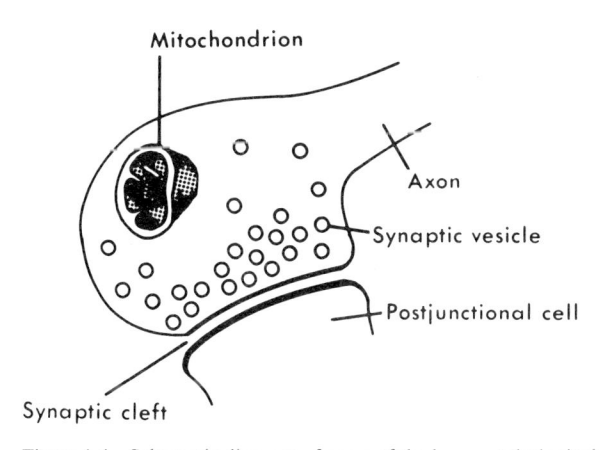

Figure 1.4 Schematic diagram of some of the key morphological features of a single synapse as demonstrated by electron microscopy. Note that the pre- and postsynaptic membranes are thickened. [Reproduced from Gardner (1975) *Fundamentals of Neurology*, 6th edn. by kind permission of the author and publisher.]

axonal ending (Fig. 1.4). The chemical transmitter passes across the presynaptic membrane and the synaptic cleft to polarize the postsynaptic membrane. Both the presynaptic and postsynaptic membranes have a proteinaceous layer on their inner surfaces. The former has presynaptic disc projections and between these are vesicle-attachment sites from which the synaptic vesicles undergo exocytosis into the synaptic cleft which contains electron-dense material and is 20–30 nm wide. Since the transmitter is stored on only one side of the cleft, transmission is unidirectional. Many thousands of synapses may be present upon the surface of a single neuron. In some parts of the nervous system, electrical (non-chemical) synapses or gap junctions are found at which there is direct current flow across the junction. Synaptic vesicles are absent in such synapses where there is loose apposition of neuronal membranes. Tight junctions, at which plasma membranes of two cells adhere, do not occur between neurons but may be seen between capillary endothelial, ependymal and Schwann cells.

Neuroeffectors are end-organs under nervous control; they include muscle and secretory glands. The highly specialized myoneural or neuromuscular junction and the control of exocrine and endocrine secretion are considered later in this book. While cardiac muscle is striated, its individual fibres are connected by specialized gap junctions or intercalated discs. For details of the nervous control of cardiac contraction and of the conducting system of the heart and that of the smooth muscle fibres in the walls of the blood vessels, all mediated by unmyelinated motor fibres of the autonomic system, the reader is referred to suitable textbooks of cardiovascular physiology. Similarly, other sources should be consulted for accounts of smooth muscle in the gastrointestinal tract and elsewhere.

RECEPTORS (STRUCTURE)

Receptors are specialized structures which respond to changes in their environment by converting mechanical, electrical, electromagnetic or chemical information which they receive into either a single electrical impulse or more often a chain of impulses. Such impulses are either conveyed into the central nervous system as sensory information or initiate a motor or effector response in the organ upon which the receptor is situated. Some receptors are arrangements of dendrites or neurons; some are not neuronal but are especially sensitive to certain specific stimuli which they are presumably designed to record. Some, such as the bipolar olfactory neurons, consist of a cell body with a single modified dendrite, while others are highly specialized and complex cells such as the retinal rods and cones. Some neuronal receptors are sensitive to chemical or physical changes occurring in the circulating blood or extracellular fluid as part of the process of homeostasis. Receptors are sometimes classified according to whether they are situated in skin (exteroceptors), in muscle and joints (proprioceptors), or in viscera (interoceptors). Many types of receptor have recently been identified and often constitute no more than specialized areas of cell membranes, such as those in postsynaptic membranes, which respond specifically to transmitter release. A good example is the acetylcholine receptor on the surface of the skeletal muscle cell. The nature and classification of receptors concerned with autonomic activity, those mediating the special senses, and those which handle somatic sensory information are considered later.

THE NEUROGLIA

The neuroglia are cells in the nervous system that neither form synapses nor conduct impulses but which are plainly metabolically active as they contain mitochondria, ribosomes, endoplasmic reticulum and lysosomes. Central gliocytes include the astrocytes, oligodendrocytes, microglia and ependymal cells, while the peripheral gliocytes are the Schwann cells. The microglia are of mesodermal origin, the remainder of ectodermal origin. The so-called macroglia are the oligodendrocytes and the astrocytes. *Oligodendrocytes* predominate in the white matter, especially in rows between bundles of nerve fibres, although they may be seen in grey matter as well. These cells play the same role in relation to the myelination of fibres in the central nervous system as do

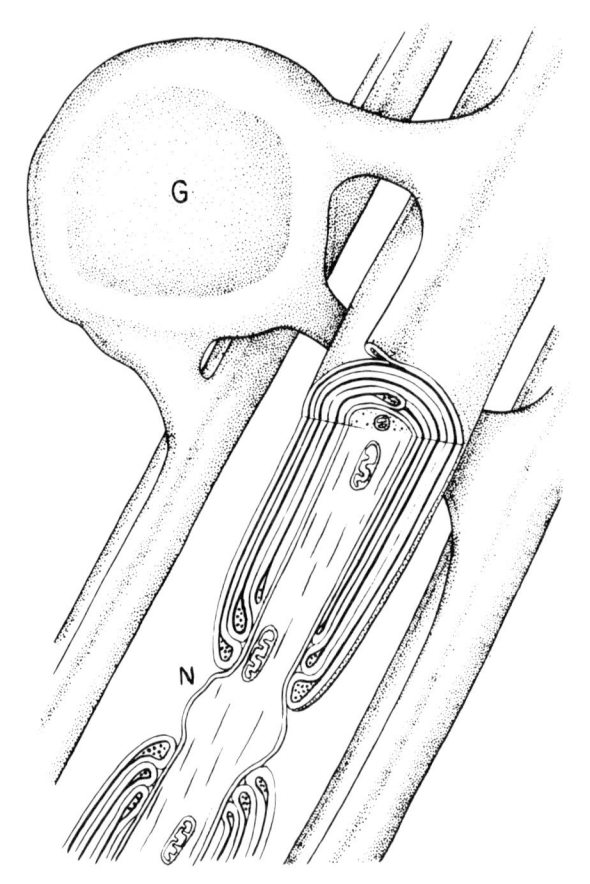

Figure 1.5 Myelinated coverings of fibres in the central nervous system. Oligodendrocyte (G) has three footlike processes going to different axons. The oligodendrocyte's cytoplasmic membrane is indicated in three dimensions in the centre of the figure to show the concentric wrappings that form myelin (dark lines). Note that the loops of glial cytoplasm end at the node of Ranvier (N), leaving it unmyelinated. [Reproduced from Patton et al (1976) *Introduction to Basic Neurology* by kind permission of the authors and publisher, and modified from Bunge et al (1961) *Biophys. Biochem. Cytol.* **10**:67 (1961).]

the Schwann cells in peripheral nerves. They do not invest but often lie in close relationship to unmyelinated fibres as well. Unlike Schwann cells, which individually myelinate a single nerve fibre between nodes, a single oligodendrocyte often myelinates several axons, again between internodes (about 1 mm) (Fig. 1.5). Oligodendrocytes are small with short processes; without special silver stains they may be difficult to distinguish from small neurons (Fig. 1.6).

The *astrocytes* are larger than oligodendrocytes and stellate in form. Most astrocytes have at least one process that forms an end-foot on the capillary endothelial cell so that these end-feet collectively form cuffs around capillaries. Similarly, other processes blend with the subpial basal lamina to form a glial limiting membrane on the surface of the brain, thus separating it from pial elements and surface vessels. There are specialized arrangements of astrocytes, to be mentioned in subsequent chapters, in the cerebellum, the retina and possibly the posterior lobe of the pituitary. The astrocytes play an important supporting role in the nervous system. They may at times be phagocytic and can proliferate to form a special type of scar (gliosis) in response to injury. They may assume abnormal sizes and shapes in response to various metabolic disturbances or infections (as in hepatic encephalopathy and multifocal leukoencephalopathy). Much remains to be learned, however, about their metabolic role and influence upon neuronal activity.

Microglia are cells of mesodermal origin, many derived from mononuclear cells which migrate from the blood vessels. When inactive they are small, stain darkly, and have few short processes (Fig. 1.6). When activated in response to disease or injury, they become macrophages.

In addition to cellular elements and blood vessels there is intercellular fluid or ground substance. Its nature and function is still unknown, although it may be pathologically increased in cerebral oedema.

EPENDYMA AND NEURILEMMA

Ependymal cells, believed by many to be neuroglial, form a single layer of cells with ciliated surfaces lining the cerebral ventricles and the central canal of the spinal cord. Specialized ependymal cells in the choroid plexuses fulfil an important role in controlling the production (part diffusion and part secretion) of the cerebrospinal fluid.

The role of the neurilemma in the formation of myelin sheaths and in investing unmyelinated fibres in the peripheral nervous system has already been mentioned. The neurilemmal sheath also fulfils an important role in directing regenerating nerve fibres after injury to a nerve. These cells possess other functions which are still poorly understood. For example, they may sometimes be phagocytic in that they ingest degenerating myelin after disease or injury.

THE NEURON AND ITS FUNCTION

Practically all nerve cells are excitable (although cochlear hair cells, retinal rods, cones and horizontal cells belong to a group of cells which do not generate impulses, and the question as to whether they are neurons is open to debate). Electrically excitable neurons respond to stimuli by undergoing transient physicochemical changes, which usually alter the resting potential of the cell and initiate a nerve

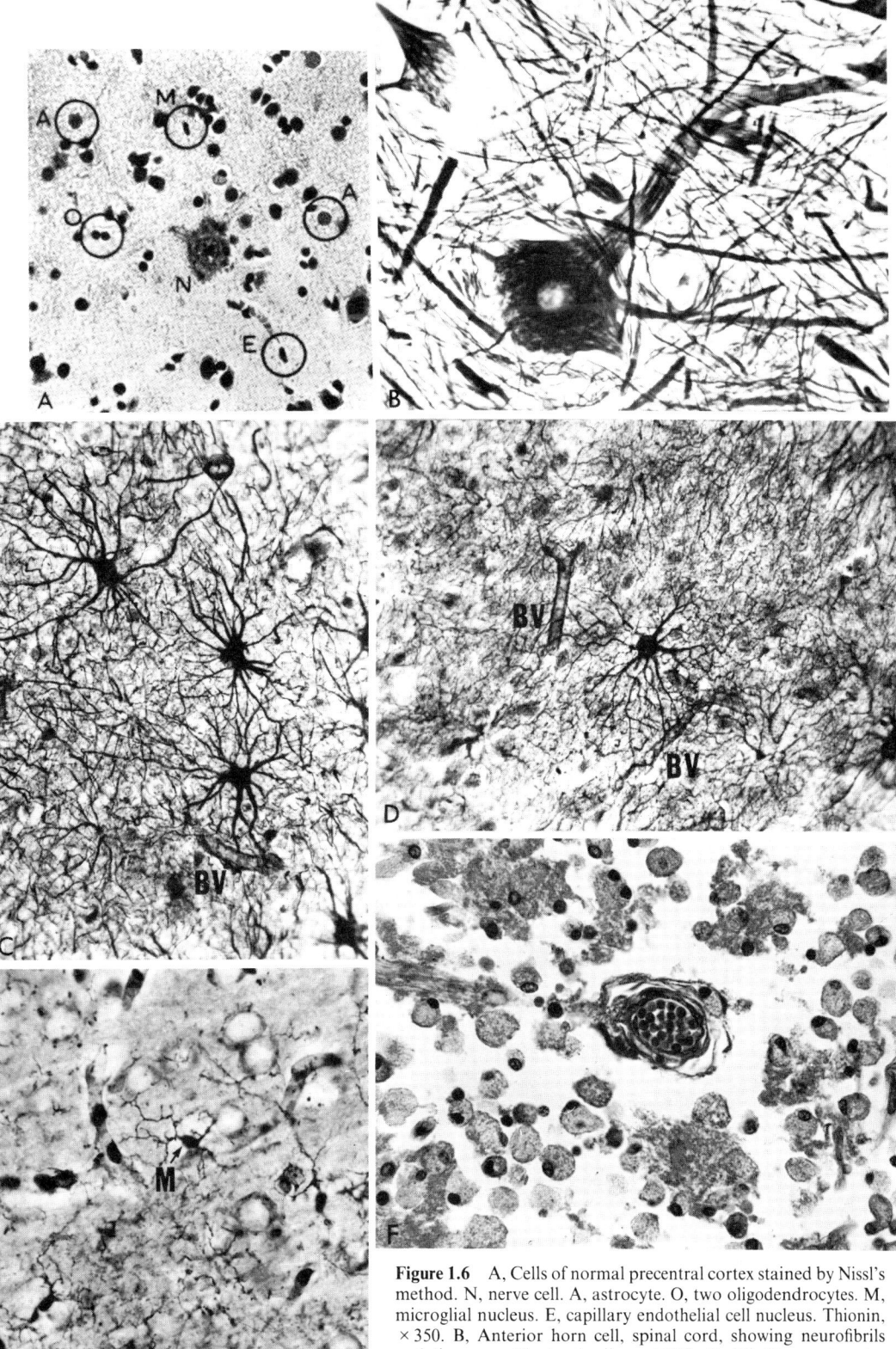

Figure 1.6 A, Cells of normal precentral cortex stained by Nissl's method. N, nerve cell. A, astrocyte. O, two oligodendrocytes. M, microglial nucleus. E, capillary endothelial cell nucleus. Thionin, ×350. B, Anterior horn cell, spinal cord, showing neurofibrils and the axon. Hortega's silver, ×350. C, Fibrillary astrocytes in the cortex. Cajal's gold sublimate, ×350. D, Protoplasmic astrocytes in the cortex. BV, Blood vessel, Cajal's gold sublimate, ×350. E, Normal microglia in the cortex of a rabbit (human cells are similar). Hortega's silver, ×450. F, Reactive microglial cells ('compound granular corpuscles' or 'gitter' cells) which are distended with phagocytosed lipid. [Reproduced from Blackwood et al (1964) *Atlas of Neuropathology*, 2nd edn, by kind permission of the authors and publisher.]

impulse. Owing to the property of conductivity, this impulse is then propagated along the cell membrane and is accompanied by an action potential which can be recorded electrically.

The membrane of the nerve cell, like that of many other cells, has a complex structure. At its centre is a matrix of phospholipid, much of it organized as a discontinuous fluid bilayer (Singer and Nicolson, 1972). Also integral to the membrane are many globular molecules of protein, so arranged that their ionic and highly polar groups protrude from the surface into the aqueous phase, while the non-polar groups are largely buried in the hydrophobic interior of the membrane. Neuronal membranes are not fixed and stable structures. On the contrary, they are labile and metabolically active, controlling not only active transmembrane transport in either direction but also relative permeability to different ions. In nerve and skeletal muscle cells, the membrane is relatively impermeable to organic cations, more generally permeable to chloride (Cl^-), relatively permeable to potassium (K^+), and much less permeable to sodium (Na^+). In the resting state, and to a lesser extent in the active state, the concentration of intracellular K^+ is high and that of Na^+ low in comparison with extracellular fluid. Most of the ions that do diffuse across the membrane pass through protein pores within it called channels. These channels, which are proteins that can be isolated and studied, are selective for the ions which each allows to pass, depending upon the size, charge and hydration energy of the ions (see Kandel and Schwartz, 1985). Thus there are, for example, sodium, potassium and chloride channels within the neuronal and muscle cell membrane. The relative permeability of different membranes to different ions depends upon the relative proportions of different channels present within it. Thus, for example, the equilibrium potential (see below) for Cl^- may be positive *or* negative in relation to the resting membrane potential, and changes in chloride conductance are often involved in inhibitory synaptic transmission. The differences in ionic concentration across the membrane result in an electrical charge with the interior of the fibre negative to the exterior in the resting state. This state of polarization can be quantified by recording the resting potential through a microelectrode inserted into the neuronal soma (or muscle cell). Normally this potential is about $-70\,mV$ in nerve and $-90\,mV$ in muscle. Transfer of ions across this membrane in response to a stimulus sufficient to excite the cell occurs through the opening of the relevant channels. Normally a state of equilibrium exists so that inward movement of one ion is balanced by a comparable outward movement of another. At equilibrium the difference in charge across the membrane for a single ion is called the equilibrium potential; it differs from the resting potential slightly because of differences between passive flux and pump flux (see later) for the different ions. In the past the resting potential was often called the resting membrane potential, since in the Bernstein membrane theory it was generally thought that depolarization and ionic shift across the membrane in response to excitation of the cell was largely dependent upon selective permeability of the membrane to different ions. It is now known that such selective permeability exists, and that passive ion transfer occurs, but in addition the propagated nerve impulse also involves a process of active transport involving the operation of the sodium (or sodium–potassium) pump and the expenditure of energy, largely derived from adenosine triphosphate (ATP).

Excitation of a neuron, leading to a propagated action potential which travels along its axon, is dependent upon the electrochemical gradients for Na^+ and K^+ ions. It is accompanied by the utilization of oxygen and glucose, the formation of carbon dioxide, and the production of heat. Energy consumption, with the conversion of ATP to ADP and phosphorus, is a recovery process needed to reestablish the electrochemical gradients for these ions. The extent to which a nerve fibre can continue to function without this recovery process depends upon the nature and diameter of the fibre. Once this potential is initiated, the wave of depolarization spreads at constant speed along the axon, its rate of conduction being dependent upon the diameter of the fibre. Thus in large-diameter axons (such as the giant axon of the squid) a velocity of 25 metres per second is achieved, but in man unmyelinated axons are all much thinner and conduction occurs much more slowly. However, in myelinated nerves the insulating quality of the myelin decreases capacitance and thus reduces the number of charges held across the membrane at a given resting potential; this allows much more rapid conduction, which again depends upon the thickness of the insulation. In such nerves conduction 'jumps' from one node of Ranvier to the next (Fig. 1.7), a process called saltatory conduction (Latin *saltare*—to hop). Conduction of the action potential is accompanied by the inward movement of sodium and the outward movement of potassium, and in less than a millisecond the polarity of the resting potential is reversed to about $+40\,mV$. An electrical 'spike' can be recorded accompanying this event (Fig. 1.8). As the peak of the potential moves on, sodium begins to move out, potassium begins to move back inwards and the resting potential is eventually restored.

The axon hillock of the neuronal soma is the impulse initiation site, with a relatively low threshold

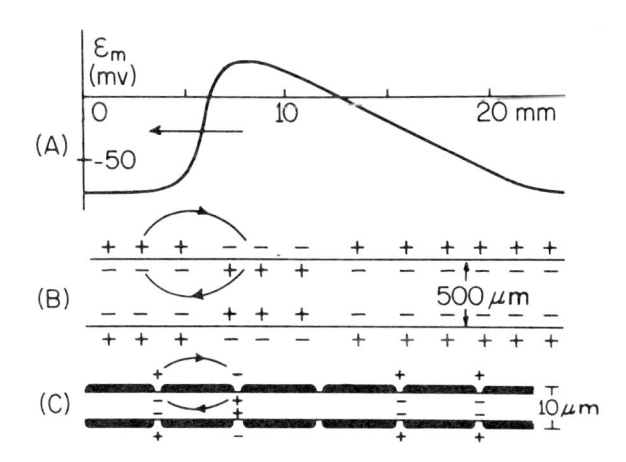

Figure 1.7 Mechanisms of conduction in unmyelinated squid axon (B) and myelinated mammalian axon (C). Trace A shows the axon potential propagating from right to left. Arrows indicate the direction of current flow through the membrane in front of the action potential. Similar current flow (not shown) occurs in the wake of the action potential, but it does not re-excite the repolarized membrane because permeability to Na$^+$ is still inactivated and the membrane is refractory. [Reproduced from Ruch and Patton (eds) (1965) *Physiology and Biophysics*, by kind permission of the authors and publisher.]

of electrical excitation. It responds to depolarization of sufficient intensity, usually produced by activity in the input region of the soma, and gives an all-or-none response (the action potential) depending upon a specific regenerative increase in the sodium conduction of the membrane (Ardley, 1978). The action potential, once generated, spreads irresistibly with constant amplitude to the termination of the axon. Thus conduction in nerves and fibre tracts is either 'on' or 'off' and is digital in nature. During the transmission of the action potential, the axon remains insensitive to a further stimulus, however strong this may be (the absolute refractory period); during the period of return to the resting potential, it again becomes excitable, but at a higher threshold (the relative refractory period). Transient hyperpolarization for a few milliseconds follows return to the resting level, producing a brief positive afterpotential (Fig. 1.8). However, subthreshold stimuli may produce, even in such structures, localized, non-propagating electrical charges which are graded in intensity until the stimulus increases so as to reach the threshold and induce the all-or-none response (Fig. 1.9). Graded responses which diminish decrementally as they spread from the site of stimulation are typically seen in nerve cell bodies and their dendrites, as well as in peripheral sensory receptors, and are much more difficult to characterize and record.

Some recent developments in neurobiology

Within the last 20 years the introduction of a number of invaluable experimental techniques of physiological investigation has greatly increased our understanding of neuronal function and of the behaviour of excitable tissues and biological membranes in particular. Thus, for example, it is now known that many neurotransmitters (see p. 13) such as acetylcholine, glutamate, GABA, glycine, etc., usually act upon the postsynaptic membrane of muscle cells and increase their permeability to cations and anions (Cull-Candy, 1984). At a molecular level the effect is visualized as a brief and transient opening of discrete ionic channels caused by transmitted molecules becoming attached briefly to membrane-bound receptors. Many channels, including those gated by receptors, produce brief rectangular current pulses when they open or close. When electrical recordings are made with intracellular microelectrodes inserted into single cells, the tiny currents produced by the opening of single ionic channels are swamped by the intrinsic membrane noise resulting from the leakage of ions across the membrane. Techniques are now available for recording such noise and for analysing the much more substantial noise associated with the activation of a large number of ionic channels. However, the *patch-clamp* technique, involving the close apposition of the polished tip of a micropipette (tip diameter 2–4 μm) against the surface membrane of a cell, now makes it possible to record from a few μm^2 of membrane. This technique yields information about single channel currents which cannot be obtained in any other way; it is particularly valuable in studying receptor-gated channels in membranes with low receptor density.

A second invaluable development has arisen from the ability to record minimal current flow in the membrane associated with movement of charged particles (the so-called '*gating currents*') which 'open the gates' for ionic flow and thus immediately precede channel opening (Aidley, 1978). The use of such measurements, combined with studies using specific toxins such as tetrodotoxin (which selectively blocks sodium channels without affecting the gating current), have made it possible to calculate, for example, sodium channel density in axonal membranes.

Thirdly, the introduction of the *voltage-clamp* technique has made it possible to clarify certain distinctive differences between the physiological behaviour of nerve cell bodies (somata) on the one hand, and of axons on the other. When a depolarizing current is injected into axons they do not show the sustained repetitive firing which is found, for example, in the somata of motor neurons. The term

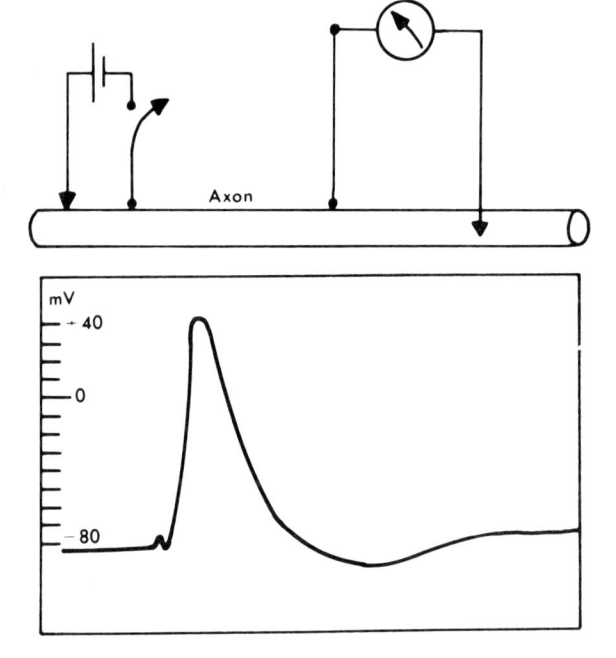

Figure 1.8 Schematic representation of a single unmyelinated nerve fibre and the action potential that can be recorded from it. In the upper figure, the axon is represented as a hollow tube. At the left, two stimulating electrodes connected to a current source are shown touching the fibre. At the right, two recording electrodes are shown (the symbol for the galvanometer represents a direct current amplifier and recording instrument). Where one of the electrodes (a microelectrode with a tip less than 1 μm in diameter) pierces the membrane, a potential difference is recorded, the interior being about -80 mV. When the switch is closed (not shown) and a brief above-threshold pulse of current is delivered, the membrane potential is reversed and the exterior becomes about $+40$ mV, for a total swing of about 120 mV. This is the beginning of the all-or-nothing response. The small deflection immediately preceding the action potential is the 'shock artifact' produced by a leakage of stimulating current down the fibre. Note also the positive after-potential. [Reproduced from Gardner: *Fundamentals of Neurology*, 6th edn, by kind permission of the author and publisher.]

'voltage clamp' (Crill and Schwindt, 1983) means that the action potential across the cell membrane is held constant by injecting currents through an intracellular microelectrode to counteract the membrane currents. Two microelectrodes are therefore required—one for recording current, the other for injecting it. This method has made it possible to study ionic conductance in the membrane of nerve cells (and incidentally also in that of skeletal muscle) and has given an insight into the active properties of central neurons that could not be obtained by any other methods. Much more information, in consequence, is now available about input–output responses of mammalian neurons and about the influence upon them of activity in ionic conductance channels first activated in the near-threshold range of the cell's membrane potential. Several putative neurotransmitters have been shown to affect the ionic current flowing through some of these newly described channels; these findings are likely to be of great importance in studying both normal and abnormal neuronal behaviour.

Finally, much new information of importance has emerged from the study of chemical mechanisms involved in the regulation of cellular processes. 'One of the most important functions of the animal plasma cell membrane is to receive extracellular messages and transduce them into intracellular messages that in turn activate appropriate cellular responses' (Rasmussen and Goodman, 1977).

Physiological studies in the late 1950s and early 1960s focused attention on the role of cyclic 3'5'-adenosine monophosphate (cAMP) as an almost ubiquitous 'second messenger' in cell activation. However, in the 1970s considerable evidence emerged to indicate that the calcium ion has an equally important role. It is now well recognized that the calcium ion and cAMP (as well as its companion nucleotide cyclic 3'5'-guanosine monophosphate or cGMP) are almost universal and closely interrelated second messengers which play a crucial role in the activation of particular cell types by specific intracellular messengers, although within this universal theme of cell activation there are a number of variations according to different cells and systems.

SYNAPSES

The arrival of a nerve impulse at a synaptic junction on a cell body may, at those electrical synapses which exist in the mature mammalian nervous system, induce a direct local depolarization in the receptor cell membrane. Such electrical synapses are found, for example, in the mesencephalic nucleus of the fifth cranial nerve, in Deiters' nucleus of the eighth nerve, and in the inferior olive. Transmission at many other mammalian synapses is chemically mediated, however, involving the release of a transmitter substance which traverses the synaptic cleft to combine with receptors at their sites on the postsynaptic membrane. It is now clear that entry of calcium ions during depolarization of the terminal membrane is an essential prerequisite for the liberation of transmitter. After a brief synaptic delay (usually of the order of 0.6–0.9 msec), the postsynaptic membrane is depolarized, leading to the generation of either an excitatory postsynaptic potential (EPSP) or an inhibitory postsynaptic potential (IPSP, see below). The time course of the synaptic potential is very brief, for example as in the case of nicotinic synapses where acetylcholine is the transmitter, but it may be

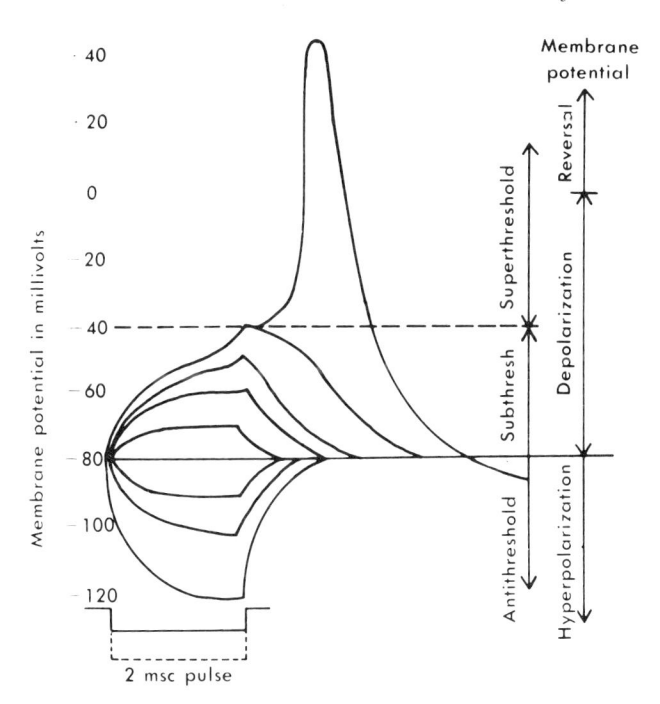

Figure 1.9 A family of curves obtained by stimulating a nerve fibre with a short current pulse of variable strength and polarity. With weak stimulation local membrane depolarization results. As the strength is increased, the local response is greater. Finally, threshold is reached and an action potential results as the membrane potential is reversed. If the polarity of the stimulating electrode is reversed, hyperpolarization results and increases with the magnitude of the stimulus. [Reproduced from Gardner (1975) *Fundamentals of Neurology*, 6th edn, by kind permission of the author and publisher; modified from Katz (1966) *Nerve, Muscle, and Synapse*.]

seconds, minutes or even longer when peptides or hormones are involved. If this EPSP is subthreshold, no action potential is generated in the postsynaptic cell, but the cell is rendered temporarily more sensitive to a subsequent stimulus (facilitation). An EPSP above threshold (about 10 mV), by contrast, causes the cell to discharge. The properties of synapses between axons and dendrites are not well understood. They have a relatively high excitatory threshold, but once excited, depolarization may be relatively prolonged. This property may apply constant stimulation to the cell body, thus being one factor involved in the repetitive activity of certain neurons. The inward flow of ions which accompanies the EPSP, due to a non-selective increase in membrane permeability to all ions, mediated by an ionic channel distinct from the sodium channel, involves current flow through a sink, which must be accompanied by comparable flow outwards through other parts of the membrane constituting a source. As distance from the sink increases, the flow of current diminishes. This decrement with distance represents a graded response. There is some similarity between the mechanism of synaptic transmission in the nervous system, with generation of an EPSP, and neuromuscular transmission in which the release of acetylcholine at the motor nerve ending produces an end-plate potential. Acetylcholine is also the transmitter at many synapses in the central nervous system. There are many other central synaptic transmitter substances in addition to acetylcholine, including noradrenaline, dopamine, serotonin, histamine and numerous amino acids, probably including glutamic and aspartic acids and many more. Adenosine may also act as a transmitter in certain spinal cord synapses. An important difference between neuromuscular and central synaptic transmission is that the former depends upon the sudden massive release of acetylcholine from a single axon to a single muscle fibre. In the central nervous system many EPSPs are subthreshold, and excitation of the target cell depends upon the summation of the output flow from many presynaptic terminals or synaptic knobs, each of which may release subliminal amounts of transmitter substance.

Neuromuscular transmission, and that at other neuroeffector junctions, is virtually always excitatory. Many synapses in the central nervous system, however, are inhibitory. Inhibition can be either presynaptic or postsynaptic. Presynaptic inhibition results from any process which reduces the amount of excitatory transmitter released from presynaptic endings, thus rendering the EPSP subthreshold. For example, some presynaptic terminals may produce prolonged subthreshold depolarization of other synaptic knobs with a consequent reduction in transmitter release. More frequently an inhibitory, rather than excitatory, transmitter substance is released which produces hyperpolarization in the postsynaptic cell. This process is generally associated with increased membrane conductance, especially to K^+ (the 'shunting' or 'short-circuiting' action which moves the membrane potential further away from the threshold). This inhibitory postsynaptic potential (IPSP) renders the cell less excitable. Thus the activity of a cell at any one time may depend upon the balance between excitatory and inhibitory activity in the synapses upon its surface. The principal known inhibitory transmitters are gamma-aminobutyric acid (GABA), glycine, and alanine. There is a fundamental difference between the K^+ channels which are gated by the action potential (voltage-gated channels) and those opened by transmitter release associated with the IPSP (chemically gated); the two classes are different pharmacologically (see below).

The passage of information through the nervous system involves alternating electrical and chemical mechanisms. In each neuron the generation of an action potential (the Hodgkin cycle relates to the circular relationship between the membrane potential and the sodium conductance underlying the upstroke of this potential) followed by propagation of the nerve impulse either induces an effector response or causes release of a transmitter substance at a synapse, which then initiates a process in another neuron. A balance exists at any one moment between excitation and inhibition, which modulates the resulting response.

RECEPTORS (FUNCTION)

Sensory receptors
Many sensory receptors can be looked upon as transducers which convert the energy to which they respond in a specific manner into an electrical response. This so-called receptor or generator potential is a graded response in that its amplitude depends upon the intensity of the stimulus. If the stimulus reaches a threshold value, it produces an all-or-none response in the form of an action potential which carries sensory information into the central nervous system. The generator potential is amplitude-modulated in that its amplitude depends upon the intensity of the sensory input. The resulting action potential, however, is frequency-modulated. Since this potential is all-or-none, it can only signify an increased intensity of stimulus by an increased firing frequency.

If a stimulus is prolonged at a steady intensity, then the frequency of discharge usually becomes progressively less and then either ceases or is maintained at a much lower frequency. This phenomenon is known as adaptation. Adaptation explains why one is conscious of the movement of a part of the body, but awareness of the posture adopted then declines until further movement occurs.

Receptors in which adaptation leads to a reduced but stable generator potential with a reduced firing rate are called tonic. In these tonic receptors the frequency of repetitive discharge is directly proportional to the magnitude of the generator potential. While a constant generator potential persists, a new spike discharge in the axon is generated as soon as the refractory period following the previous spike discharge has passed. In certain other receptors, which are called phasic (such as pacinian corpuscles and hair follicle receptors), adaptation is rapid and total so that the generator potential rapidly declines to the baseline even though the stimulus continues. These phasic receptors transduce sensory information which reaches perception only when a stimulus is changing (as in oscillatory or rhythmical stimulation)—not when it is constant. In some specialized receptors such as the muscle spindle, sensitivity may be modified by activity in motor nerve fibres which innervate components of the receptor.

Postsynaptic receptors
Certain specialized nerve cells have the faculty of responding to chemical changes in their extracellular environment; these are known as chemoreceptors. Little is known of the mechanisms involved. There are many highly specific membrane receptors, especially on postsynaptic membranes, which are capable of recognizing, or combining with and responding to, transmitter substances. Some recent progress has been made in isolating and characterizing such receptors. Thus, many specific receptors upon neuronal surfaces in the central nervous system are being identified by means of immunocytochemical techniques. Using α-bungarotoxin, which binds irreversibly to the cholinergic receptor, it has been estimated that there are about 4×10^7 acetylcholine receptors per neuromuscular end-plate. The receptor is probably a lipoprotein with a molecular weight of about 250 000; each receptor comprises five polypeptide subunits and each subunit probably contains two binding sites for acetylcholine. The cholinergic receptors may well be different in the neuromuscular junctions of smooth and cardiac muscles, in the neuroeffector junctions in secretory glands, and in the cholinergic synapses in the central nervous system and autonomic ganglia. For example, in autonomic ganglia and in certain neuromuscular junctions there are at least two types of receptors—nicotinic and muscarinic—as judged by pharmacological probes (see p. 15).

SOME NEUROPHARMACOLOGICAL PRINCIPLES

The chemical constitution, general metabolism, and regulatory control of the nervous system will be considered in subsequent chapters. However, there are certain principles of neuropharmacology related to processes of nerve conduction and synaptic transmission which can usefully be considered here. Study of the effects of various drugs and toxins is highly relevant to our understanding of normal and disordered nervous function.

The nerve impulse

The generation and conduction of the neuronal action potential were considered in detail above (p. 8). The voltage-sensitive Na^+ and K^+ channels in the neuronal membrane may be blocked by the local anaesthetic procaine and its analogues. Tetrodotoxin (from the puffer fish) and its virtually identical analogue tarichotoxin (from Western American newts) block only the Na^+ channels, leaving the K^+ channels intact. Saxitoxin (from marine diflagellates)

TABLE 1. Putative neurotransmitters in the mammalian CNS

Name	Marker enzyme	Uptake process	Receptor types	Suggested neuronal pathways
γ-Aminobutyric acid (GABA)	Glutamate/ decarboxylase	Yes	$GABA_a$ and $GABA_b$	Purkinje cell–interpositus and Deiters' nuclei Caudate–putamen–substantia nigra Retinal interneurons Hippocampal interneurons Spinal cord dorsal horns
Glycine	None known	Yes	Strychnine-sensitive	Spinal cord interneurons (e.g. Renshaw cells)
Glutamic acid	None known	Yes	Possibly three	As with GABA above; where GABA is inhibitory, glutamic acid is generally excitatory
Acetylcholine	Choline acetyltransferase	Yes (for choline)	Muscarinic and nicotinic	Skeletal motor system Preganglionic sympathetic Pre- and postganglionic parasympathetic Septal–hippocampal Striatal interneurons
Dopamine	Tyrosine hydroxylase	Yes	DA_1 and DA_2	Nigrostriatal Mesolimbic–amygdala–nucleus accumbens Tuberoinfundibular Superior cervical ganglion interneurons Retinal interneurons
Noradrenaline	Dopamine-β-hydroxylase	Yes	$\alpha_1, \alpha_2, \beta_1$ and β_2 adrenoceptors	Postganglionic sympathetic Ventral brain stem–limbocortical pathway Locus coeruleus–limbocortical pathway Brain stem–spinal cord Locus coeruleus–cerebellum Hypothalamus
Adrenaline	Phenethanolamine-N-methyl transferase	Yes	As above	Adrenal medulla parenchymal cells Pons–medulla–tractus solitarius–hypothalamus
5-Hydroxytryptamine (serotonin)	Tryptophan hydroxylase	Yes	$5\text{-}HT_1$ and $5\text{-}HT_2$	Brain stem–spinal cord Brain stem–diencephalon–telencephalon
Histamine	Histidine decarboxylase	No	H_1 and H_2	? Hypothalamus Postganglionic sympathetic fibres

[Modified from McGeer and McGeer (1973) *Prog. Neurobiol.* **2**:69 and from Iversen (1982) *Lancet*, by kind permission of the authors and publishers.]
For information on the role of other substances (including cAMP, adenosine, prostaglandins and various peptides) in neurotransmission, see pp. 17–19.

TABLE 2. Actions of drugs on synaptic and neuroeffector transmission

Mechanism of action	System	Drugs	Pharmacological effect of drug
Interference with synthesis of transmitter	Cholinergic Adrenergic	Hemicholinium α-Methyl-*p*-tyrosine	Depletion of ACh Depletion of noradrenaline
Inhibition of monoamine reuptake	Monoaminergic (non-selective) Noradrenergic Dopaminergic Serotoninergic	Imipramine, amitriptyline, cocaine Desipramine Nomifensine Zimelidine Fluoxetine	Accumulation of monoamines at extracellular sites
Blockade of transport system in storage granule membrane	Monoaminergic	Reserpine	Destruction of noradrenaline by mitochondrial MAO and its depletion in adrenergic terminals
Displacement of transmitter from axon terminal	Cholinergic	Carbachol	Cholinomimetic
	Monoaminergic	Ephedrine, tyramine Amphetamine	Sympathomimetic Dopaminergic
Prevention of release of transmitter	Cholinergic Adrenergic	Botulinum toxin Bretylium, guanethidine	Anticholinergic Antiadrenergic

TABLE 2. *Continued*

Mechanism of action	System	Drugs	Pharmacological effect of drug
Mimicry of transmitter at postsynaptic receptor (postsynaptic agonists)	Cholinergic		
	Muscarinic	Methacholine	Cholinomimetic
	Nicotinic	Nicotine	Cholinomimetic
	Adrenergic		
	Alpha	Ephedrine, phenylephrine	
	Beta	Isoprenaline	Sympathomimetic
	Beta$_2$	Salbutamol	
	Dopaminergic	Dopamine	
		Bromocriptine	Dopaminergic
		Apomorphine	
	Serotoninergic	Lysergic acid diethylamide (LSD)	Serotoninergic
	GABA-ergic		
	Non-selective	Muscimol	GAGA-ergic
	GABA$_B$	Baclofen	
Blockade of endogenous transmitter at postsynaptic receptor (postsynaptic antagonists)	Muscarinic		
	Non-selective	Atropine	
	Muscarinic M$_1$	Pirenzepine	Cholinergic blockade
	Muscarinic M$_2$	No specific antagonist	
	Adrenergic		
	Alpha (non-selective)	Phenoxybenzamine, phentolamine	
	Alpha$_1$	Prazosin, indoramin	
	Alpha$_2$	Idazoxin	Adrenergic blockade
	Beta (non-selective)	Propranolol, oxprenolol (partial agonist)	
	Beta$_1$	Practolol (partial agonist), atenolol	
	Dopaminergic		
	Non-selective	Phenothiazines (e.g. chlorpromazine)	
		Thioxanthenes (e.g. flupenthixol)	Dopamine blockade
		Butyrophenones (e.g. haloperidol)	
	D$_2$	Sulpiride	
	Serotoninergic		
	Non-selective	Methysergide, metergoline, cyproheptadine	5-HT blockade
	5-HT$_1$	Buspirone (partial agonist)	
	5-HT$_2$	Ketanserin	
	GABA$_A$	Bicuculline	GABA blockade; opening of Cl$^-$ channels
	GABA$_B$	Baclofen	Depression of Ca^{2+} current
	Histamine		
	H$_1$	Conventional antihistamines (e.g. mepyramine)	Histamine blockade
	H$_2$	Cimetidine, ranitidine	
Inhibition of enzymatic breakdown of transmitter	Cholinergic	Anticholinesterase agents [physostigmine, pyridostigmine, propylphosphofluoridate (DFP)]	Cholinomimetic
	Monoaminergic		
	Non-selective MAO inhibitors	Phenelzine, tranylcypromine	Accumulation of monoamines at certain sites
	MAO A inhibitors	Pargyline (low doses)	
	MAO B inhibitors	Selegiline	
Mimicry of transmitter at presynaptic receptor (presynaptic agonists)	Adrenergic (alpha$_2$)	Clonidine, methyldopa (and its metabolite α-methylnoradrenaline)	Reduced neurotransmitter release
	Dopaminergic	Apomorphine (low doses)	
Drugs acting indirectly through ion channels	Chloride channels	Benzodiazepines, barbiturates	Channel activation
	Sodium channels	Tetrodotoxin	Channel blocking

Extensively modified from Koelle (1968) by kind permission of the author and publisher. I am also grateful to Dr J. K. Aronson and Dr G. Goodwin for their advice and help in updating the table.

is of a chemically different structure but is also a specific Na⁺ channel blocker (Ritchie and Rogart, 1977). Tetraethylammonium ions, by contrast, block the chemically gated K⁺ but not the Na⁺ channels. This does not affect neuronal excitability but prolongs the time course of action potentials by delaying repolarization. The discovery of agents with such high specificity has been of great value in elucidating the biochemical and biophysical details of the formation and propagation of the nerve impulse.

Synaptic transmission

Very many chemical substances that can act as neurotransmitters have been identified. Table 1 lists some of the more important substances, together with the enzymes responsible for their synthesis and the parts of the nervous system at which they exercise their principal effects. In the case of most neurotransmitters there is a marker enzyme which occurs uniquely in each class of neuron and also a specific uptake process. These uptake processes, again related to transmitter-specific classes of neurons, are important in the inactivation of transmitters which are recaptured after release from neurons, and they are also valuable in research for identifying transmitter-specific cells as well as the receptors with which the transmitters interact (Iversen, 1982).

ACETYLCHOLINE

Acetylcholine is synthesized within neurons from acetyl CoA and choline through the action of choline acetylase (Fig. 1.10) and is then stored in synaptic vesicles in preparation for its release. Each vesicle contains one quantum (between 10 000 and 50 000 molecules of ACh). On the arrival of a nerve impulse, calcium ions (Ca^{2+}) enter the axonal terminal and active actin filaments, which pull the vesicles into the active zone, thus initiate the release mechanism. Approximately 300–400 quanta enter the synaptic cleft when the axon terminal is invaded by a single action potential. Magnesium ions (Mg^{2+}) may block this process. Acetylcholine released from the synaptic vesicles combines with the acetylcholine receptors in the postsynaptic membrane, but some may diffuse away to be rapidly hydrolysed by local acetylcholinesterase. This hydrolytic process is partially blocked by cholinergic drugs such as physostigmine (eserine) and its analogues, which accounts for the value of these drugs in patients with myasthenia gravis, in which some acetylcholine receptors become coated with antibody with reduced responsiveness. Nicotine applied in low concentration to motor end-plates and ganglion cells stimulates transmission, but in higher concentration blocks it. Acetylcholine can behave similarly and therefore is said to have a nicotinic effect. The block induced by high concentrations of acetylcholine, as may follow excessive medication with cholinergic drugs, produces cholinergic paralysis. The action of acetylcholine upon smooth muscle, however, resembles that of muscarine, which causes such cells to contract. This action can be blocked by atropine. Most of the synapses in the central nervous system at which acetylcholine is the transmitter are muscarinic in type. Somewhat paradoxically, while acetylcholine seems almost invariably to subserve an excitatory function, its role in the cardiac pacemaker is inhibitory.

There are a great many drugs in common clinical use which influence the activity of acetylcholine either by mimicking its action or by blocking its effects in various ways. Some of these are listed in Table 2. In the central nervous system, atropine, scopolamine, and diisopropylphosphofluoridate reduce the acetylcholine concentration and may produce confusion, hallucinations, agitation and slowing of mental processes. Oxotremorine and arecoline have the reverse effect of increasing acetylcholine concentration, thus enhancing the amplitude of physiological tremor, which then becomes overt. In recent years, cholinergic opiate receptors have also been identified upon the cell bodies of the central nervous system, where it is now evident that morphine and its analogues exert their pharmacological effects. Examples of the many drugs which produce muscular weakness or paralysis by acting at the neuromuscular junction are D-tubocurarine and suxamethonium, which are routinely used in anaesthesia. The former blocks the effect of acetylcholine by competing for the receptor site, the latter by mimicking the action of acetylcholine but by having so prolonged an effect that its action is blocked.

BIOGENIC AMINES

The principal biogenic amine transmitters are the catecholamines dopamine, noradrenaline and adrenaline (Fig. 1.11) and serotonin [5-hydroxytryptamine (5-HT)], which is an indole amine. These substances are synthesized within the neuronal soma and transported to the axon terminals. Tyrosine, produced by the hydroxylation of phenylalanine, is the precursor of catecholamine synthesis and is converted by tyrosine hydroxylase into dihydroxyphenylalanine (dopa). Decarboxylation of the latter by dopadecarboxylase produces dopamine, which is a major neurotransmitter, especially in the cells of the substantia nigra, which also contain its pigmentary derivative, melanin. In other cells, dopamine-β-hydroxylase, in the presence of oxygen and ascorbic acid, converts dopamine into noradrenaline. In the

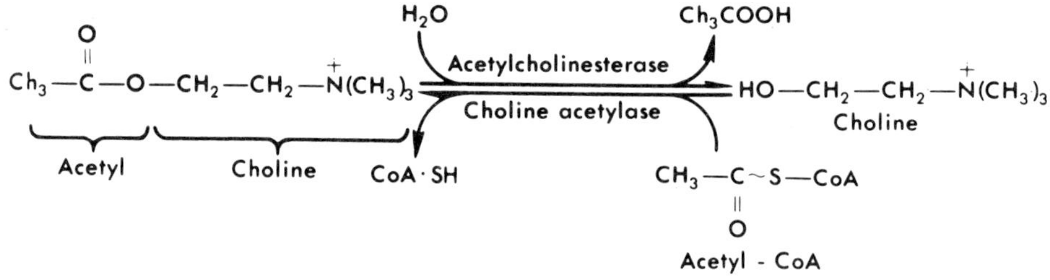

$$CH_3-\underset{\underset{O}{\|}}{C}-O-CH_2-CH_2-\overset{+}{N}(CH_3)_3 \underset{\text{Choline acetylase}}{\overset{\text{Acetylcholinesterase}}{\rightleftharpoons}} HO-CH_2-CH_2-\overset{+}{N}(CH_3)_3$$

Figure 1.10 Formation and breakdown of acetylcholine. [Reproduced from Gardner (1975) *Fundamentals of Neurology*, 6th edn, by kind permission of the author and publisher.]

adrenal medulla, noradrenaline may be converted by phenylethanolamine-N-methyltransferase into adrenaline, which then enters the bloodstream, thereby exercising its hormonal effects.

The noradrenaline-containing neurons of the brain originate from cell bodies in the pons and medulla oblongata and connect monosynaptically with various cortical areas, and especially with the limbic system and hypothalamus. Some descend into the spinal cord. These neurons appear to be involved in many functions, including sleep and wakefulness, emotion, neuroendocrine function and temperature regulation. There are three principal systems of dopamine-containing neurons: (a) the nigrostriatal system, which is largely involved in motor function, (b) the tuberoinfundibular system, which relates to hypothalamic-pituitary control, and (c) the mesolimbic-dopamine system, which is believed to play a role in the control of mental and emotional processes. As with acetylcholine, the release of these transmitter amines at nerve endings is Ca^{2+}-dependent.

The degradation of catecholamine neurotransmitters is thought to depend largely upon two enzymes, namely monoamine oxidase (MAO), which is largely intraneuronal and is released from mitochondria, and catechol-*O*-methyltransferase (COMT), which is largely extraneuronal and is probably associated with the adrenergic receptor. However, pharmacological experiments suggest that other as yet unidentified mechanisms may be involved in the destruction of noradrenaline, at least when this is released from nerve terminals. Any noradrenaline or adrenaline released into the circulation is metabolized in the liver.

Postsynaptic receptors specifically responding to dopamine and to noradrenaline and adrenaline have been recognized. The adrenergic receptors are of two types. Alpha receptors, which respond to noradrenaline and to a lesser extent to adrenaline, are probably self-regulatory in that, when activated, they inhibit the further release of transmitter. Beta receptors, by contrast, activate adenylate cyclase, which converts adenosine triphosphate (ATP) to adenosine-3,5-monophosphate (cAMP), which then activates the response in the effector cell. These receptors and their pharmacology are fully discussed in textbooks of clinical pharmacology.

Serotonin (5-HT) is synthesized from tryptophan via 5-hydroxytryptophan through successive oxidation and decarboxylation. Decarboxylation alone produces pressor agents (e.g. tyramine, tryptamine). Serotonin produces contraction in smooth muscles (e.g. in the walls of arteries). In the central nervous system serotonin is probably involved in the control of behaviour and in the regulation of sleep and body temperature. Serotonin is synthesized in certain neurons of the median raphe of the brain stem and is believed to be the neurotransmitter in some of these cells. In the pineal body, noradrenaline-induced release of cAMP can stimulate the enzymatic conversion of serotonin into melatonin, a hormone which, among other actions, produces lightening of skin pigmentation.

Many drugs are known to influence the activity of biogenic amines, with consequent profound effects upon brain function (Table 2). In general, drugs which depress the synthesis or release of noradrenaline or adrenaline have a sedative or depressant effect, whereas those which similarly depress dopamine tend to produce drug-induced parkinsonism. Reserpine, originally used in the treatment of hypertension but later as a sedative, reduces the concentration of all brain catecholamines and of serotonin. It may also produce severe depression and parkinsonism. The major tranquillizers belonging to the group, which includes the phenothiazines, thioxanthenes and butyrophenones, interact with both noradrenergic and dopaminergic neurons. It is probably the effect of blocking dopamine receptors which accounts for their antipsychotic action as well as for their tendency to produce drug-induced parkinsonism and various forms of dyskinesia. The minor tranquillizers (including the benzodiazepines), used principally to treat anxiety, appear to act by 'turning off' central noradrenergic neurons. There are two main classes of antidepressant drugs. The monoamine oxidase (MAO) inhibitors block the action of MAO in oxidatively deaminating cate-

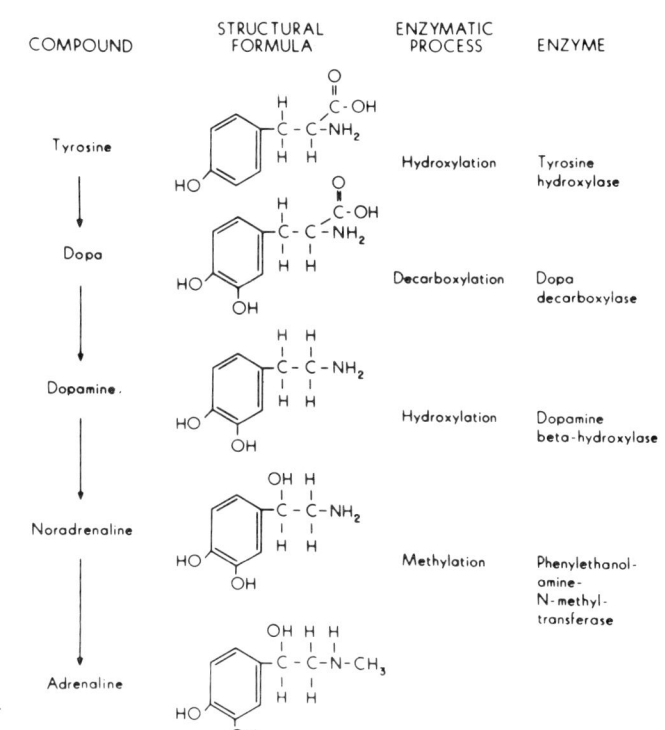

Figure 1.11 The sequential synthesis of the catecholamines. [Reproduced from Gardner (1975) *Fundamentals of Neurology*, 6th edn, by kind permission of the author and publisher.]

cholamines, thus increasing the cerebral concentration of both dopamine and noradrenaline. However, the effect of the tricyclic antidepressants such as amitriptyline and imipramine is much more selective upon noradrenergic neurons. Desipramine, for instance, is a potent inhibitor of noradrenaline uptake but has only a minimal effect upon dopamine. The tricyclic drugs also have an effect in blocking serotonin. Some of these drugs, and especially desipramine, may have a powerful stimulant effect which is beneficial in the treatment of narcolepsy. For this reason they have largely supplanted other stimulants such as the amphetamines and methylphenidate, which have also been used as appetite suppressants but which have been widely abused. Amphetamine and its derivatives interact with catecholamine-containing neurons. Increased motor activity is thought to be due to stimulation of noradrenergic neurons. The behavioural effects and amphetamine-induced psychosis may relate to its dopaminergic effect.

Another important class of drugs deserving brief consideration is that of the hallucinogenic agents such as lysergic acid diethylamide (LSD). It is still not certain whether this and related agents produce their effects by occupying serotonin receptor sites or by direct inhibition of serotoninergic neurons.

AMINO ACIDS AND POLYPEPTIDES

The neurotransmitter role of excitatory amino acids such as glutamic and aspartic acids has been inferred from the effects which are induced when these substances are applied iontophoretically to the surface of postsynaptic neurons. Both are present in high concentration in the cerebral cortex. Glutamic acid is the more powerful amino acid, but their exact localization and function and their putative receptors have not been identified. Glutamic acid may be a sensory afferent transmitter in the spinal cord, but here the polypeptide substance P is much more powerful. The latter, now isolated not only from the dorsal root ganglia but also from the hypothalamus, seems to be a neurotransmitter acting not only in primary sensory nociceptive neurons, but also in the hypothalamus–pituitary axis.

The inhibitory actions of GABA and of glycine are much better understood, and receptors for both have been identified. GABA is derived from glutamic acid by decarboxylation and appears to be the principal inhibitory neurotransmitter in the brain. In the spinal cord, however, it appears to be involved only in presynaptic inhibition. It is directly antagonized by picrotoxin and bicuculline, drugs which consequently produce convulsions in experimental animals. In the spinal cord, and probably in the brain stem, the major inhibitory postsynaptic transmitter is glycine, acting particularly at interneurons. The glycine receptors are blocked by strychnine so that poisoning with this drug causes severe muscular spasms that may be precipitated by any sensory stimulus, owing to loss of the modulating inhibitory role upon motor activity of these interneurons. Tetanus toxin, which has a similar clinical effect, blocks the release of glycine from the same inhibitory nerve endings. The effect of benzodiazepine drugs in giving muscular relaxation and in reducing spasticity appears to result from competition for the glycine receptors, where they mimic the effect of glycine.

HISTAMINE

The role of histamine in the brain and in other parts of the central nervous system is still uncertain. It is present in particularly high concentrations in post-ganglionic sympathetic fibres and in the hypothalamus, and while a neurotransmitter role has been postulated, proof is still lacking.

cAMP, ADENOSINE, AND PROSTAGLANDINS

Adenosine-3,5-monophosphate is the intracellular mediator of the action of many substances which interact with cellular receptors. It therefore plays an important part in synaptic transmission. cAMP mediates the effects of noradrenaline upon postsynaptic neurons. Adenosine can increase cAMP levels experimentally in brain slices and cultured cells by interacting with extracellular receptors linking to adenylate kinase. This and other evidence suggests that it may act as a transmitter in both the central and the peripheral nervous systems, but its function has yet to be defined. Prostaglandins (PG) are a class of chemical substances occurring naturally in many tissues and are related derivatives of prostanoic acid. The first prostaglandin to be isolated was an active acidic lipid which caused contracture of uterine muscle. It now appears that PGE_1 and PGE_2 may inhibit sympathetic nervous activity by acting first upon the release of transmitter from adrenergic terminals and then by affecting the response in the noradrenaline receptor. Similarly, while the iontophoretic application of noradrenaline or cAMP to cerebellar Purkinje cells inhibits their spontaneous firing, the simultaneous application of PGE_1 or PGE_2 inhibits the response to noradrenaline but not to cAMP. Undoubtedly, further functions for this class of substances in the nervous system are likely to be identified in the next few years.

Neurosecretory peptides and neuromodulators

Neurotransmission as described above generally denotes a process through which a substance released at a presynaptic terminal acts upon receptors on a contiguous postsynaptic neuron, directly affecting the electrical resistance of the plasma membrane within milliseconds. Neuromodulation denotes a process occurring over a longer time-scale (seconds to hours) which affects target cell responsiveness to other messengers. There are many peptides that are present in the nervous system which fulfil a secretory

TABLE 3. Categories of neuropeptides

Brain peptides	*Gastrointestinal peptides*
Hypothalamic-releasing hormones	Vasoactive intestinal polypeptide (VIP)
Thyrotropin-releasing hormone	Cholecystokinin (CCK)
Gonadotropin-releasing hormone	Gastrin
Somatostatin	Insulin
Corticotropin-releasing hormone	Glucagon
Growth hormone releasing hormone	Bombesin
Atriopeptin	Secretin
Neurohypophyseal hormones	Motilin
Vasopressin	
Oxytocin	*Others*
Neurophysins	Angiotensin
Substance P	Bradykinin
Neurotensin	Sleep peptide(s)
Methionine enkephalin	Calcitonin
Leucine encephalin	Neuropeptide Y
Dynorphin	
Pituitary peptides	
Adrenocorticotropic hormone	
endorphin	
melanocyte-stimulating hormone	

role, especially in the hypothalamus and pituitary gland. Some of these act as hormones as well as neuromodulators and some are common to the brain and the gut, while many are also vasoactive causing either constriction or dilatation of blood vessels with consequential effects upon the blood pressure. Various categories of neuropeptides are listed in Table 3. A relatively newly discovered neuropeptide is atriopeptin, present in the atrial cells of the heart but also in the brain, where it is believed to play a part in controlling cardiovascular activity as well as fluid and electrolyte balance (Standaert et al, 1985). As will be mentioned later, the role of encephalins in pain perception and control is now recognized to be of considerable importance in view of the ability of these peptides to bind opiate receptors. Dynorphin is probably one such example. Many more such endogenous ligands for receptors for psychoactive drugs are likely to be discovered.

References

Aidley D. J. (1978) *The Physiology of Excitable Cells*, 2nd edn. Cambridge: Cambridge University Press.
Blackwood et al (1964) *Atlas of Neuropathology*, 2nd edn. E. & S. Livingstone.
Bunge et al (1961) *J. Biophys. Biochem. Cytol.* **10**:67.
Catton, W. T. (1970) Mechanoreceptor function. *Physiol. Rev.* **50**:297.
Ciba Foundation Symposium 91 (1982) *Substance P in the Nervous System*. London: Pitman.
Cooper, J. R., Bloom, F. E. and Roth. R. H. (1974) *The Biochemical Basis of Neuropharmacology*, 2nd edn. Oxford: Oxford University Press.
Cull-Candy, S. C. (1984) New ways of looking at synaptic channels: noise analysis and patch-clamp recording. In Baker, P. F. (ed.) *Recent Advances in Physiology*, 10th edn, chap. 2. Edinburgh: Churchill Livingstone.
Crill, W. E. and Schwindt, P. C. (1983) Active currents in mammalian central neurons. *Trends in Neurol. Sci.* **6**:236.
Curtis, B. A., Jacobson, S. and Marcus, E. M. (1972) *An Introduction to the Neurosciences*. Philadelphia: W. B. Saunders Company.
Fitzgerald, M. J. T. (1985) *Neuroanatomy, Basic and Applied*. London: Baillière Tindall.
Gardner, E. (1975) *Fundamentals of Neurology*, 6th edn. Philadelphia: W. B. Saunders Company.
Hodgkin, A. L. (1964) *The Conduction of the Nervous Impulse*. Springfield, Ill.: Charles C. Thomas.
Hydén, H. (ed.) (1967) *The Neuron*. Amsterdam: Elsevier Publishing Company.
Iversen, L. (1982) Neurotransmitters and CNS disease: introduction. *Lancet*.
Kandel, E. R. and Schwartz, J. H. (1985) *Principles of Neuroscience*, 2nd edn. London: Edward Arnold.
Katz, B. (1966) *Nerve, Muscle, and Synapse*. New York: McGraw-Hill Book Company.
Koelle, G. B. (1968) Functional anatomy of synaptic transmission. *Anesthesiology* **29**:643.
McGeer, P. L. and McGeer, E. G. (1973) Neurotransmitter synthetic enzymes. *Prog. Neurobiol.* **2**:69.
Pappas, G. D. and Purpura, D. P. (eds) (1972) *Structure and Function of Synapses*. New York: Raven Press.
Patton, H. D., Sundsten, J. W., Crill, W. E. and Swanson, P. D. (1976) *Introduction to Basic Neurology*. Philadelphia: W. B. Saunders Company.
Peters, A., Palay, S. L. and Webster, H. de F. (1976) *The Fine Structure of the Nervous System: The Neurons and Supporting Cells*. Philadelphia: W. B. Saunders Company.
Rasmussen, H. and Goodman, D. B. P. (1977) Relationships between calcium and cyclic nucleotides in cell activation. *Physiol. Rev.* **57**:421.
Ritchie, J. M. and Rogart, R. B. (1977) The binding of saxitoxin and tetrodotoxin to excitable tissue. *Rev. Physiol. Biochem. Pharmacol.* **79**(2).
Sagar, S. M. and Martin, J. B. (1985) Peptide neurotransmitters in the brain. In Swash, M. and Kennard, C. (eds) *Scientific Basis of Clinical Neurology*. Edinburgh: Churchill Livingstone.
Schadé, J. P. and Ford, D. H. (1973) *Basic Neurology*, 2nd edn. Amsterdam: Elsevier Publishing Company.
Singer, S. J. and Nicolson, G. L. (1972) The fluid mosaic model of the structure of cell membranes. *Science* **175**:720.
Standaert, D. G., Saper, C. B. and Needleman, P. (1985) Atriopeptin: potent hormone and potential neuromediator. *Trends in Neurol. Sci.* **8**:509
Tower, D. B. (ed.) (1975) The nervous system, vol. 1. In Brady, R. O. (ed.) *The Basic Neurosciences*. New York: Raven Press.
Vogt, M. (1979) The impact on neurology of 40 years' advances in pharmacology. *Brain* **102**:445.
Watson, W. E. (1974) Physiology of neuroglia. *Physiol. Rev.* **54**:245.

Part 2: General morphology and organization

INTRODUCTION

The nervous system consists of central and peripheral components in each of which there are somatic and autonomic parts. The somatic parts are concerned with the control of movement and the recording and interpretation of sensory information; the autonomic part is concerned with the regulation of visceral activity and the maintenance of the body's internal environment.

The central nervous system (CNS) comprises the brain and spinal cord. The brain consists of two cerebral hemispheres (the cerebrum), the cerebellum, and the brain stem (mid-brain, pons, and medulla oblongata), which joins the brain to the spinal cord.

The peripheral nervous system consists of the cranial and spinal nerves, which arise from the brain and spinal cord, and of the ganglionated trunks, nerves and plexuses that form the peripheral part of the autonomic nervous system.

THE SKULL, SPINE, AND MENINGES

Development and general morphology

THE SKULL

During fetal life the brain is enclosed in a membranous capsule in order to provide for its growth. Centres of ossification soon appear and by rapid growth extend toward each other. Between the islands of bone the membrane gradually disappears as the calvarium (skull vault) is formed. At birth only small areas of membrane are left, termed the fontanelles. The anterior fontanelle usually closes last, at about the eighteenth month of life. In infantile hydrocephalus, or other conditions causing increased intracranial pressure in infancy, there may be failure of fusion or even wide separation of the sutures.

During development, ossification may (rarely) fail completely so that the calvarium is entirely membranous, or else it may be incomplete, leaving central fissures in the frontal, parietal or occipital regions, where outpouchings of the meninges (meningoceles), or less often of brain tissue (encephaloceles), may persist. Conversely, there may be premature fusion of the sutures (craniostenosis) with consequent effects upon brain growth. Developmental errors less commonly affect the cartilaginous base of the skull, but in achondroplasia the base may be shortened and flattened, with consequent prominence of frontal bones, an abnormally shaped skull, and sometimes compression of the medulla oblongata and upper spinal cord at the craniovertebral junction.

The adult calvarium is formed of two tables of bone—the inner and outer—separated by a fine layer of cancellous bone traversed by many venous channels and lakes or diploe. Major blood vessels, including the middle meningeal arteries and the intracranial venous sinuses, form grooves on the inner table. Within the cranial cavity there are three principal compartments or fossae: the anterior, which houses the frontal lobes of the cerebrum, the middle, which contains the temporal lobes, and the posterior, in which lie the cerebellum and brain stem. The structure of the base of the skull is much more complex. In the frontal, sphenoid, ethmoid and maxillary bones, the inner and outer tables of the skull are separated by air-containing cavities—the paranasal sinuses—which communicate with the nasal cavity. The petrous portions of the temporal bones, lying beneath the temporal lobes, house the structures of the internal and middle ear. The fibres of the olfactory nerves enter the cranial cavity through the cribriform plate of the ethmoid bone to enter the olfactory bulbs beneath the frontal lobes. The pituitary gland (hypophysis) lies in a midline bony cavity—the sella turcica—between the anterior and middle fossae. There are many openings or foramina in the skull base through which cranial nerves, arteries and veins enter or leave the cranial cavity, the largest being the foramen magnum, at which the medulla oblongata ceases and the spinal cord begins.

Localized hyperostosis of the skull can be significant, as it sometimes occurs as a reaction of the bone to an underlying neoplasm, such as a meningioma. However, internal hyperostosis of the frontal bones—a common radiological finding—is of no pathological significance. Enlargement of the sella turcica may be due to a pituitary neoplasm, but flattening of the sella with erosion or decalcification of its anterior and posterior margins (the clinoid processes) may be a consequence of raised intracranial pressure. Prominent convolutional markings outlining the imprints of the cerebral gyri on the inner table of the skull vault (giving an appearance of so-called 'beaten copper mottling' radiologically) may also be a consequence of raised pressure in hydrocephalus. Much more often they too are of no pathological significance. Flattening of the skull base (platybasia) may be a consequence of Paget's disease or other diseases of the bone and can cause compression of cranial nerves in their exit foramina or compression of the upper spinal cord. More often this results from a congenital defect of the occipital condyles so that there is partial invagination of the atlas vertebra into the posterior part of the foramen magnum (basilar impression of the skull).

THE SPINAL COLUMN

The vertebral body is formed from two primary centres of ossification. When only one functions, a hemivertebra may be formed. Other centres form the neural arch or lamina, the spinous process, and the transverse processes. At birth the upper and lower parts of the vertebral body are still cartilaginous and the body is separated laterally from the two halves of the neural arch or lamina by the cartilaginous neurocentral sutures. The two halves of the lamina are not yet united, although ossification is far advanced. (Ossification of the spinous and transverse processes is not complete until puberty.) Sometimes in the cervical region several vertebral bodies fuse without intervening intervertebral discs (the Klippel-Feil syndrome); this condition may be associated with other developmental anomalies of the craniovertebral junction. Fusion of the neural arch or lamina may fail to occur. Spina bifida occulta, with such failure of fusion in the arches of, for example, the fifth lumbar or first sacral vertebrae or both, may be entirely asymptomatic but can also be accompanied by various abnormalities of development of the spinal cord, the cauda equina, or both. Sometimes a dimple in the skin or a tuft of hair may overlie such a defect. A more extensive failure of fusion of the neural arches—spina bifida operta—is more often associated with overt abnormalities of the cord and its coverings (meningocele, meningomyelocele, or bifid spinal cord).

There are 7 cervical, 12 thoracic or dorsal, and 5 lumbar vertebrae, each separated by intervertebral discs which lie between their bodies. In the adult the five parts of the sacrum are normally fused together. In a coronal plane the column is straight; lateral curvature (scoliosis) is always abnormal. In a sagittal plane the column normally shows a curve convex anteriorly (lordosis) in the cervical and lumbar regions, and a curve convex posteriorly (kyphosis) in the dorsal region (Fig. 1.12). The first two vertebrae of the cervical spine—the atlas and axis—are specialized in structure. Anteroposterior movement between the head and the neck takes place largely through a sliding movement at joints between the lateral parts of the atlas and the occipital condyles. However, the body of the atlas is rudimentary, being largely replaced by a process extending upwards from the body of the axis, the so-called dens or odontoid process, which is held in position by a strong transverse ligament lying behind it but in front of the spinal canal. Much of the movement of rotating the head from side to side takes place when the atlas rotates around this odontoid process. Occasionally a developmental defect occurs in which the odontoid process is not firmly attached to the body of the axis; its retaining ligament may be defective so that its posterior displacement may compress the spinal cord. Similar dislocation of the odontoid may result from disease such as rheumatoid arthritis.

In addition to articulating with one another through the intervertebral discs the vertebrae are connected by their lateral articular processes in the neurocentral joints, each with their capsular ligaments, lying in close relationship to the intervertebral foramina through which the spinal nerves leave the spinal canal. The vertebral bodies are also attached to each other by anterior and posterior common ligaments, the laminae by the ligamenta flava, and the spinous processes by the interspinous ligaments. The spinal canal is that central cavity bounded by the vertebral bodies anteriorly and the laminae posteriorly, in which the spinal cord and cauda equina lie. The lateral and anteroposterior diameters of the canal are longer in the cervical and lumbar regions than in the dorsal region, corresponding to the cervical and lumbar enlargements of the spinal cord (see Fig. 1.12).

The intervertebral disc

The intervertebral disc is limited by two flat plates of hyaline cartilage attached to the vertebral bodies above and below it. Between these plates lies an outer fibrocartilaginous ring—the annulus fibrosus—which is attached to both the anterior and the posterior common ligaments. Within this ring is the soft gelatinous semifluid nucleus pulposus, which represents a remnant of the notochord (see Fig. 1.14). When the annulus fibrosus and the posterior common ligament degenerate or are torn, the nucleus pulposus may herniate either into an intervertebral foramen (lateral prolapse) or into the spinal canal (central prolapse).

The meninges

The brain and spinal cord are covered by three membranes or meninges which are named (from the outer one to the inner one) the dura mater, the arachnoid and the pia mater.

The *dura mater* is thick and fibrous and serves as the internal periosteum or endocranium of the bones of the skull, to which it is closely applied. The inner surface is covered with a layer of endothelial cells. Sheaths of dura mater extend outwards for a short distance as a covering for the cranial nerves as they pass through their respective foramina. Certain fibrous processes of the dura, known as septa, partially separate the cranial cavity into four compartments—the falx cerebri, the tentorium, the falx cerebelli and the diaphragma sellae. The falx cerebri descends from the cranial vault in the midline, lying between the cerebral hemispheres in the longitudinal fissure. It is attached anteriorly to the crista galli and posteriorly to the tentorium. At its superior attached border it splits into two layers to contain the superior sagittal venous sinus, and its lower free border similarly splits to contain the inferior sagittal sinus. The tentorium cerebelli forms a partition between the posterior and middle fossae of the skull, its free border surrounding the midbrain, and its attached border being fixed to the occipital and parietal bones and to the superior border of the petrous portion of the temporal bone. The posterior part of its attached border splits to enclose the transverse sinus, and the anterior part similarly encloses the superior petrosal sinus. The falx cerebelli lies in the midline between the tentorium and the internal occipital protuberance, to both of which it is attached, and its free border separates the cerebellar hemispheres posteriorly. The diaphragma sellae forms a roof to the sella turcica and contains an opening through which passes the infundibulum.

The *pia mater* is a delicate membrane lined with

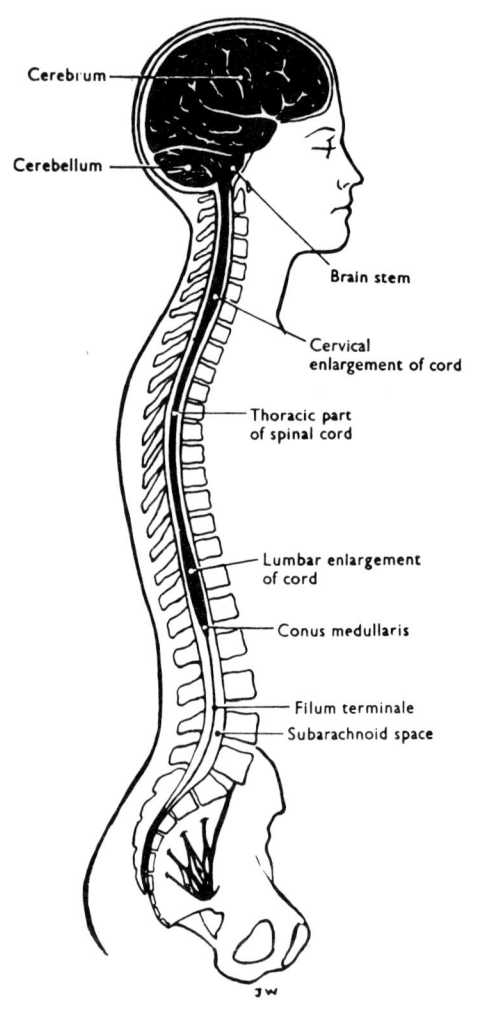

Figure 1.12 The brain and spinal cord in situ. [Reproduced from Mitchell and Mayor (1977) *The Essentials of Neuroanatomy*, 3rd edn, by kind permission of the authors and publisher.]

endothelial cells which intimately clothes the surface of the brain, dipping into the sulci.

The *arachnoid* is a similar membrane lying between the dura mater and the pia mater and bridging over the sulci. The space between the arachnoid and the pia mater, known as the subarachnoid space, contains the cerebrospinal fluid (see p. 238). Its expansions are known as the subarachnoid cisterns. One of the largest of these is the cisterna magna, which joins the median exit foramen of the fourth ventricle (the foramen of Magendie) to the spinal subarachnoid space below the foramen magnum and behind the upper cervical cord. The cerebellomedullary cistern lies between the inferior surface of the cerebellum and the posterior surface of the medulla. The cisterna pontis, continuous with this, lies anteriorly to the pons and is continued upwards into the cisterna interpeduncularis. This in turn is continued forwards into a cistern lying in front of the optic chiasm—the cisterna chiasmatis. The subarachnoid space extends for a short distance into the substance of the brain and spinal cord in sheaths accompanying arteries which penetrate the brain substance (the Virchow-Robin spaces). Between the dura mater and the arachnoid lies a potential space, the subdural space. The arachnoid and pia mater together are sometimes called the leptomeninges and the dura the pachymeninx.

The pia mater also closely invests the spinal cord and its roots and spinal nerves; the pia-arachnoid becomes continuous with the neurilemma or sheath of Schwann and with the perineurium in the intervertebral foramina. The pia also enters the substance of the spinal cord, forming numerous fine septa. The arachnoid, separated from the pia by the subarachnoid space (which, as in the cranial cavity, is traversed by numerous fine trabeculae), extends downwards as far as the second sacral vertebra. The dura mater extends a little lower; it is separated from the walls of the spinal canal by an epidural space containing fatty tissue and a plexus of veins lying on the dorsum of the vertebral bodies. Throughout the canal the spinal cord is suspended in its sheath by a series of pial tooth-like attachments (ligamenta denticulata), which are attached to the surface of the cord at each segment and laterally to the dura.

DEVELOPMENT AND GROWTH OF THE NERVOUS SYSTEM

Introduction

As the cellular mass of the human embryo increases, some areas grow at different rates, thus constituting metabolic or physiological gradients. The layer of cells on the dorsum of the early embryo constitutes the ectoderm, those lying ventrally the endoderm, and those in between the mesoderm. The nervous system originates from a midline thickening of the dorsal ectoderm called the neural plate, which first infolds to form a neural groove. This later becomes enclosed to form a neural tube (Fig. 1.13) which becomes separated from the dorsal ectoderm by a migrating layer of mesoderm. The mesoderm surrounding that part of the enclosed neural tube that ultimately becomes the spinal cord subsequently forms the vertebral laminae. The bodies of the vertebrae form around the longitudinal notochord, which lies ventral to the neural tube (Fig. 1.14). The rostral end of the tube expands irregularly to form fore-, mid-, and hind-brain vesicles from which the brain is ultimately derived. The ectodermal cells in the dorsolateral margins of the neural groove form

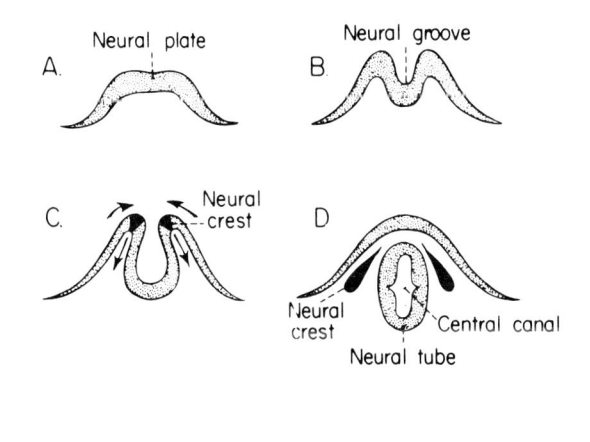

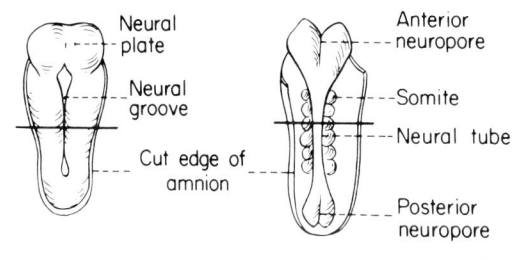

Figure 1.13 Above: Formation of neural tube. A, Neural plate develops. B, Neural groove forms. C, Neural groove deepens and neural crests appear at the lip margin. D, Neural groove becomes neural tube with the neural crests at its sides.

Below: Two dorsal views of this development are shown. At the left, the stage represented shows both the neural plate and the groove being formed. At the right, the neural groove has not finished closing over into a tube and shows anterior (rostral) and posterior (caudal) neuropores. The horizontal lines represent the approximate levels of sections C and D. [Reproduced from Patton et al (1976) *Introduction to Basic Neurology*, by kind permission of the authors and publisher.]

the specialized neural crest cells which migrate away from the enclosed neural tube to form the peripheral parts of the somatic and autonomic nervous systems, including the ganglia of the posterior roots, cranial nerves and autonomic systems. In relation to the developing brain other specialized ectodermal cells form placodes from which parts of the special sense organs and some cranial ganglia are developed.

The notochord seems responsible for the induction (the initiation of differentiation) of the segmented part of the nervous system from the midbrain downwards, while the nonsegmented forebrain is induced by the cephalic mesoderm. The adult nervous system retains some semblance of a tubular structure, the tube being represented in the mature spinal cord by its central canal, and in the brain by its ventricular system. The regional specificity which determines the development of the individual paths of the nervous system from the ectoderm is now thought to result from a gradient of inducing factors released by the underlying mesoderm. There is some evidence that such inducers may be peptides with a molecular weight of less than 1000.

If the neural tube fails to close rostrally during development, it gives rise to anencephaly or other less profound cerebral malformations, depending upon the location and extent of the failure. If the failure of closure occurs more caudally, spina bifida and related malformations result.

Cellular differentiation

The primitive neuroblast is the precursor cell of all neurons. (Some authorities dislike the term 'neuroblast' since, unlike other blast cells, the primitive cells from which neurons arise do not divide, but it is reasonable to retain the term provided this point is accepted.) Some of these primitive cells migrate outwards from the neural crests along with developing nerve roots, often retaining their central connections, to form the posterior root ganglia, the paraspinal sympathetic ganglia, the visceral autonomic plexuses, the medulla of the adrenal gland, and other chromaffin cells (as in the glomus jugulare). The specialized neuroectoderm of the primitive neural plate gives rise not only to neuroblasts but also to spongioblasts from which the glia is derived, and it also produces the ependyma, which forms the internal lining of the neural tube. There is good evidence that large neurons develop first, that motor cells develop before sensory cells, and that interneurons develop last, while glial cells develop after neurons (see Schacher, 1981). Further differentiation in the neural tube produces an inner mantle layer adjacent to the ependyma, and from this the spinal and cerebral grey matter are ultimately derived. The outer marginal layer is relatively cell-free and constitutes the framework into which the processes of the developing nerve cells grow. Myelination begins at about the fourth month of life, ultimately leading to the formation of fibre tracts.

The spinal cord

Through cellular proliferation the spinal part of the neural tube increases in length and thickness, but its growth lags behind that of the developing vertebral column so that the mature spinal cord is shorter than the column. In the mantle zone two groups of cells appear—the basal and alar laminae (Fig. 1.15)—separated by a groove, the sulcus limitans. The cells of the basal lamina subserve functions which are primarily efferent (e.g. the anterior horn cells, which are motor effectors, and the lateral column cells, which are autonomic effectors), whereas those of the alar lamina, which form the posterior grey matter, are largely afferent (concerned with somatic and vis-

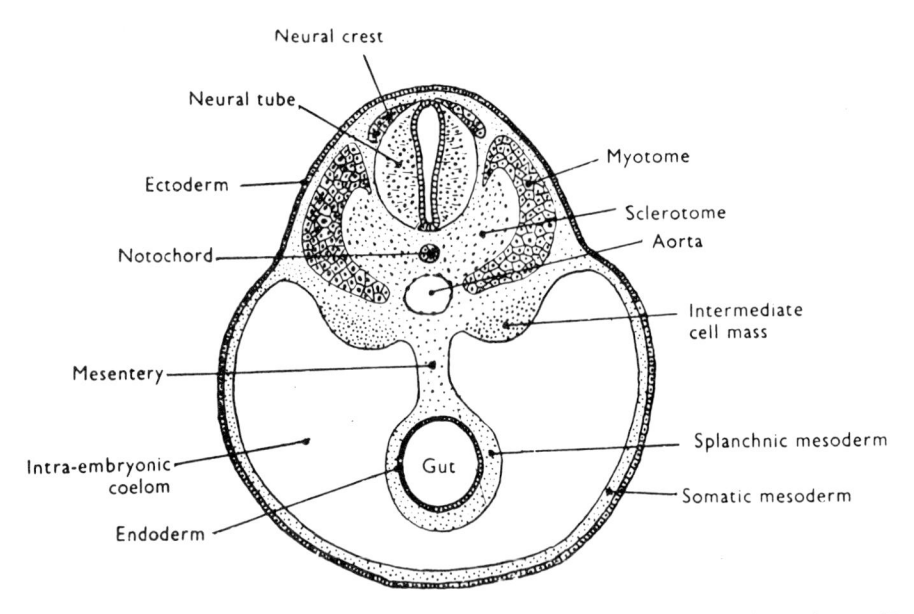

Figure 1.14 Cross section through a human embryo about 4 weeks old, showing the neural tube and neural crests. [Reproduced from Mitchell and Mayor (1977) *The Essentials of Neuroanatomy*, 3rd edn, by kind permission of the authors and publisher.]

ceral afferent activity). Some processes of basal neuroblasts form the motor or anterior roots of cranial and spinal nerves. Alar neurons form connections with the centripetal axonal branches of the unipolar neurons which have previously migrated outwards to form the posterior root ganglia. They also form intrasegmental connections with other neurons in the same cord segment, as well as intersegmental and suprasegmental relationships. The latter connections enable these cells ultimately to play an important role in the processing of sensory information.

Synapse formation and trophic interaction

In the neuromuscular system it is clear that functioning motor neurons greatly influence the chemosensitivity of the muscle fibre membrane (acetylcholine receptors are confined to the region of the motor end-plate but spread along the membrane after denervation). The presence of muscles in the periphery also has a profound influence upon neuronal development and growth so that some 'pathfinding' by developing neurons appears to be guided by chemical signals from the periphery. Nerve growth factor has been shown to provide a trophic signal in the development of the autonomic nervous system and many neurobiologists believe that many more growth factors will be discovered in the future. The specificity of synapses within many parts of the nervous system is not in doubt, but we are only just beginning to learn about the processes which, for example, determine that the axon of a cell should know during development where to go, and once it has arrived, how to stop and form an appropriate connection (see Kandel, 1981).

The brain

The fore-, mid- and hindbrain vesicles—the prosencephalon, the mesencephalon and the rhombencephalon respectively—are initially divided from each other and from the spinal cord by shallow sulci (Fig. 1.16). With increasing growth three flexures appear: the cephalic (or mesencephalic), the pontine and the cervical (at the junction with the spinal cord). With rapid growth of the forebrain (Fig. 1.17), the upper part of its basal portion, the diencephalon, forms large upward and lateral pouches on either side, each of which (a telencephalon) ultimately develops into a cerebral hemisphere, including half of the cerebral cortex, the central white matter and the basal ganglia. During this process, migrating immature cells move outwards past the primitive marginal zone to form the cortical plate from which the grey matter of the cortex is developed. The telencephalon grows so rapidly that it ultimately overlaps the other parts of the brain. The two hemispheres are joined by various white commissures of which the corpus callosum is the most important, and with increasing cellular growth and proliferation of cells the surface becomes deeply enfolded to form the gyri and sulci (Fig. 1.18).

In the mesencephalon and prosencephalon there

Structure and function of the nervous system 25

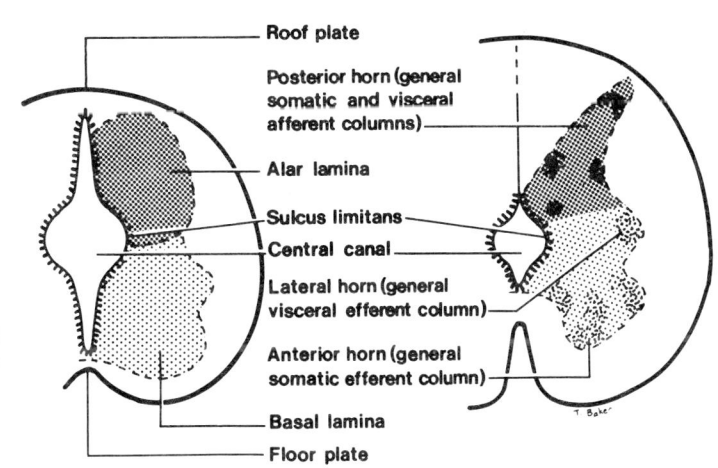

Figure 1.15 A diagram showing the alar and basal laminae in the embryonic spinal cord and the columns of cells developed in them. [Reproduced from Mitchell and Mayor (1977) *The Essentials of Neuroanatomy*, 3rd edn, by kind permission of the authors and publisher.]

are ependymal, mantle and marginal zones, as in the spinal cord. A modified upward extension of the sulcus limitans divides the mantle layer into ventral (or basal) and dorsal (or alar) laminae. Efferent and afferent columns of cells develop in these respective laminae, but are each separated by additional intermediate columns of cells (the visceral or branchial columns) which ultimately innervate structures derived from the branchial arches. All of these columns become divided into individual groups of cells or grey nuclei of the individual cranial nerves. The mesencephalon becomes the midbrain, but the rhombencephalon is ultimately divided into the metencephalon (pons and cerebellum) and the myelencephalon (medulla oblongata). In the metencephalon the edges of the alar plates are called the rhombic lips. These give rise to the cerebellar plates, from which the cerebellum is derived. In each lip there is a layer of specialized cells—the external granular layer—which later migrates internally to form the deeper (cellular) layers of the cerebellar cortex.

The ventricular system and central canal

The tubular characteristics of the developing neural tube are maintained into adult life, forming the cerebral ventricular system and the central canal of the spinal cord (Figs. 1.19 and 1.20). The *cerebrospinal fluid* (CSF), formed by the choroid plexuses within the lateral ventricles, leaves the latter through the interventricular foramina of Monro, and then traverses the third ventricle. CSF leaves the latter by the aqueduct of Sylvius to enter the fourth ventricle, making its exit into the subarachnoid space through the lateral foramina (of Luschka) and the median foramen (of Magendie). The circulation and absorption of the CSF is considered later (p. 238). In the subarachnoid space over the brain and spinal cord, the fluid acts as a protective supporting cushion for the nervous system, but it also possesses other nutritive functions, relating especially to the transport of substances into and out of the nervous parenchyma. The ventricular system and central canal are lined by a layer of ependymal cells. The central canal of the spinal cord remains patent and contains CSF in infancy, but in the normal adult it is effectively no more than a potential space. The central canal can

Figure 1.16 Development of the forebrain, midbrain, and hindbrain. The two sketches at the top also show the ventricles. A side view of the developing central nervous system is shown below. [Reproduced from Patton et al (1976) *Introduction to Basic Neurology*, by kind permission of the authors and publisher.]

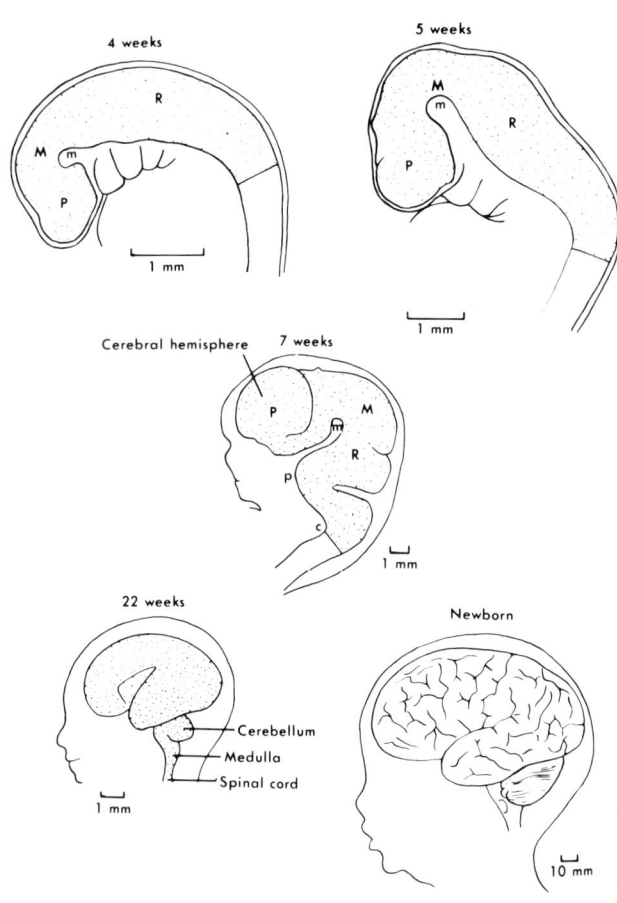

Figure 1.17 The development of the external form of the human brain. P, prosencephalon. M, mesencephalon. R, rhombencephalon. m, mesencephalic (cephalic) flexure. p, pontine flexure. c, cervical flexure. [Reproduced from Gardner (1975) *Fundamentals of Neurology*, 6th edn, by courtesy of Dr Ronan O'Rahilly and by kind permission of the author and publisher.]

become dilated in hydromyelia and/or syringomyelia if CSF which cannot leave the exit foramina of the fourth ventricle is driven downwards into it.

THE BLOOD SUPPLY OF THE BRAIN AND SPINAL CORD

The cerebral arterial circulation

The intracranial blood supply is derived from the two internal carotid arteries and the two vertebral arteries, which unite anteriorly to form the basilar artery. The circle of Willis, situated at the base of the brain, is formed by anastomoses between the internal carotid arteries, the basilar artery and their branches. The basilar artery divides into the two posterior cerebrals which are joined to the two internal carotids by the posterior communicating arteries. The internal carotids give off the two anterior cerebral arteries, which are then united by the single anterior communicating artery, thus completing the circle.

Extracranial arterial disease, in the aorta and in the common carotid, internal carotid, and vertebral arteries in the neck, often produces symptoms of cerebrovascular insufficiency. Hence anomalies in the origin and formation of the arteries themselves, and of the circle of Willis, and the efficacy of collateral channels must all be considered in the pathogenesis of cerebrovascular disease. The principal intracranial arteries and their areas of distribution are shown in Fig. 1.21.

THE COLLATERAL CHANNELS

The internal carotid and vertebral arteries share the blood supply to their own half of the brain in such a way that there is normally no interchange of blood between them. Their respective streams meet in the posterior communicating artery at a 'dead point' at which the pressures of the two are equal, but the two blood supplies do not mix. However, if both internal carotid or, alternatively, both vertebral arteries are occluded, blood passes backwards or forwards from the pair which are still patent. Similarly, if one internal carotid or one vertebral artery is occluded, blood

Figure 1.18 A, Sagittal view of an adult brain specimen. B, Lateral view of an adult brain specimen. C, Ventral view of an adult brain specimen. [Reproduced from Patton et al (1976) *Introduction to Basic Neurology*, by kind permission of the authors and publisher.]

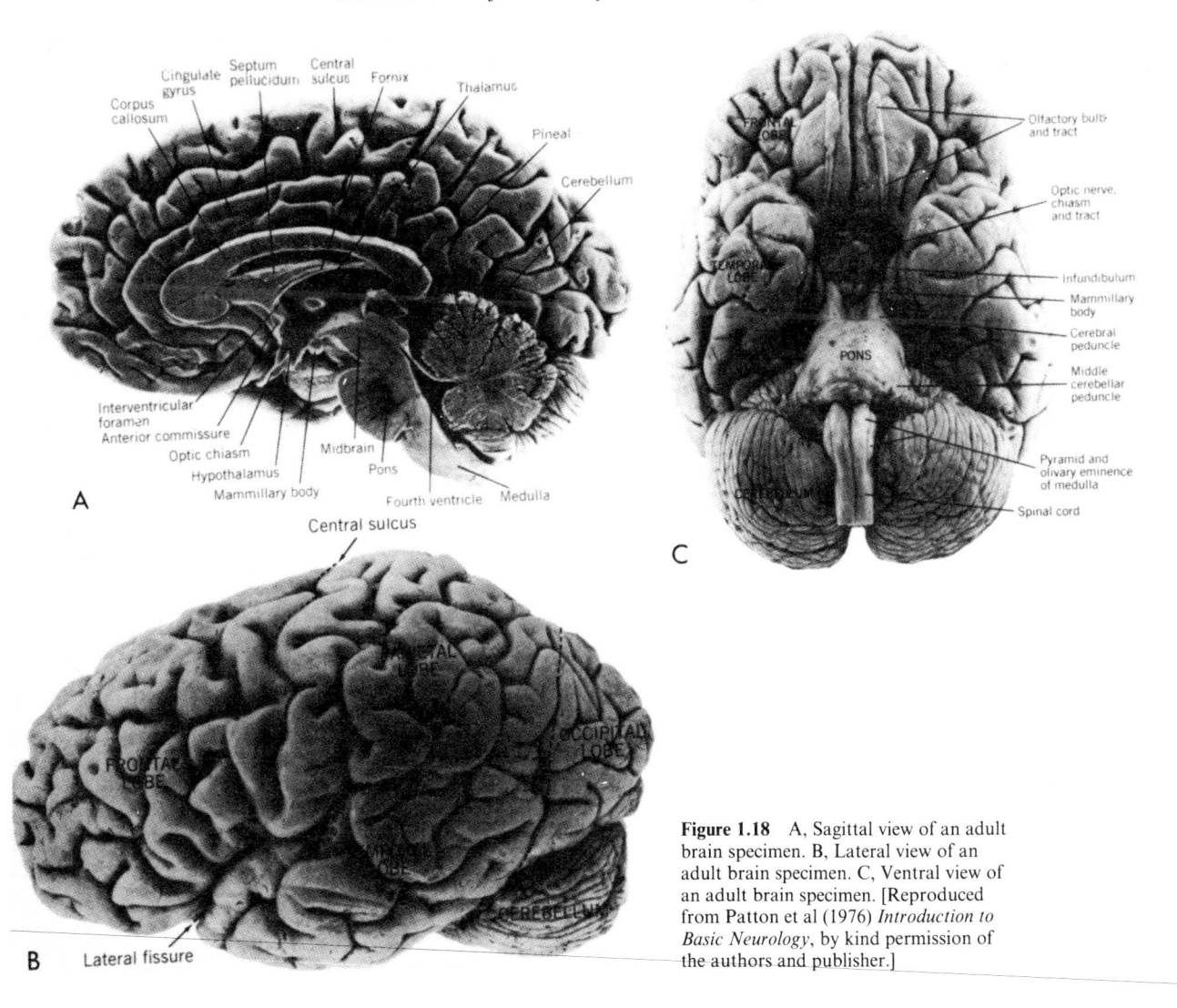

crosses the midline so that the area that would otherwise be deprived of blood is supplied by its contralateral fellow. Normally, the two streams from the vertebral arteries remain unmixed, each on its own side of the basilar artery.

The circle of Willis is the principal collateral channel helping to preserve circulation to the cerebral hemispheres if one of its principal feeding arteries is occluded. But when there is occlusion of one internal carotid artery in the neck, important collateral channels may be established via the external carotid circulation, with reverse flow through the ophthalmic artery. Less beneficial and indeed detrimental to the brain-stem circulation is the reverse flow down one vertebral artery into the distal subclavian artery ('subclavian steal') that may follow proximal occlusion of one subclavian artery. In the cerebral cortex, areas of infarction due to occlusion of major arterial branches are limited by collateral flow through the profuse meningeal arterial anastomoses which exist at watershed areas between the anterior, middle and posterior cerebral areas of supply. However, perforating vessels which supply the internal capsule and basal ganglia are genuine end-arteries.

CEREBRAL BLOOD FLOW

The extent and patency of the collateral channels are factors of importance in limiting the size of the area of infarction which results from arterial occlusion. Another factor of importance is the ability of the cerebral blood vessels to compensate rapidly for sudden changes in blood supply. These changes can

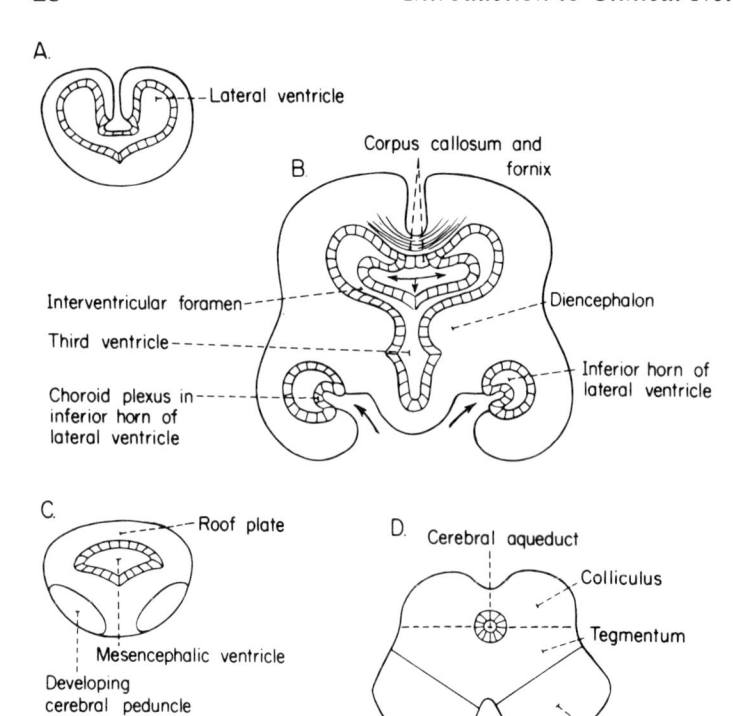

Figure 1.19 A and B, Frontal sections through the developing forebrain, showing portions of lateral and third ventricles and choroid plexus. The arrows in B are in the subarachnoid space, marking sites at which blood vessels will invaginate to form the choroid plexus of the lateral and third ventricles. The continuity of the ventricular system is illustrated in Fig. 1.20. C and D, The developing midbrain, showing the formation of the cerebral aqueduct, colliculi, tegmentum, and cerebral peduncles. [Reproduced from Patton et al (1976) *Introduction to Basic Neurology*, by kind permission of the authors and publisher.]

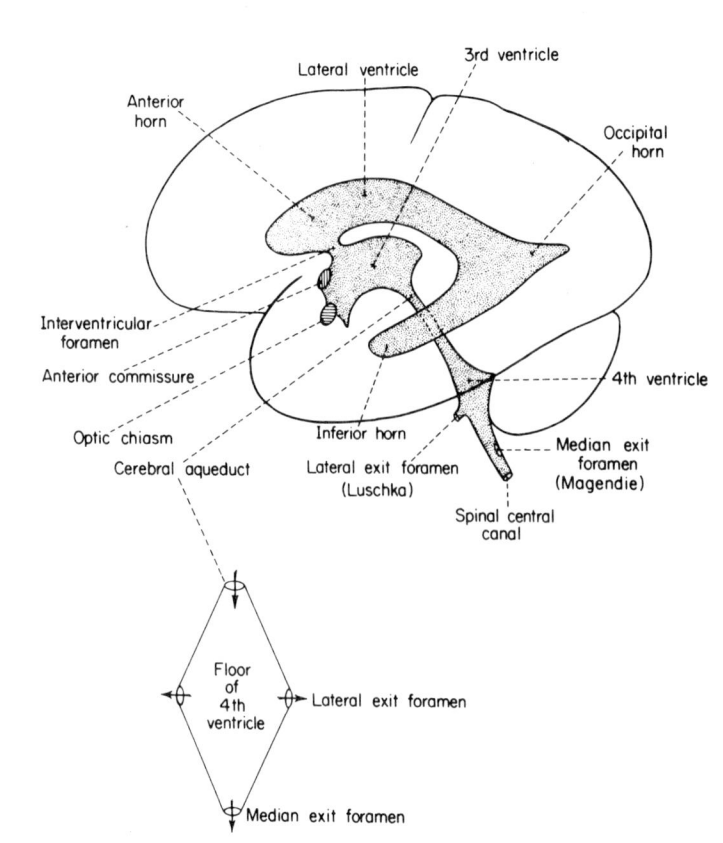

Figure 1.20 Above: Lateral view of adult ventricular system in situ. Below: The arrows in the posterior view of the floor of the fourth ventricle indicate the flow of cerebrospinal fluid: into the fourth ventricle from the cerebral aqueduct and out through the two lateral and one median exit foramina. [Reproduced from Patton et al (1976) *Introduction to Basic Neurology*, by kind permission of the authors and publisher.]

be assessed by using the many methods now available to measure cerebral blood flow (CBF). Since Kety and Schmidt introduced the nitrous oxide method, many other techniques have been utilized. Cerebral 'transit time' can be measured by calculating the time taken for a radioactive bolus injected into the internal carotid artery to reappear in the jugular vein, but such measurements are of little diagnostic value. An electromagnetic flow meter can be used to measure flow in the carotid artery, but requires surgical exposure of the vessel. Others have used hydrogen gas and have measured hydrogen and other variables by means of electrodes inserted into the carotid artery and jugular vein, or have injected radioactive erythrocytes and studied the dilution curve in the jugular bulb. More commonly, use is made of a radioactive inert gas such as xenon-133 or krypton-85, either inhaled or injected into the internal carotid artery. With the latter technique by using scintillation crystals placed laterally over the head it is possible to measure regional blood flow in different areas of the cerebral hemisphere. Calculations may also be applied to compare flow in the cortex and in the white matter of the brain. Even greater precision and sophistication has more recently been added by the use of such techniques as computed tomography (CT scanning) after intravenous sodium isothalamate (a method of measuring cerebral blood volume), positron-emission computed tomography (PET scanning) which assesses regional flow but also oxygen and glucose utilization, single-photon emission tomography, and emission-computed tomography after inhalation of ^{133}xenon. Using such methods it is possible to measure CBF in millilitres of blood per 100 grams of brain per minute, a ratio (mean arterial BP/CBF) indicative of cerebral vascular resistance (CVR) and another parameter indicating cerebral oxygen utilization (arteriovenous O_2 difference/CBF).

Normal cerebral blood flow is about 55 ml/100 g/min, representing approximately 750 ml/min in the average adult, or 15% of resting cardiac output. This flow diminishes with increasing age. The CBF is controlled by the perfusing pressure (which in normal subjects corresponds to the mean arterial blood pressure) and by the cerebrovascular resistance. The ability of the brain to keep CBF relatively constant despite variations in these parameters is known as *autoregulation*, a facility which is highly developed under normal conditions but which may be profoundly altered by cerebrovascular disease. Cerebral vasomotor innervation appears to play a minor part in autoregulation. A rise in intravascular pressure may cause some constriction of pial arterioles, while a fall causes dilatation. The major factor controlling cerebrovascular resistance in both man and animals is the CO_2 tension of the arterial blood. Inhalation of gas containing more than 3.5% CO_2 causes a significant increase in CBF. Changes in O_2 tension tend to have the reverse effect in that inhalation of O_2 causes vasoconstriction and hypoxia tends to cause dilatation.

In patients with hypertension and cerebral atherosclerosis, consistent reductions in the overall CBF may occur; such reductions tend to be greater in patients with symptoms and signs of cerebral ischaemia. When angiography demonstrates occlusion of a major vessel (internal carotid or middle cerebral) on one side, the total CBF is generally reduced more on the affected side of the head, but in some cases, depending presumably upon the efficacy of the collateral circulation and the patency of small vessels, there is a general reduction of the CBF, even in the clinically uninvolved hemisphere. A similar unilateral reduction in CBF through the internal carotid circulation has been reported in the prodromal phase of a migraine attack.

Not surprisingly, it has been suggested that cerebral ischaemia should be treated by the inhalation of CO_2. However, several workers have found that inhaled CO_2 does not increase CBF in patients with occlusion of major vessels and that cerebral oxygen utilization may actually be reduced, possibly because diseased small cerebral vessels are unresponsive.

Local hypoxia and tissue acidosis around an area of infarction may cause vasomotor vascular paralysis, vasodilatation, and loss of autoregulation, which may in turn result in excessive blood flow around the periphery of such an area (the 'luxury perfusion syndrome'). This phenomenon may give rise to venous engorgement (red venous blood) and sometimes even haemorrhage, extending the area of initial damage. Inhaled CO_2 would be likely to increase flow into such areas and would therefore be harmful. This process not only causes local tissue damage but also tends to divert blood away from an ischaemic focus ('intracerebral steal syndrome'). Fortunately such hyperaemic foci with loss of autoregulation usually persist for only 2 or 3 days, though occasionally they last much longer. Autoregulation may be temporarily impaired over the entire affected hemisphere.

Hypocapnia (loss of CO_2 with consequential reduction in blood bicarbonate) induced by hyperventilation may be effective in restoring autoregulation in patients in whom it was lost. Hyperventilation and hypocapnia seem not to cause cerebral ischaemic hypoxia in patients with cerebral ischaemia. On the contrary, they may increase local flow by producing vasoconstriction in the normal collateral channels, thus increasing the perfusion pressure to the ischaemic area. There is also some evidence to suggest that centres in the brain stem

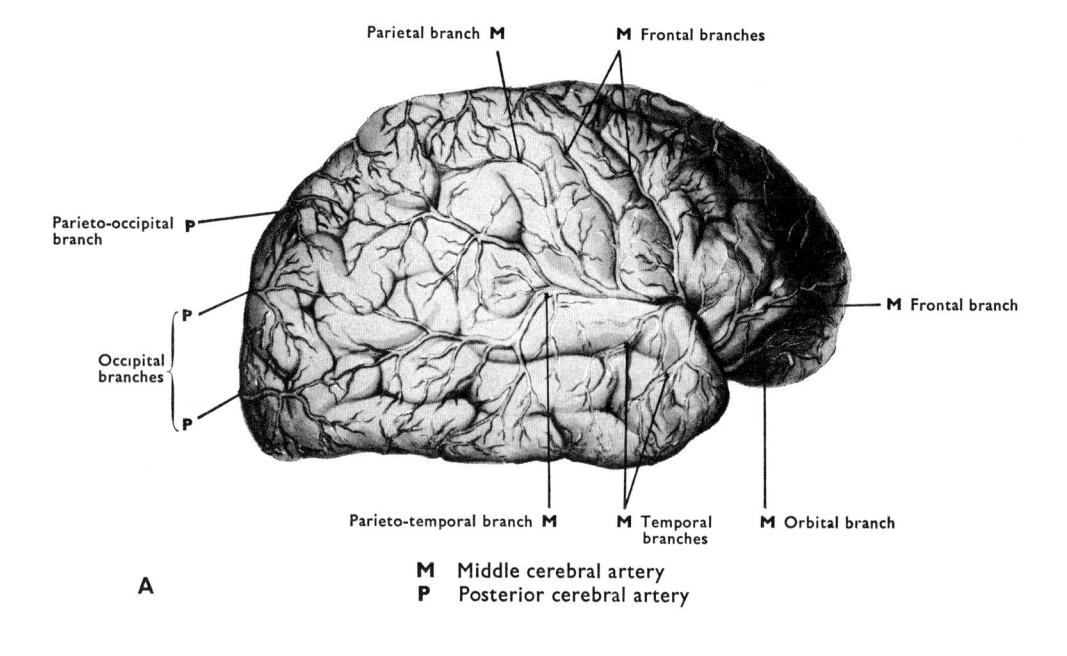

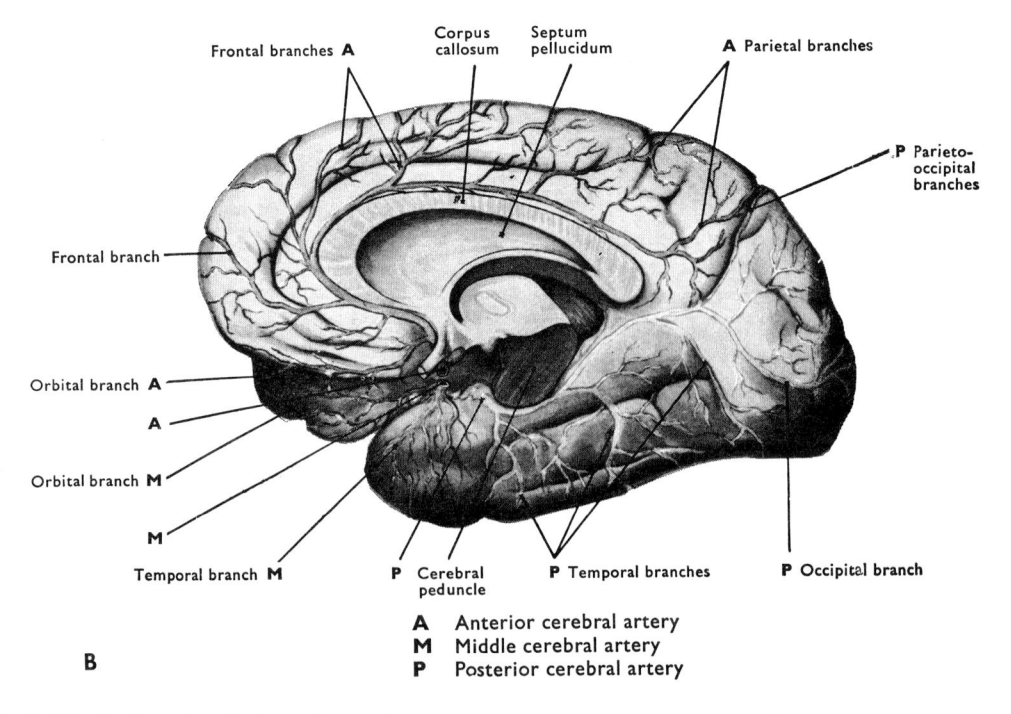

Figure 1.21 A, Distribution of cerebral arteries on the superolateral surface of the right cerebral hemisphere. B, Distribution of cerebral arteries on the median and tentorial surfaces of the right cerebral hemisphere. C, Arteries of the base of the brain. [Reproduced from Walton (1985) *Brain's Diseases of the Nervous System*, 9th edn, by kind permission of the publisher.] (*Illustration continued on the opposite page*)

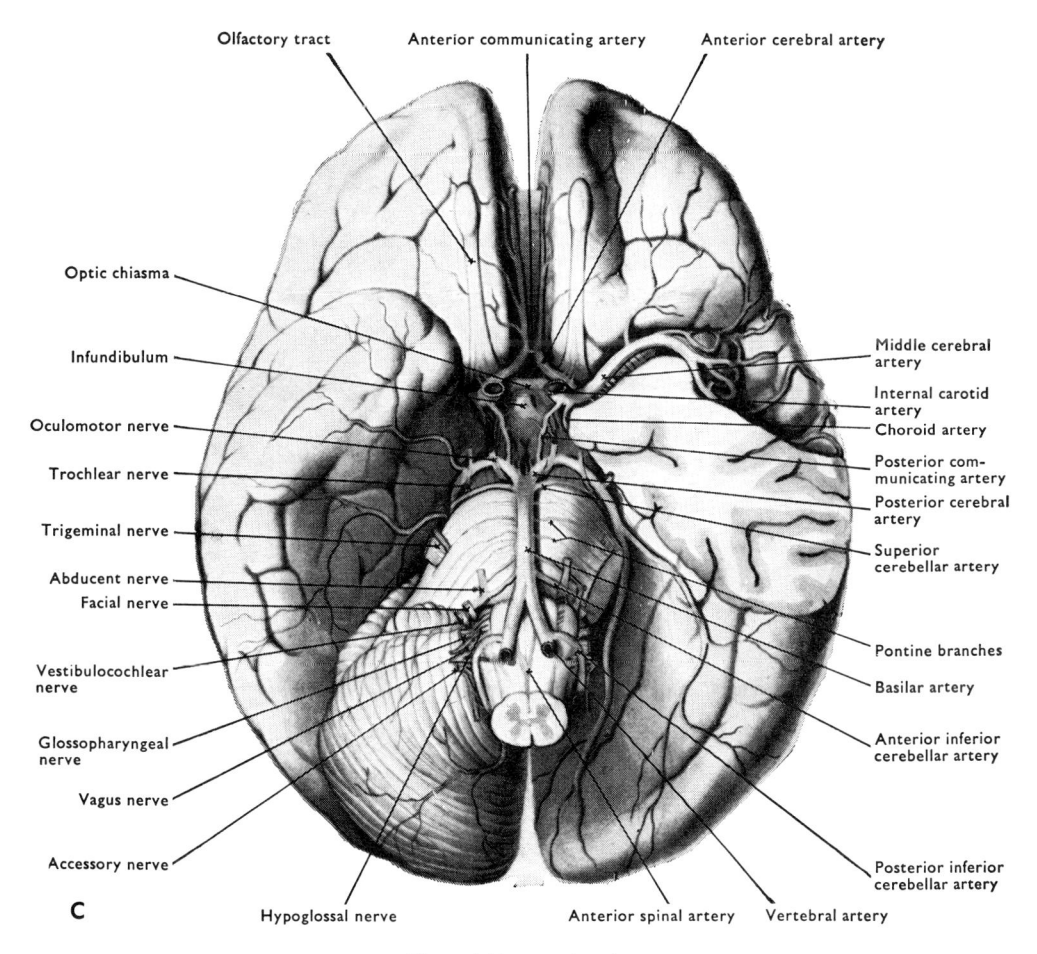

Figure 1.21. *continued*

may exercise a neurogenic controlling effect upon CBF and metabolism.

Blood flow in extracranial arteries

While angiography (see p. 266) is the traditional method of demonstrating occlusion or stenosis of extracranial vessels, in which disease (especially of the carotids and vertebrals in the neck) may cause various neurological manifestations, several non-invasive techniques have been used increasingly of late, including CT scanning, oculoplethysmography, carotid phonoangiography and especially directional Doppler ultrasonography. The latter is a useful, safe and atraumatic method which is invaluable in demonstrating such lesions.

THE BLOOD-BRAIN BARRIER

All vessels within the central nervous system are surrounded by a thin covering formed by the processes of astrocytes. The plasma in the vessels is separated from the nervous tissue by the endothelium of the capillaries and their basement membranes, external to which is the extracellular space of the nervous system. The blood–brain barrier consists of the endothelial lining cells, the basement membrane and the perivascular processes of astrocytes. Intravenous injection of trypan blue stains only the astrocytic processes; the dye does not reach the nervous parenchyma except where the barrier is incomplete, as in the pineal, pituitary and choroid plexuses, for example. Injected large molecules (ferritin, horseradish peroxidase) cannot pass the tight junctions of the capillary endothelial cells in either direction. However, gases, water, glucose, electrolytes and amino acids diffuse freely across the blood–brain barrier into the intracellular space (glial cells and neurons) and into the extracellular space of the brain. Acute cerebral lesions, whether due to trauma, inflammation or infarction, increase the permeability of the barrier and thus alter the extra- and intracellular concentrations of protein, water and electrolytes.

The cerebral venous circulation

THE VENOUS SINUSES

The intracranial venous sinuses are spaces lying between layers of the dura mater and are lined with endothelium. They receive blood from the veins of the brain and drain directly or indirectly into the internal jugular vein. They communicate with the meningeal veins and, by means of emissary veins, with the veins of the scalp. The major sinuses and veins are depicted in Fig. 1.22.

Thrombosis of the intracranial venous sinuses is usually due either to the extension of infection from neighbouring structures or to direct injury. Rarely, it occurs in the absence of any evident local cause. These two varieties of sinus thrombosis are rather unsatisfactorily distinguished as 'secondary' and 'primary' respectively.

'Primary' sinus thrombosis is rare and is most frequently seen at the extremes of life, especially during the first year. It occurs in wasted, debilitated infants, especially as a complication of congenital heart disease or gastrointestinal infection, and later in life in individuals suffering from severe anaemia, exhausting infections such as enteric fever, or emaciating diseases such as carcinoma and tuberculosis. It has also been described as a complication of oral contraceptive medication and in pregnancy and the puerperium. The principal predisposing factors appear to be anaemia, increased coagulability of the blood, low blood pressure, and dehydration.

'Secondary' sinus thrombosis may be the result of direct injury of a sinus through fracture of the skull or surgical operation in its vicinity. Infection may spread to the sinuses from an area of osteomyelitis of a cranial bone. The transverse sinus may thus become infected from mastoiditis, or through the jugular vein from the fauces. Infection may spread from the transverse to the superior sagittal sinus. The latter and the cavernous sinus may be directly infected from frontal sinusitis or from infection of the other paranasal sinuses. Owing to the comparatively free communication between the intracranial venous sinuses and the superficial veins of the face and scalp, cutaneous sepsis may also cause intracranial sinus thrombosis. The cavernous sinus is especially liable to become infected as a result of pyogenic infections in the neighbourhood of the upper lip. Though sinus thrombosis may be the only manifestation of infection, it may be associated with extradural, subdural or intracerebral abscess, or localized or diffuse leptomeningitis.

The blood supply of the spinal cord

ARTERIAL SUPPLY

The spinal cord is richly supplied with blood (Fig. 1.23). There are two posterior spinal arteries, each derived from the corresponding vertebral or posterior inferior cerebellar artery and passing downwards upon the side of the medulla oblongata and throughout the whole length of the spinal cord, where they lie either in front of or behind the dorsal nerve roots. The single anterior spinal artery is formed by the union of branches from each vertebral artery, and descends throughout the length of the spinal cord in the anterior median fissure. The spinal arteries are reinforced by segmental arteries which enter the intervertebral foramina and are derived from the vertebral, intercostal and lumbar arteries. The spinal cord is thus surrounded by an arterial wreath, which unites the spinal arteries and sends branches horizontally inwards to supply the white matter and the greater part of the posterior horns of the grey matter. The anterior horns of grey matter are supplied by branches of the anterior spinal artery which are distributed to the anterior horn on each side alternately. Blood from the anterior spinal artery supplies the whole of the cord except the posterior columns and a variable part of the posterior horns; the posterior arteries supply the remainder. Descending branches also supply the cauda equina.

Methods of measuring spinal cord blood flow in animals have been devised, and experimental work has confirmed that motor or sensory activity causes temporary vasodilatation and increased blood flow in the relevant portions of the cord and cauda equina.

Syndromes of spinal cord ischaemia and/or infarction may result from embolism or occlusion of the anterior spinal artery due to atheroma, aortic disease or a drop in perfusion pressure, and may complicate aortography. Posterior spinal artery occlusion due to intrathecal phenol injection has also been described. In general, the motor neurons and the central grey matter are more vulnerable to ischaemia than is the white matter.

VEINS

The spinal veins derived from the substance of the spinal cord terminate in a plexus in the pia mater. Longitudinal channels pass upwards into the intracranial venous sinuses. Segmental veins pass outwards along the nerve roots to join the internal vertebral venous plexus, in which blood also flows upwards to the intracranial venous sinuses. The posterior half of the cord is drained by the posterior medullary veins. The anterior medullary group can

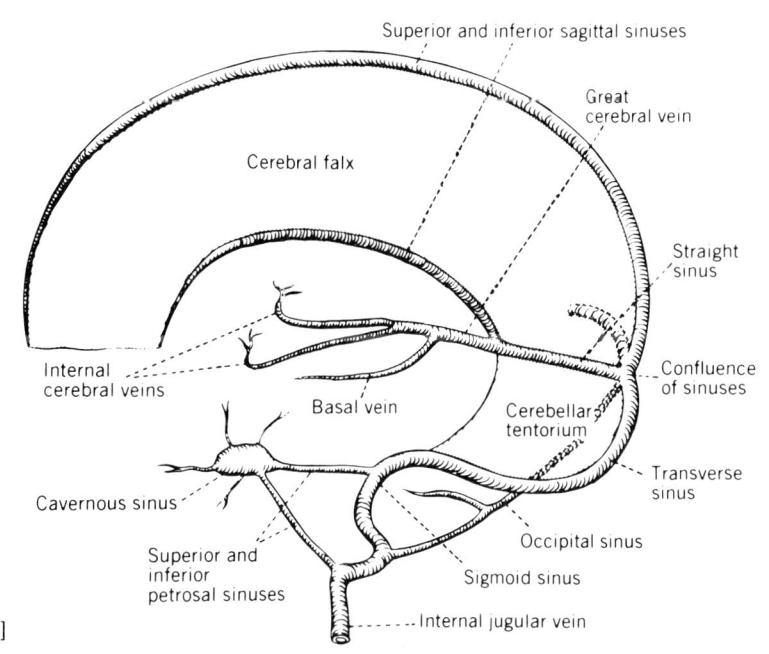

Figure 1.22 Diagram of major cerebral sinuses receiving the cerebral veins. [Reproduced from Patton et al (1976) *Introduction to Basic Neurology*, by kind permission of the authors and publisher.]

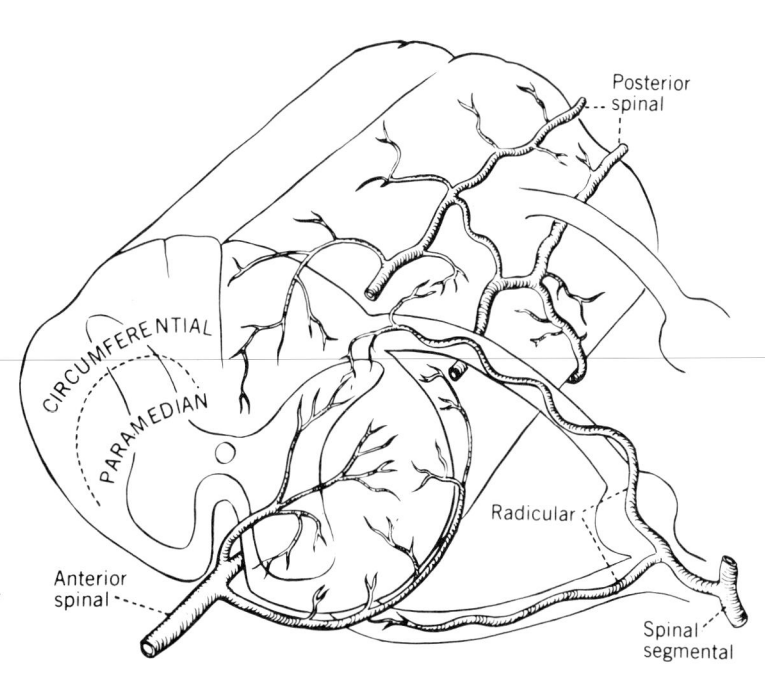

Figure 1.23 Arterial supply to the spinal cord. [Reproduced from Patton et al (1976) *Introduction to Basic Neurology*, by kind permission of the authors and publisher.]

be divided into one lateral and two medial groups, and the anatomical pattern helps to explain the clinical features of venous infarction of the cord. Venous drainage through the intervertebral foramina is relatively unimportant, but thrombophlebitis may reach the spinal veins by this route.

THE CEREBRUM

General morphology

The general morphology of the cerebral hemispheres has been illustrated in Fig. 1.18. The longitudinal

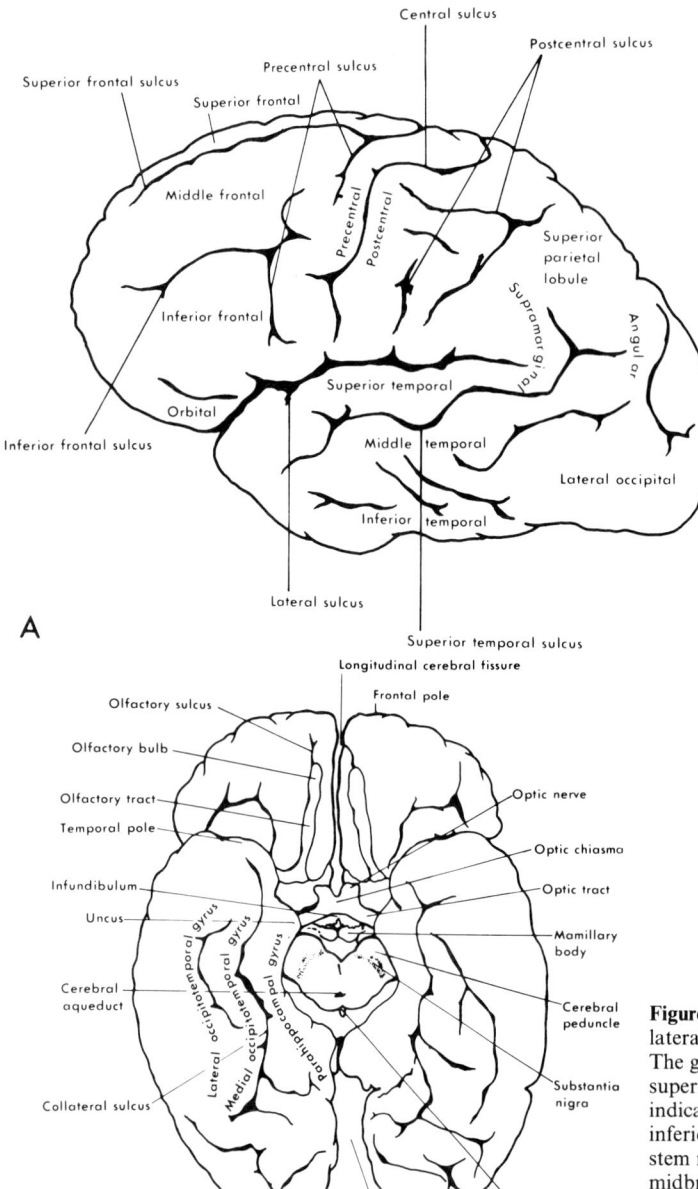

Figure 1.24 A, Outline sketch of the lateral surface of the cerebral hemisphere. The gyri are directly labelled (except the superior frontal) and the sulci are indicated by lines. B, Outline sketch of the inferior aspect of the brain, with the brain stem removed by a section through the midbrain. [Reproduced from Gardner (1975) *Fundamentals of Neurology*, 6th edn, by kind permission of the author and publisher.]

fissure which separates the two hemispheres is largely occupied by a fold of dura mater, the falx cerebri. The convolutions are called gyri, the fissures between them the sulci, and many of both are named (Fig. 1.24). The frontal lobe lies anterior to the central or rolandic sulcus, and the temporal lobe lies below the lateral sulcus (fissure of Sylvius), in the depths of which is the insula. The parietal lobe lies behind the central sulcus, but the division between it on the one hand and the posterior part of the temporal lobe on the other is less well defined, and the transition between both of these and the occipital lobe is somewhat arbitrary, not being defined by any single sulcus. The frontal precentral gyrus is especially concerned with the control of movement, the postcentral gyrus of the parietal lobe with somatic sensation, the middle part of the superior temporal gyrus with hearing, and the striate cortex of the occipital pole with vision. The prefrontal cortex plays a part in the control of intellect and personality, the orbital cortex

Structure and function of the nervous system 35

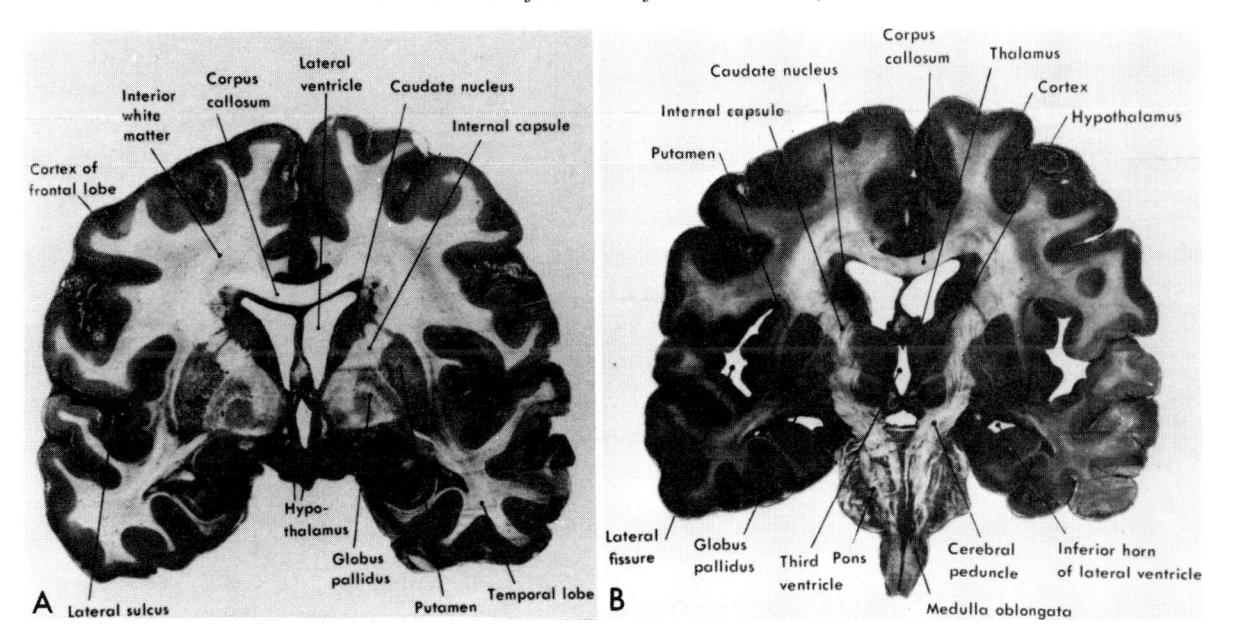

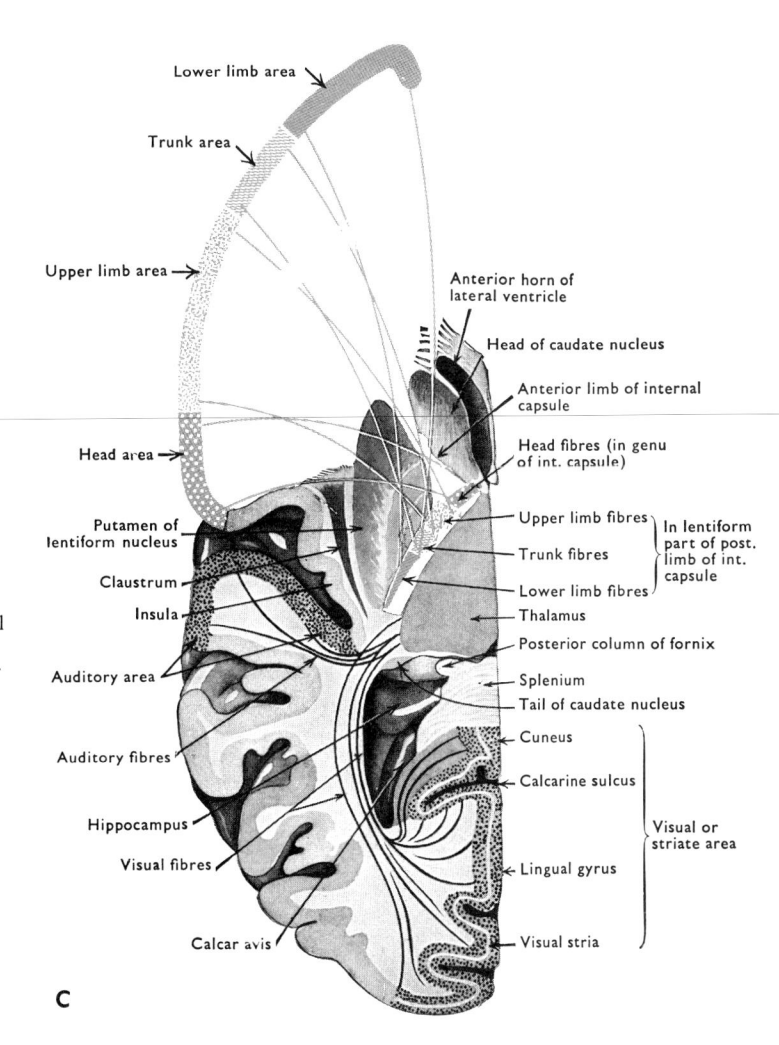

Figure 1.25 A, Photograph of a coronal slice of brain, stained by a Berlin blue reaction that accentuates the grey matter and leaves white matter relatively unstained. B, Photograph of a coronal slice of brain, posterior to that of Fig. 1.25A, and stained by the same method. C, Diagram of motor, auditory and visual areas of left hemisphere and their relations to the internal capsule. [A and B reproduced from Gardner (1975) *Fundamentals of Neurology*, 6th edn, by kind permission of the author and publisher; C reproduced from Walton (1985) *Brain's Diseases of the Nervous System*, 9th edn, by kind permission of the publisher.]

(and especially its cingulate gyrus) in visceral and emotional activity, and the medial temporal cortex (especially the hippocampal gyrus and related structures) in controlling the sense of smell and in memory function. In man, specialized functions relating to speech production and perception and various executive and cognitive skills (praxis and gnosis) reside in one cerebral hemisphere (usually the left hemisphere in right-handed persons) which is known as the dominant hemisphere. Deep in the cerebral cortex are numerous myelinated fibre tracts and pathways which form the central white matter of the hemisphere and which join the various cortical areas to one another. In addition, there are ascending and descending tracts connecting with the central grey matter of the various basal ganglia and other nuclei and with the brain stem and spinal cord. Tracts also cross the midline to the opposite hemisphere in various commissures, of which the corpus callosum is the most important. The principal grey nuclei in the depths of each cerebral hemisphere are the thalamus and hypothalamus; the caudate and lenticular nuclei, which together form the corpus striatum; the globus pallidus; and the putamen (Fig. 1.25). The internal capsule is an important collection of myelinated fibre tracts, connecting the central white matter above with the cerebral peduncle below.

THE CEREBRAL CORTEX

The cerebral cortex or pallium is the layer of grey matter covering the cerebral hemisphere. Man is distinguished from the lower vertebrates and invertebrates by the massive development of the neocortex of the forebrain. The phylogenetically primitive paleocortex (largely olfactory) and archicortex (largely embodied in man in the so-called limbic system, including the hippocampus) together form the so-

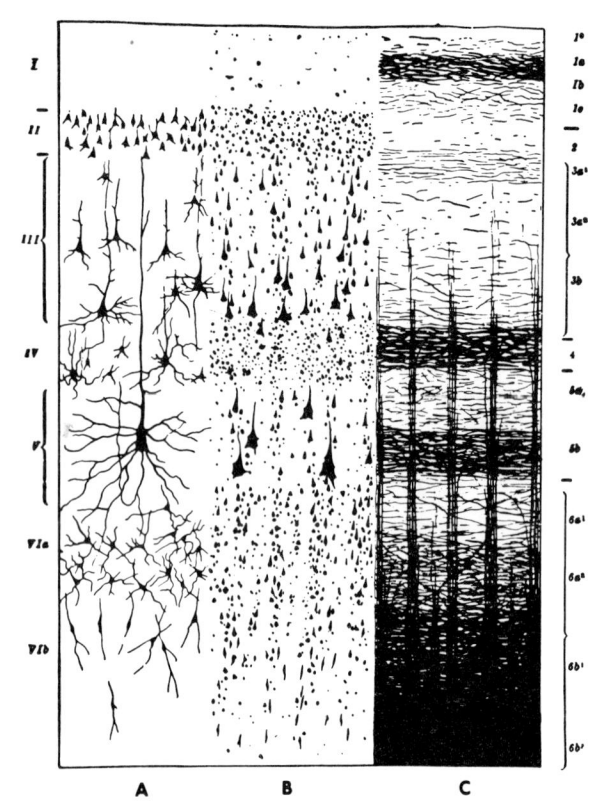

Figure 1.26 Schematic diagram showing the structure of the cerebral cortex obtained by (A) Golgi stain, (B) Nissl stain, and (C) myelin stain. [Reproduced from Ranson and Clark (1959) *The Anatomy of the Nervous System: Its Development and Function*, by kind permission of the authors and publisher.]

called rhinencephalon, or 'smell brain', though these areas subserve many other functions in man relating to memory and emotion in addition to smell. Man's neocortex has a surface area of 2000 cm^2 and varies in thickness from 2 to 4.5 cm. Many different cell

TABLE 4. The layers of homotypical neocortex*

Layer	Chief type of cell	Other features	Axonal distribution of predominant cell
1. Molecular layer (plexiform layer)	Occasional horizontal and stellate cells	Cell poor; it is an important synaptic field	Throughout layer 1
2. Outer granular layer	Small and medium-sized pyramidal cells	Also contains stellate cells	Intracortical and to white matter
3. Pyramidal cell layer (outer pyramidal layer)	Medium and large pyramidal cells	Also contains stellate cells	To white matter
4. Inner granular layer	Stellate cells (granule cells)	Main termination of specific afferent fibres	Intracortical
5. Ganglionic layer (inner pyramidal layer)	Small to giant pyramidal cells	Giant cells mostly limited to precentral gyrus	To white matter
6. Fusiform cell layer (layer of polymorphic cells)	Fusiform cells	Other cells of different shapes and sizes (hence the term polymorphic)	To white matter

*Reproduced from Gardner (1975), by kind permission of the author and publisher.

types are present in the cortex and are usually arranged into six layers (see Fig. 1.26 and Table 4). The way in which the cells are arranged within these layers varies greatly from one area of the cortex to the other; the study of the architecture of these cellular arrangements is known as *cytoarchitectonics*. Brodmann, many years ago, produced a cytoarchitectural map of the cortex, divided into numbered areas.

Three principal types of cortical neurons have been identified, namely pyramidal, stellate and fusiform cells. Pyramidal cells have a soma varying in diameter from 15 to 10 μm; the largest are the so-called Betz cells. Each pyramidal cell has an apex with a long dendrite projecting towards the cortical surface, a basal dendritic arborization, and axons which project away from the cortex into white matter. It is believed that all the axons of the Betz cells (which are about 25 000 in number) contribute to the corticospinal (pyramidal) tract and supply distal limb motor neurons. Relatively few of the other axons reach the pyramidal tract without the intervention of interneurons. The Betz cell axons probably contribute about 2.5% of the one million fibres in each such tract.

Stellate cells, as their name implies, have a star-shaped dendritic tree confined to the cortex. The fusiform cells of the deepest cortical layer lie with their bodies perpendicular to the cortical surface. They have short dendrites leaving each pole, and are to be contrasted with horizontal cells of the superficial cortical layer which have bodies lying parallel to the surface and dendrites running in a similar direction.

Myelin stains of the cortex reveal horizontal bands of myelinated fibres traversing layers 4 and 5 (the lines of Baillarger), the outer one in the visual cortex (Brodmann's area 17) being so prominent that it gives a visible striation (the line of Gennari), this being known as the striate cortex. When all six cortical layers can be easily identified, the cortex is called homotypical; when the layers are less distinct, it is called heterotypical. In the precentral motor cortex (area 4), layers 2 and 4 are poorly defined (agranular cortex). In some areas where sensory information is recorded (the postcentral gyrus, area 3, or the occipital striate cortex, area 17), layers 3 and 4 contain few pyramidal cells and the density of stellate or granular cells in layers 2 and 4 is increased (granular cortex). In some cortical areas groups of cells in various cortical layers, interconnected by vertical axons or dendrites, seem to form cell columns; these often function as units in information processing. All cortical cells gradually decrease in number with increasing age after 20 years of age; the decrease is greatest in large neurons, less in small neurons and least in glial cells (Henderson et al, 1980).

Some axons leaving the cortex constitute corticofugal fibres which project to the basal ganglia, thalamus, brain stem, cerebellar grey nuclei and spinal cord, while others form commissural fibres travelling to the opposite hemisphere. Yet others form association fibres and project to other parts of the cortex; some are short and remain cortical but others are long and form prominent tangential subcortical tracts (the arcuate or U-fibres which are especially prominent in the posterior parts of both hemispheres).

The electrical activity of the cortex

Cortical neurons have many properties similar to those of spinal cord nerve cells, which have been studied more extensively (p. 8), but there are some important differences. The resting potential of cortical neurons is about -60 mV, but has marked fluctuations presumably resulting from constant bombardment through synaptic connections with other cells. Many cortical neurons also show graded excitatory or depolarizing postsynaptic potentials (EPSPs) and inhibitory, hyperpolarizing postsynaptic potentials (IPSPs), but the IPSPs are often larger and of longer duration than those recorded in the spinal cord. A bewildering and complex array of connections (somatodendritic, axodendritic and many more) interlink the neurons of the cortex. For example, the pyramidal cells may be excited or inhibited by afferent fibres, by interneurons, and by recurrent collaterals. Few generalizations about the physiological activity of cortical neurons are yet possible.

The electrocorticogram (ECoG) is the record of the spontaneous electrical activity of the cerebral cortex measured through an electrode applied to its surface. The electroencephalogram (EEG—see p. 254) is the record of the electrical activity of the brain studied with electrodes applied to the intact skull. Sensory-evoked potentials induced by a sensory stimulus applied to a peripheral receptor may be recorded over the area of cortex where the afferent impulses are received. These evoked potentials, which represent synchronous potential changes in the neuronal population underlying the recording electrode, can now be recorded through the intact skull, representing peripheral stimuli of somatic, visual or auditory origin. In clinical practice, the recording of such evoked potentials, demonstrating abnormalities of pattern, amplitude and latency of the response, can give invaluable information concerning the integrity of secondary pathways.

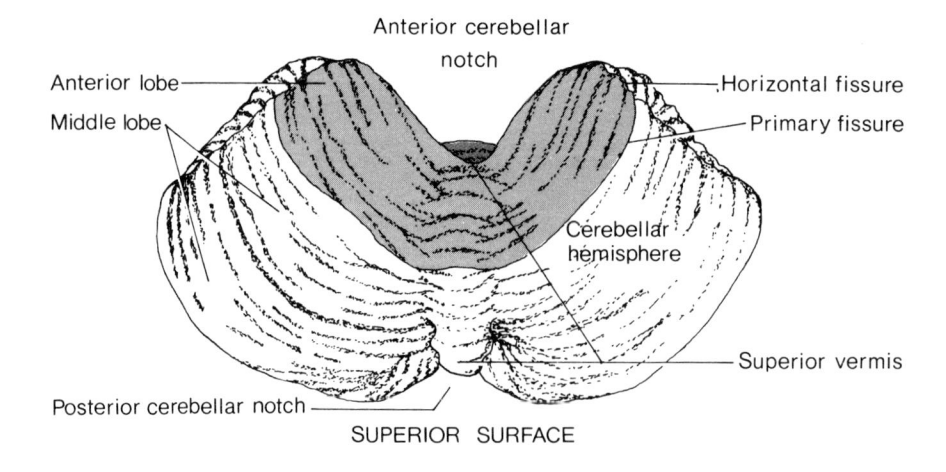

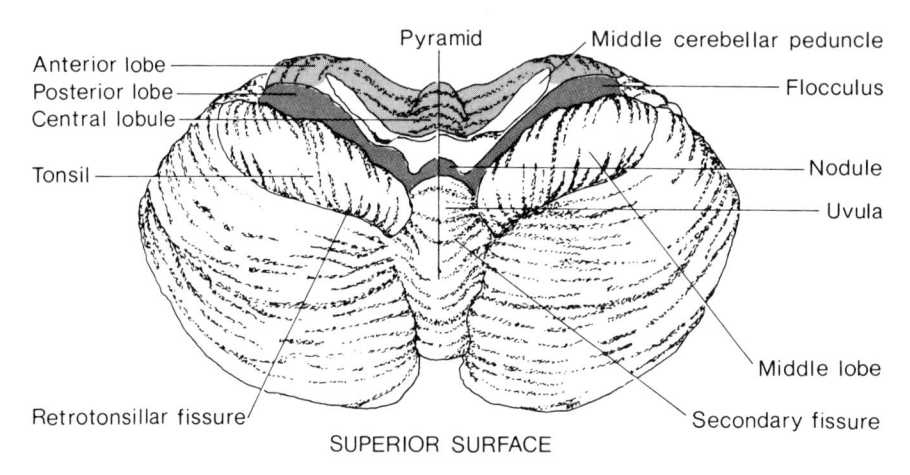

Figure 1.27 The superior and inferior surfaces of the cerebellum. Various authorities have advocated complex cerebellar subdivisions, but here the older and adequate subdivision into three main lobes has been retained. [Reproduced from Mitchell and Mayor (1977) *The Essentials of Neuroanatomy*, 3rd edn, by kind permission of the author and publisher.]

THE CEREBELLUM

The cerebellum is responsible for modulating afferent somatic sensory information and for correlating this with the motor output from the cerebrum and brain stem in order to coordinate movements of greater precision. Function and dysfunction resulting from cerebellar disease are considered in Chapter 8.

General morphology

The cerebellum occupies the greater part of the posterior cranial fossa, being separated from the cerebral hemispheres above by a fold of dura mater—the tentorium cerebelli—whose free medial border virtually encircles the midbrain. It consists of two cerebellar hemispheres united by the median vermis. On its inferior surface is a midline hollow—the vallecula—into which the inferior part of the vermis projects. The surface anatomy of the cerebellum is illustrated in Fig. 1.27, and its relationship to the pons and medulla, which lie in a shallow anterior groove, is illustrated in Fig. 1.28. The superior, middle and inferior cerebellar peduncles, which join the cerebellum to the brain stem, can also be seen.

In contrast to the brain stem (see below) with its external white matter and internal grey nuclei, the cerebellum, like the cerebrum, has a core of white matter and an outer cortex of grey matter. Deep in the white matter lie a series of grey nuclei—the lateral or dentate (Fig. 1.28), the intermediate and the medial or fastigial. The intermediate and medial nuclei are sometimes called the roof nuclei. (Indeed, some include the dentate nuclei under the latter term.) Axons from the cells of the cortex and the nuclei connect cortex to cortex (association fibres),

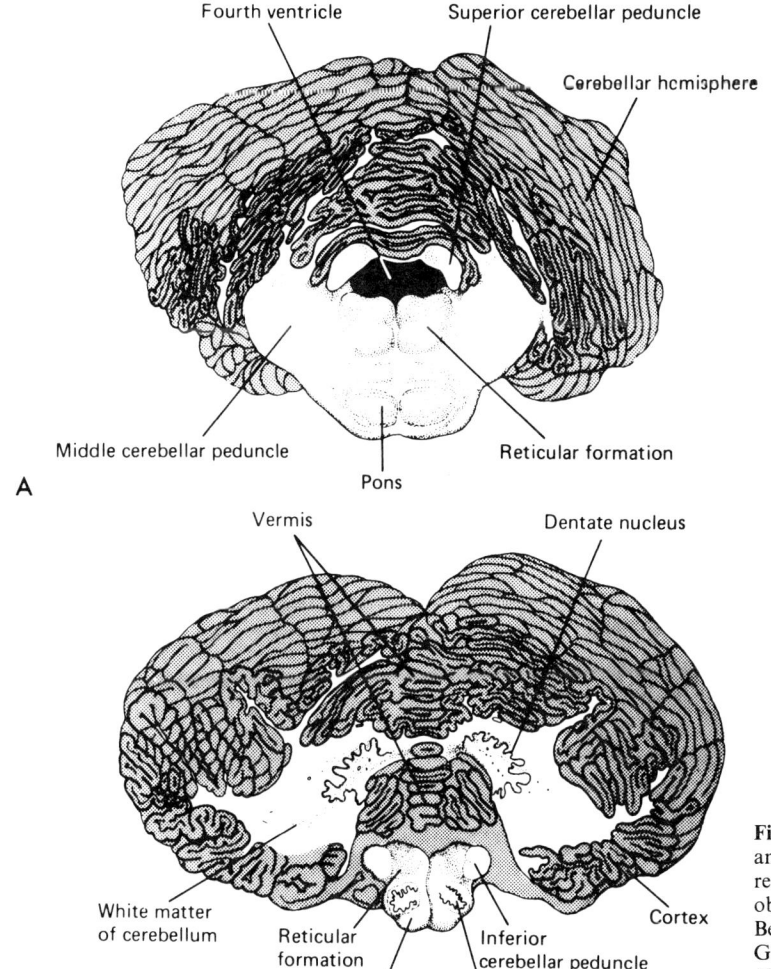

Figure 1.28 A, Transverse slice of pons and cerebellum, stained by a Berlin blue reaction. B, Transverse slice of medulla oblongata and cerebellum, stained by a Berlin blue reaction. [Reproduced from Gardner (1975) *Fundamentals of Neurology*, 6th edn, by kind permission of the author and publisher.]

cortex to nuclei, and vice versa, and cerebellum to brain stem or spinal cord (projection fibres). There are also some commissural fibres from the nuclei (but not from the cortex) connecting hemisphere to hemisphere. Thus, efferent fibres from the dentate nuclei make up most of the superior cerebellar peduncles. The physiological characteristics as well as the function and dysfunction of the cerebellum are considered later (see 'The motor system', p. 158), but some comments on cellular structure and organization can usefully be given here.

Cellular structure and organization

The cerebellar cortex, unlike the cerebrum, is of uniform thickness and shows a consistent cellular and synaptic organization throughout (Fig. 1.29). In the deepest part of the outer molecular layer lie the Purkinje cells with related basket, Golgi and stellate cells. Beneath these is the granular layer, made up largely of small granular neurons.

The Purkinje cells have an extensive dendritic arborization (Fig. 1.30) in the molecular layer; their axons project into white matter but give off collaterals to other Purkinje cells and Golgi cells. Two main types of afferent fibres enter the cerebellum through the inferior and middle peduncles. Mossy fibres, derived from many sources, synapse with granule cells, forming synaptic glomeruli in islands of the granular layer. Axons of granule cells enter the molecular layer and bifurcate, forming parallel fibres which synapse with many Purkinje cell dendrites, thus enabling a single mossy fibre to influence the activity of many Purkinje cells. Mossy fibre input to granular cells is excitatory, and each Purkinje cell may receive synaptic input from up to

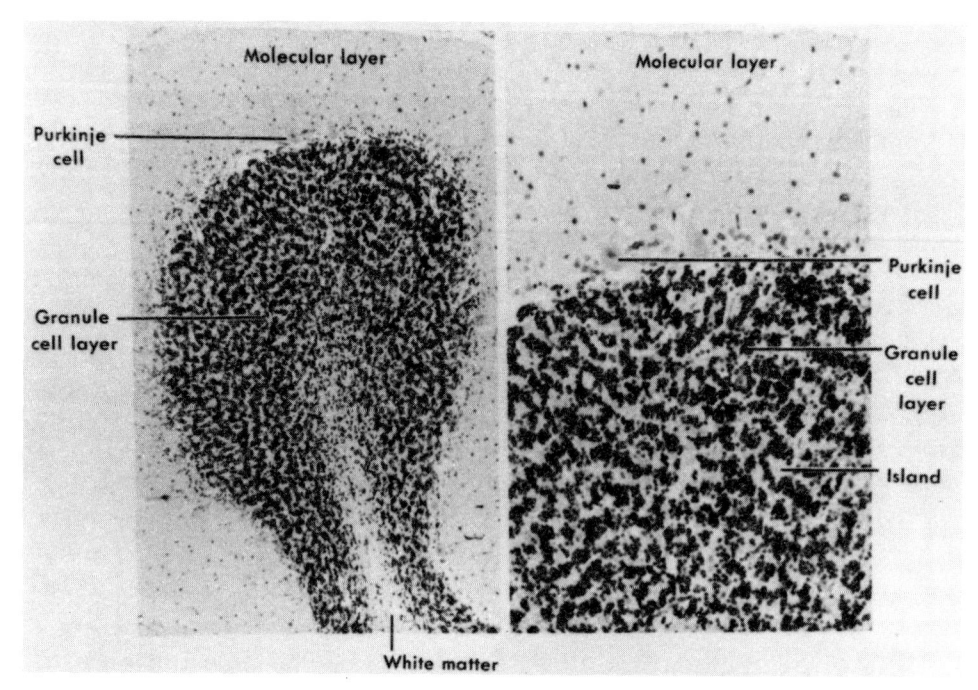

Figure 1.29 Photomicrographs of cerebellar cortex, haematoxylin and eosin stain. Note the clear areas or 'islands'. Ordinary stains fail to show the complex synaptic glomerulus that occupies each island (see Fig. 1.33). Note also that this histological stain fails to show the details of the Purkinje cells. Magnifications about ×100 (left section) and ×250 (right section). [Reproduced from Gardner (1975) *Fundamentals of Neurology*, 6th edn, by kind permission of the author and publisher.]

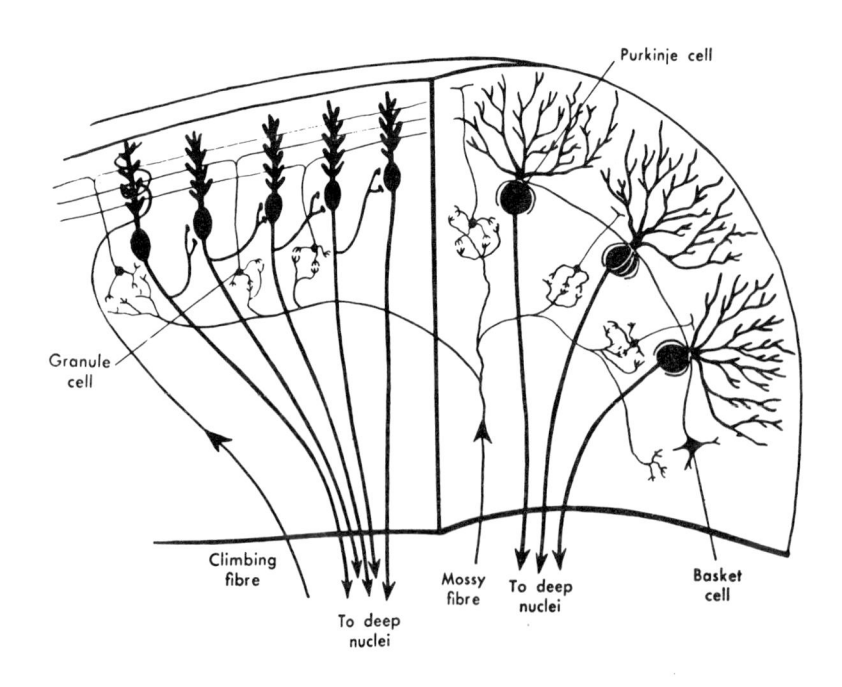

Figure 1.30 Diagram of cells in a folium of the cerebellum. The Purkinje cells have a large dendritic tree across the plane of the folium, and hence in the view on the right are much more extensive than in the plane parallel to the length of the folium on the left. Mossy fibres synapse with many granule cells in the cerebellar glomeruli. The axons of granule cells enter the molecular layer and divide, each branch running lengthwise in the folium as a 'parallel' fibre, synapsing with Purkinje cells and basket cells. Climbing fibres synapse directly with Purkinje cells. Axons of Purkinje cells have recurrent branches to adjacent Purkinje cells and to other cells (not shown). [Reproduced from Gardner (1975) *Fundamentals of Neurology*, 6th edn, by kind permission of the author and publisher.]

100 000 parallel fibres from granular cells, allowing a finely graded excitatory input which evokes repetitive firing in the form of single spikes with the production of action potentials in Purkinje cells. The stellate and basket cells, by contrast, are inhibitory interneurons which inhibit Purkinje cell activity. The Golgi cells fulfil a similar inhibitory role upon granule cells by synapsing with their dendrites.

Climbing fibres arise from the inferior olives in the medulla and synapse with the dendrites of not more

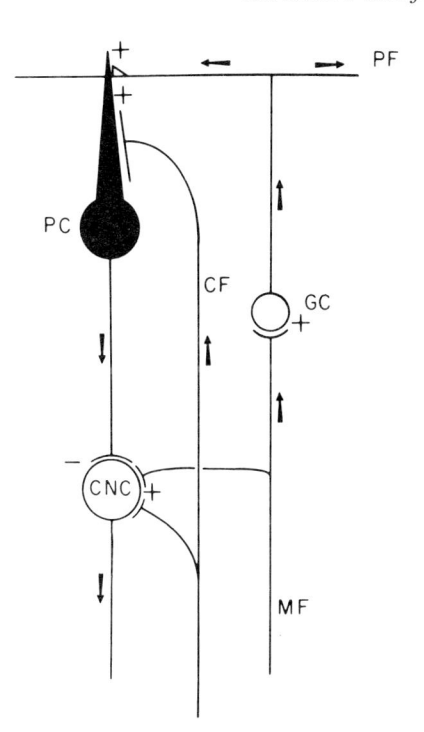

Figure 1.31 Basic neuronal circuit of the cerebellum. PC, Purkinje cell. PF, parallel fibre. GC, granule cell. MF, mossy fibres. CF, climbing fibres. CNC, cerebellar nuclear cell. Cortical interneurons are omitted. Plus sign (+) indicates excitatory synapses, and minus sign (−) signifies inhibitory synapses. [Reproduced from Patton et al (1976) *Introduction to Basic Neurology*, by kind permission of the authors and publisher.]

than 10 Purkinje cells (Fig. 1.31). Excitation through climbing fibres, in contrast to that evoked through parallel fibres, evokes complex spike discharges. It has been suggested that the climbing fibre system is concerned with the control of rapid, phasic movement, whereas that of the mossy fibre system is involved in the control of slow tonic movements.

THE BRAIN STEM

General organization

The midbrain, pons and medulla oblongata together constitute the brain stem, which is largely made up of ascending, descending and decussating myelinated fibre tracts which join the different parts of the brain and the spinal cord, together with other tracts which interconnect various nuclei of the cranial nerves as well as other nuclei (the substantia nigra and red nucleus of the midbrain and the inferior olivary nuclei) which play important roles in the control of movement and, therefore, are related to the extrapyramidal motor and cerebellar systems. Other nuclei, such as the superior and inferior colliculi of the midbrain (visual and auditory) and the gracile and cuneate nuclei of the medulla (somatic sensory), constitute important relay stations in sensory pathways. As was noted in the section on embryology, the nuclear groups receiving primary afferent fibres from the cranial nerves are generally situated in the posterolateral part or the tegmentum of the brain stem, while the efferent (largely motor) neurons are situated more anteriorly. Instead of forming continuous columns of cells as in the anterior horns of the cord, they are divided into discrete nuclei (Fig. 1.32). Diagrammatic representations of the various structures seen in sections of the brain stem at different levels are shown in Fig. 1.33.

The reticular formation of the brain stem contains, in a physiological rather than an anatomical sense, both activating and inhibitory systems concerned with sleep, consciousness and arousal, with activation and inhibition of movement, and with control of behaviour and memory via connections with the cerebral limbic system. This formation is continuous above with the intralaminar nuclei of the thalamus, which constitute a part of the system. The reticular formation is represented by a group of cells and fibres which form the central portion or core of the brain stem. It receives multisynaptic inputs from the spinal cord, and its axons project both to the spinal cord and to more rostral structures in the brain. Within the reticular system of the medulla oblongata are small groups of neurons that constitute the respiratory and cardiac centres which exercise profound controlling influences through somatic and autonomic efferent fibres upon the respiratory and cardiovascular systems. There is also a less well defined centre controlling peristaltic and other motor and secretory activity in the gastrointestinal tract, sometimes loosely referred to (because of one of its functions), as the vomiting centre. Many of the specific functions of the reticular system will be considered later.

The cranial nerves are comparable in many respects to spinal nerves except that some are purely motor and some are purely sensory, unlike spinal nerves, each of which contains motor components (anterior roots) and sensory components (posterior roots). The second or optic nerve is in fact a myelinated fibre tract extruded from the central nervous system during development, and the olfactory bulb and tract (the first nerve) is somewhat similar as its ganglion cells lie in the nasal mucosa. These and the eighth (vestibulocochlear) nerves are discussed later (see 'The special senses', p. 125), as are the third (oculomotor), fourth (trochlear) and sixth (abducens) nerves, which are concerned with ocular movement and the pupillary reactions. The fifth

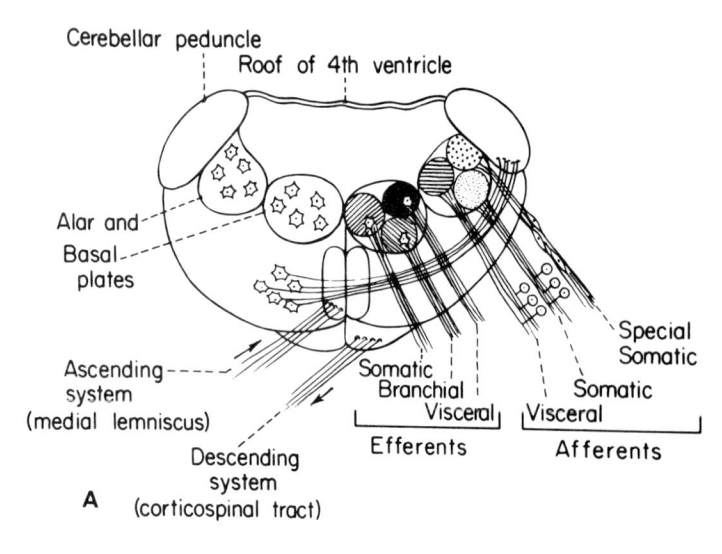

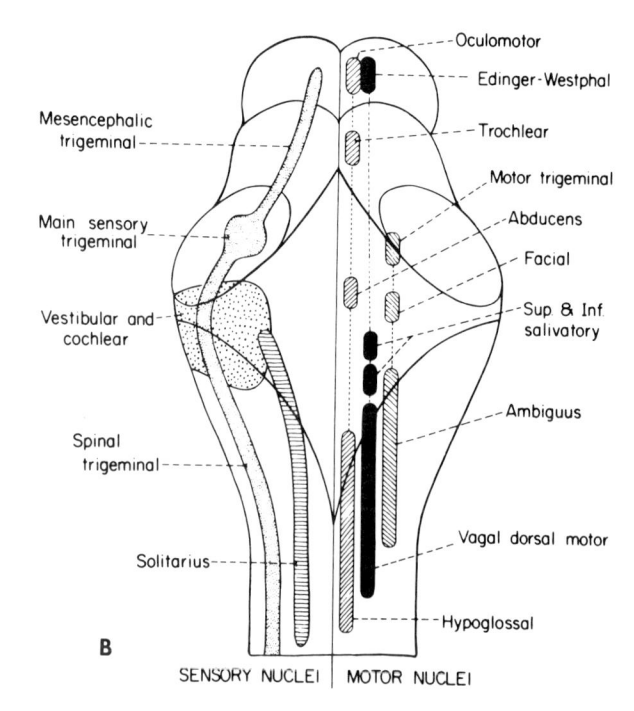

Figure 1.32 Schematic cross-section of the brain stem, showing approximate location of motor nuclei and sensory receiving nuclei of cranial nerves and their respective efferent and afferent fibres. On the left side the primitive alar and basal plates have not yet divided into subgroups of nuclei as they have on the right. Contralateral input to the cerebellum is also indicated, as well as fibres ascending in the medial lemniscus and corticospinal fibres descending to the pyramids. The cranial nerves can be grouped according to the functional categories of their efferent and afferent fibres and associated brain stem nuclei. B, Cranial nerve nuclei in surface projection on a schematic posterior view of the brain stem. The cerebellum has been removed by a cut through the cerebellar peduncles, so that the floor of the fourth ventricle is revealed. Caudally, the medulla is severed at about the transition to the spinal cord. Rostrally, the superior and inferior colliculi of the midbrain are included. The cranial nerve sensory nuclei are shown on the left side and the motor nuclei on the right. These motor and sensory nuclei are grouped according to the functional categories indicated in A. [Reproduced from Patton et al (1976) *Introduction to Basic Neurology*, by kind permission of the authors and publisher.]

(trigeminal) nerve has a sensory root and ganglion (gasserian), which carries somatic sensation from the face, and a motor root, which innervates the muscles of mastication (temporales, masseters and pterygoids). The seventh (facial) nerve is motor to the facial muscles, but also includes the chorda tympani, which carries taste from the anterior two-thirds of the tongue. The eleventh (spinal accessory) nerve innervates the sternomastoid and trapezius, and the twelfth (hypoglossal) nerve innervates the muscles of the tongue. The ninth or glossopharyngeal nerve is motor to the stylopharyngeus and to some circular fibres of the upper pharyngeal muscle, thus playing a part in the control of swallowing; it also carries taste from the posterior one-third of the tongue. The tenth or vagus nerve innervates the muscles of the soft palate, pharynx and larynx but also carries the principal cranial parasympathetic outflow to the lungs, heart and abdominal viscera.

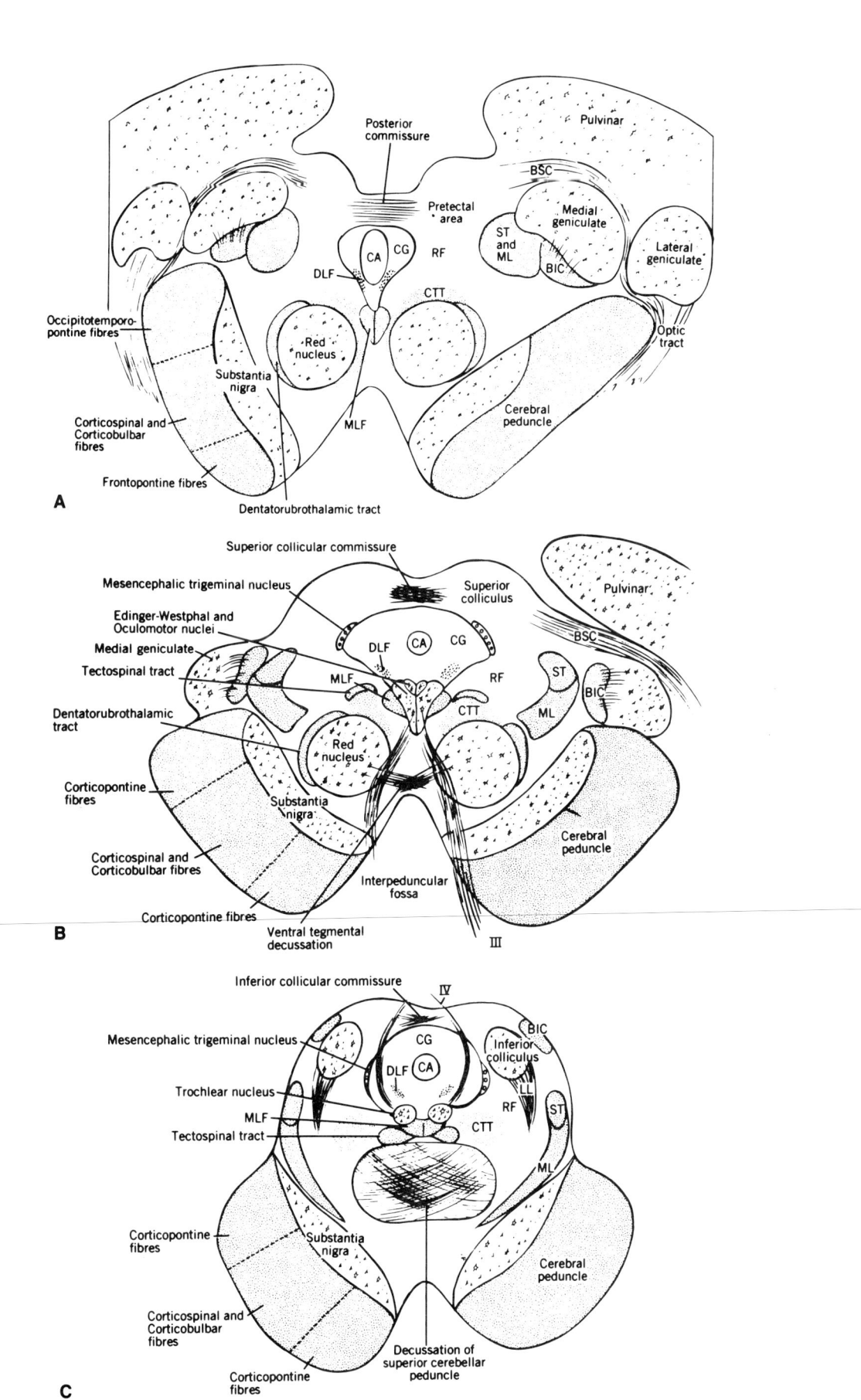

Figure 1.33 *See legend on page 46.*   *Illustration continued on the following page*

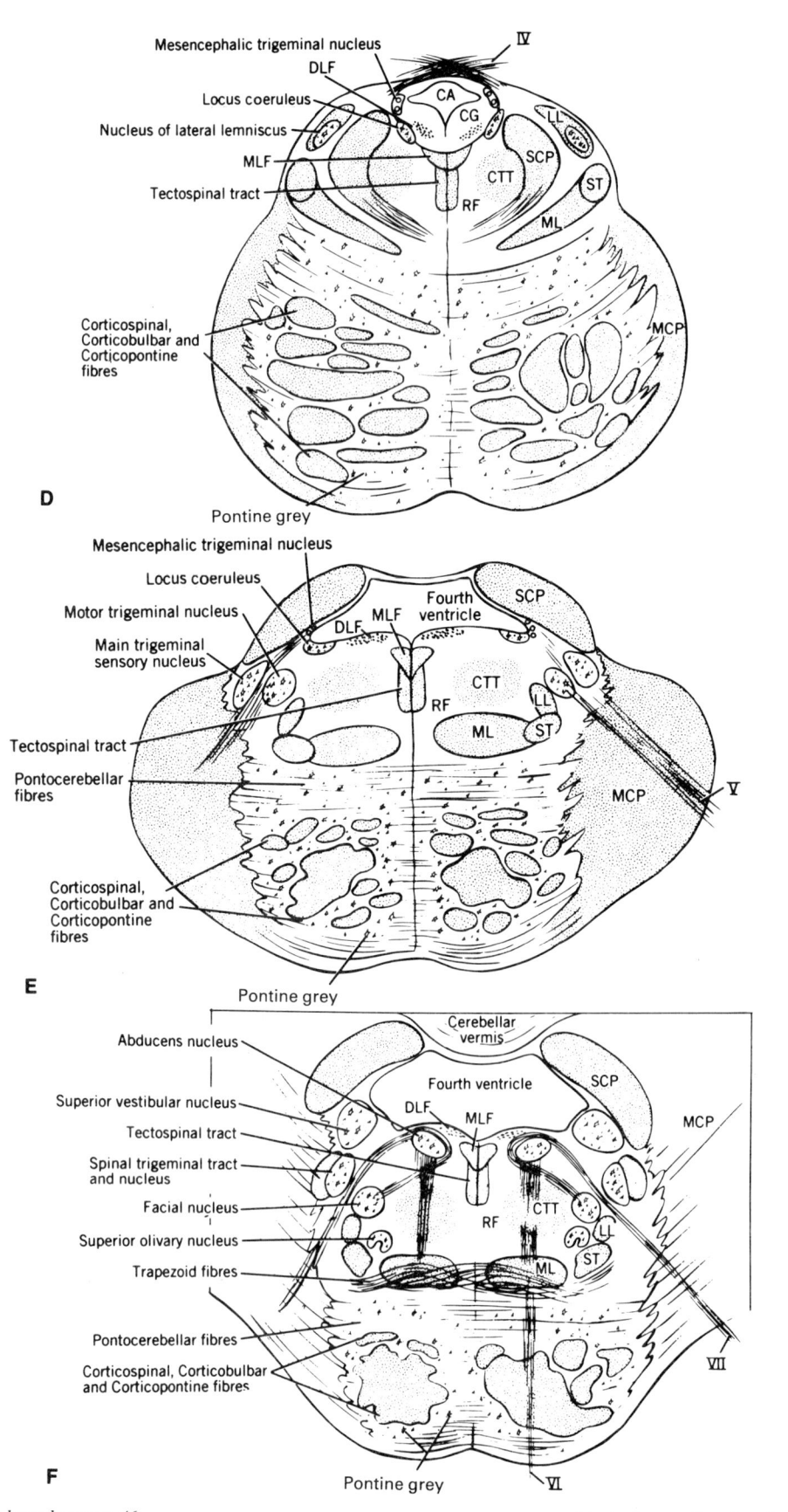

Figure 1.33 *See legend on page 46.*

Illustration continued on the opposite page

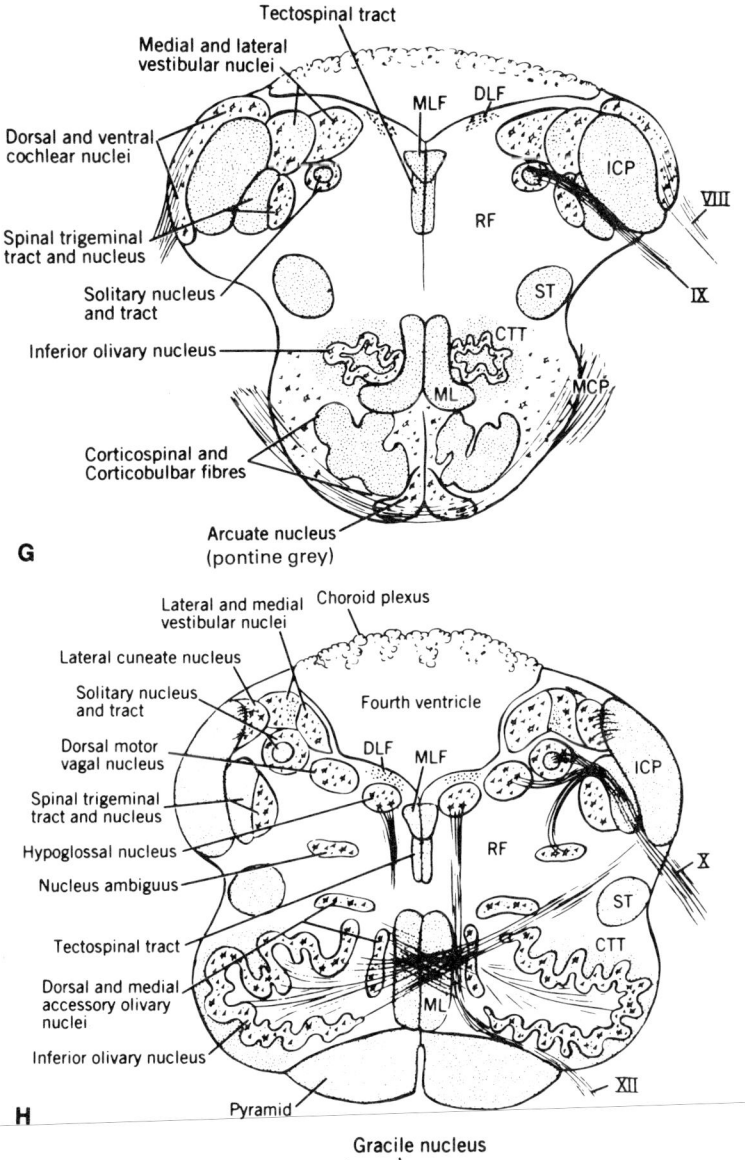

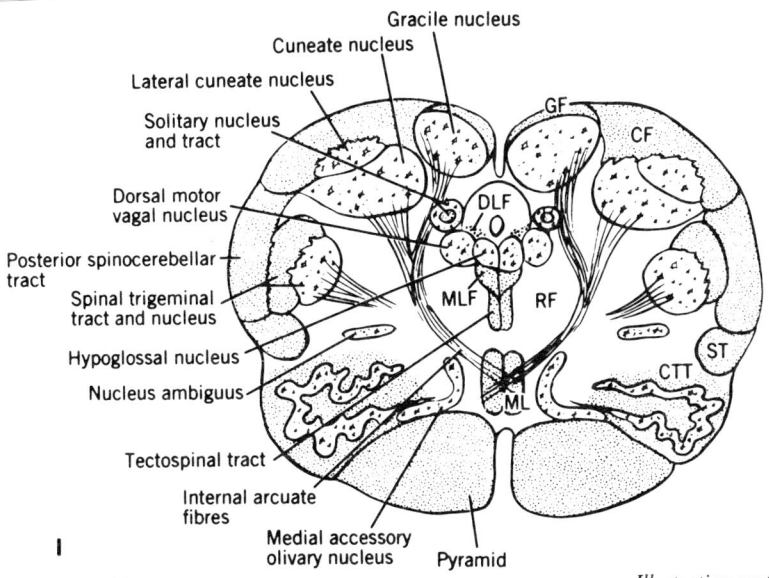

Figure 1.33 *See legend on page 46.*

Illustration continued on the following page

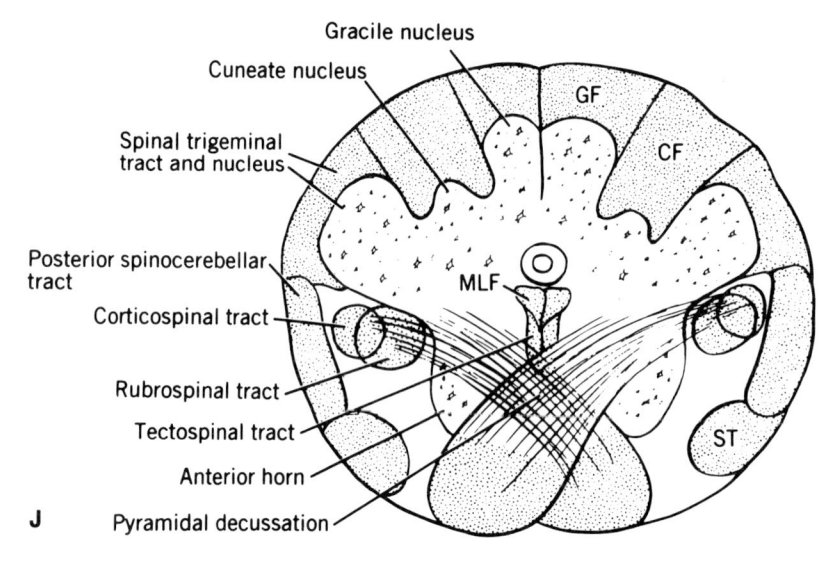

Figure 1.33 A, Region of transition between the midbrain and the diencephalon. The spinothalamic and medial lemniscal fibres are intermingled here before entering the thalamus. The optic tract enters the lateral geniculate, sending some of its fibres beyond it as the brachium of the superior colliculus (BSC) to the pretectal region. The brachium of the inferior colliculus (BIC) is entering the medial geniculate. The posterior commissure is interconnecting the pretectal region on the two sides. The central tegmental tract (CTT) contains a variety of descending fibre systems from the red nucleus and the reticular formation (RF) throughout the tegmental field of the brain stem. In the cerebral peduncle, the corticospinal and corticobulbar fibres separate two groups of corticopontine fibres, designated occipitotemporopontine and the frontopontine. CA, cerebral aqueduct. CG, central grey matter. CLF, dorsal longitudinal fasciculus. ML, medial lemniscus. MLF, medial longitudinal fasciculus. ST, spinothalamic tract. B, The midbrain at the level of the superior colliculus and oculomotor nerve (III). Fibres of the oculomotor nerve are exiting into the interpeduncular fossa. The medial lemniscus (ML) is in the lateral part of the tegmental field. The brachium of the corticospinal tract is intermixed somewhat with the rubrospinal fibres. The posterior column fibres—the cuneate and gracile fasciculi—are reaching the cuneate and gracile nuclei. The spinothalamic fibres are in the anterolateral part of the field. The spinal trigeminal tract and nucleus will overlap with the posterolateral fasciculus and the substantia gelatinosa of the posterior grey matter of the spinal cord caudal to this section. Some of the anterior grey matter of the cervical spinal cord appears just lateral to the pyramidal decussation. CF, cuneate fasciculus. GF, gracile fasciculus. ST, spinothalamic tract. C–J show further successive sections of the brain stem continuing caudally. [Reproduced from Patton et al (1976) *Introduction to Basic Neurology*, by kind permission of the authors and publisher.]

THE SPINAL CORD AND GANGLIA

General morphology

The spinal cord begins where the medulla oblongata ends at the foramen magnum and extends to the lower border of the first lumbar vertebra. It terminates in a thin fibrous extension of the pia mater—the filum terminale—which lies in the cauda equina, eventually fusing with the coccygeal dura mater and thus in a sense tethering the cord. The tapering terminal portion of the cord is known as the conus medullaris.

There is a posterior median longitudinal groove on the surface of the cord—the posterior median sulcus—with two less clearly defined posterior intermediate sulci lateral to it and a deep anterior fissure (the anterior median fissure) in the depths of which lies the anterior spinal artery. The central grey matter of the cord, in which lies the central canal, is approximately H-shaped but varies considerably in its extent and shape in different segments, being considerably larger in the cervical and lumbar enlargements. It is surrounded by myelinated columns of fibres that are organized into columns or funiculi—the anterior, lateral and posterior—which, like the grey matter, vary in configuration depending upon the segmental level at which a transverse section is examined. A spinal cord segment is that portion of the cord giving rise to a single spinal nerve on each side. Since the cord is much shorter than the spinal column, the individual segments of the cord do not correspond to the vertebrae in relation to which they lie. For example, the sixth dorsal segment of the cord lies approximately at the level of the fourth dorsal spinous process, while all of the lumbar, sacral and coccygeal segments occupy the part of the cord beneath the tenth dorsal and the first lumbar vertebrae inclusive. The segmental organization of the cord is illustrated in Fig. 1.34 and the appearance of the cord in transverse section at different levels is shown in Fig. 1.35.

Structure and function of the nervous system

prioceptive sensation rostrally, the gracile from the lower limbs, and the cuneate from the upper limbs. The more important tracts in the lateral columns are the lateral corticospinal (pyramidal, motor efferent), spinocerebellar, and lateral spinothalamic (sensory afferent for pain and temperature sensation). There is also an anterior corticospinal tract and an anterior spinothalamic, which conveys crude touch sensation (Fig. 1.36). In the rostral cervical cord one may also find the lower part of the spinal accessory (eleventh cranial nerve) nucleus and a downward extension of the medial longitudinal fasciculus, an important interconnecting pathway that is largely confined to the brain stem and is principally concerned with the coordination of ocular movement and binocular vision.

The spinal nerve and ganglia

The spinal nerves are formed by the fusion of the posterior roots, which enter the cord close to the posterior horns of the grey matter, with the anterior roots, which emerge from the surface of the cord close to the anterior horns. The anterior roots are wholly efferent, containing both somatic and visceral efferent fibres arising from the anterior horn and intermediolateral cells respectively. Similarly the posterior roots receive both somatic and visceral afferents, but their pseudounipolar ganglion cells lie in the posterior root ganglia (Fig. 1.37).

Each spinal nerve, containing afferent and efferent fibres, divides into a posterior ramus, which innervates the muscles and skin of the back, and an anterior ramus, which supplies the anterior body wall, the limbs, and other appendages. The individual muscles or muscle groups innervated by a single anterior root may be referred to in developmental terms as myotomes. With the exception of the intercostal muscles, each of which is supplied by a single dorsal segment, most muscles of the trunk and limbs receive contributions from several spinal nerves because of the arrangements of the various plexuses. Similarly, cutaneous areas that send sensory afferents to a single cord segment are called dermatomes. On the trunk, despite substantial overlap, a segmental arrangement of dermatomes is well preserved (see p. 202), but sensory segmentation in the limbs is much less clear-cut. In the autonomic system, preganglionic efferent fibres travel to the various sympathetic and parasympathetic ganglia via white rami communicantes, while some of the postganglionic fibres which arise from the latter re-enter peripheral nerves via grey rami in order to travel distally to effector organs.

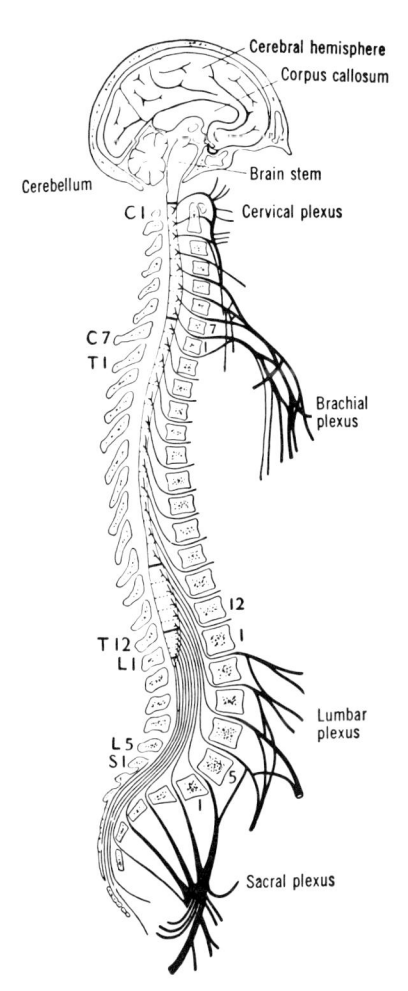

Figure 1.34 Drawing of the brain and cord in situ. The brain is shown sectioned in the median plane. Although not illustrated, the first cervical vertebra articulates with the base of the skull. The letters along the vertebral column indicate cervical, thoracic, lumbar and sacral vertebrae. Note that the cord ends at the upper border of the second lumbar vertebra. [Reproduced from Gardner (1975) *Fundamentals of Neurology*, 6th edn, by kind permission of the author and publisher.]

In the spinal cord grey matter the posterior horns are particularly concerned with the reception of afferent fibres of various kinds, and many cells within them are interneurons (see below), whereas in the anterior horns the neurons are almost wholly efferent. The intermediolateral grey matter in the dorsal region gives rise to sympathetic efferent fibres and in the sacral region to parasympathetic efferents. In the dorsal region there is a lateral horn occupied by a column of cells from which the dorsal spinocerebellar tract arises.

The posterior columns of grey matter, divided in the cervical cord into the gracile (medial) and cuneate (lateral) fasciculi, largely convey fine tactile and pro-

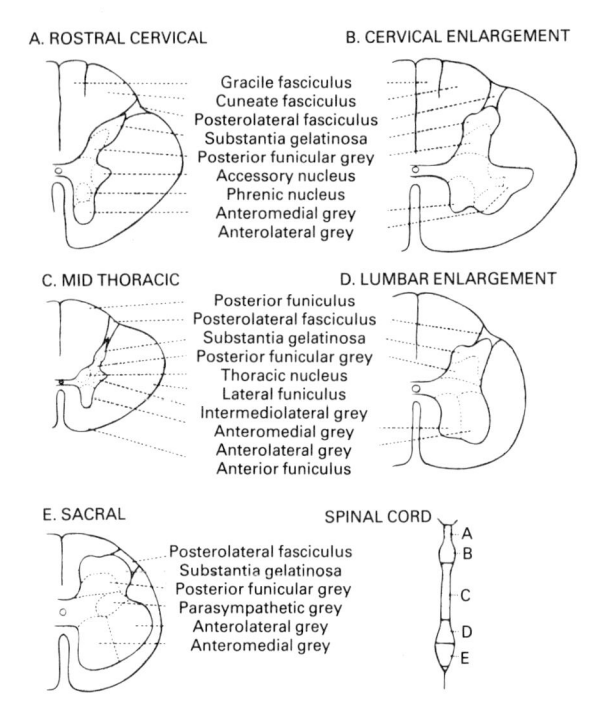

Figure 1.35 Grey matter and white matter of the spinal cord, as seen in representative cross sections. The inset at the lower right indicates the approximate level in the spinal cord for each of the sections. [Reproduced from Patton et al (1976) *Introduction to Basic Neurology*, by kind permission of the authors and publisher.]

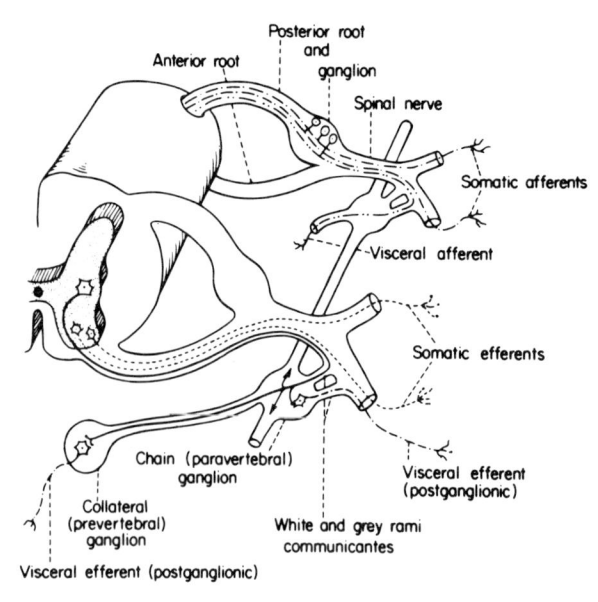

Figure 1.37 Diagram of spinal cord, spinal nerves and sympathetic components, emphasizing the route taken by somatic efferent and afferent fibres, and visceral efferent and afferent fibres. For clarity, afferent paths are shown in the upper and efferent paths in the lower spinal nerve. [Reproduced from Patton et al (1976) *Introduction to Basic Neurology*, by kind permission of the authors and publisher.]

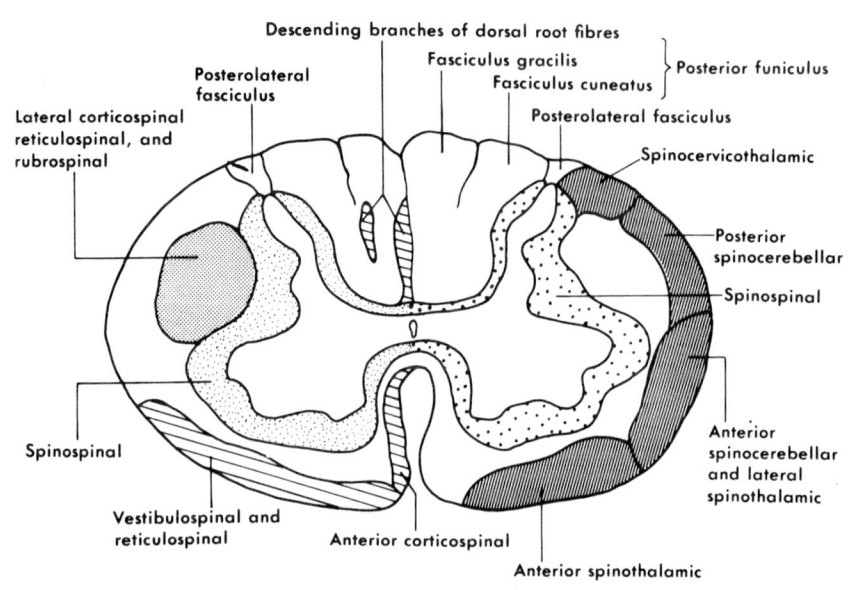

Figure 1.36 The main tracts of the spinal cord. Ascending tracts are shown on the right side and descending tracts on the left. [Reproduced from Gardner (1975) *Fundamentals of Neurology*, 6th edn, by kind permission of the author and publisher.]

Motor and sensory organization in the spinal cord

The primary afferent neurons of the posterior roots enter the spinal cord in a series of rootlets, the thinly myelinated fibres and the unmyelinated ones becoming grouped more laterally, while the heavily myelinated fibres are destined for the posterior columns more medially. In the posterolateral fasciculus that caps the posterior horn, many of the former fibres give off ascending and descending collaterals, some long and ascending to the medulla, and some short which later enter the posterior horns to synapse with a variety of interneurons at different segments. As a result afferent input at one level can be rapidly transmitted to many different cord segments. Some fibres then traverse the posterior horns intact in order to synapse with motor neurons, forming a simple reflex arc. Others synapse with interneurons in the posterior horn. In the posterior horn of grey matter itself, many poorly defined layers of cells have been identified, including the substantia gelatinosa and the nucleus proprius. The role of these cells, of the ascending, descending, commissural and interneuronal connections that they make, and their function in modulating various forms of sensation and movement and reflex activity are considered later (see 'The motor system' and 'The sensory system', pp. 158 and 194).

The principal cells of the anterior horn are the large alpha motor neurons, which innervate the voluntary muscles, and the small gamma motor neurons, which innervate the intrafusal fibres of the muscle spindles. There are also interneurons which, through recurrent axons synapsing with anterior horn cells, produce an inhibitory 'negative feedback' that limits the discharge of alpha motor neurons. The number of alpha motor neurons in different segments of the cord and on the two sides is remarkably constant in different individuals and throughout life (except for evidence that there is a progressive decline in number in advanced age). The neurons are organized consistently into groups which can be shown to innervate specific muscles and muscle groups. Physiologically, too, alpha motor neurons innervating flexor muscles can be distinguished in certain aspects of their behaviour from those which have an extensor function (Chapter 8). The heavily myelinated fibres of the anterior roots which carry the axons of the alpha motor neurons traverse the peripheral nerves to end at a neuromuscular junction or end-plate upon a single striated muscle fibre. A single anterior horn cell (alpha neuron), its axon, and the many muscle fibres which it supplies form one motor unit. The anatomy and physiology of the motor unit and of the neuromuscular junction and voluntary muscle will be considered under 'The motor system' (p. 158).

The peripheral nerves

Strictly speaking, the peripheral nervous system begins in the anterior and posterior roots as they enter or leave the cord. Outside the cord, in the intervertebral foramina and more peripherally, the nerves are invested by Schwann cells. However, peripheral nerves are commonly regarded as those which are formed from single spinal nerves, or groups of nerves, or those which emerge from the brachial and lumbosacral plexuses. The structure of unmyelinated and myelinated fibres, including Remak and Schwann cells, has already been considered (p. 3), and is further shown in Fig. 1.38. The myelin sheath is concentrically laminated with a periodicity of about 18 nm. This periodicity refers to the distance between the major dense lines between which is a less electron-dense intraperiod line. The clear space on either side of the intraperiod line is believed to contain hydrophobic lipids of the membrane. The number of myelin lamellae and hence the thickness of the sheath is related to the diameter of the axon, and so too is the internodal length (the distance between individual nodes of Ranvier). In an adult limb nerve fibre with an axonal diameter of about $12 \mu m$, each internodal length is about 1.0 mm, but there is much variation between different nerves. In many areas small pockets of Schwann cell cytoplasm split the major dense line of the myelin sheath, and sometimes a series of such clefts is seen at a point where the myelin sheath shows funnel-shaped clefts. These may be points at which substances pass from the Schwann cell cytoplasm through the myelin into the axon. They are especially frequent in young and regenerating nerves.

A characteristic compound nerve action potential can be recorded along the course of a mixed motor and sensory peripheral nerve following supramaximal electrical stimulation. This is divided into the A wave (the largest), which has three components—alpha, beta and gamma, conducting at 90, 50 and 30 m/s respectively; a small B wave with a velocity of 10 m/s; and a C wave (the smallest) with a velocity of about 2 m/s. The velocity of conduction can be correlated precisely with axonal diameter in unmyelinated fibres and with myelin sheath thickness in myelinated fibres. The fibres of largest diameter conduct most rapidly. On this basis, the fibres of peripheral nerves can be divided similarly into A, B and C fibres depending upon their axonal and myelin sheath diameter and their speed of conduction. The A fibres are the largest, the alpha wave being produced by alpha motor neurons ($10-18 \mu m$ in diameter) and by group Ia sensory fibres from the muscle spindles and tendon organ receptors. The beta wave is produced by group II sensory fibres ($6-12 \mu m$ in diameter) such as those from the Pacinian

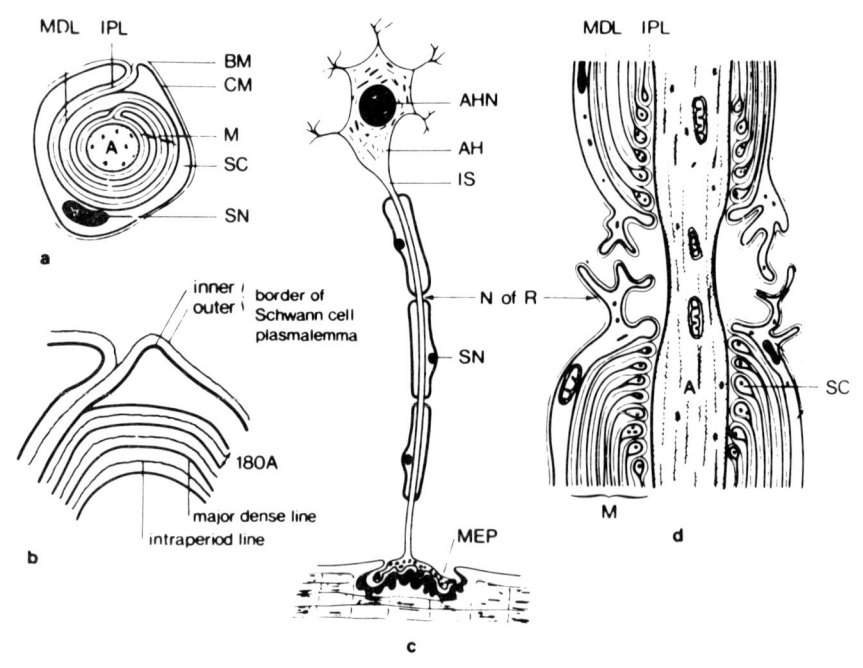

Figure 1.38 Diagrams of the structure of a myelinated nerve fibre.

a, Formation of the myelin sheath (M) by wrapping of the Schwann cell (SC) membrane (CM) around the axon (A). SN, Schwann cell nucleus. MDL, major dense line. IPL, intraperiod line. BM, basement membrane.

b, High power drawing of the inner mesaxon to show the formation of the major dense line from the union of two inner borders of the Schwann cell plasmalemma, and the intraperiod line by the union of two outer borders of the Schwann cell plasmalemma.

c, Diagram of an α-motor neuron. The anterior horn cell (AH), with its nucleus (AHN) and initial segment (IS), lies in the spinal cord. The axon is invested with Schwann cells separated by nodes of Ranvier (N of R), and the terminal ramification lies in the motor end-plate (MEP).

d, Diagram of the structure of a node of Ranvier. The interdigitating processes from adjacent Schwann cells almost occlude the nodal gap. Schwann cell cytoplasm (SC) lies superficial to the myelin sheath, and also in pockets splitting the major dense lines where the myelin becomes applied to the axon. [Reproduced from Bradley (1974) *Disorders of Peripheral Nerves*, by kind permission of the author and publisher.]

corpuscles, and the gamma wave is produced by gamma motor neurons innervating intrafusal muscle fibres in the spindles and by group II afferents from the spindles (4–8 μm in diameter). The B potential is derived from small myelinated fibres 2 to 6 μm in diameter, which include slow gamma efferents and group III sensory afferents from pain and hair receptors. Finally, the C potential comes from unmyelinated fibres (0.2–3 μm in diameter), which are mainly group IV pain and temperature afferent fibres and postganglionic fibres of the autonomic nervous system. In a sensory nerve such as the sural nerve, unmyelinated fibres outnumber the myelinated ones by about four to one. A diagram of a transverse section of a nerve is shown in Fig. 1.39.

Each large mixed nerve comprises thousands of nerve fibres grouped into fasciculi, each surrounded by a sheath of perineurium, consisting of three or four layers of specialized cells which form a blood–nerve barrier, similar in certain respects to the blood–brain barrier and acting as a major barrier against the passage into nerves of substances of large molecular weight. The blood–nerve barrier is less efficient in the spinal nerve roots, which may account for the selective involvement of the latter in some disease processes, especially the autoimmune polyneuropathies. Within the fasciculi are strands of endoneurial connective tissue, while the fasciculi themselves are bound together by the collagen of the epineurium. Blood is supplied to peripheral nerves by small vasa nervorum. Blockage of these arteries resulting from disease or compression may give rise to infarction of peripheral nerves or to various forms of ischaemic neuropathy.

Structure and function of the nervous system

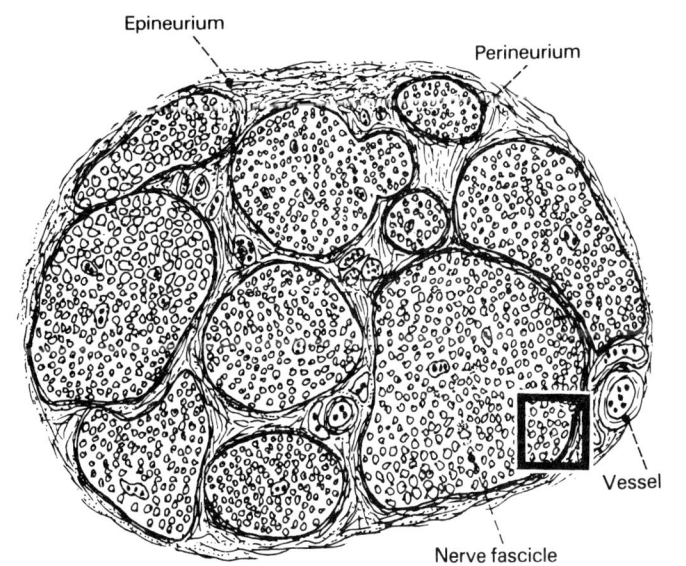

Figure 1.39 A, Diagrammatic representation of a nerve trunk in transverse section shown as if the myelin sheath of individual axons were stained with osmic acid. The small, irregular, dark circles represent the myelin sheaths surrounding each axon, but are not intended to indicate the marked variation in axonal diameter and myelin sheath thickness seen in different fibres in most nerves.

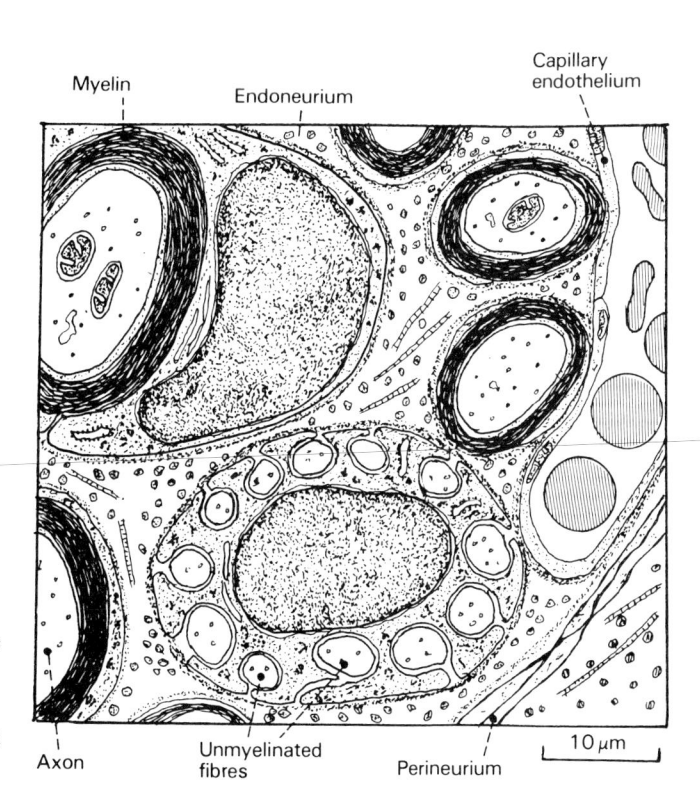

Figure 1.39 B, One edge of a single nerve fascicle (an enlargement, as seen with the electron microscope, of the rectangle in A). [Reproduced from Fitzgerald (1985) *Neuroanatomy, Basic and Applied*, by kind permission of the author and publisher.]

References

Bradley, W. G. (1974) *Disorders of Peripheral Nerves.* Oxford: Blackwell Scientific Publications.

Brodal, A. (1969) *Neurological Anatomy in Relation to Clinical Medicine,* 2nd edn. New York, Oxford University Press.

Cervos-Navarro, J., Betz, E., Ebhardt, G., Ferszt, R. and Wüllenweber, R. (1978) *Pathology of the Cerebrospinal Microcirculation* (Advances in Neurology, vol. 20). New York: Raven Press.

Clarke, E. and Dewhurst, K. (1972) *An Illustrated History of Brain Function.* Oxford: Sandford Publications.

Clarke, E. and O'Malley, C. D. (1968) *The Human Brain and Spinal Cord.* Berkeley and Los Angeles: University of California Press.

Curtis, B. A., Jacobson, S. and Marcus, E. M. (1972) *An Introduction to the Neurosciences.* Philadelphia: W. B. Saunders Company.

Fitzgerald, M. J. T. (1985) *Neuroanatomy, Basic and Applied.* London: Baillière Tindall.

Gardner, E. (1975) *Fundamentals of Neurology,* 6th edn. Philadelphia: W. B. Saunders Company.

Henderson, G., Tomlinson, B. E. and Gibson, P. H. (1980) Cell counts in human cerebral cortex in normal adults throughout life using an image analysing computer. *J. neurol. Sci.* **46**:113.

Kandel E. R. (1981) Synapse formation, trophic interactions between neurons and the development of behaviour. In Kandel, E. R. and Schwartz, J. H. (eds) *Principles of Neuroscience,* chap. 43. London: Edward Arnold.

Lenman, J. A. R. (1975) *Clinical Neurophysiology.* Oxford: Blackwell Scientific Publications.

Meyer, A. (1971) *Historical Aspects of Cerebral Anatomy.* Oxford: Oxford University Press.

Mitchell, G. A. G., and Mayor, D. (1977) *The Essentials of Neuroanatomy,* 3rd edn. Edinburgh: Churchill Livingstone.

Patton, H. D., Sundsten, J. W., Crill, W. E. and Swanson, P. D. (1976) *Introduction to Basic Neurology.* Philadelphia: W. B. Saunders Company.

Pearlman, A. L. and Collins, R. C. (eds) (1984) *Neurological Pathophysiology,* 3rd edn. Oxford: Oxford University Press.

Peters, A., Palay, S. L. and Webster, H. de F. (1976) *The Fine Structure of the Nervous System: The Neurons and Supporting Cells.* Philadelphia: W. B. Saunders Company.

Ranson, S. W. and Clark, S. L. (1959) *The Anatomy of the Nervous System: Its Development and Function.* Philadelphia: W. B. Saunders Company.

Schacher, S. (1981) Determination and differentiation in the development of the nervous system. In Kandel, E. R. and Schwartz, J. H. (eds) *Principles of Neuroscience,* chap. 42. London: Edward Arnold.

Schaumburg, H., Spencer, P. S. and Thomas, P. K. (1983) *Disorders of Peripheral Nerves* (Contemporary Neurology Series, Vol. 24). Philadelphia: F. A. Davis Company.

Singer, S. J. and Nicolson, G. L. (1972) The fluid mosaic model of the structure of cell membranes. *Science* **175**:720.

Walton, J. N. (1985) *Brain's Diseases of the Nervous System,* 9th edn. Oxford: Oxford University Press.

Wilkinson, J. L. (1985) *Neuroanatomy for Medical Students.* Bristol: Wright.

2

SOME GENERAL PRINCIPLES OF VALUE IN INTERPRETING THE PATHOPHYSIOLOGY OF THE NERVOUS SYSTEM

INTRODUCTION

The preceding material on the nervous system has provided an outline of the structure and function of this system in man, and of its component structures in general terms. The chapters which follow will consider in greater depth the pathophysiology of its individual components, such as the motor and sensory systems, for example. This chapter aims, by contrast, to help the reader to understand some of the principles which govern the genesis of those neurological symptoms and signs which will be considered later in more detail to indicate the means by which some such disorders of function are produced and how they can be recognized and interpreted.

SOME IMPORTANT PATHOPHYSIOLOGICAL INFLUENCES

The nervous system cannot be considered in isolation, for without adequate oxygen and nutrients, which depend in turn upon efficient circulatory and respiratory activity, the nervous system cannot survive. The converse is also true, for the activity of the autonomic nervous system exercises a profound influence upon the behaviour of the heart and circulation, upon respiratory activity, upon the gastrointestinal system, and upon endocrine activity. These complex interrelationships, and the homeostatic mechanisms upon which the normal functioning of the human body depends, have been elucidated increasingly by anatomical and physiological studies, but there still remain many unanswered questions. Upon what, for instance, does the ability of the brain to control thought processes depend? Mental disease is often present when all available investigative techniques fail to demonstrate any abnormality in cerebral structure or function, and mental influences on bodily systems can be profound.

Disorders of the mind sometimes initiate and often accentuate symptoms of physical disease, while conversely some organic diseases are regularly accompanied by psychological manifestations. The basis of these relationships may be obscure, but their importance must be recognized by all doctors. Disease is an abstraction, however well defined in pathological or biochemical terms a disease process may be. It is the patient who suffers from the disease who is real and who shows a personal and individual reaction to it. The pathological process may be influenced by his genetic constitution, by the condition of other organs or systems apart from that primarily affected, and by his state of mind.

Many organic disorders regularly produce consistent clinical manifestations independent of the personality and constitution of the individual. The syndrome resulting from division of one median nerve, for instance, is not usually modified significantly by the patient's mental state. But if the nerve lesion is incomplete, say due to transient compression, the severity of the resultant symptoms and the rate of the recovery can be influenced by factors other than the physical process, resulting in restoration of normal conduction in the damaged fibres. Much will depend upon the nature of the lesion. If it was an industrial injury, involving a claim for financial compensation, the patient's disability may be excessive and his recovery unduly delayed.

Many functions, such as those concerned with speech, seeing and hearing, with the control of movement, and with the appreciation of sensation, are subserved by the passage of impulses along pathways which have been clearly delineated. They can be disordered by a defect of development (a congenital abnormality). They may be rendered abnormal by a pathological process, whether it results from inherited factors (genetically determined illness) or is acquired. The lesions so produced give rise to symptoms and signs depending upon their situation and character and the functions of the pathways involved. Many subsequent chapters deal in detail with these functions and with the means by which abnormalities can be recognized, the lesions responsible localized, and their nature determined. The pathophysiological effects of these processes are not immutable; the resultant disease or dysfunction can be greatly influenced by the personality, constitution and mental state of the affected individual. Some patients are physically and mentally less perfect than others and yet show no obvious defect; but constitutionally they are less able to resist stress and may be disturbed by environmental influences that would leave others relatively unaffected. The effects of fatigue, of ageing, and of other influences not easily measured scientifically must also be noted. Are the patient's headaches due to emotional tension or to an intracranial tumour? Is his suspicion that he has malignant disease well founded or is he suffering from cancer phobia? Do his insomnia and anxiety stem from constitutional inadequacy, or are they the result of underlying physical disease? These are some of the many questions which the doctor often needs to answer, questions which require for their elucidation all his reserves of experience and understanding.

In discussing pathophysiology we must also consider the use of the term 'functional' as utilized in medicine to identify the nature of an illness, since its usage is a common source of misconception. True functional disorders are those diseases in which the function of an organ is disordered, but which do not result from any evident structural or biochemical change in the organ or system involved. In neurology, so-called 'idiopathic' epilepsy is a reasonable example, though it is likely that in this and many other states of altered function, some as yet unidentifiable biochemical or physical abnormality is present. However, the term 'functional disorder' as conventionally used is not usually applied to such diseases, but rather to symptoms and signs which result from emotional disorder. When a symptom or syndrome is regarded as functional, this usually means that it has no physical cause and, by implication, that its origin is psychological. Thus, headaches due to nervous tension are 'functional', as is loss of the voice (hysterical aphonia) in the young singer facing her first professional engagement. In other words, anxiety reactions, symptoms due to mental or emotional fatigue, and symptoms manifesting a subconscious desire to escape from stress (hysteria) are usually so identified. But it would be incorrect to include in this category deterioration of intellectual function (dementia) resulting from physical disease of the brain.

Functional disorders, therefore, are those in which clinical manifestations are due not to physical disease but to mental processes, whether conscious or subconscious. These processes may, in turn, cause physical changes in bodily function. The increased heart rate, perspiration, and insomnia which commonly accompany anxiety are good examples. Hence, the clinical use of 'functional', if not strictly correct semantically, is useful and hallowed through usage, provided its meaning is appreciated and it is not regarded as a final diagnosis. For if a disorder is accepted as 'functional' it must be decided whether the patient's disability is due to conscious anxiety, to hysteria, or even to psychosis. Its nature, and if possible its cause, must be determined if treatment is to be effective. The distinction between organic and functional disease is often difficult, and even when there is clear evidence of physical disease its effects are often accentuated or distorted by concurrent psychological factors. The converse is also true, in that symptoms which by their very nature are plainly functional (this is especially true of hysterical manifestations) are commonly an initial manifestation of organic disease (multiple sclerosis or brain tumour are important examples) and only too easily obscure the early physical features of the illness. As they presumably result often from conscious or subconscious anxiety about the illness and are invariably accentuated if the doctor fails to recognize the significance or even the actual presence of the organic infrastructure, it is not surprising that in such circumstances diagnostic error is all too easy. The doctor must strive not only to recognize and interpret the symptoms and signs of physical disease but also to understand the potential effect upon them of mental and emotional factors and vice versa.

SOME PATHOPHYSIOLOGICAL FOUNDATIONS OF NEUROLOGICAL DIAGNOSIS

In order to forecast the outcome of a patient's illness and to advise treatment, accurate diagnosis is usually necessary. In many disorders of the nervous system the physical signs indicate the anatomical localization of the lesion or process responsible for abnormalities of function, while the history of the illness reveals the detailed evolution of the patient's symptoms and often suggests the nature of the pathological change.

The intelligent interpretation of physical signs demands an adequate knowledge of neuroanatomy and neurophysiology as outlined in the preceding chapter on the structure and function of the nervous system. In several chapters which follow we shall deal with disorders of various systems and will consider how these are produced and recognized, and how the lesion or process responsible can be localized and identified.

Most symptoms and signs resulting from nervous disease can be classified as positive or negative. Positive symptoms may be produced by irritation of a part of the nervous system, causing it to behave abnormally, or by the release of a primitive pattern of activity normally suppressed in the adult human brain. Focal epilepsy resulting from pressure upon the cerebral motor cortex is an example of the former, involuntary movements occurring in disease of the basal ganglia of the latter. Negative symptoms, by contrast, are those produced by temporary or permanent loss of function, so that an activity, normally present, is lost. Paralysis of a limb is one such symptom. The law of dissolution of Hughlings Jackson is useful. This suggests that those functions and skills most recently acquired during evolution and training may be the first to be lost in cerebral cortical disease, whereas primitive activities and instinct survive longer. A similar principle applies to temporary disturbances of cerebral function produced, for example, by anaesthetics or other drugs. A naturalized foreigner may revert to using his native tongue during recovery from anaesthesia, and only when recovery is more complete is he able to utilize the language of his adopted country. Man differs from the primate in his ability to move individual fingers in order to perform fine movements. Thus, gripping an object by means of opposition of the thumb and other fingers can be called the 'precision grip'. The primate depends more upon the 'power grip', produced by flexion of all fingers. In an early lesion of the hand area of the motor cortex or of its efferent corticospinal or pyramidal fibres in man, the 'precision grip' is impaired, as is discrete movement of the individual fingers, while the 'power grip' is still normal.

Disordered function depends not only upon the localization of pathological change but also upon its acuteness, its extent, and the effects it has upon contiguous nervous tissue and upon interconnected though anatomically remote structures. An acute cerebral lesion may have greater effects than its anatomical extent would lead one to expect, for around the lesion the activity of surrounding brain tissue may be disturbed by oedema, ischaemia or haemorrhage, and other related pathophysiological changes. An acute lesion can produce a state of 'shock' or temporary loss of function in related areas of the brain or spinal cord. This is seen in the patient with an acute hemiplegia that is initially flaccid and is only later spastic. In a patient with an acute transverse spinal cord lesion, the limbs below the level of the lesion are initially flaccid and totally paralysed but, as shock wears off, spasticity develops. By contrast, slowly developing lesions of equal extent produce fewer symptoms and physical signs, as it is only the structures actively compressed or invaded by the lesion whose function is disturbed. Those structures surrounding the lesion have more time to adapt to its presence. Other forms of adaptation also occur, particularly in the cerebral cortex, for here it may be possible for a function lost through a cortical lesion to be 'adopted', though usually much less efficiently, by an unaffected and often contiguous area of the brain. This type of adaptation occurs more readily in children than in adults, for the younger the patient the greater the flexibility and plasticity of cerebral organization. In the spinal cord there is much less opportunity for this type of reorganization than in the brain. In the peripheral nerves opportunities for such an adoption of function are almost non-existent. However, these nerves are able to regenerate effectively after injury, whereas clinically effective regeneration does not occur within the spinal cord or brain.

DEGENERATION AND REGENERATION IN THE NERVOUS SYSTEM

An adult nerve cell, once destroyed, can never be replaced. With increasing age there is a progressive fall-out of certain cortical and spinal neurons. In elderly individuals it is common to find within the cerebral cortex neurofibrillary tangles and so-called senile argyrophilic plaques (Fig. 2.1), which develop in relation to degenerating neurons. Such lesions, if seen in profusion in the cerebral cortex at a relatively early age, are virtually diagnostic of presenile dementia. The changes seen at a later stage in senile dementia are similar, but it is the age at which they are found and their profusion which is important, as they almost invariably occur in some degree as a result of normal ageing processes.

When certain processes of a nerve cell are destroyed, the cell body may nevertheless survive. But if the axon of an anterior horn cell is divided, the Nissl substance in the cell of origin at first aggregates and is later dispersed to the periphery (chromatolysis), while the nucleus shifts also towards the periphery (Fig. 2.2). These changes are more easily

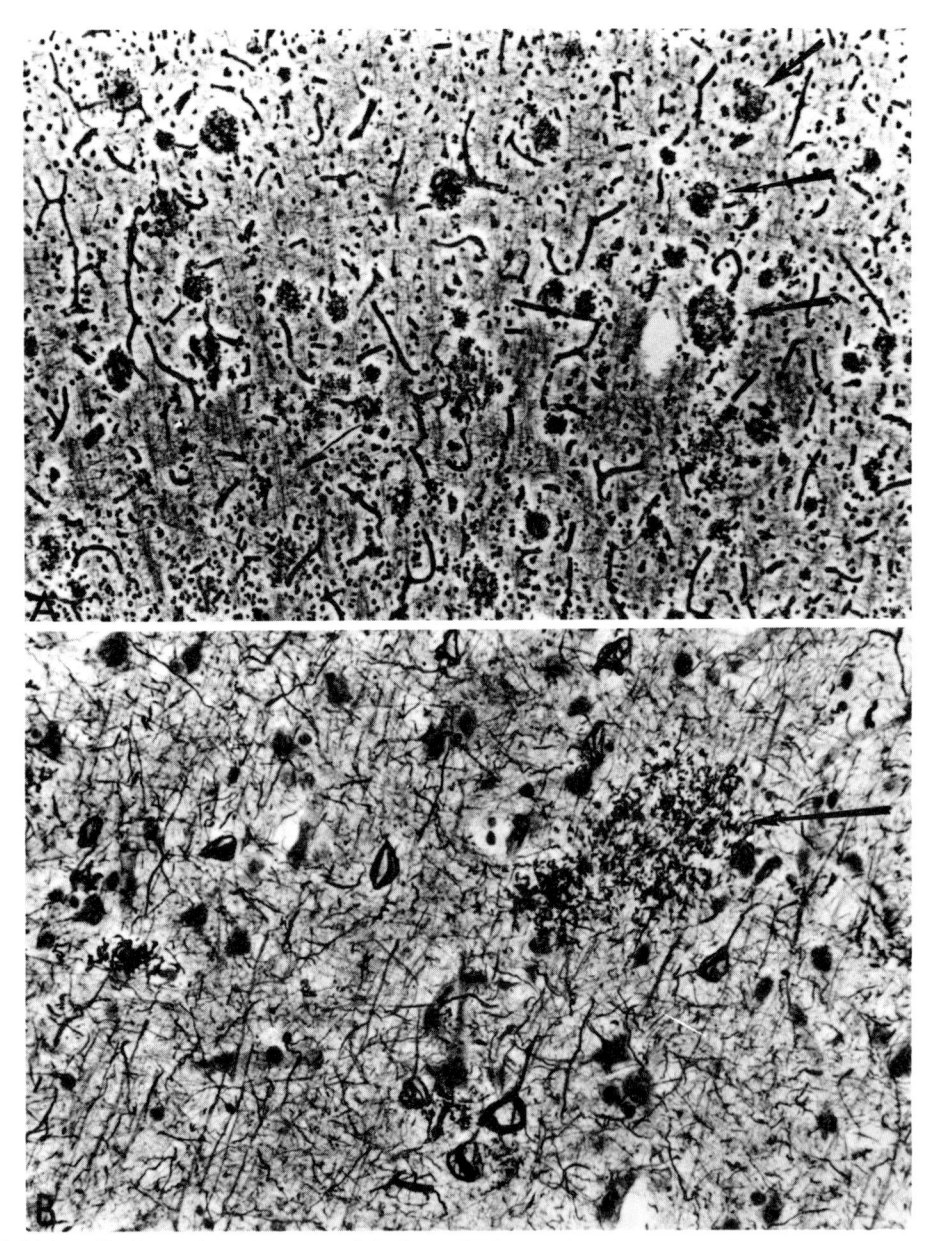

Figure 2.1 A, Multiple senile plaques (some are arrowed) in the cerebral cortex in a case of senile dementia; Von Braunmühl, × 100. B, A higher power view of a large senile plaque (arrow) and of multiple neurofibrillary tangles in a case of senile dementia; von Braunmühl, × 400 (Illustration kindly provided by Professor B. E. Tomlinson).

seen in large cells that have abundant Nissl substance. The severity of the changes is related to the distance of the axonal lesion from the parent cell body, being more severe when the lesion is close. It is less common for cells with bodies and processes confined to the central nervous system to survive axonal section, so that these cellular changes can sometimes be used to locate the cells of origin of degenerating axons in a peripheral nerve or in a specific fibre pathway.

An axon severed from its cell body undergoes wallerian (orthograde) degeneration. Within a few days the terminal part of the axis cylinder swells. Later it becomes beaded and then disintegrates. This process of swelling and progressive disintegration then moves slowly proximally ('dying back of the axon'). If the axon is myelinated, the myelin sheath begins to break down within a few days and the neurilemmal cells then proliferate, subsequently ingesting or enfolding both the disintegrating axis cylinder and the myelin within Schwann cell processes. In addition to distal

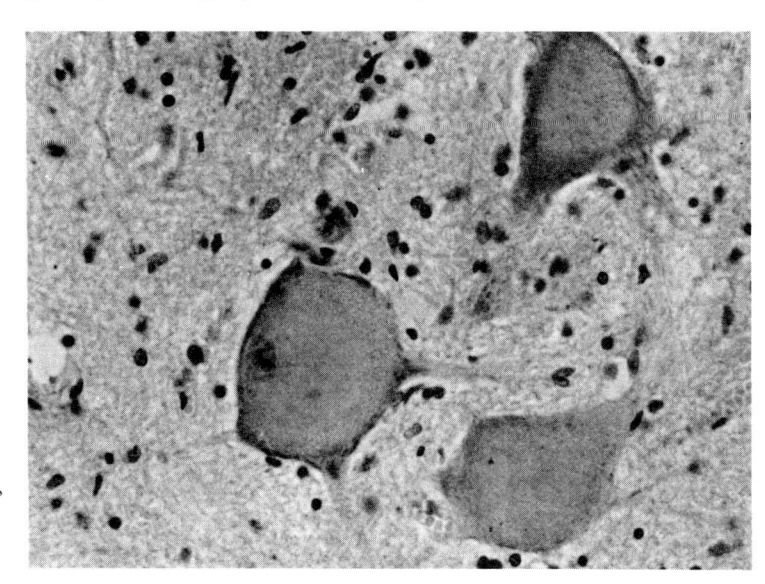

Figure 2.2 Chromatolysis of an anterior horn cell. The cell is swollen and rounded, the Nissl substance is accumulated at the periphery, and the nucleus is eccentric. H & E, × 350.

or orthograde degeneration of the axon, retrograde degeneration extending proximally from the point of degeneration of the axon backwards towards the cell body or soma occurs. Histiocytes have a phagocytic role and proliferating connective tissue cells also play a part in the degenerative process. Similar axonal changes occur in the central nervous system, except that gliosis results from astrocytic proliferation and the microglia act as phagocytes. Exceptionally, within some parts of the central nervous system, retrograde degeneration can be transneuronal (extending across synapses).

In peripheral nerves, soon after an axon is divided, its tip begins to grow out distally into the surviving neurilemmal sheath, which directs its growth. This distal growth occurs only when the cell body survives, and the chromatolytic process is then reversed. Growth occurs at a rate of a millimetre or two a day at first, but after a few weeks it slows down. Myelin gradually re-forms until eventually the axon re-establishes distal contact. Although profuse axonal sprouting may be seen in the brains or spinal cords of very young animals and infants after injury, it is doubtful whether this is ever effective, as the axonal sprouts rarely, if ever, make functional contact with any other neuron or effector organ.

In clinical neurology there are many disease processes that cause demyelination in peripheral nerves or in the central nervous system but which initially leave the axon intact, though it is incapable of conducting normally. In peripheral nerves such demyelination may begin at or close to the nodes of Ranvier (perinodal demyelination) and can then spread to involve one or many internodal distances. Subsequently, if the disease process is reversed, remyelination may occur. In such cases the regenerated myelin sheath is often abnormally thin and the internodal distances are often irregular and much shorter than normal. Such a demyelinating neuropathy usually causes marked slowing of conduction in peripheral nerves, but as the disease process recovers this may eventually return to normal. However, there is some evidence that Na^+ channels may spread into the demyelinated internodal region, thus helping, at least in part, to support conduction. Demyelination within the central nervous system also affects conduction in the parent axon. The process by means of which remyelination occurs in the central nervous system is less well understood, but presumably accounts for the remissions which may occur in demyelinating disorders such as multiple sclerosis.

PATHOLOGICAL REACTIONS IN THE NERVOUS SYSTEM

Pathological changes in the nervous system can be classified into three broad groups: (a) focal lesions, which cause a localized disturbance of function, (b) diffuse or generalized disorders (whether of infective, metabolic, toxic, vascular or other aetiology) that affect nervous and supporting elements throughout the nervous system, and (c) systemic nervous diseases, in which the pathological process shows a predilection for a particular neuronal structure or group of structures, such as the anterior horn cells, the cerebellum and its connections, or the corticospinal (pyramidal) tracts.

Some focal lesions and diffuse disorders affect nervous tissue more-or-less by accident and are not primarily neurological diseases. Thus cerebrovascular disease, which may produce a focal cerebral lesion such as a haemorrhage or an infarct, is usually a complication of atherosclerosis and/or hypertension, whereas the diffuse pathological changes involving the brain in syphilis represent only one component of the widespread changes resulting from the infection. In the systemic nervous diseases, by contrast, as in motor neuron (motor system) disease, there is clearly some unknown factor which causes the pathological process to be confined to a particular group of nerve cells or fibre pathways. The tissues of the nervous system vary in their susceptibility to many different noxious influences. Thus ischaemia affects nerve cells more severely than it does fibres, while plaques of demyelination have a more profound influence upon white matter. There are also differences in the effects of ischaemia, compression and various toxins upon nerve fibres, depending upon their diameter and degree of myelination and thus secondarily upon whether they conduct motor or sensory impulses.

Virtually every pathological lesion of the nervous system can be categorized under one of the following headings:

1. Developmental disorders
2. Traumatic (physical or chemical injury)
3. Inflammatory { infective / allergic or postinfective (hypersensitivity) } { acute / subacute / chronic }
4. Neoplastic { benign / malignant { primary / secondary } }
5. Degenerative { vascular / other, or of unknown aetiology }
6. Metabolic and endocrine

Many of the important nervous lesions of developmental origin give gross disorders of anatomical development and configuration. Examples are anencephaly, hydrocephalus due to stenosis of the aqueduct of Sylvius, and arteriovenous malformations or angiomas of the brain or spinal cord. Trauma to the nervous system produces necrosis, haemorrhage, and subsequent scar formation, the scar consisting of proliferated neuroglial cells and fibrils (gliosis) and of mesenchymal fibrous tissue derived from fibroblasts in the supporting tissue of the blood vessels. Among the acute inflammatory disorders are the meningitides, which produce the typical pathological change of inflammation and exudation in the meninges (Fig. 2.3). Meningitis, if severe, can also give rise to superficial degenerative changes in the underlying nervous tissue or to more extensive ischaemic changes in the nervous parenchyma resulting from an obliterative endarteritis of the blood vessels which traverse the subarachnoid space (Fig. 2.3B). Chronic granulomatous meningitides (tuberculosis, cryptococcosis, sarcoidosis) commonly produce these effects but can also cause hydrocephalus as a result of blockage of the cerebrospinal fluid circulation or multiple cranial nerve lesions owing to involvement of nerve trunks in the inflammatory process in the subarachnoid space. Pyogenic infection of the substance of the brain and spinal cord usually begins as a diffuse suppuration, but localization and abscess formation generally follow with the formation of a capsule.

Many of the so-called neurotropic viruses, such as those which give rise to virus encephalitis and anterior poliomyelitis, are polioclastic, that is they show an affinity for nerve cells. Inflammatory changes, with perivascular cellular infiltration and degeneration of nerve cells, are therefore seen in the grey matter of the brain and spinal cord. Sometimes inclusion bodies are found within the nucleus or cytoplasm of infected cells. The virus of herpes zoster, for example, shows a particular affinity for the cells of the posterior root ganglia. By contrast, that of herpes simplex can give an acute necrotizing encephalitis, especially involving the temporal lobes. The virus can be identified in a biopsy sample of necrotic brain by immunofluorescent methods and/or electron microscopy.

Syphilis is still an important chronic infection of the central nervous system. The meningovascular form gives meningeal inflammation and endarteritis of cerebral and spinal arteries. In general paresis there are degeneration of nerve cells, gliosis and minimal inflammatory changes in the cerebral cortex. In tabes dorsalis the most prominent change is gliosis and meningeal fibrosis at the entry zone of the posterior spinal nerve roots, with secondary ascending degeneration of the posterior columns of the spinal cord (Fig. 2.4). In allergic or postinfective encephalomyelitis, in contrast to the virus infections, inflammatory changes predominate in the white matter, giving perivascular collections of inflammatory cells and patchy myelin loss. The pathological changes in the latter group of diseases show some resemblance to those observed in the demyelinating diseases of unknown aetiology, such as multiple sclerosis, in which there are foci of demyelination known as plaques (Fig. 2.5) throughout the white matter of the brain and spinal cord. This primary lesion, in which the axis cylinders are initially preserved, is eventually replaced by a glial scar.

In the systemic autoimmune diseases such as polyarteritis nodosa and systemic lupus erythematosus, granulomatous vascular lesions may involve the central and/or peripheral nervous system, causing multifocal infarctions of the brain or infarcts in

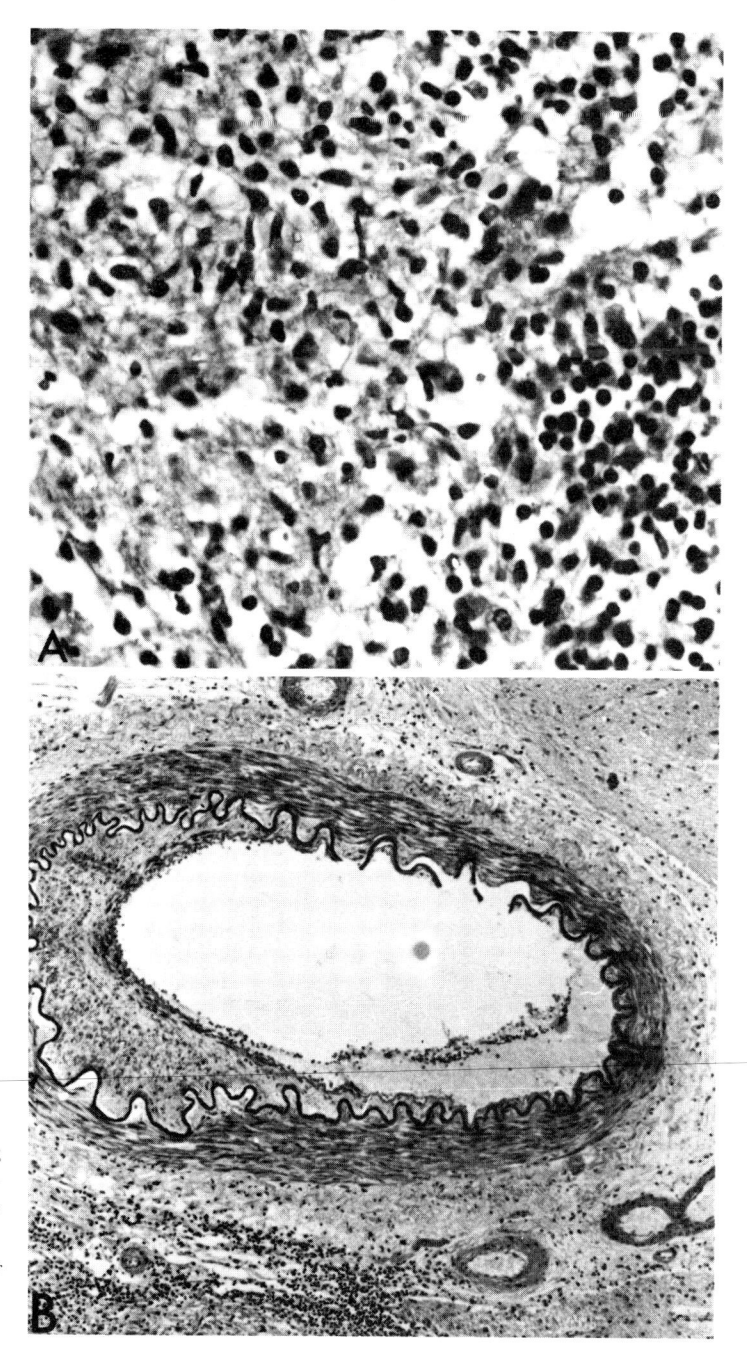

Figure 2.3 A, Tuberculous meningitis; collections of lymphoid and epithelioid cells in the subarachnoid space. H & E, ×400. B, Endarteritis in tuberculous meningitis. H & E, ×64. [Reproduced from Walton (1985) *Brain's Diseases of the Nervous System*, 9th edn, by kind permission of the publisher.]

peripheral nerves with resultant polyneuropathy or mononeuritis multiplex. Other granulomatous arteritides (including cranial, temporal or giant-cell arteritis) can sometimes have similar effects.

Most of the benign tumours which affect the central nervous system are extracerebral and extramedullary, lying outside the brain or spinal cord, though within their bony encasements. The two most common tumours are the meningioma, which arises from cells of the arachnoid membrane, and the neurofibroma or neurilemmoma, which grows from the sheath of Schwann of the cranial nerves, spinal roots or peripheral nerves. These neoplasms compress and distort but do not invade nervous tissue. The gliomas are the largest group of malignant tumours of the central nervous system. These are infiltrating and invasive tumours whose relative malignancy depends upon whether the principal constituent cell of the

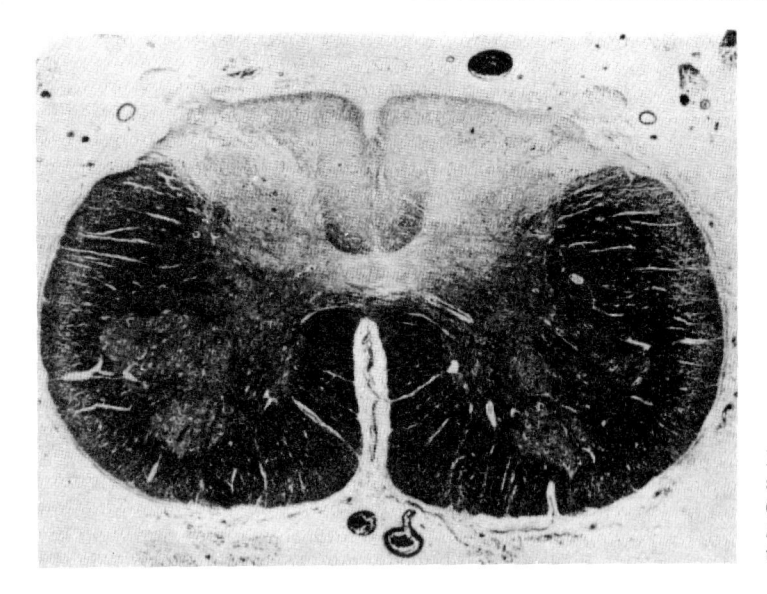

Figure 2.4 Tabes dorsalis; section of spinal cord. [Reproduced from Walton (1985) *Brain's Diseases of the Nervous System*, 9th edn, by kind permission of the publisher.]

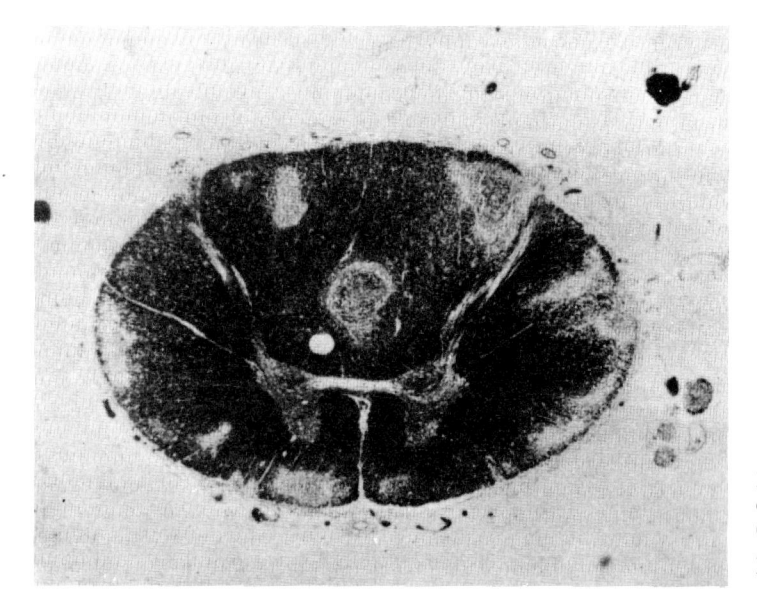

Figure 2.5 Multiple sclerosis: spinal cord, T9. [Reproduced from Walton (1985) *Brain's Diseases of the Nervous System*, 9th edn, by kind permission of the publisher.]

tumour is a relatively mature astrocyte or one of its more rapidly multiplying primitive precursors. Metastatic malignant tumours are also common. Cancer of the lung, breast and kidney and the malignant melanoma are among those which most often metastasize to the brain.

Vascular disorders of the nervous system are common. Bleeding into the subarachnoid space (subarachnoid haemorrhage) produces an aseptic meningeal inflammation comparable in its effects to meningitis, and in some cases a degree of meningeal organization or so-called arachnoiditis may result. Rarely, chronic bleeding into the subarachnoid space can give rise to haemosiderosis of the meninges, with consequent degeneration of the superficial parts of the brain, cranial nerves and spinal cord. Haemorrhage in the nervous parenchyma produces an area of necrosis which is eventually walled off by gliosis and fibrosis. If it is small, the necrotic area is absorbed and a scar results, but more often a cavity is left which is filled with clear straw-coloured fluid containing bilirubin. An infarct, too, shows an area of central ischaemic necrosis. Within 24 hours, activated microglial cells (the histiocytes or scavengers of the nervous system) invade the necrotic area and become distended with fatty remnants of the necrotic myelin which they have ingested. A minute infarct, produced by embolic occlusion of a tiny cortical vessel, gives little more histologically than a small cluster of activated microglial cells, whereas a large infarct shows an extensive central area of necrosis surrounded by distended phagocytes ('gitter' cells—Fig. 1.6F) and proliferating astrocytes. A large infarct may eventually be represented by a contracted glial scar or by a cavity, while multifocal infarction due to occlusion of small arteries or arterioles, occurring usually in hypertensive patients, sometimes leads to the formation of multiple small cavities or lacunes ('status lacunosus').

There are many degenerative disorders of the nervous system of unknown aetiology but with relatively specific neuropathological changes. In motor neuron disease, for instance, the cells of the motor nuclei of the brain stem, the anterior horn cells of the spinal cord, and the corticospinal (pyramidal) tracts show progressive degeneration. In Huntington's chorea there is selective degeneration of the caudate nucleus and the nerve cells of the frontal cortex. But in these and many other disorders, although the anatomical distribution of pathological change is well defined, their nature is little understood. The brain damage which follows cerebral anoxia or ischaemia has generally been attributed to a failure of energy metabolism, secondary disturbances of local blood flow, or the release of toxic free radicals. However, there is now some evidence that the neurotoxic effect of synaptically-released excitatory amino acids plays a crucial role in these processes (Meldrum, 1985). Nevertheless, we still do not know why anoxia affects particularly the cells of the deepest layer of the cerebral cortex, the Ammon's horn area of the hippocampus, and the cerebellar Purkinje cells, nor why deficiency of vitamin B_{12} damages selectively the sensory fibres of peripheral nerves, the posterior columns of the cord, and the corticospinal (pyramidal) tracts. Many metabolic disorders seriously disturb nervous function but produce relatively little pathological change. In hypoglycaemia the changes are similar to those of anoxia, while in hepatic failure there is astrocytic proliferation, particularly in the basal ganglia. The pathological changes in many forms of polyneuropathy are also non-specific, consisting either of segmental loss of myelin, beginning near the nodes of Ranvier (demyelinating neuropathies), or of swelling and fragmentation of axis cylinders in the peripheral nerves (neuropathies due to axonal degeneration).

CONSTITUTION AND HEREDITY

Readers should understand the basic principles of genetics and human inheritance. Many neurological disorders, and particularly some of those referred to above as 'degenerative' in character, are inherited in a strictly mendelian manner. A disease resulting from a dominant gene situated on one of the autosomes—an autosomal dominant trait—is passed on by an affected individual to half of his or her children of either sex if penetrance or expressivity of the gene is complete. Examples of disorders inherited in this way are Huntington's chorea and facioscapulohumeral muscular dystrophy. A recessive gene produces its effect only if it is paired with a similar gene lying on the other chromosome of the pair. Such an autosomal (non sex-linked) recessive trait therefore produces clinical effects only when two unaffected heterozygotes marry. Hence there is usually no past history of the disease in the family unless there has been intermarriage between relatives (consanguinity). In such families, the statistical likelihood is that the disease will affect one in four of a series of brothers and sisters (a sibship). Freidreich's ataxia, hepatolenticular degeneration and limb-girdle muscular dystrophy are examples of diseases that are usually inherited in this way. Only rarely does a carrier of a single recessive gene show signs of disease (a manifesting heterozygote).

A single abnormal recessive gene can produce an effect, however, if it is situated on the X chromosome. Such a condition occurs in males and is carried by females who are usually unaffected, although sometimes they demonstrate certain clinical or biochemical effects of the gene, presumably due to inactivation of the normal X chromosome (as proposed in the Lyon hypothesis) and are then called manifesting carriers. Such features may be helpful in carrier detection. It is then known as a sex-linked or X-linked recessive trait. The disease may have affected maternal uncles and would be expected to appear by probability in half the male children of an apparently unaffected female carrier. Diseases inherited in this manner include colour blindness, haemophilia, and the Duchenne type of muscular dystrophy. Any inherited disease can appear anew in a family if a previously normal gene has undergone a process of spontaneous change or mutation.

Advances in molecular genetics have recently led to the introduction of techniques which will ultimately bring major benefit to those suffering from many inherited diseases. DNA recombinant studies are making possible chromosomal mapping and the development of gene-specific markers. This applies not only to the X chromosome, where characterization of the Duchenne muscular dystrophy gene is imminent, making possible precise carrier detection and antenatal diagnosis through chorionic biopsy, but also to other chromosomes. Thus, flanking markers have been identified for Huntington's chorea on chromosome 4, and the same now seems to be the case with dystrophia myotonica (chromosome 19).

Apart from diseases which are clearly inherited by the mechanisms described above, there are many other disorders of the nervous system in which genetic influences are important, though less clearly defined. In epilepsy and in multiple sclerosis, for example, multiple family members are affected more often than could be accounted for by chance, though no clear pattern of inheritance emerges. Recent work suggests that specific histocompatibility antigen (HLA) patterns may imply an inherited susceptibility. It is important to consider not only the environmental influences but also the constitutional influences which may have a bearing upon each patient's disease.

THE APPROACH TO THE PATIENT

A systematic approach to each patient with symptoms suggesting disease of the nervous system is an essential preliminary to accurate diagnosis. The question should first be asked, where is the lesion or systemic process responsible for these symptoms and signs? Is it extracerebral, in the skull or meninges, in the cerebral cortex, in the white matter, in the brain stem, or in the cerebellum? If the clinical picture indicates a disorder of the spinal cord or of the lower motor neuron, is the lesion in the spinal column, the meninges, the spinal cord, the spinal roots, the plexuses, the peripheral nerves, the motor end-plates, or the muscles? In each case could it be congenital, traumatic, inflammatory, neoplastic, degenerative or metabolic? Is there disease in the heart, great vessels, lungs or other organs which could be responsible? Are emotional or psychological factors contributing to the patient's disability? While the answers to many of these questions are often self evident, it is well that they should be asked, since it is only through such a comprehensive approach to patients with neurological disease that the doctor will eventually acquire the skill and experience which will allow him to discard the irrelevant information and concentrate upon those salient facts which lead to accurate diagnosis.

THE NOSOLOGY OF NERVOUS SYSTEM DYSFUNCTION

Pathophysiology implies the study of normal function and the ways in which it may be disordered. Later we will deal in depth with the mechanisms which underlie the production of symptoms and signs (collectively entitled nosology) of dysfunction in various components of the nervous system. The remainder of this chapter will deal briefly with reasons why diagnosis is the ultimate aim and with the clinical methods used in recognizing and interpreting the symptoms and signs that will lead to the correct diagnosis.

Symptoms and signs of neurological dysfunction

THE AIM OF DIAGNOSIS

In neurology, prognosis and treatment usually depend upon an accurate diagnosis, arrived at from an analysis of symptoms and signs combined with information obtained from the appropriate ancillary investigations. In some disorders, such as epilepsy and migraine, appraisal of the patient's symptoms is all-important in reaching a diagnosis, and physical examination is usually negative. Conversely, in other conditions the history may be uninformative and diagnosis depends upon a meticulous physical examination. Usually the history and examination are mutually interdependent, one throwing light upon the significance of the other. The individual symptoms and signs which can result from nervous system dysfunction are so many that a planned approach to each patient is needed, so designed that complaints which at first seem irrelevant are not ignored but are fitted into place so that the patient and his disease are viewed as a whole.

Diagnosis is not, however, an end in itself. The doctor will be assessed by his patients not upon his flair for diagnosing rare disease, but upon his understanding of their needs, of their hopes and fears, and of the intensely personal problem which their illness presents. The correct management of two identical cases of disabling neurological disease will be quite different if the sufferers differ widely in attitude, emotional constitution and domestic environment. There are many such chronic and crippling progressive disorders which pose serious problems to both patient and doctor. They present a challenge which requires tact, sympathy and understanding, as well as diagnostic skill and ingenuity in changing circumstances. These qualities cannot be learned from a textbook but are derived from continuing contact and communication with patients and their relatives both in the hospital environment and in their homes. Diagnosis, then, is only the beginning, and need not always be strictly accurate for management to be correct, provided the broad pattern of the patient's disease is recognized. On the other hand, there are many conditions, such as meningitis, subdural haematoma and spinal tumour, in which diagnosis must be made early if death or severe disability is to be avoided.

Some useful terms in neurological pathophysiology

There are many important neurological terms, largely derived from Greek and Latin, which are in common use in neurological medicine but which are often used loosely or incorrectly. The prefix *a-* means absence of; the prefix *dys-*, disturbance of; *hyper-*, increased; and *hypo-*, decreased. If the Greek suffix *-phasis* is taken to denote conceptual aspects of speech function, then *aphasia* is used to denote loss of this function, and *dysphasia* when the disorder is less severe. Similarly, *aphonia* is loss of the ability to phonate, *anarthria* means inability to articulate and *dys*arthria slurring or indistinct articulation. *Atrophy* or *hypotrophy* of muscle means wasting; *hypertrophy*, enlargement; *hypoaesthesia* (often shortened to hypaesthesia), reduced sensation; and *hyperpathia*, increased sensitivity to painful or unpleasant sensory stimuli.

In much the same way, *ataxia* means unsteadiness or lack of coordination, *apraxia* or *dyspraxia* loss or impairment of acquired motor skills, and *agnosia* loss of the ability to recognize and interpret sensory information. The suffix *-plegia* means paralysis and *-paresis* weakness. Thus a *monoplegia* is a paralysis of one limb, a *monoparesis* weakness of one limb. Similarly a *hemiplegia* means paralysis of one arm and leg on the same side of the body, *tetraplegia* or *quadriplegia* paralysis of all four limbs, and *paraplegia* paralysis of the lower limbs only. The term *diplegia* is often used to identify a form of spastic weakness of all four limbs affecting the lower limbs, as a rule more severely than the upper limbs.

Eliciting symptoms of neurological dysfunction

After listing the principal symptoms of which the patient complains, it is usual to note in chronological order a description, taken from the patient's own words, of how they developed. Once the patient has described his complaints it is then important for the sake of completeness to ask leading questions which have until then been avoided assiduously, so as not to present the suggestible patient with additional symptoms which he may then profess to have. These should relate to some of the principal symptoms of nervous disease. Has there been, for instance, any pain or headache, or any loss or impairment of consciousness, either brief or prolonged? Have there been visual symptoms such as impairment of sight or diplopia, or has the patient noticed any change in speech or swallowing? Are memory, behaviour and concentration unimpaired? Have deafness, tinnitus, giddiness or unsteadiness been experienced, or any involuntary movements of the head, trunk or limbs occurred? It is also wise to enquire specifically about weakness, paralysis or clumsiness of the limbs (though few patients would overlook such striking complaints) and about numbness, tingling, 'pins and needles' or other unusual sensations. And one must know whether control of the vesical or anal sphincters and/or of sexual function has been impaired and whether there have been any more general symptoms such as breathlessness, weight loss (or gain), anxiety, depression, sleeplessness, anorexia or vomiting.

Having elicited one or more symptoms, this knowledge alone is usually insufficient. If the complaint is of headache, for instance, much more must be known. Where in the head is it situated, and does it spread? What is its character? When does it or did it begin? How long does it last and how often does it occur? Is there any warning of its onset? Does anything seem to precipitate it or aggravate it once it has begun, and does anything relieve it? Are there associated symptoms of anxiety or of visual disturbance, vomiting or other physical problems? This kind of enquiry can be applied, with minor modification, to almost any symptom of nervous disease, but should not be learned by rote. An inquisitive approach in which each symptom is scrutinized and carefully analysed is better. Such critical enquiry and appraisal is more revealing and profitable to both doctor and patient than a carefully ordered routine learned by heart. Nevertheless, the enquiry must be comprehensive. While the experienced doctor may reach the core of the problem with a few well-chosen questions, there are no short cuts for the beginner. Experience, and experience alone, will teach which symptoms may safely be discarded as irrelevant and which are crucial.

The patient's own testimony can sometimes be unreliable or unavailable. In the unconscious patient, for example, one must interview relatives and others who may possess the essential information, and it is equally important to have independent evidence about patients who have suffered lapses of consciousness or mental and behaviour disorders.

It is also necessary to assess the patient's previous health. Have there been serious accidents or illnesses in the past, or any unusual sequelae of the common childish ailments? Was there any evidence that the patient was born by a difficult labour or with perinatal problems? Or was there a history of 'brain fever', or blackouts or head injury in childhood? Social and occupational details are also important. What was the patient's standard of education and what occupations has he followed? Are his domestic circumstances satisfactory or are there financial and/or personal difficulties? And what evidence is available about his physical and emotional constitution? Was he excessively nervous or overprotected as a child? Did he wet the bed or walk in his sleep? And has he changed employment frequently? What are his interests and hobbies, and have these changed? Such enquiries can yield valuable information, indicating perhaps the possibility of brain injury, encephalitis, febrile convulsions, or meningitis in childhood, or alternatively, deterioration in intellect, change in personality, or lifelong personality disorder (psychopathy) with failure to adjust to the demands of society. Such information may cast light upon the nature and significance of many symptoms, as may details concerning the consumption of alcohol, tobacco and drugs.

The family history too is important, as some neurological disorders are clearly inherited, and in others inherited predisposition may play a part. One must enquire about nervous or mental disease in siblings, parents and more distant relatives. If further cases of disease come to light, then a pedigree is needed. Important disease in other systems in family members should also be noted.

This guide to eliciting symptoms of nervous disease is merely an outline, but these general principles are important. The amplified descriptions of symptoms and symptom complexes which appear in subsequent chapters will help to stress important inter-relationships between individual symptoms.

Eliciting signs of neurological dysfunction

The clinical examination of the nervous system depends much upon establishing a carefully itemized routine. The method outlined below is one which the author has found to be satisfactory in practice.

THE MENTAL STATE

Disease of the brain can profoundly affect behaviour and awareness, so that assessment of the mental state is of great importance. Individual manifestations will be considered and defined in subsequent chapters. Here specific abnormalities will not be considered in detail, but brief information will be given about certain common abnormalities which may be sought.

First, the patient's state of awareness must be assessed. Is he comatose or semicomatose (see p. 86), confused or disorientated, or is he alert and well orientated in time and place? Is his mood normal, or is he euphoric or elated, depressed, anxious or agitated? Are his behaviour and social adjustment normal or is he antisocial and amoral, or dirty in his habits and blandly unconcerned? Does he show disordered thought processes with ideas of persecution (paranoia) or other delusions? Are there visual or auditory hallucinations? While some such questions can be answered through careful observation and by questioning the patient, simple but more formal tests may be required to assess memory, intellect and powers of abstract thought. To assess attention, concentration and immediate recall, the patient should be asked to repeat a series of numbers forwards and then backwards. The normal individual can easily remember seven figures forwards and five backwards. Similarly, he is asked to subtract serial sevens from 100 and the number of mistakes made as well as the time taken are recorded. This tests the ability to calculate and gives some information about intellect.

Usually one can tell whether remote memory is intact when taking the history. In assessing recent memory and the ability to record and retain new impressions it is helpful to ask the patient for details of his last meal or to give him a name, an address and the name of a flower to remember. He should be asked to repeat these several minutes later. He can also be asked to repeat a standard sentence such as one of the Babcock sentences, namely, 'One thing a nation must have to be rich and great is a large, secure supply of wood'. Most normal individuals can repeat this correctly by the third attempt. In testing the patient's ability to think in an abstract manner, one may seek interpretation of common proverbs or a fable. A defect of abstract thinking will be apparent, for instance, in the individual who suggests that people who live in glass houses should not throw stones as they would break the glass. Finally, in assessing the patient's intellectual state, it is usual to ask for the names of recent US presidents, prime ministers, monarchs, etc., the names of six large cities, or European capitals. For accurate assessment of minor changes, detailed psychometric testing by a psychologist is required.

PRAXIS AND GNOSIS AND THE BODY IMAGE

Praxis is the ability to perform purposive skilled movements. If this function is impaired, those skills most recently acquired in the course of growth and development may be the first to be lost. In testing this function the patient is asked to perform moderately complex movements, such as those involved in dressing, shaving, opening a box of matches and striking one, and constructing a model with toy bricks. Inability to perform these movements in a patient without obvious motor weakness, ataxia or sensory impairment may indicate a disorder of praxis known as apraxia.

Gnosis is the ability based upon the reception of sensory stimuli, either visual, tactile or auditory, to recognize the nature and significance of objects. An agnosia for spoken speech gives a form of sensory or receptive aphasia (see p. 74), while inability to recognize musical sounds is called amusia. In clinical practice the term agnosia is most often used for defects of visual or tactile recognition. This may relate to articles in the patient's environment, but can also be concerned with the parts of his own body. In testing these functions he is asked to interpret humorous drawings or pictures which tell a story, or to identify objects such as a coin placed in the hand. He should also be asked to identify parts of the body, for example one ear, a knee, or individual fingers in himself and in the examiner. The patient's awareness of his own body and of its relationship to external space is known as the body image, and a loss of awareness of a part of the body image is a form of agnosia or impairment of gnosis. This can also involve an inability to distinguish right from left (right–left disorientation), a possibility which should be borne in mind when testing.

SPEECH

The function of speech can be subdivided into first the higher or cortical control of speech, and second the lower or peripheral mechanisms which control phonation and articulation. Reading and writing are closely allied to other speech functions, as is the ability to calculate. An inability to express one's thoughts in words, when the mechanisms of phonation and articulation are intact and understanding of the spoken word is preserved, is known as motor, expressive (or Broca's) aphasia, and a failure to understand the spoken word is called sensory, receptive (or Wernicke's) aphasia. These and related functions are readily tested by asking the patient to name a series of common objects of progressive difficulty (hand, mouth, pen, radiator, spectacles, stethoscope, etc.) and by giving a series of simple commands, or seeking answers to simple questions. A patient with slight motor aphasia may be accurate in his speech but yet at a loss for simple words, while one with sensory aphasia may fail to obey commands or name simple objects; or else he may use inappropriate words in his reply to questions, as words to him, like symbols, have lost their meaning and significance. When the answers to these questions have been recorded, the patient should then be asked to read, interpret and perhaps paraphrase a short passage from a book and to write down his name and address and some of his outstanding symptoms. He should also be asked to copy in writing a short passage and then to write to dictation. Finally, the ability to do a number of simple sums should be tested.

A patient with complete paralysis of the muscles of articulation may be well able to understand and interpret the spoken and written word and to express himself fluently in writing. If he cannot make a sound, this is called aphonia, but if the sound is uttered and cannot be moulded into words, this is anarthria. Complete anarthria is uncommon, but slurring or indistinctness of speech due to disease or dysfunction of the motor pathways controlling articulation is more common and is called dysarthria. The patient should be asked to repeat a number of set phrases which may demonstrate dysarthria; 'British constitution' and 'Methodist episcopal' are good examples of phrases in common use.

THE SKULL AND SKELETON

Inspection and palpation of the skull is an essential part of the neurological examination. The size and shape of the skull and any asymmetry should be noted, as should the presence of abnormal bony protuberances or points of tenderness. Auscultation in the temporal fossae and over the globes of both eyes should also be carried out, and the patient should be asked to stop breathing so that the presence or absence of a cranial bruit or murmur may be recorded. It is also necessary to listen for a bruit over the carotid, vertebral and subclavian arteries in the neck. Cranial bruits are often heard in normal children, but if one is heard unilaterally this is more likely to be significant. In the remainder of the skeleton any bony deformities (abnormal spinal curvature, pes cavus, etc.) should be noted, as should any limitation of movement in the spinal or limb joints.

Restricted flexion of the neck with pain in the occipital region and in the back of the neck itself (neck stiffness) is elicited by placing a hand under the head of the supine patient and attempting to flex the head until the chin touches the anterior chest wall. Neck stiffness is occasionally due to disease of the cervical spine, but is much more often due to meningeal irritation, as in meningitis or subarachnoid haemorrhage. Rarely it is due to herniation of the cerebellar tonsils through the foramen magnum. Other signs of meningeal irritation include Kernig's sign (pain and restriction of extension of the leg at the knee when the thigh is flexed to 90° upon the trunk) and Brudzinski's sign (sharp flexion of the upper and lower limbs induced in infants with meningitis when neck stiffness is being elicited). Limitation of straight leg raising with pain down the back of the thigh may also be due to meningeal irritation but is more often a consequence of compression of one of the nerve roots which form the sciatic nerve, as by a prolapsed intervertebral disc.

THE SPECIAL SENSES

The sense of smell (the olfactory nerve) should be tested in each nostril independently with the other occluded. Camphor, coffee, peppermint and oil of cloves are convenient test substances. When there is a possibility that total bilateral loss of the sense of smell (anosmia) is being feigned, the patient should also be asked to smell concentrated ammonia solution. This volatile substance stimulates trigeminal and not olfactory nerve endings in the nasal and pharyngeal mucosa, and the patient with organic anosmia usually reacts briskly. Failure to respond to the stimulus gives some support to the view that the alleged anosmia may be factitious.

Taste should be tested on either side of the tongue, first on the anterior two-thirds, then on the posterior third where accurate assessment is very difficult. The four modalities of taste which can be recognized are sweet (sugar), salt (salt), bitter (quinine), and sour or acid (citric acid or vinegar). The tongue should be protruded and dried and held with gauze while a fine brush dipped in a solution of one of the test agents is applied to the surface. The patient should then be asked to point to one of four cards on which these four modalities are listed. Taste sensation from the anterior two-thirds of the tongue is carried in the chorda tympani (facial nerve) and from the posterior one-third of the tongue in the glossopharyngeal nerve.

Vision (the optic nerve)

In testing vision it is usual to begin by testing visual acuity in each eye independently, the other being covered. Usually, Snellen's test types are used, and the patient is asked to read, at a distance of 6 m (20 feet), the letters on the card. Each line of type is numbered and the acuity is recorded as 6 or 20 over the number of the lowest line of type which can be read accurately; for instance, 6/6 or 20/20 is normal. If the patient normally wears spectacles the acuity should then be recorded when they are worn, the so-called corrected acuity. This test is appropriate to distance vision, whereas near vision is tested with Jaeger's reading card, in which case acuity is expressed as from J1 to J6, J1 being normal and J6 showing severely impaired acuity. When vision in one or both eyes is so severely impaired that none of the test types can be seen, sight is recorded as limited to 'counting fingers', 'hand movements' or 'light perception' only. In patients who claim to be blind and in whom hysteria is suspected, it may be of value to see whether blinking occurs at the threat of a blow, or if unilateral blindness is thought to be of emotional origin, printed words with alternate letters of different colours may be presented to a patient with coloured glasses applied over each eye alternately, and it is a relatively easy matter to determine that the visual loss is not genuine.

Colour vision is rarely impaired as a result of disease, but colour-blindness is present from birth in about 8% of males and in occasional females, being inherited as an X-linked recessive trait. This function is tested most satisfactorily with the Ishihara charts, with which full instructions are supplied.

The visual fields must next be tested, first on confrontation. The patient and the examiner sit face to face and the patient is instructed to gaze steadily at the bridge of the examiner's nose. One eye is then covered and a convenient test object (the examiner's finger, or preferably a pin with a white head) is brought into the patient's field of vision from all angles, the patient being instructed to say 'now' whenever it first comes into view. The procedure is then repeated with the other eye. In this way, gross defects in the peripheral visual fields may be detected and must then be confirmed by accurate charting on a perimeter. Even the perimeter, however, is not accurate enough to plot in full the important area of central vision around the fixation point, which is subserved by the macular area of the retina. To examine this area fully, particularly if small scotomas (small areas of visual loss) are to be detected, central vision must be charted on the Bjerrum screen. Patients with central scotomas, due to disease of the macula or the nerve fibres from this area, may have greatly reduced visual acuity and may be unable to read, even though the peripheral fields as charted on the perimeter are full. The visual field for large objects is larger than that for small objects, and for white objects it is more extensive than for red. A scotoma for red may sometimes be detected before one for white can be found.

The optic discs and fundi are next inspected, after dilatation of the pupils with a mydriatic agent if necessary. The optic disc is normally faintly pink in colour but its temporal half is usually somewhat paler. A deep physiological cup into which the vessels dip may give a mistaken impression of pallor of the central and temporal areas of the disc until a pink rim of normal-appearing disc is seen to its temporal side. Some blurring of the nasal margin of the disc is common in many normal individuals, and sometimes only the extreme temporal margin is clear-cut. In papilloedema, or swelling of the optic nerve head, not only are the disc margins blurred and sometimes impossible to define, but the vessels may be seen to be 'heaped up' in the centre of the disc. In addition, no physiological cup is present, the veins are distended, and there may even be haemorrhages and exudates in the surrounding retina. In optic atrophy, by contrast, the disc is flat and dead-white in colour, with clearly defined and often irregular margins. In examining the fundus, abnormal pigmentation, white patches of retinal degeneration, haemorrhage, hard white exudates, vascular changes (arterial narrowing, 'nipping' of veins at arteriovenous crossings, micro-aneurysms) and any other abnormality should be noted and described if present. Retinal angiography with fluorescein has proved to be invaluable in distinguishing some of these abnormalities.

Any abnormal position of the globe of either eye, such as proptosis (asymmetrical protrusion), exophthalmos (uniform protrusion) or enophthalmos (sunken eye) must also be recorded, as must the state of the eyelids and pupils. Drooping of the eyelids, or ptosis, may be observed, or alternatively lid-lag, revealing white sclera above the cornea on downward ocular movement. The size, equality or otherwise, and regularity of the pupils should now be examined, together with the response on shining a bright light into the eyes; the effect upon the other pupil (the consensual reaction) as well as the direct reaction should be observed. Changes occurring on accommodation-convergence, i.e. when transferring the gaze rapidly from a distant to a near object (such as a finger placed a few inches from eyes), are also tested. The afferent pathway for the pupillary reflex to light is in the optic nerve, the efferent pathways in the parasympathetic constrictor fibres of the oculomotor nerve and the dilator fibres of the ocular sympathetic.

Ocular movements (the oculomotor, trochlear, and abducent nerves) are now examined. The patient is asked to follow an object with both eyes, such as a finger which is moved quickly from right to left and then up and down in front of the eyes. If diplopia (double vision) occurs in any direction of gaze this should be noted, as well as the position of the two images in relation to one another. Any deviation of the ocular axes during movements is also recorded, as well as the presence or absence of nystagmus, an oscillatory or rotatory movement which is a most important physical sign. If the eyes give one or two sharp jerks only, at the extremities of lateral gaze, then these movements (nystagmoid jerks) are of no significance, but if the 'to and fro' movement occurs three or more times, this constitutes nystagmus. Its character and direction should also be carefully observed, as well as the ocular movements which produce it. It should be noted whether it is phasic (with a quick phase in one direction, slow in another), whether it is present on fixation or only in certain directions of gaze, and whether it is equal in the two eyes or worse in one than in the other. Forms of nystagmus and their cause are considered in detail under 'The special senses' (p. 125).

In certain cases, it is not the movement of one or the other eye which is defective, but movement of the two eyes together—laterally, upwards or downwards. These are movements which are necessary for the maintenance of binocular vision. Such defects of conjugate ocular movement have considerable localizing value and should, if present, be carefully defined. Similarly, disease may cause loss of the ability to converge the ocular axes when watching an object approach the bridge of the nose, so this should be tested for. There are several reflexes involving ocular movements which are commonly used in clinical practice. Thus, in eliciting oculocephalic reflexes the movements of the eyes are recorded on flexion or lateral movement of the head and neck (the 'doll's head' manoeuvre), while optokinetic nystagmus elicited by asking the patient to watch a rotating striped drum also gives useful information. Electronystagmography and other techniques of recording ocular movement precisely are now being more widely used in clinical practice and are considered later.

Hearing and labyrinthine function (the auditory and vestibular nerves)

An approximate assessment of the efficiency of a patient's hearing can be obtained by recording the distance at which a whispered voice or the ticking of a watch can be heard in each ear, with the other ear temporarily occluded. If comparison with a normal subject suggests that one or both ears are deaf, it is necessary to decide whether the deafness is due to disease in the middle ear (middle-ear or conductive deafness) or in the cochlea or auditory nerve (nerve, sensorineural or perceptive deafness). This may be determined by testing with a 256- or 512-frequency tuning fork. Normally, air conduction is better than bone conduction, and in nerve deafness this principle is still true, though hearing by either means may be greatly diminished. In middle ear deafness, by contrast, bone conduction is better. Descriptions of the Rinne test and Weber test are given on p. 150.

Clinical assessment of labyrinthine function may be difficult, but in patients with vertigo it is reasonable to make sudden alterations in the position of the head to see whether this produces nystagmus or vertigo. For instance, a patient may be asked to lie down suddenly and the head is then turned sharply to one side or the other. This test for postural vertigo is particularly useful in patients who complain of giddiness brought on by change in posture. Details of this technique, of caloric tests, and of other methods of testing the function of the labyrinths and central vestibular connections are given on p. 153.

THE MOTOR SYSTEM

In the patient who is able to walk, observation of the gait is foremost in examination of the motor system, as certain neurological diseases produce striking abnormalities. The hemiplegic patient tends to drag or to circumduct his weak and spastic leg, while the arm is commonly flexed at the elbow and lies across the abdomen when he walks. The patient with a spastic paraparesis shows a stiff and clumsy mode of progression in which both feet seem to drag along the ground. The festinant gait of parkinsonism is even more striking. The patient shuffles along with short hurried steps, the head bowed and the back bent, as if he were having continually to press forwards to prevent himself from falling on his face. By contrast, the individual with cerebellar ataxia walks on a wide base, the feet abnormally far apart. He staggers occasionally from side to side and if asked to stop suddenly or to turn, he is very unsteady and may even fall. Equally characteristic is the 'clopping' or slapping gait seen in unilateral or bilateral footdrop resulting from weakness of the dorsiflexors of the feet. The walk of the patient with pelvic girdle weakness due to muscular dystrophy (or to other forms of myopathy or spinal muscular atrophy) is characterized by a waddle, protuberant abdomen and accentuated lumbar lordosis. Another important abnormality of gait is the high-stepping unsteady demeanour of the patient with sensory ataxia, as in tabes dorsalis, who slaps his feet down hard as if he is not sure where they are in space.

Having observed the gait, it is then necessary to note specific abnormalities of posture or involuntary movements that cannot be corrected or prevented by willed effort on the part of the patient. If involuntary movements are present, their situation, nature, amplitude, rhythmicity and frequency should be assessed. It is also important to note whether changes in posture are permanent or temporary and whether they are influenced by volitional activity.

To examine the neuromuscular system it is usual first to inspect the muscles, noting the presence or absence of atrophy (a reduction in muscular bulk), hypertrophy (muscular enlargement) or fasciculation (involuntary twitching of isolated bundles of muscle fibres). Next, contractures or irreversible shortening of muscles and tendons, possibly resulting in skeletal atrophy or deformity, should be sought before proceeding to an examination of muscular power.

Beginning with the motor cranial nerves, the muscles of mastication (temporals, masseters, and pterygoids), supplied by the motor division of the fifth or trigeminal nerve, are tested by asking the patient to clench the teeth or to move the jaw from side to side against resistance while the bulk and firmness of the muscles on the two sides are compared. The seventh or facial nerve is first tested by inspection of the face and then by asking the patient to close the eyes tightly and to show the teeth. Inability to bury the eyelashes on one side may be a significant physical sign, while differences in power between the upper and lower facial muscles should be noted. Similarly the fact that emotional movement of the face, as in smiling, is normal, while volitional movement on command is impaired may be important. Movement of the palate on saying 'ah' may reveal a disorder of one of the vagus nerves, and if the uvula moves to one side this implies weakness of the opposite side of the palate, possibly resulting from a lesion of this nerve. Similarly, atrophy and weakness of one trapezius and sternomastoid may imply disease of the ipsilateral spinal accessory nerve, while atrophy and fasciculation of the tongue and deviation to one side when it is protruded indicates a lesion of the twelfth or hypoglossal nerve on the side to which the tongue protrudes.

Most of the trunk and limb muscles may be tested individually if necessary. Rational application of simple anatomical knowledge will indicate how each may be tested, but unless there is striking atrophy of single muscles or muscle groups, such a detailed examination is rarely necessary. In a routine examination it is usual to test representative groups of muscles, which are contracted against resistance from the examiner. These include those which abduct the shoulder, flex and extend the elbow, and extend and flex the fingers (the grip) in the upper limbs. The upper and lower abdominal muscles may be compared in the recumbent patient by noting whether the umbilicus deviates upwards or downwards on lifting the head. In the lower limbs it is usual to test hip flexion, flexion and extension at the knee, and dorsi- and plantar flexion of the feet.

In view of subjective variations from one examiner to the next, no single method of assessing the power of individual muscles is perfect. One widely used method gives numerical gradings from 0 to 5 to identify degrees of power, as given below:

0 No contraction
1 Flicker or trace of contraction
2 Active movement, with gravity eliminated
3 Active movement against gravity
4 Active movement against gravity and resistance
5 Normal power

Grades 4−, 4 and 4+ may be used to indicate movement against slight, moderate and strong resistance respectively.

If examination reveals weakness of one or more major muscle groups it is then sometimes necessary to examine the power of individual muscles in order to determine whether the pattern of weakness indicates, for instance, disordered function of a single peripheral nerve or nerve root.

In certain cases it is also necessary to test for muscular fatigability. In patients with myasthenia gravis, for example, an initial contraction may be powerful, but if the movement is repeated several times it becomes progressively weaker. By contrast, in myotonia, muscular contraction is usually powerful, but on relaxing (say after making a fist) the fingers 'uncurl' abnormally slowly. Direct percussion of a myotonic muscle gives a 'dimple', which slowly disappears. This phenomenon must be distinguished from myoidema, a localized ridge which forms after a direct blow upon a muscle belly and which is usually seen in malnourished, cachectic or hypothyroid patients.

The tone of the limb muscles is next tested by noting and comparing the resistance which the muscles show to passive movement at the shoulder, elbow, knee and ankle joints. This may be a very difficult examination as some patients find it almost impossible to relax the limb being tested and try to help by carrying out the movements themselves. If tone is reduced (hypotonia) the limbs are limp, 'floppy', and excessively mobile with little resistance, whereas if tone is increased (hypertonia) the limbs may be spastic, in which case there is a severe initial resistance which suddenly 'gives' (clasp-knife rigidity). Alternatively, the tone may be increased throughout the entire range of movement (plastic or lead-pipe rigidity) or it may be intermittently normal and increased (cog-wheel rigidity). In spastic limbs, a muscle under stretch may show clonus (rapid intermittent involuntary contraction and relaxation). This can best be seen at the ankle on sudden dorsiflexion of the foot, at the knee on pushing sharply downwards against the upper border of the patella, and sometimes on sudden extension of the fingers.

Tests for coordination are performed next in order to seek signs of cerebellar disease. The patient should be asked to alternately touch his nose and the examiner's finger with the tip of his index finger, and any tremor or past-pointing should be noted. In the lower limbs, the heel–knee test, in which the heel of one foot is placed on the opposite knee and then moved smoothly down the shin, is used. Other valuable tests which may reveal the clumsy incoordinate movements of cerebellar disease include rapid tapping with the fingers or toes on a convenient surface, 'playing the piano' on a table top, or rapid alternating pronation and supination of the hands and forearms.

There are several primitive reflexes which, present in the newborn, disappear with maturation but which may persist in infants with cerebral palsy. Some may reappear in adults suffering from diffuse degenerative brain disease. The tonic neck reflex is elicited by turning the head and neck to one side. Extension of the limbs occurs on the side towards which the head is turned. In the normal infant this reflex is no longer obtainable after the sixth month. It is typically present in adults with severe cerebral or brain-stem lesions, resulting in a 'decerebrate' state. The grasp reflex of the hand (a similar reflex can sometimes be elicited in the foot) is one of reflex flexion of the thumb and fingers, causing grasping of an object, when the palmar surface of the fingers or distal part of the palm is stroked. This reflex is the result of a lesion of the upper part of the contralateral frontal cortex, and if present unilaterally, may therefore be of some localizing value. The sucking reflex of the normal neonate and the closely related snout reflex (a pout or snout evoked by a sharp tap on the closed lips) may reappear in adults with diffuse brain disease or with bilateral corticospinal tract lesions in the upper brain stem or above. For the interpretation of other infantile automatisms the reader is referred to texts on paediatric neurology. In normal adults the contraction of both orbicularis oculi muscles (blinking) induced by a tap on the centre of the forehead above the nose (the glabellar tap sign) quickly habituates if the tap is repeated, but in patients with parkinsonism the blinking continues to occur rhythmically in time with the taps.

Finally, the deep and superficial reflexes are tested. First the jaw jerk is elicited by placing a finger across the patient's chin, with the mouth slightly open, and then tapping sharply downwards on the finger. A brisk contraction of the masseters is a positive jaw jerk, which is present in about 10% of normal individuals but which is exaggerated when there is bilateral corticospinal tract disease in the upper brain stem. In the upper limbs the biceps jerk is elicited by a blow on a finger which is placed across the patient's biceps tendon with the elbow flexed, the radial jerk is elicited by a brisk tap on the tendon of the brachioradialis as it traverses the lateral aspect of the lower end of the radius, and the triceps jerk is elicited by tapping the tendon of the triceps just above its insertion into the olecranon, again with the elbow flexed. To produce a finger jerk the examiner's fingers are tapped as they lie in contact with the palmar aspect of the tips of the patient's fingers, which should be partially flexed. Like the jaw jerk the finger jerk is present in some normal individuals and in those who are tense. If it is present on only one side, however, this may be significant. A concomitant flexion of the terminal phalanx of the thumb occurring when the finger jerk is elicited usually indicates that this reflex is exaggerated. Similar flexion of the terminal phalanx of the thumb occurring when the terminal phalanx of the middle finger is flicked sharply downwards between the examiner's finger and thumb (Hoffmann's sign) may also indicate corticospinal tract dysfunction, particularly if present on one side only. In the lower limbs the knee jerk is elicited by a blow on the patellar tendon with the knee in a semiflexed position, while the ankle jerk is obtained by tapping the Achilles tendon while the foot is passively dorsiflexed. Sometimes reinforcement (Jendrässik's manoeuvre) is necessary to bring out these reflexes. The patient is asked to grip an object or to clasp the hands together firmly when any tendon is about to be tapped, as this generally has the effect of producing a state of partial tension in his muscles (with increased gamma efferent discharge to the muscle spindle) so that all stretch reflexes are increased.

The first of the superficial reflexes to be tested are usually the abdominals. To elicit these, brisk strokes are made downwards and inwards in each quadrant of the abdomen with a sharp instrument such as the point of a pin, which should cause the umbilicus to move towards the stimulus. The superficial anal reflex consists of contraction of the external sphincter when the skin around the anus is stroked, while the cremasteric reflex consists of elevation of one testis on stroking or scratching the inner aspect of the upper thigh. The value of the anal and cremasteric reflexes, save in lesions of the cauda equina, is limited in clinical neurological practice. Finally, one of the most important reflexes is the plantar response. A firm stroke is made along the sole from the heel to the base of the fifth toe, along the outer side of the foot. Plantar flexion of all the toes is a flexor or normal response, while dorsiflexion of the great toe with plantar flexion and 'fanning' of the other toes is the extensor or Babinski response.

To assess the integrity of the parasympathetic outflow from the second and third sacral segments of the spinal cord, it may be necessary to elicit the anal sphincter reflex (contraction of the internal sphincter around the examiner's finger) or the bulbocavernosus reflex (contraction of bulbocavernosus elicited by pinching the glans penis).

When eliciting the deep tendon and abdominal reflexes, the patient must be resting comfortably and the muscles being tested should be relaxed. It is best to compare each reflex on one side of the body with the corresponding reflex on the opposite side of the body, observing any asymmetry of response. Conventionally, each reflex is recorded as −, +, + + or + + +, depending upon its activity, while the plantar responses are recorded as ↓ (flexor), ↕ (equivocal) or ↑ (extensor).

THE SENSORY SYSTEM

The different modalities of sensation should be tested independently as they follow different pathways in the spinal cord and brain. The perception of pain may conveniently be tested by a pin prick and that of touch with a fine wisp of cotton wool. Abnormalities of sensory perception should be sought on the face, trunk and limbs by exploring representative areas with the two types of stimuli mentioned. The corneal reflexes, evoked by touching each cornea with a fine wisp of cotton wool, should also be elicited. If an area of diminished pain sensation (hypalgesia) or touch sensation (hypaesthesia) is discovered, or even one of apparent hypersensitivity (hyperpathia), this should be outlined by applying repetitive stimuli from within to without the area and vice versa, asking the patient to say when a change occurs. The area of sensory change should then be charted on a drawing of the human body, each modality being recorded separately. If pain loss is found, then temperature perception should be tested within the same area using test-tubes filled with hot and cold water.

The finer and more discriminative aspects of sensibility should also be tested. Thus the patient may be asked to identify objects placed in the hands or to identify figures drawn on his skin when his eyes are closed. He is also asked to state the direction of movement each time the terminal phalanx of a finger or the great toe is moved passively upwards or downwards; any defects in position and joint sense so elicited are recorded. The appreciation of vibration should also be tested with a 128-frequency tuning fork over bony prominences such as the sternum, elbow, knuckle, anterosuperior iliac spine, patella and external malleolus. The ability to perceive whether the tips of the fingers or the soles of the feet are being touched with one or two points can also be tested. The normal threshold for two-point discrimination on the tips of the fingers is 2–3 mm, while on the sole of the foot it is 2–3 cm. Another useful test for eliciting very minor defects of sensation is to touch similar points on opposite limbs, sometimes independently and sometimes together, while asking the patient to say which has been touched. A patient who can perceive stimuli which are applied independently may feel the stimulus on only one side when both are touched at the same time. This phenomenon is known as tactile inattention.

Testing of sensory function carries many pitfalls for the unwary, and needs considerable practice and experience before it can be accurately performed. One reason for this is that suggestible individuals may easily produce spurious areas of cutaneous sensory loss, and hypalgesia is one of the commonest neurological signs of hysterical origin. Furthermore, many less intelligent patients find it difficult to understand what is being required of them, while the more intelligent may appreciate sensory changes that are the result of unintentional variation in intensity of stimulus rather than organic disease.

SIGNS OF DISEASE IN OTHER SYSTEMS

The human body does not function as an isolated nervous system, and neurological symptoms and signs often depend upon primary disorders of other systems. Cerebral infarction, for instance, can be a sequel of myocardial infarction, a brain abscess may be the result of bronchiectasis, or a confusional state may result from uraemia due to renal disease. Even though the patient's symptoms and physical signs may indicate disease or dysfunction of the nervous system, examination of the patient as a whole must be no less assiduous, for the essential clue to the nature of the patient's illness may lie elsewhere.

Discussion and differential diagnosis

A detailed clinical history and a physical examination recorded in meticulous detail are of no value unless they can be correctly interpreted, and it is upon this interpretation that treatment depends. It is at this stage that experience plays the greatest part, but experience can be acquired only if the student or young doctor learns to sift through the accumulated data, discarding the irrelevant and tabulating the significant. He must therefore at this stage apply his powers of inductive and deductive reasoning in order to decide first the location and secondly the nature of the pathological changes responsible for the patient's disease. He should be expected to tabulate in order of likelihood the possible diagnoses which he is considering, and must then decide which ancillary investigations, if any, are required in order to establish whichever is correct. For the history and examination are but a means to an end, the end being diagnosis, upon which management of the patient depends.

References

Adams, R. D. and Victor, M. (1985) *Principles of Neurology*, 3rd edn. New York: McGraw-Hill.

Bickerstaff, E. R. (1980) *Neurological Examination in Clinical Practice*, 4th edn. Oxford: Blackwell Scientific Publications.

Blackwood, W., Doods, T. C. and Sommerville, J. C. (1964) *Atlas of Neuropathology*, 2nd edn. Edinburgh: Churchill, Livingstone.

Davison, A. N. and Thompson R. H. S. (eds) (1981) *The Molecular Basis of Neuropathology*. London: Arnold.

Duchen, L. W. and Adams, J. H. (1985) *Greenfield's Neuropathology*, 4th edn. London: Edward Arnold.

Emery, A. E. H. (1983) *Elements of Medical Genetics*, 6th edn. Edinburgh: Churchill Livingstone.

Emery, A. E. H. (1984) *An Introduction to Recombinant DNA*. Chichester and New York: John Wiley.

Gordon, N. (1976) *Clinics in Developmental Medicine* (Paediatric Neurology for the Clinician), **59/60**. Philadelphia: J. B. Lippincott Company.

Holmes, G. (1968) *An Introduction to Clinical Neurology*, 3rd edn, revised by W. B. Matthews, Edinburgh: Churchill Livingstone.

de Jong, R. N. (1979) *The Neurologic Examination*, 4th edn. Hagerstown, Md: Harper and Row.

Klein, R. and Mayer-Gross, W. (1957) *The Clinical Examination of Patients with Organic Cerebral Disease*. London: Cassell & Co.

Lance, J. W. and McLeod, J. G. (1981) *A Physiological Approach to Clinical Neurology*, 3rd edn. London: Butterworth.

Matthews, W. B. (1976) *Practical Neurology*, 3rd edn. Oxford: Blackwell Scientific Publications.

Mayo Clinic (1981) (Section of Neurology) *Clinical Examinations in Neurology* 5th edn. Philadelphia: W. B. Saunders Company.

McKusick, W. A. (1964) *Human Genetics*. Englewood Cliffs, N. J: Prentice-Hall.

Medical Research Council (1976) *Aids to the Examination of the Peripheral Nervous System*. London: H.M.S.O.

Meldrum, B. S. (1985) Excitatory amino acids and anoxic/ischaemic brain damage. *Trends in Neurol. Sci.* **8**:47.

Paine, R. S. and Oppé, T. E. (1966) (Neurological Examination of Children) *Clinics in Developmental Medicine* **20/21**. London: The Spastics Society and Heinemann.

Patten, J. (1977) *Neurological Differential Diagnosis*. London: Harold Starke.

Reitan, R. M. and Davison, L. A. (1974) *Clinical Neuropsychology: Current Status and Applications*. Chichester: John Wiley & Sons.

Spillane, J. D. and Spillane, J. A. (1982) *An Atlas of Clinical Neurology*, 3rd edn. Oxford: Oxford University Press.

Swash, M. and Kennard, C. (eds) (1985) *Scientific Basis of Clinical Neurology*. Edinburgh and London: Livingstone.

Walton, J. N. (1982) *Essentials of Neurology*, 5th edn. London: Pitman Medical.

Walton, J. N., (1985) *Brain's Diseases of the Nervous System*, 9th edn. Oxford: Oxford University Press.

Zacks, S. I. (1971) *Atlas of Neuropathology*. New York: Harper & Row.

3

HUMAN VERBAL COMMUNICATION AND CONCEPTUAL ASPECTS OF MOVEMENT AND SENSORY PERCEPTION

INTRODUCTION

To understand the means by which the function of speech is developed and controlled and the ways in which it may be disordered is an endeavour which defeats many doctors. Even less comprehensible to some are the functions of praxis and gnosis, the first of which is concerned with the performance of complex willed movements, and the second with the recognition of sensory information (visual, auditory and tactile). Admittedly the anatomical and physiological organization of these functions is complex and still poorly understood. The many views expressed concerning localization of speech function within the cerebral hemispheres, along with the profusion of minutely varying disorders of speech which have been described, each with its own title, have added to the confusion. And yet, at the risk of oversimplification, it can be said that appreciation of a number of simple basic principles can bring clarity to what has long been a difficult field. First it is necessary to understand something of the way in which speech and other higher cerebral functions are acquired and developed and then to mention some of the ways in which they are disordered by disease.

THE ORGANIZATION OF SPEECH

Control of speech in the cerebral cortex

The young infant takes his first step towards the acquisition of speech function when he begins to associate particular sounds with particular objects in his environment. These sounds are subsequently organized into words, which are symbols used to identify the objects concerned. Nouns, therefore, are acquired first, and subsequently conceptual or abstract powers of thought are developed with the utilization of adjectives, verbs and adverbs to qualify these nouns or to describe activities instead of things. As the psychological concept of a word symbol is developed, so too the proprioceptive sensory impulses derived from the muscles of articulation come to be unconsciously associated with the expression of the word concerned, so that the child appreciates that certain specific movements of the larynx, lips and tongue will result in the production of this word. Gradually, as additional words are acquired these symbols lose some of their importance as individual entities but acquire new significance or meaning from their association with other words. In this way grammar and syntax develop and meaningful phrases and sentences are built up. When the child begins to read, visual symbols take their place alongside the appropriate sounds, and in the process of writing (visual speech) these same symbols acquire new associations in proprioceptive sensations derived from the fingers of the writing hand. Similarly, in learning a new language the words utilized in a foreign tongue develop associations with words of the same meaning in the individual's native language. Words have now acquired new and abstract meanings and are utilized not only for the communication of thoughts to others, but also for so-called 'internal speech' or the conscious logical process of abstract thought. Speech, therefore, is the communication of meaningful thoughts through the use of symbols which are usually written or spoken words.

Not all thought, however, is verbal. Some depends upon the construction of visual or auditory images within the mind, but the more complex problems are generally dealt with by the thinker in verbal form. The scientist or the musician may, by contrast, think in terms of mathematical or chemical formulas or of musical sounds, but these too are symbols, either auditory or visual, which are comparable to the written or spoken word. Similarly, meaning may be conveyed by facial expression or gesture (so-called silent language). In reading Braille print, the blind utilize tactile information instead of visual information.

It is therefore apparent that many sensory and motor activities are concerned in the understanding and production of words, whether spoken or written, and in the understanding of other auditory, kinaesthetic or visual symbols. Thus, in order to speak a sentence it is necessary first for the person concerned to formulate the thought he wishes to express, then to choose the appropriate words (a choice which depends upon his acquired knowledge of the significance of these symbols), and then to control the motor activity of the muscles of phonation and articulation, a process which involves the reception and correlation of proprioceptive sensory impulses from the muscles concerned. If the message is to be written rather than spoken, sensory impulses from the hand and arm are also involved. Similarly, in the understanding of speech, whether spoken or written, the accurate recording of auditory or visual stimuli is essential before the significance of the symbols utilized can be appreciated.

In the human brain those areas of the cerebral cortex which are particularly concerned with the production or understanding of spoken or written verbal symbols must have connections with those which control the motor activity of the muscles of articulation and writing and with the areas dealing with the reception of auditory and visual stimuli. These connections are achieved by means of a profusion of subcortical association fibres which not only pass between various areas of cortex in one cerebral hemisphere but also communicate, via the corpus callosum, with comparable cortical areas in the other hemispheres. The process of learning of speech, as of other functions, appears to depend upon the repeated passage of impulses along stereotyped pathways in these association tracts, a process which involves a progressive facilitation of the synapses that are traversed, so that the ease of passage of impulses is greatly increased. The function of memory and the ability to recall words or other symbols, as well as the emotional responses or visual images evoked by particular words or phrases, appears to depend upon the reactivation, either involuntarily or at will, of association pathways in which the necessary information has been 'stored'.

The function of speech cannot be said to be 'localized' in any particular part of the brain, as so many different cortical areas and association pathways are concerned in its integration. It is, however, true that in nearly all persons (93% of the population) who are right handed, the overall control of speech function is subserved by the left cerebral hemisphere. In about 60% of the remaining 7% who are left handed or ambidextrous, the left hemisphere remains dominant and controls this faculty, but in others it is controlled from the right side. Furthermore, the area of the dominant hemisphere which lies at the posterior end of the inferior frontal convolution (Broca's area), just in front of that part of the motor cortex controlling movements of the muscles of articulation, is particularly concerned with production of the spoken word. Similarly the posterior third of the superior temporal convolution on this side (Wernicke's area) exercises important influences upon the understanding and interpretation of word symbols. An important association pathway which connects Broca's area with Wernicke's area is the external capsule and arcuate fasciculus, which passes around the posterior end of the sylvian fissure and runs forward in the white matter in the inferior parietal lobe. It passes deep to the angular gyrus and in this area makes connections with visual association fibres. After division of the corpus callosum and other commissural connections in a right handed person, speech can deal only with conceptual information that reaches the left cerebral hemisphere. The right hemisphere is then isolated from verbal expression (a so-called disconnection syndrome).

The peripheral neuromuscular control of speech

There are two essential processes—phonation and articulation—by which the voluntary musculature is able to convert the thought conceived in the cerebral cortex into the spoken word. Phonation, the production of sound, results from the controlled passage of a column of air across the vocal cords, and the sound so produced is increased by resonance in the sounding-box of the larynx and pharynx. The sound is then modified by movements of the lips and tongue which subserve the function of articulation. These processes can be disturbed by lesions of the motor pathways which control the voluntary muscles concerned. The clinical features so produced are discussed below.

APHASIA

Although the term 'aphasia', if strictly interpreted, means absence of speech, it is usually utilized instead of the more correct 'dysphasia' to identify any disorder, however mild, of the use of words as symbols. Aphasia occurs in various forms and degrees, depending upon the location, extent and severity of the cerebral lesion that is responsible.

A word means more to the nervous system than any one of the innumerable ways in which it can be pronounced or written. Its basis is a combined neurophysiological and psychological concept (called a word-schema by Brain) through which its meaning is evoked. Classification of aphasic disorders is still largely empirical, though there is reasonable correspondence between modern anatomical and functional classifications.

The classification of aphasia

Modified from Geschwind (1970) the principal varieties of aphasia and related disorders can be classified as follows (Walton, 1985)

1. *Broca's aphasia* (expressive or motor aphasia, anterior aphasia)
2. *Wernicke's aphasia* (sensory or receptive aphasia) pure word deafness (auditory aphasia)
3. *Global or total aphasia*
4. *Conduction aphasia* (central aphasia of Goldstein, syntactical aphasia)
5. *The posterior* (*association*) *aphasias*
   a. the syndrome of the isolated speech area
   b. nominal, anomic or amnestic aphasia
6. *Related disorders of language:* agraphia, alexia, acalculia, amusia

BROCA'S APHASIA (MOTOR OR EXPRESSIVE APHASIA)

This results from a lesion in the neighbourhood of Broca's area. In its severest form the patient loses the power to speak completely or may say little more than 'yes' or 'no'. He nevertheless understands fully the spoken word, and will readily obey commands. His inability to express his thoughts in words may be the cause of severe distress and it is often apparent that he is well aware of what he wishes to say, but is unable to find the appropriate words. The writing of words, a form of motor speech, is usually similarly affected (agraphia). When the aphasia is less severe, the patient uses far fewer words than his normal vocabulary would allow, and these are utilized hesitantly and sometimes repetitively (perseveration) with slurring and long pauses, but nevertheless the words which are used are appropriate to the thoughts being expressed. Occasionally in polyglots or immigrants there is loss of the ability to utilize the language of the adopted country with preservation of fluent expression in their native tongue, but more often all the languages which the patient knows, including his native tongue, are equally impaired. In addition, even when speech can no longer be utilized at will to express the patient's thoughts, emotional expression such as the use of expletives in response to an appropriate stimulus may be unimpaired. The conveying of meaning by gesture is preserved, but reading aloud produces the same difficulty and poverty of expression as in spontaneous speech.

WERNICKE'S APHASIA (SENSORY OR RECEPTIVE APHASIA)

This is essentially an inability to appreciate the significance of words, whether spoken or written. The patient with this condition, which is generally produced by a lesion in the neighbourhood of Wernicke's area of the dominant cerebral hemisphere, shows a complete failure to comprehend the meaning of words which he hears or sees. The appreciation of musical sounds may also be lost (amusia). The patient still has words at his command, and his speech is often fluent and voluble, but he uses words inappropriately so that what he says or writes may be agrammatical and unintelligible. This form of speech disorder has sometimes been called jargon aphasia. Paraphasia (word or letter substitutions or incorrect word usage) is invariable and is either literal (the use of incorrect vowels or consonants within a word) or verbal (the use of incorrect words). Repetition of words offered by the examiner is impaired, as is the naming of objects. Handwriting is usually normal, but the content of spontaneous writing is often paraphasic, though copying may be normal. The patient often lacks insight and is frustrated by his inability to communicate. Word deafness (auditory aphasia) is a fractional form of receptive aphasia in which the patient is totally unable to understand the meaning of words spoken to him, but yet his own speech, reading and writing are normal and he himself is able to use words appropriately. However, even though his own speech is normal he finds it difficult to understand what he himself says and cannot repeat words or write to dictation. The lesion responsible is thought to lie in the subcortical white matter deep in the superior temporal gyrus. Similarly, in word blindness the patient cannot recognize written words or letters. In 'pure' word blindness it is only the ability to recognize verbal symbols which is impaired, but sometimes the patient is also unable to appreciate the significance of numbers and even of colours. The lesion here is also subcortical but more posterior.

GLOBAL APHASIA

Both of the major syndromes described above are seen in clinical practice, but mixed aphasia is equally common. Thus, when a large lesion of the dominant hemisphere involves both Broca's and Wernicke's areas there is impairment of both the expression and comprehension of speech, so-called global aphasia.

CONDUCTION APHASIA

Conduction or central aphasia results from lesions of the arcuate fasciculus, which divide the association fibres between Broca's and Wernicke's areas. The patient's speech is copious, but paraphasic errors (use of incorrect words or sounds as parts of individual words) are common. Object naming is impaired as in nominal aphasia (see under next heading), and the patient has difficulty in reading aloud. The speech content is similar to that of Wernicke's aphasia, but the patient can understand both written and spoken language.

THE POSTERIOR (ASSOCIATION) APHASIAS

Lesions in or near the angular gyrus of the dominant hemisphere can interrupt connections between Wernicke's area and most other areas of the brain while leaving intact the association pathway to Broca's area via the arcuate fasciculus and external capsule.

A large lesion can produce the so-called syndrome of the isolated speech area in which speech is fluent but paraphasic, while object-naming, spontaneous writing and comprehension of both oral and written language are impaired. Repetition of words spoken by the examiner is normal but the patient may demonstrate echolalia (see below). If the lesion is less extensive, speech may be fluent with only occasional paraphasia, and comprehension of written and spoken language and repetition are normal, though spontaneous writing is impaired. In such cases the most striking abnormality is often difficulty in naming people and objects (anomia—nominal or amnestic aphasia), although the patient is well aware of their nature and significance. In other words it is the association between a particular object and a particular word which is lost. The patient, when shown a pencil, for instance, is unable to recall the word 'pencil', though he will say and demonstrate that the object is used for writing and will recognize that the word 'pencil' is correct when it is offered to him. This sign most often results from a cortical lesion just posterior to Wernicke's area.

RELATED DISORDERS OF LANGUAGE

Other lesions of association pathways can give rise to the fractional disorders of speech known as agraphia, alexia and acalculia. Agraphia, the inability to write, is simply a form of Broca's aphasia and can result from lesions near Broca's area but also from a lesion of association pathways when spoken speech is unimpaired. Similarly, alexia, the inability to understand the written word, is a form of receptive aphasia but can occur (usually with agraphia) as a result of focal lesions in the angular or supramarginal gyri of the dominant parietal lobe.

Pure alexia without agraphia has also been called pure subcortical word blindness or visual aphasia, as the patient cannot recognize words, letters or colours but can visualize colours. He cannot copy but can write and speak normally and spontaneously. The lesion responsible usually involves the visual cortex of the dominant hemisphere and the splenium of the corpus callosum, thus separating the intact visual cortex from Wernicke's and Broca's areas. A contralateral homonymous hemianopia is invariably present.

Pure alexia with agraphia (visual asymbolia or cortical word blindness) is usually due to lesions in the region of the dominant angular gyrus which divide the pathways between the visual association and speech areas. The patient cannot read, copy or write spontaneously.

Acalculia, or the inability to calculate, is a closely related phenomenon in which the patient cannot appreciate the symbolic significance of figures. A patient with Broca's aphasia may be unable to carry out mental arithmetic, but loss of the ability to use mathematical symbols, either verbal or written, is more often seen in lesions of the dominant parietal lobe. Amusia, a defect of musical expression or appreciation, can be either expressive (in association with Broca's aphasia) or receptive (in association with Wernicke's aphasia).

It is thus apparent that the organization of speech function in the dominant hemisphere is a complex mechanism, depending not so much upon 'localization' in specific cortical areas but upon a large series of neuronal pathways and cell stations in which patterns of speech and related functions are stored and can be recalled at will. Pathological lesions may impair these functions by destroying cell stations or their intercommunicating pathways, and many types of speech disorders are thus produced.

Examination of a patient with aphasia

Examination of a patient with aphasia requires patience and a systematic approach. The following scheme of investigation fulfils all ordinary clinical requirements (Walton, 1985):

1. Is the patient right- or left-handed and, if the latter, did he write with the right hand?

2. What was his state of education with regard to reading, writing and foreign languages?
3. Does he understand the nature and use of objects, and can he understand pantomime and gesture, or express his wants thereby?
4. Is he deaf? If so, to what extent and on one or both sides?
5. Can he recognize ordinary sounds and noises?
6. Can he comprehend spoken language? If so, does he at once attempt to answer a question?
7. Is spontaneous speech good? If not, how is it impaired? Does he make use of paraphasias, either literal or verbal recurring utterances, or jargon?
8. Can he repeat words uttered in his hearing?
9. Is his sight good? Is there hemianopia or impaired visual acuity?
10. Does he recognize written or printed speech and obey a written command? If not, does he recognize words, letter or numerals?
11. Can he write spontaneously? What mistakes occur in writing? Is there paragraphia? Can he read his own writing some time after he has written it?
12. Can he copy written words, or transcribe from print into writing? Can he write numerals and perform simple mathematical calculations?
13. Can he read aloud?
14. Can he name at sight words, letters, numerals and common objects?
15. Can he write from dictation?
16. Can he match an object with its name, spoken or written, when a series of objects and names is presented to him?

Conclusions

In general, a fluent aphasic syndrome with paraphasia suggests that Broca's area is intact and suggests a posterior lesion, whereas speech which is slow, telegraphic and dysarthric indicates one situated anteriorly. Impaired comprehension and repetition suggest Wernicke's aphasia, while good comprehension and poor repetition indicate conduction aphasia. Conversely, good repetition and poor comprehension favour a lesion in the angular gyrus region isolating the speech area. In global aphasia spontaneous speech, writing, reading, comprehension, repetition and object naming are all impaired, while in nominal aphasia the object naming is abnormal but comprehension is good and spontaneous speech relatively unaffected. Comprehension should not be tested simply by asking the patient to obey commands, as an individual with apraxia (see p. 78) may understand the command but be unable to comply.

Associated neurological signs may also be helpful. A contralateral hemiparesis is usually present in Broca's aphasia, less often in Wernicke's, whereas a visual field defect is commonly present in association with Wernicke's aphasia and rarely with Broca's. Kertesz and Poole (1974) have found that an aphasia quotient, based upon numerical scores for fluency, comprehension, repetition, naming and information, can form a useful basis of clinical classification.

DYSARTHRIA

Complete loss of speech function due to a disorder of the neuromuscular mechanisms responsible for articulation is known as *anarthria*. It is quite different from aphasia in that the patient's understanding of speech and his reading and writing are intact, but he is unable to speak owing to the fact that the muscles of the lips and tongue cannot control the movements of the expired air in order to form words. Anarthria is rare, but *dysarthria*, or impaired articulation, is relatively common. The speech of a dysarthric patient is slurred and indistinct, but his use of words is appropriate and his understanding unimpaired. The muscles responsible for articulation are those of the face (supplied by the seventh or facial nerve), the larynx and pharynx (supplied by the tenth or vagus nerve), the jaw (supplied by the motor root of the fifth or trigeminal nerve), and the tongue (supplied by the hypoglossal nerve). Lesions giving rise to dysarthria can be classified as (a) upper motor neuron lesions, (b) disorders of coordination and of the extrapyramidal system, (c) lower motor neuron lesions, (d) lesions of the myoneural junction, and (e) myopathic lesions.

A unilateral lesion involving one corticospinal or pyramidal tract, for example, in the motor cortex of one cerebral hemisphere, will sometimes give dysarthria, though this is not usually severe unless the lesion is extensive. Bilateral corticospinal tract lesions are usually necessary to produce dysarthria of the upper motor neuron type, as occurs in patients with bilateral damage to the motor cortex or lesions of the upper brain stem. Total anarthria and often dysphagia can occur in a patient who has a hemiplegia due to a unilateral cerebral infarct and then develops a second one on the opposite side. There is often pathological emotional lability in such cases, with inappropriate laughing and crying (pseudobulbar palsy). Dysarthria can also result from lesions of the nervous pathways that influence, without directly promoting, muscular activity. Thus, disorders of the cerebellar system may cause incoordination of the articulatory muscles, resulting in jerky or explosive speech with undue separation of syllables (e.g. 'scanning' speech, occasionally seen in multiple sclerosis). Extrapyramidal disorders such as Parkinson's disease give rigidity of the muscles subserving speech, as of the limbs, and the speech therefore becomes slow, quiet and monotonous.

Lower motor neuron lesions, as in patients with motor neuron disease affecting the bulbar musculature (progressive bulbar palsy), or in patients with polyneuritis (e.g. after diphtheria), bulbar poliomyelitis or syringobulbia, can also give dysarthria. Depending upon the severity and extent of the muscular atrophy and weakness, the speech is slurred and indistinct and eventually becomes unintelligible. Usually dysphagia, or other evidence of weakness of the bulbar musculature, is also present.

A similar type of dysarthria, again due to weakness of the articulatory muscles, is seen in myasthenia gravis, and here the slurring increases markedly with fatigue. In patients with myotonia, stiffness of the tongue may give a distinctive stiff or strangled quality to the speech, while in facioscapulohumeral muscular dystrophy, inability to close the lips makes it impossible for the patient to pronounce labials, so that a characteristic dysarthric speech is produced.

PALILALIA AND ECHOLALIA

Palilalia is a rare syndrome characterized by an increasingly rapid repetition of stereotyped words or phrases. It is usually seen in cases of postencephalitic parkinsonism, and less often in general paresis or pseudobulbar palsy. Echolalia, by contrast, is the repetition of sounds or words made by others and is thus seen during the normal development of speech in infants. Nevertheless, it too can be pathological if observed in adults, as in cases of general paresis or Gilles de la Tourette's syndrome (recurrent compulsive utterances and gestures, with multiple tics). It can also take the form of parrot-like repetition of a word or phrase in posterior or association aphasia (see above).

MUTISM

Mutism is the total inability to speak, sometimes seen in a person without any demonstrable organic disease of the central nervous system. It can occur in psychotic patients, such as schizophrenics, and is an occasional manifestation of hysteria. Mutism combined with the loss of volitional movement of the trunk and limbs occurring in a patient who nevertheless appears to be conscious (akinetic mutism) is a rare result of an upper brain-stem lesion.

APHONIA

Patients with aphonia have lost the ability to phonate but are still able to articulate, so that they speak in a whisper. While aphonia may be the result of disease of the larynx and vocal cords (laryngitis, tumour or paralysis of the vocal cords), it is most often a hysterical manifestation, the unconscious motivation being usually an attempt to escape from a stressful situation. Thus it may occur in a young singer on the evening of her first professional engagement. Often it is necessary to inspect the vocal cords in order to establish the diagnosis of hysterical aphonia and to exclude organic disease, but apart from a history of previous hysterical manifestations or of recent stress, the most useful diagnostic pointer is that the patient is still able to phonate when coughing.

SPEECH DISORDERS IN CHILDHOOD

Developmental disorders of speech form a small but important group of disorders in which accurate diagnosis is of paramount importance as many children with these disorders may be wrongly regarded as suffering from mental handicap when in fact many respond to appropriate treatment.

Deafness

The totally deaf child will remain completely mute unless properly trained, as the normal channel for acquiring speech (i.e. through hearing) is not available to him. Usually the diagnosis becomes apparent when it is observed that the child, who has caused concern to his parents through his failure to speak, also fails to respond to external noise. High-tone deafness is more difficult to diagnose because the child with this condition does acquire speech, though this is unintelligible to any but his parents as he fails to utilize those vowel sounds and consonants (e.g. *e* and *t*) that depend upon high tones for their recognition. Audiometry is necessary for confirmation of the diagnosis, and special techniques are available for use in young children.

Developmental dysarthria

Dysarthria in childhood can be a manifestation of local developmental abnormalities, such as cleft palate, or of cerebral palsy, in which case there are usually other neurological signs which indicate its nature. There is, however, a small group of children in whom dysarthria, associated with incoordinate or clumsy movements of the tongue and palate, is the only neurological abnormality. The condition may be due to a congenital apraxia (see below) of the muscles of articulation. Cases of this type respond well to long-continued speech therapy.

Developmental receptive aphasia

Congenital word deafness or auditory imperception is a rare form of speech defect, much commoner in males than females, in which the patient fails to acquire normal speech function although he is not deaf. He responds to sounds, yet shows no interest or attention when spoken to. After a number of years many such patients acquire a vocabulary of their own which, though meaningful to them, is incomprehensible to all except their nearest relatives. This type of defective speech was formerly identified by the now obsolete terms 'idioglossia' and 'lalling'. It may be difficult to distinguish such speech from the defective speech of high-tone deafness except by audiometry.

Developmental dyslexia

Developmental dyslexia, or reading defect, is much commoner than receptive aphasia, being seen most often in left-handed children. It occurs in various degrees of severity, and can either be sporadic or inherited as a dominant trait. In broad terms it appears to be due to a defect in the establishment of speech function in one of the cerebral hemispheres, and is often associated with 'mirror-writing' (writing from right to left with reversals of words and letters, as if viewed in a mirror). It commonly occurs in children who are in other respects intelligent. The printed word is wrongly pronounced, a dictated word wrongly spelled, and writing is usually abnormal. Many normal children, particularly in families in which one parent is left handed or ambidextrous, pass through a temporary phase of mirror-writing, at least of certain letters, when first learning to write.

Dyslalia

Dyslalia is a benign and not uncommon form of speech disorder occurring in childhood. The child develops speech at the normal age and speaks fluently though unintelligibly as he tends to substitute one consonant for another in many words. This is now thought to be a syndrome of multiple aetiology. In some cases the child imitates the defective articulation of other family members, in some there is mild mental handicap, and in yet others the condition appears to be a mild and rapidly reversible form of developmental dysphasia or developmental dysarthria. Usually these children acquire normal speech within 3–12 months of beginning speech therapy, but without treatment the abnormal speech pattern may persist for many years.

Stammering

Stammering is a disorder of articulation characterized by the repetition of sounds or syllables and by prolonged pauses which punctuate speech. It is much more common in boys than in girls. Dentals (t,d), labials (p,b) and gutturals (k) are the sounds which seem most difficult to pronounce, and severe facial grimacing may accompany the attempt to utter words containing these letters. While many have suggested that this condition is of psychogenic origin, the fact that it is very common in left-handed children and particularly in shifted sinistrals (those who are naturally left handed but who have been persuaded to write with the right hand) suggests that it has an organic basis and, like reading defects, it may be related to an incomplete localization of speech function in a cerebral hemisphere. It has a strong familial incidence and sometimes occurs in children with mild developmental dysarthria or apraxia or other features of minimal cerebral dysfunction. It can be present from the age of 2 or 3 years, but quite often begins at the age of 6–8 years when a child who has previously spoken fluently is beginning to read and write. While many stammerers seem shy and introspective, this mental attitude is most probably the result rather than the cause of their disability. Certainly there is no evidence that stammering is a result of organic brain disease, though it may develop for the first time in some adult patients with mild Broca's aphasia. It is more properly regarded as a functional disorder of the organization and establishment of speech function. It can often be controlled to some extent by the use of syllabic speech.

APRAXIA

Apraxia is the inability to carry out a willed voluntary movement despite the fact that the motor and sensory pathways concerned in the control of the movement are intact. In other words no actual paralysis, ataxia or sensory loss may be present. Thus a patient who is asked to put out his tongue may be completely unable to do so on request, though a moment later he will spontaneously lick his lips. Hence the condition can be regarded as a loss of acquired motor skills, or an inability to reactivate those nervous pathways in which the memory and technique of specific movements (praxis) have been recorded and 'stored'. Sometimes when apraxia is incomplete it is clear that the concept of a movement is imperfect as its component parts are correctly carried out but incorrectly combined. It can be considered to be a defect of the 'association' areas or fibres concerned with the ideomotor or conceptual control of volitional motor activity. The supramarginal gyrus of the dominant parietal lobe appears to contain an important cell station in this organization of movement, and lesions of this area commonly produce bilateral apraxia. A lesion between this cortical area and the motor cortex of the left cerebral hemisphere will lead to apraxia of the right limbs, while a lesion of the corpus callosum dividing those fibres which are passing to the right motor cortex will give rise to left-sided apraxia.

Apraxia of the lips and tongue is relatively common, while in the extremities apraxic disturbances may be revealed as an inability to dress or undress (dressing apraxia) or to construct models from blocks or letters with matches (constructional apraxia). Dressing apraxia is usually associated with lesions of the non-dominant parietal lobe, and constructional apraxia with dominant hemisphere lesions. Apraxia of gait is usually seen as a consequence of bilateral frontal lesions, especially in demented patients. Oculomotor apraxia, involving eye movements (see p. 143), has also been described.

AGNOSIA

Presumably, visual, auditory and tactile stimuli are perceived in the occipital, temporal and postcentral areas of the cortex, respectively, as crude physical phenomena which acquire significance only when related to past sensory experiences that have been collated and 'stored' as sensory memories in the appropriate association areas of the cortex. This process of recognition of the significance of sensory stimuli is known as *gnosis*. Lesions of the appropriate association areas of the cerebral cortex impair this faculty of recognition even though the primary sensory pathway is intact; thus, the primary sensory modalities of fine touch, tactile discrimination, vision and hearing are preserved. The syndrome so produced is called agnosia. Visual agnosia is an inability to recognize objects seen, in a patient who is not blind. Auditory agnosia is a failure to appreciate the significance of sounds in a patient who is not deaf (a condition which shows some resemblance to Wernicke's aphasia). A patient with tactile agnosia (often called astereognosis) cannot identify objects which he feels. Usually an agnostic defect involves only one sense, e.g. vision or hearing or touch, so that a patient who cannot recognize a pen, and may not even see that it is an object with which to write, will name it at once if it is placed on his hand. Conversely, one with tactile agnosia will identify visually an object which was unrecognized when he held it. One form of congenital indifference to pain is thought to be due to a developmental agnosia for painful sensations (pain asymbolia). Visual agnosia is usually a consequence of lesions of the dominant parieto-occipital lobe, while auditory agnosia is caused by temporal lobe lesions.

THE BODY IMAGE

A constant stream of sensory impulses from the special senses, skin, muscles, bones and joints informs us of the condition and situation of the parts of our body in relation to each other and in relation to our external environment. From these stimuli we build up almost unconsciously an image of our body which is continually varying. Certain parts of the body such as the hands and mouth play such important roles in our everyday activity, and are so well endowed with highly developed sensory receptors, that their share of the body image is proportionally much greater than, say, the small of the back. A skilled craftsman or the driver of a motor vehicle becomes so attuned to the use of his tools or vehicle that in a sense these become a part of his body image and he then unconsciously relates himself plus the tool or vehicle and not himself alone to his environment. This concept of the body image is 'stored' in the association areas of the parietal lobes, and when the performance of motor skills is included it becomes clearly related to the function of praxis mentioned above. Certain lesions of the parietal lobe tend to distort the body image so that the patient is unable to distinguish right from left (right–left disorientation). One relatively specific clinical symptom-complex called Gerstmann's syndrome, usually associated with lesions of the dominant angular gyrus, is characterized by finger agnosia (inability to name or select individual fingers), agraphia, acalculia and right–left disorientation, often with constructional apraxia. He may neglect one entire side of his body and the whole of extrapersonal space on that side (autotopagnosia) and may even deny that the contralateral limbs are paralysed and sometimes attempts to throw them out of bed. This is one specific variety of denial of illness (anosognosia). Denial of blindness is often called Anton's syndrome. Visual disorientation with loss of the ability to find one's way around, even in familiar surroundings, is called topographical agnosia. Often, the patient with a parietal lobe lesion will perceive normally sensory stimuli applied independently to the two sides of the body, but if bilateral stimuli are simultaneously applied, one may be ignored (tactile inattention). Similarly, visual inattention may occur when objects are presented individually or simultaneously in the

DEVELOPMENTAL APRAXIA AND AGNOSIA

Specific learning defects other than developmental dyslexia have been recognized increasingly in recent years and appear to be the result of either minimal brain damage due to birth injury or defective physiological organization of cerebral dominance. In contradistinction to the dyslexics, these so-called 'clumsy' children, who often demonstrate minor involuntary movements resembling chorea and who are often wrongly regarded as being mentally retarded, usually show a higher verbal score than performance score on the Wechsler intelligence scale for children. Defects of sensory perception as well as of skilled motor activity are often recognized in some of these children. They often improve to some extent as they grow older, but many require patient individual instruction in the particular skills such as writing in which they are defective.

DISCONNECTION SYNDROMES

The term disconnection syndrome was introduced to identify disorders of higher cerebral function which result from the interruption of association pathways between different parts of the cerebral hemispheres and between one hemisphere and the other. Several such syndromes (e.g. conduction aphasia and the syndrome of the isolated speech area) have already been described earlier in this section. However, much additional information concerning the interhemispheric transfer of information has been derived from experiments in animals and from surgical procedures or disease in man interrupting the fibres of the corpus callosum. Surgical section of this structure has been performed by some neurosurgeons for the treatment of intractable epilepsy. Such patients appear superficially normal, even though their cerebral hemispheres are functioning independently. If a right-handed patient, after the operation, has an object placed in his right hand or projected upon his right visual field, he can name it, but similar information presented on the left may not be recognized or named. This defect is due to an inability to transfer information recorded in the right hemisphere to speech centres on the left side. Similarly, infarction of the anterior four-fifths of the corpus callosum due to occlusion of both anterior cerebral arteries allows the patient to read in both visual fields as visual information can be transferred between the occipital lobes across the intact posterior one-fifth of the corpus callosum. However, in such a patient an object held in the left hand cannot be named as there is no means by which tactile information recorded in the sensory cortex of the right hemisphere can be conveyed to Wernicke's area on the left. Similarly, such a patient cannot write with the left hand or comply with verbal commands to perform specific movements with this hand as verbal concepts or instructions formulated or received and interpreted in the left hemisphere cannot be conveyed to the motor area of the cortex on the right. A number of other fractional disconnection syndromes have been described.

CONCLUSIONS

An understanding of the many complex disorders of speech, movement and recognition occurring in patients with cerebral lesions depends upon a working knowledge of the means by which these functions are organized and controlled in the brain. These functions depend not upon the activity of isolated specific cortical areas but upon a complex network of association fibres joining a series of cortical cell stations. Lesions in varying situations will affect these individual functions in various ways, often giving fractional disorders of function to which certain specific names have been applied. It is, however, necessary to understand the whole before identifying the particular, and from this understanding, information of considerable value in the localization of cerebral lesions may be derived. Disorders may also occur in the peripheral neuromuscular mechanisms subserving speech. Here again, a systematic analysis of the patient's symptoms and signs will aid in identifying the situation and nature of the lesion or lesions responsible.

References

Critchley, M. (1964) *Developmental Dyslexia*. London: Heinemann.
Critchley, M. (1970) *Aphasiology*. London: Edward Arnold.
Critchley, M. (1975) *Silent Language*. London: Butterworth.
Critchley, M. (1979) *The Divine Banquet of the Brain*. New York: Raven Press.
Dimond, S. J. (1979) Tactual and auditory vigilance in split-brain man. *J. Neurol. Neurosurg. Psychiat.* **42:**70.
Eagles, E. L. (ed.) (1975) Human Communication and Its Disorders. In Tower, D. B. (editor-in-chief) *The Nervous System*, Vol. 3. New York: Raven Press.
Fredericks, J. A. M. (1969) Disorders of the body schema. In Vinken, P. J. and Bruyn, G. W. (eds) *Handbook of Clinical Neurology*, vol. 4, chap. 11. Amsterdam: North-Holland.
Gazzaniga, M. S., Bogen, J. E. and Sperry, R. W. (1965) Observations on visual perception after disconnexion of the cerebral hemispheres in man. *Brain* **88:**221.

---

opposite visual fields. Less severe disturbances can result in inaccurate localization of tactile or visual stimuli.

Geschwind, N. (1965) Disconnexion syndromes in animals and man. *Brain* **88**:237, 585.

Geschwind. N. (1970) The organization of language and the brain. *Science* **170**:940.

Geschwind, N. (1974) Selected papers on language and the brain. In *Boston Studies on the Philosophy of Science*, vol. XVI. Dordrecht, Holland and Boston: D. Reidel Publishing Company.

Gubbay, S. S. (1976) *Clumsy Children*. London: W. B. Saunders Company.

Kertesz, A. (1986) Language, cognition and higher cerebral function. In Walton, J. N., Beeson, P. B. and Bodley Scott, R. (eds) *The Oxford Companion to Medicine*. Oxford: Oxford University Press.

Kertesz, A. and Poole, E. (1974) The aphasia quotient: the taxonomic approach to measurement of aphasic disability. *Canad. J. Neurol. Sci.* **1**:7.

Lhermitte, F. and Gautier, J. C. (1969) Aphasia. In Vinken, P. J. and Bruyn, G. W. (eds) *Handbook of Clinical Neurology*, vol. 4, chap. 5. Amsterdam: North-Holland.

Morley, M. (1972) *The Development and Disorders of Speech in Childhood*, 3rd edn. Edinburgh: Churchill Livingstone.

Patton, H. D., Sundsten, J. W., Crill, W. E. and Swanson, P. D. (1976) *Introduction to Basic Neurology*. Philadelphia: W. B. Saunders Company.

Rose, F. C. (ed.) (1984) *Progress in Aphasiology* (Advances in Neurology) vol. 42. New York: Raven Press.

Subirana, A. (1969) Handedness and cerebral dominance. In Vinken, P. J., and Bruyn, G. W. (eds) *Handbook of Clinical Neurology*, vol. 4, chap. 13. Amsterdam, North-Holland.

Walton, J. N. (1985) *Brain's Diseases of the Nervous System*, 9th edn. Oxford: Oxford University Press.

Weinstein, E. A. and Friedland, R. P. (eds) (1979) Hemi-inattention and hemisphere specialization. In *Advances in Neurology*, vol. 18. New York: Raven Press.

4

CONSCIOUSNESS AND ITS DISORDERS

INTRODUCTION

Consciousness is a state or faculty which almost defies definition. It implies a state of awareness of one's self and of one's surroundings. It encompasses many recurring sensory experiences combined with emotions, ideas and memories which are the product of thought processes. The cerebral cortex clearly plays an important role in maintaining and determining the content of the conscious state, but cortical control of motor or sensory activity is by no means autonomous. Such mechanisms can be activated or suppressed through the activity of the reticular substance of the upper brain stem and thalamus and by hypothalamic mechanisms. This reticular-hypothalamic complex exercises important influences upon the state of awareness. Disturbances of consciousness are largely dependent upon lesions, either functional or structural, of these areas of the brain or of the pathways which connect them to the cortex.

The term 'arousal' refers to a state of awareness or wakefulness that is roughly the converse of sleep, while various disorders of consciousness are known as clouding of consciousness (or confusion), stupor and coma. While the content of consciousness is essentially a cortical function, the thalamocortical projection system is important in the control of cortical activity. Specific thalamic nuclei project to specific sensory areas of the cortex. In addition there are a series of non-specific thalamic nuclei, including the intralaminar nuclei, the septal or midline nuclei, and the reticular thalamic nucleus. While stimulation of the specific nuclei produces an evoked electrical cortical response confined to the appropriate sensory area, stimulation of the non-specific nuclei gives a widely distributed surface negative response of long latency associated with desynchronization of electroencephalographic (EEG) activity (see p. 254). These non-specific thalamic nuclei may act in a sense as pacemakers of cortical activity. They in turn are controlled by the neurons of the reticular activating system (Fig. 4.1), which are situated in the reticular formation in the upper pons and midbrain, extending also into the posterior hypothalamus. A downward projection of the reticular formation into the medulla also involves control centres for respiration and vasomotor tone, while other parts of the system are concerned with control of temperature and gastrointestinal secretions. The cells of this reticular system form a diffuse reticulated network made up of neurons of many different shapes and sizes, many of which have axons projecting caudally into the spinal cord and cerebellum, others projecting rostrally. Stimulation of the reticular activating system causes activation of the EEG and arousal, while depression of its activity or destructive lesions cause varying degrees of unresponsiveness. The ascending activating mechanism controls the thalamocortical system and hence the state of consciousness, and, as will be seen later (p. 102), it also plays a part in the evocation of memory patterns.

Drugs which tend to produce unconsciousness, such as anaesthetics and hypnotics, may selectively depress the ascending reticular alerting system, while those which cause wakefulness have the opposite, facilitatory effect upon it.

Plum (1972) and Plum and Posner (1980) have summarized certain principles relating to the pathophysiology of consciousness as follows:

1. Lesions which destroy the reticular formation

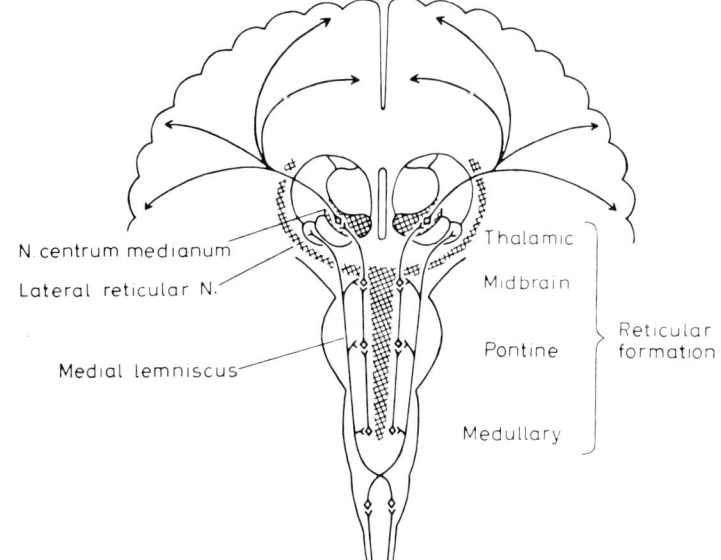

Figure 4.1 The ascending reticular activating system. The reticular formation extends rostrally to include the lateral reticular nucleus of the thalamus, the midline and intralaminar nuclei, and part of the centrum medianum, which project diffusely to the cerebral cortex as the unspecific afferent system, responsible for the maintenance of consciousness. The reticular formation of the medulla, pons and midbrain receives collaterals from ascending specific sensory pathways. [Reproduced from Lance and McLeod (1980) *A Physiological Approach to Clinical Neurology*, 2nd edn, by kind permission of the authors and publisher.]

below the lower third of the pons do not produce coma.
2. Above this level a lesion must destroy both sides of the paramedian reticulum to interrupt consciousness.
3. The arousal effects of reticular stimulation upon behaviour and the EEG are separable in that bilateral lesions of the pontine tegmentum producing coma may be associated with a normal 'waking' EEG.
4. Sleep is an active physiological process, not a mere failure of arousal, and is clearly separable from stupor and coma.
5. Sleeping and waking can occur in man even after total bilateral destruction of the cerebral hemispheres.

A lesion or dysfunction of the reticular system produces stupor or coma only if it:

a. affects both sides of the brain stem
b. is located between the lower third of the pons and the posterior diencephalon and
c. is either of acute onset or is large in its extent

SLEEP

Sleep is a periodic physiological depression of function of those parts of the brain concerned with consciousness, induced by the appropriate state of the reticular system. As sleep deepens, there is a transition in the EEG from normal alpha waves to bursts of more rapid waves (spindles), followed by the development of slow random waves. Four stages have been recognized of so-called slow-wave or orthodox sleep (Fig. 4.2). Sleep is an active physiological process during which some neurons show decreased activity while others show increased activity. An important part of normal sleep is the so-called 'rapid eye movement' (REM) phase during which most dreams occur. This phase, also called 'paradoxical sleep', occurs shortly after falling asleep and again shortly before waking and seems to be the most important stage in relieving fatigue. Paradoxical sleep occurs about every 90 minutes throughout the night, occupying in total about 20–25% of a night's sleep in the healthy adult. Features of paradoxical sleep include changes in blood pressure, heart rate and respiration, increased cerebral blood flow, occasional myoclonic jerks, and repetitive bursts of conjugate eye movement (REM). While severe nightmares usually occur during paradoxical sleep, sleepwalking, enuresis and night terrors in childhood more often occur during orthodox sleep. The term 'paradoxical' is used because the individual seems to be in relatively light sleep, but in fact REM sleep is deeper than stage IV of slow-wave sleep, as measured by the arousal threshold. A disordered relationship may occur between the REM and non-REM phases of sleep in various disorders of brain function. Insomnia, particularly in the elderly, is usually associated with brief awakenings and with a reduction in the proportion of paradoxical sleep. In drug withdrawal syndromes (e.g. delirium tremens), the patient tends to alternate between wakefulness and fitful sleep of which up to 100% is paradoxical. Barbiturate anaesthetics produce EEG changes similar to those accompanying normal sleep. Though sleep-like states

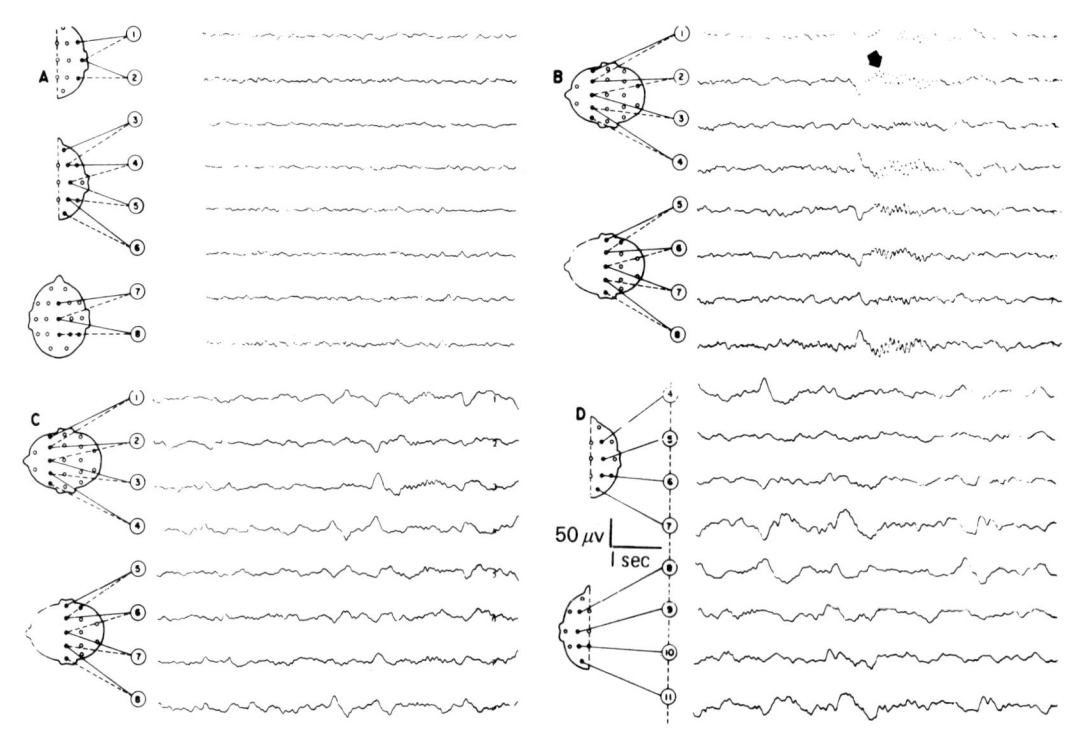

Figure 4.2 Sequential EEG records showing (A) Stage I, (B) Stage II, (C) Stage III, and (D) Stage IV of slow-wave sleep. The arrow in B illustrates sleep spindles. [Reproduced from Patton et al (1976) *Introduction to Basic Neurology*, by kind permission of the authors and publisher.]

can be induced by electrical stimulation of an area in the diencephalon, it is an oversimplification to regard this, as some have, as a 'sleep centre'.

During sleep, not only is consciousness lost, but certain bodily changes occur. As a rule, the pulse rate, blood pressure and respiratory rate fall in orthodox sleep but rise in the paradoxical phase. The eyes usually deviate upwards and the pupils are contracted but usually react to light. The tendon reflexes are abolished and the plantar reflexes may become extensor.

Some advances have been made in the neuropharmacology of sleep. Neurons of the median raphe of the brain stem contain large quantities of 5-hydroxytryptamine (5-HT), and lesions of these neurons in animals produce insomnia that can be reversed by giving a 5-HT precursor. Drugs such as *p*-chlorophenylalanine, which block 5-HT synthesis, decrease both REM and slow-wave sleep. In addition, destruction of noradrenaline-containing neurons of the locus coeruleus suppresses REM but not slow-wave sleep. Reserpine, which depletes both 5-HT and noradrenaline gives insomnia, but if a 5-HT precursor is then given, slow-wave sleep is re-established but REM sleep is not. Many peptides, including arginine vasotocin and β-endorphin, have been shown to induce drowsiness, and three more specific peptides (DSIP or delta sleep-inducing peptide, SPS or sleep-promoting substance, as well as Pappenheimer's factor 'S') have also been isolated so that the neurochemical basis of normal sleep seems complex and as yet incompletely understood (Parkes, 1985).

A number of disorders of the sleep rhythm are known. Some are semiphysiological and of no serious pathological significance, while others are produced by organic lesions in the neighbourhood of the midbrain and hypothalamus. Many of the less ominous disorders can be regarded as resulting from 'uneven' activity of the various parts of the reticular-hypothalamic complex, so that in a sense the activity of one part of the brain may be suppressed or reactivated before another.

Disorders of sleep

SLEEP PARALYSIS

This is a condition in which the patient, when falling asleep, or more commonly on waking, finds himself totally unable to move, though motor activity returns immediately if he is touched. This experience can be very alarming, but movement generally returns spontaneously within a minute or less and the condition is of no serious significance. A series of visual or other hallucinations (so-called hypnagogic hallucinations) which are of brief duration, though sometimes terrifying in character, may occur as the patient is falling asleep. This condition seems to be due to transient reactivation of association areas of the cerebral cortex. Night terrors in children are probably similar. Nocturnal myoclonus, a sudden jerk of the voluntary musculature that occurs when drifting into sleep, is also essentially physiological and presumably results from a sudden transient reactivation of the motor system. Myoclonic jerks occurring repeatedly in sleep, however, must often be regarded as pathological as some such patients develop epileptic seizures.

INSOMNIA

Insomnia is a common disorder of sleep which occurs so frequently in the elderly that it is difficult to know when it should be considered pathological. In younger patients it usually results from anxiety, an emotional disturbance which influences the reticular-hypothalamic system. Somnambulism, or sleepwalking, is also related to emotional stress and can be regarded as a reactivation of complex coordinated muscular movements occurring while consciousness remains impaired.

NARCOLEPSY

Another relatively common disorder, narcolepsy, appears to result from a functional disturbance occurring in the reticular activating system. Patients suffering from this condition experience attacks of almost irresistible sleep which develop during the day, most often in the afternoon. The attacks often occur in circumstances conducive to drowsiness, such as after a heavy meal, in a lecture, or during a monotonous activity (as when driving a car). Such sleep is usually immediately of the REM type and in many such patients the REM/non-REM ratio of nocturnal sleep is abnormal. The desire to sleep can be resisted if the patient gets up and moves around, but if he is sitting down the somnolence is overwhelming. The patient can be aroused with ease, as from normal sleep. Males are affected more often than females, and the condition usually begins in adolescence or early in adult life. There is a very close association of the narcolepsy–cataplexy syndrome (see below) with possession of the HLA leucocyte antigen DR$_2$. It is generally benign, and can be regarded as an exaggeration of physiological drowsiness occurring under appropriate circumstances. Most but not all patients with true narcolepsy also suffer *cataplexy*, episodes of sudden loss of power in the voluntary muscles which cause the patient to go 'weak at the knees' and even to slump suddenly to the ground. He may be unable to move a muscle for several seconds or even for as long as a minute. These attacks are commonly precipitated by sudden emotion such as laughing, crying, fear or excitement. The condition can be regarded as a transient inactivation of that part of the reticular substance controlling motor activity and is again an exaggeration of a common physiological reaction, as normal people sometimes become 'weak with laughter'. It has been postulated that narcolepsy and cataplexy may be due to an inborn error of metabolism involving 5-HT and/or other brain amines, but this remains unproven. Drugs such as the amphetamines (now outmoded), methylphenidate and tricyclic antidepressant remedies such as desimipramine are usually successful in treatment.

IDIOPATHIC HYPERSOMNOLENCE

Often confused with narcolepsy but different in its clinical and electrophysiological features (sleep is immediately of the orthodox or non-REM type), this condition of pathological daytime drowsiness is not uncommon and in a sense suggests that the 'set' of the reticular activating system is more towards depression than towards arousal of consciousness. Affected patients often sleep abnormally heavily during the night and may easily fall into a heavy and prolonged sleep during the day. Serotonin antagonists such as dimethysergide are often helpful in treatment, whereas drugs which are effective in the narcolepsy–cataplexy syndrome (see above) are not.

OTHER DISORDERS

Organic lesions in the region of the third ventricle and hypothalamus or upper brain stem give rise very rarely to symptomatic narcolepsy. More often they produce symptomatic *hypersomnia*, in which the patient sleeps for long periods, is difficult to rouse, and may then be confused for a variable period of time. The *pickwickian syndrome*, believed to be of hypothalamic origin, is characterized by obesity, pathological daytime somnolence (orthodox sleep) and nocturnal periodic breathing with hypercapnia. It is now known that sleep *apnoea*, defined as cessation of airflow at the nostrils and mouth lasting for at least 10 seconds, may occur up to 10 times a night in normal subjects but only during REM sleep. More severe and potentially dangerous episodes which are more prolonged and occur more frequently can result from neurological disorders associated with alveolar hypoventilation (such as muscular dystrophy or motor neuron disease), autonomic dysfunction (the

Shy–Drager syndrome), brain-stem lesions, or Ondine's curse, in which primary insensitivity of the respiratory centre of unknown cause impairs respiratory reflex drive so that breathing becomes almost wholly voluntary and no longer automatic. There is also a non-neurological primary apnoea syndrome which is essentially obstructive (the pharynx fails to open fully during inspiration but abdominal and thoracic inspiratory movements continue to occur despite occlusion of the upper airway). Many of the latter patients are obese, snore very loudly and have daytime hypersomnolence. *Akinetic mutism* is a syndrome which can follow injury to the upper brain stem and in which the patient is apparently asleep, with a relaxed musculature. Although his eyes may open and follow objects moving in his field of vision or he may respond to sounds, he cannot speak or be aroused by powerful sensory stimuli. There are usually paramedian lesions of the reticular substance of the upper brain stem. This condition must be distinguished from the so-called locked-in syndrome in which the patient is alert and wakeful but mute and tetraplegic owing to the presence of a low or midpontine lesion. The locked-in syndrome usually results from bilateral destruction of the medulla or basis pontis, and less often from lesions of both cerebral peduncles.

Certain other lesions of the midbrain and contiguous areas, and particularly those of encephalitis lethargica (now rarely, if ever, seen), produce reversal of the sleep rhythm so that the patient sleeps by day but is awake and restless at night. Disorders of this type cease to be physiological variants and are closely related to the pathological states of stupor and coma that can result from structural or metabolic disorders affecting similar areas of the brain.

STUPOR

Stupor is a disorder of consciousness in which the patient gives every appearance of being asleep but from which he cannot be fully aroused. He may open his eyes and on vigorous stimulation will show some responses which indicate a degree of awareness of his surroundings. Whereas lethargy is a state of drowsiness and indifference in which greater than normal stimulation is needed to produce a response, in stupor the subject can be aroused only by vigorous and continuous external stimulation. *Parasomnia* is a term occasionally used to describe a form of stupor resembling sleep but in which the patient remains confused when aroused. The condition of akinetic mutism (sometimes called 'coma vigil') referred to earlier can be regarded as a specific form of stupor. The patient in this state retains cycles of self-sustained arousal, seeming to be vigilant but with little or no vocalization. Though immobile and incontinent, he shows few signs of damage to descending motor pathways and makes only rudimentary movements in response to noxious stimuli, being thus in a state of 'motionless, mindless wakefulness'.

While stupor sometimes results from injury, compression or disease of the upper brain stem and hypothalamus, it can also occur as an effect of drug intoxication, metabolic disorders, anoxia or severe infections, although in these conditions delirium, to be described later, is more common. Subdural haematoma, giving rise to brain-stem compression, is a common cause of stuporous states.

COMA

Coma was once defined as complete unconsciousness with no response to sensory stimuli, even at the reflex level. In other words the comatose patient would not show even reflex withdrawal following a painful stimulus. A patient who was semicomatose, however, while seeming to be completely unconscious with no awareness of his surroundings, would respond to painful stimuli by groaning or by withdrawing the affected part. Less severe disturbances of consciousness were then described as severe, moderate or mild confusion, or simply as 'clouding of consciousness'. In more modern parlance, the term 'semicoma' is little if ever used, though 'confusion' is still employed, while coma has been redefined as 'a state of unarousable psychological unresponsiveness in which the subjects lie with the eyes closed . . . they show no psychologically understandable response to external stimulus or inner need' (Plum and Posner, 1980). *Delirium* (see p. 90) is a state of confusion with an overlay of excitement. Various scales, of which the Glasgow coma scale is one, have been used to define the severity or depth of coma.

Coma can result from many conditions, some of which are primarily cerebral disorders, while others are generalized metabolic disturbances. The disturbance of consciousness, whether due to a structural or a biochemical lesion, is produced by a disorder of function in the reticular system. The commoner causes of stupor and coma are listed in Table 5.

Mechanisms of stupor and coma

While closed head injury may induce coma as a consequence of severe and extensive laceration or contusion of brain substance, the principal mechanism of concussion appears to be a shearing strain which temporarily inactivates the reticular forma-

TABLE 5. The common causes of stupor and coma

SUPRATENTORIAL LESIONS (causing upper brain stem dysfunction)
  Cerebral haemorrhage
  Massive cerebral infarction
  Extradural haematoma
  Subdural haematoma
  Cerebral tumour
  Cerebral abscess

INFRATENTORIAL LESIONS (compressing or destroying the reticular formation)
  Pontine haemorrhage
  Cerebellar haemorrhage
  Brain-stem infarction
  Posterior fossa tumour
  Cerebellar abscess

METABOLIC PROCESSES OR OTHER DIFFUSE LESIONS
  Anoxia
  Hypoglycaemia
  Deficiency disorders
  Renal or hepatic failure
  Disorders of electrolytes and/or ionic equilibrium
  Poisoning, intoxications
  Infectious or autoimmune disorders
    Meningitis
    Encephalitis
  Head injury, including concussion and contusion
  Postepileptic states

Modified from Plum and Posner, 1980.

produces its effects by compressing the anterior cerebral vessels, consequentially increasing frontal lobe oedema. In uncal herniation, compression of the trunk of the third nerve against the free edge of the tentorium often produces unilateral pupillary dilatation, followed by ptosis and ultimately a complete third nerve palsy. Persisting uncal herniation can give rise to haemorrhages in the median raphe of the brain stem, resulting in irreversible coma. Subtentorial lesions, by contrast, may compress the brain stem directly, or else they may cause either upward displacement of the midbrain and cerebellum through the tentorial notch, or downward cerebellar tonsillar herniation. Any form of herniation may be accentuated, with disastrous effects, if cerebrospinal fluid is removed by lumbar puncture. This is particularly hazardous if tonsillar herniation (a cerebellar pressure 'cone') is present. Destructive brain stem lesions, on the other hand, cause coma through direct damage to the reticular formation, as do inflammatory processes such as encephalitis. Ischaemia and hypoxia affect the reticular substance directly, while postepileptic stupor appears to depend upon a temporary suppression of synaptic transmission in this system and/or in the pathways which connect it to the cortex.

tion. Diffuse damage to neurons and to the cerebral white matter may occur in severe cases. Some motor and sensory accompaniments of severe brain stem lesions which affect the reticular system as well as other ascending and descending pathways have been mentioned with reference to the locked-in syndrome. Other important syndromes, including the so-called decerebrate and decorticate states, are described later in the chapters on 'The motor system' (p. 158) and 'The sensory system' (p. 194). Cerebral metabolism and its disorders, many of which also cause stupor or coma, are considered in detail beginning on p. 213, while the pathophysiology of increased intracranial pressure is described on p. 238.

There are certain important principles which govern the production of stupor or coma as a consequence of supratentorial or infratentorial mass lesions (Fig. 4.3). Diffuse cerebral oedema may cause compression of the upper brain stem through symmetrical downward pressure. A localized space-occupying lesion or unilateral oedema (e.g. after extensive infarction) produces a similar effect upon the reticular substance, either as a consequence of uncal herniation through the tentorial hiatus or, less often, as a result of herniation of cerebellar tonsils through the foramen magnum (Fig. 4.3). Cingulate gyrus herniation beneath the falx cerebri, by contrast,

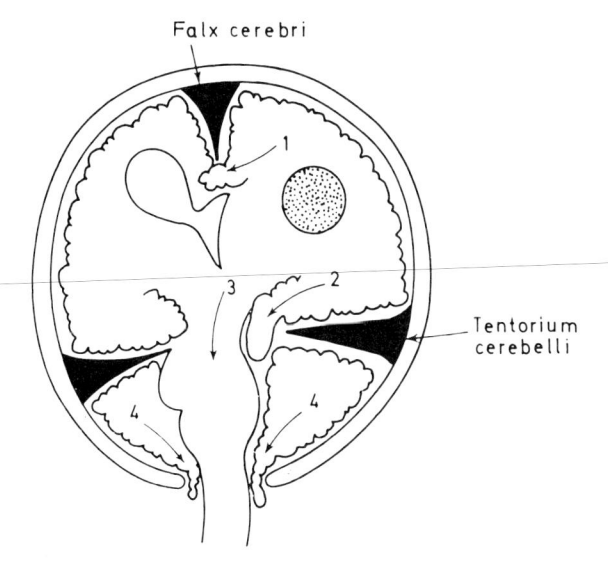

Figure 4.3 Effect of expanding supratentorial lesions on cerebral structures. (1) The cingulate gyrus may be herniated beneath the falx cerebri (cingulate herniation), (2) a portion of the temporal lobe may be compressed between the brain stem and the margin of the tentorial notch, or (3) the brain stem may be displaced downwards through the tentorial opening (central herniation). (4) In expanding infratentorial lesions, or after injudicious lumbar puncture in the presence of raised intracranial pressure, the cerebellar tonsils may herniate through the foramen magnum. [Reproduced from Lance and McLeod (1980) *A Physiological Approach to Clinical Neurology*, 2nd edn, by kind permission of the authors and publisher.]

Some specific causes of stupor and coma and their recognition

In examination of the comatose patient the head must be inspected for evidence of recent or past injury and the tongue inspected for scars resulting from previous epileptic fits. The smell of alcohol or acetone on the breath, or foetor (in uraemic or hepatic coma) may be of diagnostic value. Cervical rigidity suggests either meningitis or intracranial haemorrhage, while a bruit over the cranium or in the neck may be indicative of a vascular malformation or arterial stenosis. Skin changes, as manifested by cyanosis (in respiratory insufficiency), a cherry-red colour (in carbon monoxide poisoning), purpura (in various blood diseases), spider naevi (in hepatic cirrhosis), the typical changes of Addison's disease or hypothyroidism, or scars of previous injections (in drug addicts), may give a clue to the cause of the coma.

Changes in the respiratory rate and volume should also be noted. Periodic (Cheyne–Stokes) respiration, in which hyperpnoea alternates with apnoea, usually indicates a central cerebral or high brain-stem lesion. Brain-stem lesions can also give central neurogenic hyperventilation, apneustic breathing (a pause at full inspiration), or ataxic respiration in which random deep and shallow breaths occur. The latter type of breathing is most often found in medullary lesions. At its worst, when a medullary lesion causes the respiratory centre to be insensitive to normal chemical stimuli but conversely it becomes hypersensitive to some sedative drugs, the patient, who can breathe adequately when instructed to do so, hypoventilates progressively and may even stop breathing completely when asleep. Autonomous breathing is a rare syndrome resulting from a lesion of the cervicomedullary junction, causing paralysis of the chest and limbs; there is retention of spontaneous breathing, but the patient is unable either to take a breath or to stop breathing voluntarily.

Examination of the pupils is also important. Midbrain lesions may result in pupils of medium size which react neither to light nor to other stimuli, while lesions of the pontine tegmentum more often give small fixed pupils which may be pinpoint in pontine haemorrhage. Pinpoint pupils also result from opiate intoxication, while atropine-like drugs and cerebral anoxia cause pupillary dilatation. A fixed dilated pupil on one side usually indicates a third-nerve lesion which, in the comatose patient, may indicate uncal herniation. A unilateral Horner's syndrome can be seen in lateral medullary infarction.

Examination of the ocular movements can be useful. In lesions of the cerebral hemispheres, oculocephalic reflexes (which occur on head rotation) are normal, and caloric stimulation of the ears gives normal evoked nystagmus. These reflexes are lost when there is an extensive brain-stem lesion involving the pons. A massive frontal lesion can, however, produce deviation of the eyes towards the side of the lesion, while a pontine lesion can cause conjugate deviation of the eyes to the opposite side, with absence of oculocephalic and caloric responses. Skew deviation of the eyes results from a pontine or cerebellar lesion, while downward conjugate deviation implies damage to the midbrain.

Clearly, examination of other systems to exclude disease in the heart, lungs, liver and kidneys is obligatory in any comatose patient, and estimations of the blood sugar, urea and electrolytes and of the P_{CO_2} and P_{O_2} are usually indicated. Electroencephalography, echoencephalography (but more especially computerized axial tomography), and/or nuclear magnetic resonance may give valuable information with no risk to the patient.

The differential diagnosis of the causes of coma is a difficult but common clinical problem. An adequate history from friends or relatives who have observed the progress of the illness leading to coma eases the diagnostic problem. But when a patient is found comatose and no accurate history of the onset is available, diagnosis may bristle with difficulties. Head injury is generally identified by the history, but even if this is lacking there is usually some external evidence of laceration or contusion. In cases of subdural haematoma, however, the causal injury may have been trivial and the patient may gradually have become drowsy and eventually comatose over a period of weeks or months. Some patients with this condition are stuporous rather than comatose. In subarachnoid haemorrhage a history of sudden onset with severe headache and neck stiffness and the presence of blood-stained cerebrospinal fluid is revealing. The clinical picture of primary cerebral haemorrhage is not dissimilar, however, though in such cases a profound hemiplegia is usually present from the onset. When cerebral thrombosis is the cause, the onset is generally more gradual with less severe clouding of consciousness, though if the infarct is extensive the patient can be comatose and hemiplegic, a clinical picture which differs little from that of cerebral haemorrhage. The onset of cerebral embolism is abrupt, and there is often clinical evidence of a source of emboli, generally in the heart (mitral stenosis, bacterial endocarditis, myocardial infarction). Encephalitis and meningitis, being inflammatory disorders, are usually accompanied by fever, and the patient's comatose state is usually the end result of an illness which has lasted for a day or longer, with headache, neck stiffness (in meningitis particularly), drowsiness and confusion. In such individuals cerebrospinal fluid examination is of the greatest importance. The onset of herpes simplex encephalitis may be explosive. The clinical picture can mimic that of a space-occupying lesion in one temporal lobe and it is usually necessary to perform computed axial tomography first before it is judged safe to do a lumbar puncture (if, indeed, the latter is thought to be indicated).

Sudden coma is uncommon in patients suffering from cerebral tumour, most of whom have experienced previous headache, focal fits or the gradual development of paralysis. Papilloedema will often be present. In patients with cerebral abscess, too, the onset is generally gradual and there is often an evident focus of infection in the middle ear, nasal sinuses, skin or lung. The relatively uncommon hypertensive encephalopathy is generally recognized through the retinal and urinary changes of malignant hypertension combined with the blood pressure reading. Recognition of the coma that follows an attack of epilepsy rests upon the absence of physical signs and a history of previous fits.

Anoxia as a cause of coma will generally be identified by a history of carbon monoxide poisoning, or by a history of partial drowning, difficult general anaesthesia or chronic pulmonary insufficiency. A history of the latter is generally present in patients with severe hypercapnia. Acute alcoholism will be suspected from the smell of alcohol on the breath and confirmed by urine or blood-alcohol estimation, but it should be remembered that intoxicated patients are particularly liable to suffer head injury, while cerebrovascular catastrophes sometimes occur during an alcoholic debauch. Deep, hissing, 'acidotic' respiration with acetone in the breath, glycosuria, hyperglycaemia and ketonuria will usually establish a diagnosis of diabetic coma, while a pale, sweating, flaccid patient with bilateral extensor responses may be shown by blood-sugar estimation to be suffering from hypoglycaemia due either to insulin administration or a tumour of the pancreatic islet cells. Patients with uraemia tend to have deep acidotic breathing like that in diabetic coma, but the breath has a uriniferous smell, and hypertension, retinal changes and albuminuria are usually present. Liver disease is easily overlooked as a cause of coma, but the patient will usually have shown previously the characteristic 'flapping' tremor of the outstretched hands (asterixis) and there may be jaundice, dark urine and stigmata of hepatic cirrhosis, such as 'liver palms' and cutaneous spider naevi. Hypoventilation in chronic pulmonary disease can give an encephalopathy leading to stupor, especially after the administration of oxygen in some patients with cor pulmonale. Asterixis and myoclonus sometimes occur. The diagnosis depends upon measurement of the blood gases. Hyponatraemia or water intoxication can cause delirium leading to coma either due to inappropriate ADH secretion (often in patients with carcinoma) or rarely as a result of renal failure or compulsive water drinking. Hypernatraemia causes delirium less often, occasionally occurring in children with severe diarrhoea, in diabetes insipidus, or as a result of excessive saline administration. These disorders are diagnosed by measurement of the serum sodium or osmolality.

Other rare causes of comatose states include malaria, heat stroke, Addison's disease, myxoedema and hypopituitarism. In the latter two conditions, hypothermia is a common cause of coma and the rectal temperature may be less than 96°F (36°C). Drug intoxication must also be remembered as an increasingly common cause of a type of coma which may show no specific clinical features, especially if barbiturates, anticonvulsants or neuroleptic drugs have been taken in an attempt to commit suicide. Salicylates, by contrast, tend to produce a characteristic deep cyanosis with hyperpnoea, while opiates give characteristic pinpoint pupils. In any patient with coma of unknown cause, when no history is available, poisoning should be borne in mind and the patient's belongings should be searched for a bottle or carton which may have held the offending tablets. It will sometimes be necessary to wash out the stomach or, more often, to screen the blood and urine for the presence of barbiturates and other drugs.

Finally, psychogenic unresponsiveness (Plum and Posner, 1980) must also be considered. In so-called hysterical trance the patient usually shows some response to external stimuli (e.g. vigorous contraction of orbicularis oculi on attempting to open the patient's eyes or elicit the corneal reflex). The caloric, oculocephalic and other reflexes and the EEG are all normal, while there are no 'hard' abnormal neurological signs on examination (although some knowledgeable patients with the Munchausen syndrome who cleverly feign illness have been known to simulate convincingly an extensor plantar response). The diagnosis of catatonic stupor can be more difficult but catatonia (where the limbs maintain a posture passively imposed by the examiner), if present, is diagnostic.

The diagnosis of brain death

The diagnosis of brain death has assumed increasing importance in recent years. It is difficult to decide in patients with brain damage whether it is justifiable to maintain life indefinitely with assisted respiration and other supportive means. It is also difficult to decide that the cerebral lesion is irreversible, that death is imminent, and that preparations may properly be made to remove viable organs, especially the kidneys, heart, lungs and liver for subsequent transplantation. Plum (1972) gave a series of clinical criteria of brain death then employed at the Cornell, New York, Hospital Medical Center, and while this question continues to be a fertile source of ethical and medico-legal controversy, these represent a useful guide to current practice:

1. *The nature and duration of coma*
   a. The cause must be unequivocally structural disease (e.g. trauma, neoplasm, etc.) or of clearly known anoxic origin.
   b. There must be no chance that depressant drugs or hypothermia contribute to the clinical picture.
   c. Signs of absent brain function must persist for at least 12 hours under direct observation.
2. *Cerebral cortical function must be absent*
   a. Behavioural or reflex responses above the foramen magnum level to noxious stimuli applied anywhere on the body must be lacking.
   b. The EEG (properly recorded) must be isoelectric for 60 minutes at an amplitude of 50 μV/cm.
3. *Brain-stem function must be absent.*
   a. The pupils must be fixed to a strong light stimulus and must show no evidence of peripheral third nerve injury.
   b. Oculovestibular responses must be absent.
   c. There must be no motor activity whatever in structures innervated by cranial nerves.
   d. Spontaneous respiration must be absent. If the patient is on a respirator, there must be no breathing movements despite the patient being removed from the respirator for 3 minutes (receiving diffusion oxygen) and having a normal arterial PCO$_2$ at the start.
   e. The circulation may be intact.
   f. Purely spinal reflex responses may be retained.

Following a controversial BBC television programme in the United Kingdom in 1980 the criteria originally published by the Conference of Medical Royal Colleges and Faculties of the UK in 1976 were revised. Essentially the British criteria now in use correspond almost exactly to those listed above except that in the UK the tests must be carried out independently by two medical practitioners with expertise in the field, the tests must all be repeated with consistent results, and an EEG is no longer considered to be essential (Pallis, 1983).

DELIRIUM AND CONFUSION

There are many physical illnesses which are accompanied by mental symptoms of varying degree, most of which take the form of clouding of consciousness, with or without other more specific manifestations. This group of disorders is sometimes referred to as the symptomatic psychoses. They occur not only as a symptom of cerebral lesions but also in a variety of infective and metabolic disorders (see 'Cerebral metabolism and its disorders', p. 213). Although not primarily diseases of the nervous system, they may profoundly affect its function, even though they do not always produce histological changes in the brain that can be identified by present techniques. The clouding of consciousness or lack of awareness which results is sometimes no more than the minimal disinterest and 'fuzziness' in the head which accompanies mild influenza, but it can take the form of a severe psychotic reaction with grossly disturbed consciousness and bizarre disorders of thought.

Delirium is a term which has been used to identify a state of severely clouded consciousness in which the patient is disorientated in time and place, and in which his attention span is brief. His thought processes are disordered so that he cannot appreciate his present circumstances and relate them to past experiences. He may be living in a fantasy world peopled by the products of his imagining. Hence, delusions or false imaginary ideas are frequent, as are hallucinations, usually visual, which can be vividly real and frightening and which may result in an intense fear reaction with restless or even violent behaviour. Fluctuation in the mental and physical state is common, so that periods of shouting and restlessness alternate with periods of apparent somnolence, punctuated by low muttering. Commonly, the speech is slurred. Drowsiness is often most frequent during the day, while the patient becomes excited, hallucinated and uncontrollable at night. The stage of true delirium is often preceded by a period of restlessness and irritability, insomnia, lack of concentration, and abnormal elation or euphoria, a stage which may last for several hours or days depending on the cause. Frequently, there are associated motor manifestations. The patient is tremulous, and spontaneous twitching or jerking of the voluntary musculature occurs, even in sleep. Often a return to restful sleep is the first sign of resolution of the delirium, but even after apparent recovery, delusions may persist and often have a paranoid character, encompassing ideas of persecution or ill treatment.

Delirium occurs in classical form in patients with chronic alcoholism after a debauch or after the withdrawal of alcohol and is then known as delirium tremens. The condition which follows withdrawal of barbiturates or amphetamines in patients who have been taking excessive amounts of these drugs over a long period is similar, and is often characterized in addition by the occurrence of drug-withdrawal convulsions. Less severe and specific delirious states, differing only in detail but not in overall pattern, are seen in patients with encephalitis or meningitis, in severe infections such as septicaemia or typhoid fever, in metabolic disorders such as liver disease and pernicious anaemia, in some cases of bronchogenic carcinoma without cerebral metastases, sometimes during treatment with ACTH or cortisone, and in many other disorders. Mild delirium, observed particularly at night, is a common manifestation of febrile illnesses in childhood.

When the mental disturbances are less striking yet the patient shows only fluctuating awareness, with incoherence of thought and variable disorientation ('Where am I?') but usually without frank delusions or hallucinations, the condition is often referred to as confusion or a confusional (or organic reaction) state of mild, moderate or severe degree. This differs from delirium only in detail and indeed these disorders may merge with each other so that the delirious patient often passes through a phase of confusion during recovery. In recovery from a head injury, for instance, the patient may be delirious and later confused as consciousness is slowly restored. Hence some authorities have suggested that the term confusion should be discarded and that the condition to which it refers is better referred to as subacute delirium. For convenient clinical usage it is probably justifiable to retain the terms 'delirium' to identify the severe disturbance and 'confusion' the less severe, provided it is appreciated that there is no essential difference between the two.

Derangement of memory is a feature of many of the grades of disordered consciousness referred to earlier and is responsible for some of the spatial and temporal disorientation which is so frequent. Disturbances of memory and intellect are considered in the next chapter (p. 102).

TRANSIENT DISORDERS OF CONSCIOUSNESS

One of the commonest problems which a doctor is called upon to solve is the significance of brief disorders of consciousness, commonly referred to as 'blackouts'. Are these fits or faints? That is, are they epileptic or syncopal or, less commonly, of metabolic or emotional origin? No distinction can be more important for social and occupational reasons, and at times none can be more difficult to make with confidence.

Epilepsy

Epilepsy is difficult to define in view of the many guises which it may assume. It usually takes the form of a recurrent disorder of consciousness which is characteristically transient, ceases spontaneously, and which is often preceded or accompanied by motor or sensory phenomena. Though a definition of this type would embrace most cases of epilepsy, it could unfortunately also be utilized to describe certain cases of syncope and other conditions which are certainly not epilepsy and which must be distinguished from it. Furthermore, loss of consciousness is not invariable in some attacks which are unquestionably epileptic.

PATHOPHYSIOLOGY OF EPILEPSY

The resting membrane potential of the neuron is primarily determined by the electrochemical gradient for K^+ ions. All epileptic attacks are due to depolarization of groups of neurons. The localized application of acetylcholine (ACh) to the cerebral cortex of animals can precipitate localized uncontrolled discharge of neurons, giving the clinical manifestations of focal epilepsy. Microlectrode recording from the cerebral cortex in such circumstances demonstrates a 'burst' type of firing pattern of single cortical neurons, which appears to play a major part in the genesis of the epileptic spike in the EEG. Intravenous injection of ACh can, by contrast, precipitate generalized convulsions. Local or general electrical stimulation (as in electroconvulsion therapy in man) may have a similar effect, as do various convulsant or analeptic drugs. By contrast, inhibitory neurotransmitters, of which the most important is gamma-aminobutyric acid (GABA), may increase the electrochemical gradient for Na^+ across the neuronal membrane, giving rise to hyperpolarization and thus rendering the cell less excitable. In fact there are two types of GABA receptor: $GABA_a$ which, when stimulated, decreases the action potential amplitude by increasing Cl^- conductance, and $GABA_b$ which directly inhibits secretion due to a tonic depression of Ca^{2+} currents. Thus, GABA acts as a natural anticonvulsant and since GABA and ACh have opposite effects upon cortical neuronal excitability, an imbalance between the two could be one factor predisposing to seizure production. Pyridoxine deficiency in infancy is known to precipitate seizures, and this substance is essential for the synthesis of GABA. The relatively recent discovery of two specific receptor sites—one a GABA/chloride-ionophor/

benzodiazepine-receptor complex, the other a specific phenytoin receptor (see Spero, 1982)—has suggested that receptor/drug interaction as well as the GABA/ACh balance may be important in pathophysiology. This balance and the excitability of the neuron may be affected by many metabolic influences, including pyrexia, hypoxia, hypocalcaemia, hypoglycaemia, water intoxication and alkalosis, and by various drugs, toxins or drug withdrawal. For example, 20–25% of cerebral metabolic activity is concerned with the maintenance of the membrane potential of neurons. A reduction in oxygen and glucose supply tends to depolarize neuronal membranes by reducing oxidative metabolism. Ouabain is a drug which blocks the sodium pump and allows K^+ to diffuse out from the cell, increasing neuronal excitability, whereas rises in serum K^+ due to any cause can increase the tendency to convulse, even in normal animal brains. The hippocampus and so-called epileptic foci are particularly sensitive to alterations in serum K^+.

The so-called epileptic neuron is not, however, just 'uninhibited' as, in addition, the potentials which can be recorded from its soma and dendrites are of abnormally high amplitude and occur with greater frequency than normal. The formation of an epileptic 'focus' in the cortex may depend upon local glial proliferation, which interferes with the metabolic activity of contiguous neurons and which may also separate the cells functionally from modulating and inhibitory influences. Histological study of experimental and naturally occurring epileptic foci in animals and man, identified neurophysiologically, has shown loss of neuronal perikarya, distortion of dendrites, and loss of dendritic spines. It has also been suggested that cortical irritation produced by blood or its breakdown products in the CSF, to quote but one example of an epileptogenic lesion, may interfere with enzymatic action, causing local deficiency of Na^+-K^+-activated ATPase or impairment of the synthesis of inhibitory neurotransmitters.

The aetiology of epileptic attacks

The clinical varieties of epilepsy and their differential diagnosis and management are considered in detail in standard neurology texts, but a brief commentary is necessary here in order to understand some physiopathological principles. Cases of epilepsy can be divided into two broad groups: so-called *idiopathic epilepsy* and *symptomatic epilepsy*. In idiopathic epilepsy there is no evidence of any organic brain lesion being responsible for the attacks, nor do these attacks usually have a focal onset in any part of the body. In symptomatic epilepsy, on the other hand, the attacks are a symptom of organic disease of the brain. Some suggest that seizures occurring as a result of overt brain disease should not be regarded as epilepsy, and that this term should be reserved for the 'idiopathic' condition. This view, however, is untenable, as the nature of the seizures may be similar in the two types, and many patients once considered to be suffering from idiopathic epilepsy are being found to have the symptomatic variety, with previously unsuspected cerebral lesions being responsible for the attacks. Many apparently normal individuals would suffer fits if their brains were subjected to a pathological or biochemical insult of sufficient severity. The tendency towards seizures, the so-called 'convulsive threshold', shows considerable variation from one person to another. Those with a very high threshold would never suffer a convulsion, no matter how severe the stimulus, while those in whom it is low are often the 'idiopathic' epileptics who have attacks without apparent cause. It is difficult to draw a clear line of demarcation between the epileptic and the non-epileptic in those whose 'convulsive threshold' falls between these two extremes. Not more than about 50% of patients with penetrating brain injuries develop post-traumatic epilepsy. It seems reasonable to regard all epileptiform seizures as epilepsy, but always to look for an organic cause and to regard the patient as a case of idiopathic epilepsy only if the search is negative. How assiduous this search should be depends upon the age of the patient and the severity and frequency of the attacks. With present techniques of investigation, many patients with symptomatic epilepsy are probably wrongly diagnosed as suffering from the idiopathic variety, and there are many who believe that, ideally, all patients presenting with epilepsy, certainly in later life, should be examined by computed tomography (CT) scanning (see p. 258) in order to exclude the presence of an unsuspected cerebral lesion. The convulsive threshold is clearly constitutional, and a hereditary factor is certainly important as many epileptics have epileptic or otherwise unstable relatives. No clear pattern of inheritance emerges, however, and the chances that an epileptic may have a child who is similarly affected are not very great statistically if the other partner of the marriage is normal.

In addition to the so-called convulsive threshold, the resistance of the brain to the spread of the epileptic discharge is an important variable. It is a property which may be independent of the convulsive threshold. If this resistance is low and spread is rapid, a focal lesion will give a generalized convulsion with immediate loss of consciousness and no localizing features. If the resistance is high, the epileptic manifestations will remain localized to the appropriate area of the body (focal or jacksonian epilepsy) and consciousness may be comparatively unimpaired throughout the attack. When resistance is intermediate between these two extremes, the onset of the fit may be focal, but it will then develop into a generalized seizure. Some of the important causes of symptomatic epilepsy are given in Table 6.

The clinical classification of epileptic seizures

Traditionally, attacks of epilepsy, whether idiopathic or symptomatic, have been divided into major epilepsy (grand mal), minor epilepsy (petit mal), focal (jacksonian) epilepsy, temporal lobe (psychomotor) epilepsy, and myoclonic attacks. However, increasing knowledge has shown that these descriptive classifications are unsatisfactory for several reasons. For instance, there are many forms of minor epilepsy which are not true petit mal. In epilepsy of focal onset, depending upon the site of origin in the brain, many motor, sensory, behavioural and psychomotor manifestations may be noted. If the epileptic discharge spreads rapidly to become generalized, a major attack may occur and the focal symptoms then constitute merely the aura or warning of the major attack. Temporal lobe epilepsy is now becoming more generally known as complex partial epilepsy (Penry and Daly, 1975). A more up-to-date classification is given in Table 7.

The pathophysiology of the commoner types of seizures

The petit mal 'absence' is a transient interruption of consciousness lasting for only a few seconds, beginning almost invariably in childhood, and accompanied sometimes by flickering of the eyelids and less often by brief jerky movements of the hands. Attacks usually recur frequently throughout the day. They can often be precipitated by flickering light and are thought to be due to a synchronous discharge arising in the reticular substance (Fig. 4.4), though the cause is not understood. The attacks are usually accompanied by a wave-and-spike discharge in the EEG (Fig. 4.5). Slow, irregular wave-and-spike discharges, by contrast, may be associated with many diffuse brain diseases and with an atypical 'petit mal variant', often occurring in children with diffuse brain damage.

A major epileptic fit or convulsion ('grand mal') leads to an abrupt loss of consciousness which may or may not be preceded by a warning or aura. There may be a momentary cry followed by a tonic phase of generalized muscular rigidity in which the tongue may be bitten. The patient, if standing, will fall to the ground and often injures himself. The tonic phase passes, usually within a few seconds, to be followed

TABLE 6. **Some important causes of symptomatic epilepsy***

LOCAL CAUSES
(a) *Focal intracranial lesions sometimes associated with increased intracranial pressure*
  Intracranial tumour; cerebral abscess; subdural haematoma; angioma or haematoma
(b) *Inflammatory and demyelinating conditions*
  Meningitis; all forms of acute and subacute encephalitis and many encephalopathies; toxoplasmosis; neurosyphilis; multiple sclerosis; cerebral cysticercosis
(c) *Trauma*
  Perinatal brain injury and/or haemorrhage; head injuries of childhood and later life
(d) *Congenital abnormalities*
  The various forms of cerebral palsy; cerebral malformations
(e) *Degenerations and inborn errors of metabolism*
  The neuronal storage disorders; diffuse sclerosis and the leukodystrophies; encephalopathies of infancy and childhood, including 'infantile spasms'; tuberous scleroses and the other phacomatoses; Pick's disease; Alzheimer's disease; progressive myoclonic epilepsy; subacute spongiform encephalopathy; Creutzfeldt–Jakob disease
(f) *Vascular disorders*
  Atheroma of cerebral arteries, intracranial haemorrhage, thrombosis, embolism; eclampsia; hypertensive encephalopathy; cerebral complications of connective tissue (collagen) diseases; polycythaemia; intracranial aneurysm; acute cerebral ischaemia from any cause

GENERAL CAUSES
(a) *Exogenous poisons*
  Alcohol; absinthe; thujone; cocaine; strychnine; lead; chloroform; ether; insulin; amphetamines; camphor; leptazol; antihistamines; intrathecal penicillin; pyridoxine analogues; some amino acids; some anaesthetics (e.g. cocaine and lignocaine); water-soluble contrast media used intrathecally such as metrizamide; organophosphorus and organochlorine compounds used as insecticides, and fluoracetic acid derivatives; monoamine oxidase inhibitors, imipramine, and its derivatives; and *withdrawal* of alcohol, barbiturates, and other drugs
(b) *Anoxia*
  Asphyxia; carbon monoxide poisoning; carbon dioxide intoxication; nitrous oxide anaesthesia; profound anaemia
(c) *Disordered metabolism*
  Uraemia; hepatic failure; water intoxication; high fat intake; porphyria; hypoglycaemia; hyperpyrexia; alkalosis; hyperkalaemia; pyridoxine deficiency
(d) *Endocrine disorders*
  Parathyroid tetany; idiopathic hypoparathyroidism, and pseudohypoparathyroidism; hypoadrenalism; pituitary dysfunction including Cushing's disease and hypopituitarism; hyperthyroidism and myxoedema
(e) *Conditions associated particularly with childhood*
  Rickets; acute infections ('febrile convulsions')

*Walton (1985)

by the clonic phase of generalized jerking or convulsive movements in which there may be incontinence of urine and less often of faeces. The clonic phase actually represents recurring phases of inhibition interrupting the initial tonic phase (Fig. 4.6). There is often then a variable period of postepileptic

TABLE 7. Classification of seizures*

1. *Generalized*
   a. Tonic–clonic (grand mal)
   b. Tonic
   c. Atonic
   d. Absence (petit mal)
   e. Atypical absence
   f. Myoclonic

2. *Partial (focal)*
   A. Without impairment of consciousness (simple partial seizures)
   B. With impairment of consciousness (complex partial seizures)
      a. With motor signs (e.g. Jacksonian, versive)
      b. With somato- or special sensory symptoms (e.g. olfactory, visual)
      c. With autonomic features (e.g. epigastric sensations)
      d. With psychic symptoms (e.g. fear, déjà vu)
      e. With automatisms (complex partial seizures only)

3. *Partial seizures secondarily generalized*
   i.e. clinical or electrical evidence of focal discharge, during or after the generalized seizure

4. *Unclassifiable*
   Seizures which cannot be classified because of incomplete data

*Marsden and Reynolds (1982) and Walton (1985)

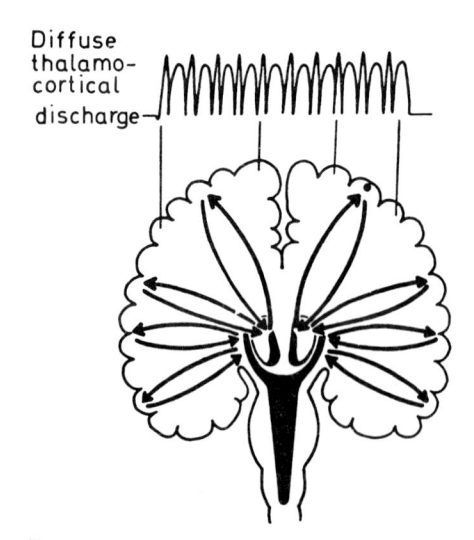

Figure 4.4 Diffuse thalamocortical discharge, associated with impairment of consciousness. This may be triggered by extension of epileptic activity from a cortical focus (secondary centrencephalic epilepsy) or it may occur spontaneously in patients with the centrencephalic trait of petit mal epilepsy. [Reproduced from Lance and McLeod (1980) *A Physiological Approach to Clinical Neurology*, 2nd edn, by kind permission of the authors and publisher.]

EEG (Fig. 4.7). If it spreads further, motor, sensory or behavioural symptoms and signs may result, depending upon the function of that part of the cortex in which it originates. Jacksonian attacks, which can sometimes be long-lasting without loss of consciousness, are one form of focal epilepsy, but so too are all the complex variants of partial seizures such as those formerly classified as temporal lobe epilepsy. These attacks often demonstrate a progressive 'march' of symptoms (such as the spread of paraesthesiae from tongue to face and hand to arm), reflecting the spread of discharge across contiguous areas of the cortex. The discharge may spread across the corpus callosum to produce a 'mirror focus' in the opposite hemisphere (Fig. 4.8*A*) or else it spreads to the reticular substance, initiating a corticothalamocortical discharge (Fig. 4.8*B*) which often then precipitates a major seizure. The length of time taken for this spread to occur usually determines whether or not the major attack has an aura with focal characteristics. During a major attack the EEG shows diffuse high-frequency discharges (Fig. 4.6).

A major convulsion is associated with a marked increase in cerebral oxygen consumption, with carbon dioxide production, sodium loss, potassium gain, and increased cerebral and venous lactate. It is followed by cerebral and systemic acidosis. If such attacks are severe, prolonged and frequent, hypoxia may damage various neuronal groups in the deepest laminae of the cortex and in the Ammon's horn area of the hippocampus. Such damage may in turn create new epileptic foci or can sometimes lead to intellectual and memory impairment.

Akinetic attacks are seizures in which consciousness is lost and postural tone is temporarily inhibited so that the patient falls, but there are no tonic or clonic motor accompaniments and consciousness is quickly restored.

Tonic seizures are episodes in which the patient assumes an abnormal dystonic posture for a few seconds or minutes. For example, a patient's limbs may be generally extended and rigid with the back arched, resembling the decerebrate posture. Such a seizure usually implies the presence of a lesion of the midbrain, such as local compression, and is usually of serious import; it is also sometimes seen in severe cases of cerebral palsy. Less severe tonic attacks, as occasionally seen, for example, in multiple sclerosis, presumed to be dependent upon an intrinsic brainstem plaque of demyelination, may simply take the form, say, of transient, rigid, abnormal posturing of one arm and hand. Consciousness is usually retained in tonic seizures.

Myoclonus is a sudden shock-like contraction of a group of muscles that produces a rapid, jerky movement, usually involving one or more limbs. This may

confusion or drowsiness followed by a period of normal sleep, or else consciousness may be quickly restored. Most if not all grand mal attacks are thought to arise locally in the cortex. When such a focal discharge remains very localized it may produce no symptoms, but a focal spike may be evident in the

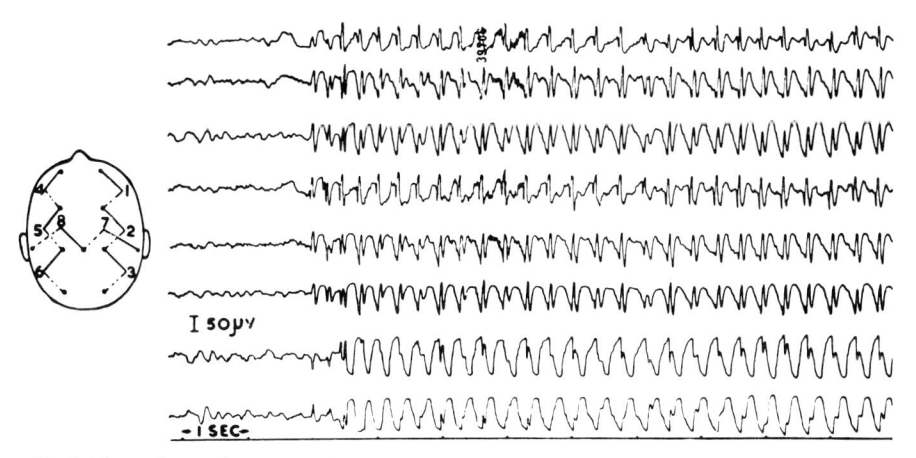

Figure 4.5 Generalized, bilaterally synchronous and symmetrical 3 Hz wave-and-spike discharges during a petit mal attack in an 18-year-old male. [Reproduced from Walton (1985) *Brain's Diseases of the Nervous System*, 9th edn, by kind permission of the publisher.]

be physiological when it occurs when falling asleep (nocturnal myoclonus). The sudden jerk or startle response that occurs in normal individuals as a consequence of a loud noise or any unexpected physical or emotional stimulus is similar. However, myoclonic jerking occurring in the waking state must be construed as a form of epilepsy. Generalized myoclonus may be sufficiently severe and abrupt to cause falling,

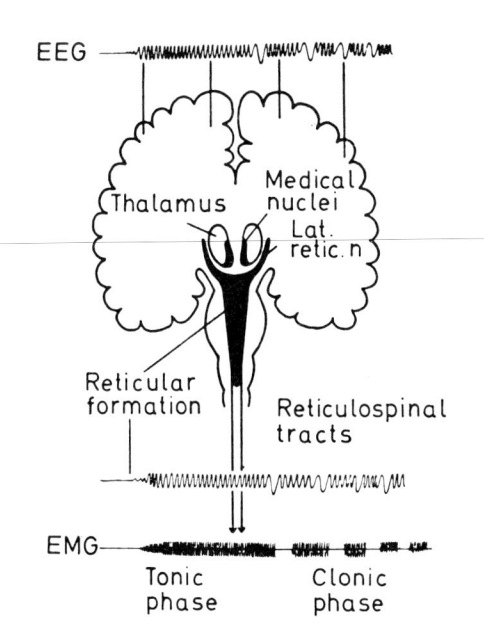

Figure 4.6 Grand mal seizure. The high-frequency EEG discharge of the tonic phase is later interrupted by slow waves that inhibit cerebral activity and permit brief periods of muscular relaxation, responsible for the clonic phase of the seizure. [Reproduced from Lance and McLeod (1980) *A Physiological Approach to Clinical Neurology*, 2nd edn by kind permission of the authors and publisher.]

and some workers have regarded such episodes as being comparable to an incipient grand mal attack terminated abruptly by active inhibition. In patients with severe and generalized myoclonus, there is evidence of disordered function of the reticular substance in that sensory stimuli of all kinds produce a greatly enhanced electrical response in the relevant area of sensory cortex. It is thus an expression of hyperexcitability of the nervous system, in which there is abnormal synchronous and repetitive firing of neuronal circuits in response to physiological stimuli. Characteristically, the spike discharges in the EEG seen in many patients with this phenomenon are synchronous with the myoclonic jerks when recorded electromyographically, while the subsequent slow wave corresponds to the period of inhibition and muscular relaxation (Fig. 4.9). There may be some analogy in a physiological sense between myoclonus and the many varieties of so-called reflex epilepsy in which petit mal and/or major seizures can be elicited by a variety of sensory stimuli, including flickering light, reading, television, music, olfactory stimuli and voluntary movement. In patients who suffer major attacks preceded by a powerful sensory (e.g. olfactory) aura, application of the relevant sensory stimulus (e.g. a strong-smelling substance) during the aura may prevent the subsequent development of a major attack, presumably because the physiological sensory stimulus inhibits the 'march' of the attack. Postepileptic confusion or stupor, or postepileptic paralysis (Todd's paralysis) in the limbs affected by a focal seizure are probably due to persisting subclinical epileptic discharge. The refractory period of the relevant neurons is far too short to suggest that neuronal 'exhaustion' could account for these prolonged phenomena.

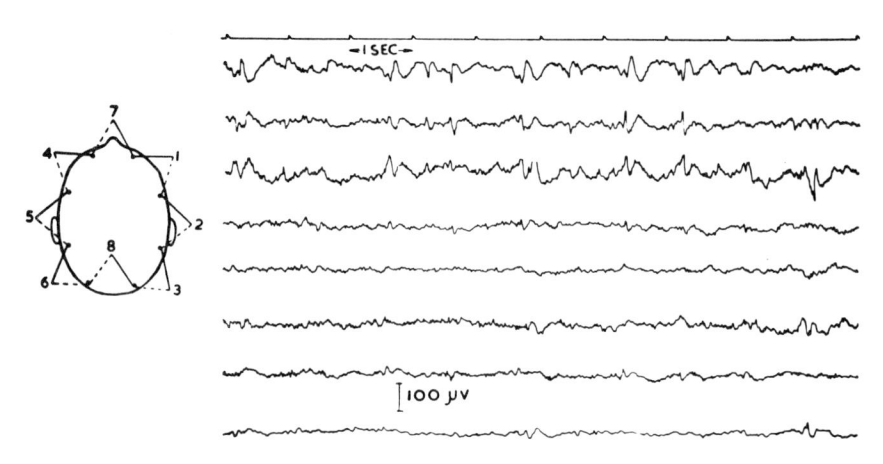

Figure 4.7 Temporal lobe epilepsy in a 30-year-old male. Focal sharp and slow waves in the right temporal region. [Reproduced from Walton (1985) *Brain's Diseases of the Nervous System*, 9th edn, by kind permission of the publisher.]

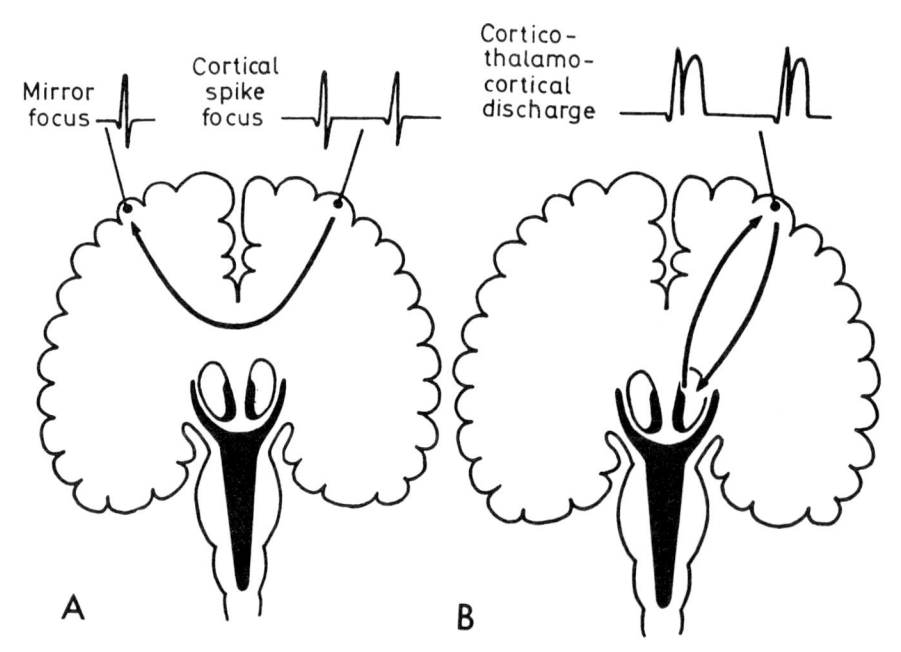

Figure 4.8 A, Focal cortical epilepsy. A potentially epileptic discharge may remain localized to one area of the cortex, or propagate via the corpus callosum to the contralateral hemisphere, forming a mirror focus. Although such focal abnormalities are apparent in the EEG, the patient may remain free from seizures. B, Focal cortical epilepsy. A cortical discharge may spread locally through association fibres or extend to the reticular formation of thalamus and brain stem (black areas in diagram). Such corticocortical or thalamocortical circuits are the probable basis of localized spike-and-wave patterns and overt focal seizures. [Reproduced from Lance and McLeod (1980) *A Physiological Approach to Clinical Neurology*, 2nd edn, by kind permission of the authors and publisher.]

Syncope and other brief disorders of consciousness

It is sometimes difficult to differentiate clinically between simple faints or syncopal attacks and epileptic seizures. Syncope is most common in young patients, particularly in adolescent girls. It is often produced by long periods of standing in one position, by an emotional shock (the 'sight of blood'), or by 'stuffy' atmospheres. It is particularly liable to occur in early pregnancy, and it can develop at any age in patients with uraemia or blood loss, or with heart block (the Stokes–Adams syndrome). Rarely, syncope of whatever cause can result in transient epileptic manifestations, including transient twitching of the limbs and urinary incontinence, if cerebral anoxia is sufficiently prolonged. Any cardiac

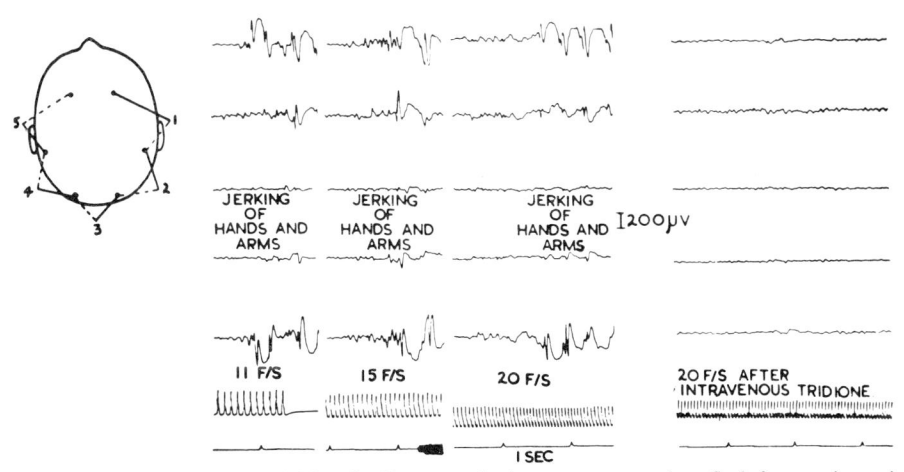

Figure 4.9 Myoclonic epilepsy in a 19-year-old female. Photomyoclonic response at various flash frequencies and subsequent effect of intravenous tridione. [Reproduced from Walton (1985) *Brain's Diseases of the Nervous System*, 9th edn, by kind permission of the publisher.]

lesion that diminishes cardiac output (e.g. aortic stenosis, auricular fibrillation, paroxysmal tachycardia or other arrhythmias) can be associated with recurrent fainting, as can chronic bronchitis and emphysema in that severe bouts of coughing with fixation of the chest wall in expansion may so impair venous return to the heart that episodes of cough syncope result. Carotid sinus syncope occurs in those in whom turning of the head or pressure upon the neck causes abnormal slowing of the heart rate or even asystole due to increased sensitivity of the carotid sinus. Rarely, fainting results from stenotic lesions of the carotids and vertebral vessels which reduce the blood supply to the brain. Micturition syncope is not uncommon, particularly in the elderly male patient during the night.

Syncope is due to cerebral ischaemia, resulting usually from pooling of blood in the skin and viscera. Generally the patient feels a 'swimming in the head' and a sensation of heat. He then begins to perspire and is usually able to reach a place of safety before consciousness is lost. The loss of consciousness is generally brief. The patient's skin is pale, cold and clammy, and his pulse is thin and rapid, but occasionally it is slow. The aura of a syncopal attack is usually much longer than that of an epileptic seizure. There are generally emotional or physical precipitating factors. Injury is uncommon and convulsive movements and incontinence are rare. The attacks usually occur when the subject is standing, not when he is sitting or lying down. Often they are brought on by standing up abruptly. These are the principal points upon which differential diagnosis is based. Syncope due to transient postural hypotension is particularly likely to occur after a hot bath, overindulgence in alcohol, after sympathectomy, in patients with spinal cord lesions impairing pressor reflexes (e.g. in tabes dorsalis) and in those taking hypotensive drugs or certain tranquillizers (particularly phenothiazines).

Chronic orthostatic hypotension (the Shy–Drager syndrome), a rare condition which is often familial, is due to degeneration in the autonomic nervous system (see p. 122). The blood pressure falls as soon as the patient assumes the upright position. Since the compensatory reflexes are impaired, there is no pallor, sweating or tachycardia, and consciousness is lost. Recovery occurs as soon as the patient lies down.

So-called vasovagal attacks have been described in which the patient becomes flushed and his pulse is slowed, while gastric or cardiac discomfort may occur. There is considerable doubt as to whether attacks of this nature ever occur in a stereotyped manner. It now seems improbable that they should be afforded separate identification, as they are merely one form of syncopal attack.

Drop attacks are episodes in which the patient's legs give way and he falls but does not lose consciousness. They are commonest in elderly women and are probably due to transient inhibition in the brain-stem reticular substance. They have been attributed to brain-stem ischaemia, but their cause is unknown.

Hysterical convulsions are generally bizarre and florid with more violent and varied and less stereotyped movements than occur in epilepsy. Tongue-biting, injury and incontinence do not occur unless the patient has been asked about incontinence so often that he eventually obliges. Usually there are other manifestations of hysteria. In young women, hysterical attacks may take the form of sudden falling with apparently transient loss of consciousness and without convulsive movements. Similar attacks are not uncommon in some male patients who develop a so-called accident neurosis after minor injury. When these attacks occur in young women who have also had genuine attacks of epilepsy, differential diagnosis can be very difficult. Hysterical hyperventilation (rapid panting respiration), which is often accompanied by panic and which leads to paraesthesiae in the lips and tongue and even to tetany, can also give rise to syncope and is often misdiagnosed. The tetany which occurs as a result of hyperventilation is due to alkalosis resulting from loss of carbon dioxide in the expired air. Other disorders associated with tetany which reduce the serum ionized calcium (repeated vomiting, dietary alkalosis, rickets and osteomalacia, hypoparathyroidism and malabsorption) do not usually give rise to attacks of loss of consciousness. In idiopathic hypoparathyroidism, however, attacks of epilepsy are common. The typical carpopedal spasms of tetany with other evidence of neuromuscular excitability (positive Chvostek's and Trousseau's signs) usually ensure that attacks of this nature are not confused with focal epilepsy, and estimation of the serum calcium will be diagnostic.

Spontaneous hypoglycaemia can give rise to attacks of lightheadedness, fatigue, sweating, paraesthesiae, giddiness, and even confused and irrational behaviour. Rarely, major epileptic convulsions result, particularly in those patients who have a tumour of the islets of Langerhans, with excessive insulin production (organic hyperinsulinism). When reactive or functional hyperinsulinism is the cause, due to an excessive fall in blood sugar following the peak produced by a high carbohydrate meal, or after rapid gastric emptying (such as may follow gastrectomy or gastroenterostomy), the symptoms are as a rule less severe. Nevertheless this condition, too, must be considered in determining the cause of transient disturbances of consciousness.

References

Adams, R. D. and Victor, M. (1985) *Principles of Neurology*, 3rd edn. New York: McGraw-Hill Book Company.
Beresford, H. R., Posner, J. B. and Plum, F. (1969) Changes in brain lactate during induced cerebral seizures. *Arch. Neurol.* **20**:243.
British Medical Journal (1973) Mute of malady. *Br. Med. J.* **1**:753.
Davison, A. N. and Thompson, R. H. S. (eds) (1981) *The Molecular Basis of Neuropathology*. London: Arnold.
Dement, W., Rechtshaffen, A. and Gulevich, G. (1966) The nature of the narcoleptic sleep attack. *Neurology* **16**:18.
Efron, R. (1957) The conditioned inhibition of uncinate fits. *Brain* **80**:251.
Emery, A. E. H. (1984) *An Introduction to Recombinant DNA*. Chichester and New York: John Wiley.
Falconer, M. A. (1974) Mesial temporal (Ammon's horn) sclerosis as a common cause of epilepsy: aetiology, treatment, and prevention. *Lancet* **ii**:767.
Hobson, J. A. and Brazier, M. A. B. (eds) (1979) *The Reticular Formation Revisited* (IBRO Monograph Series, vol. 6). New York: Raven Press.
Janz, D. (1969) *Die Epilepsien*. Stuttgart: Georg Thieme Verlag.
Johnson, R. T., Lambie, D. G. and Spalding, J. M. K. (1984) *Neurocardiology* (Major Problems in Neurology), vol. 13. Philadelphia: W. B. Saunders.
Lance, J. W. and McLeod, J. G. (1981) *A Physiological Approach to Clinical Neurology*, 3rd edn. London: Butterworth.
Marsden, C. D. and Reynolds, A. (1982) Neurology. In Laidlaw, J. and Richens, A. (eds) *Textbook of Epilepsy*, 2nd edn. Edinburgh: Churchill Livingstone.
Meldrum, B. S. (1982) Pathophysiology. In Laidlaw, J. and Richens, A. (eds) *Textbook of Epilepsy*, 2nd edn. Edinburgh: Churchill Livingstone.
Pallis, C. (1983) *An ABC of Brain Stem Death*. London: British Medical Journal.
Parkes, J. D. (1985) *Sleep and its Disorders* (Major Problems in Neurology), vol. 14. Philadelphia: W. B. Saunders.
Penfield, W. and Jasper, H. (1954) *Epilepsy and the Functional Anatomy of the Human Brain*. Edinburgh: Churchill Livingstone.
Penry, J. K. and Daly, D. D. (1975) *Complex Partial Seizures and Their Treatment* (Advances in Neurology, vol. II). New York: Raven Press.
Plum, F. (1972) Organic disturbances of consciousness. In Critchley, M., O'Leary, J. L. and Jennett, W. B. (eds) *Scientific Foundations of Neurology*. London: Heinemann.
Plum, F. (1979) The pathogenesis of stupor and coma. In Beeson, P. B. and McDermott, W. (eds) *Textbook of Medicine*, 15th edn. Philadelphia: W. B. Saunders Company.
Plum, F. and Posner, J. B. (1980) *Diagnosis of Stupor and Coma*, 3rd edn. Oxford: Blackwell Scientific Publications, and Philadelphia: F. A. Davis Company.
Porter, R. J. (1984) *Epilepsy: 100 Elementary Principles* (Major Problems in Neurology), vol. 12. Philadelphia: W. B. Saunders.
Spero, L. (1982) Epilepsy. *Lancet* **ii**:1319.
Sutherland, J. M. and Eadie, M. J. (1980) *The Epilepsies: Modern Diagnosis and Treatment*, 3rd edn. Edinburgh: Churchill Livingstone.
Swash, M. and Kennard, C. (eds) (1985) *Scientific Basis of Clinical Neurology*. Edinburgh and London: Livingstone.
Teasdale, G. and Jennett, W. B. (1974) Assessment of coma and impaired consciousness. *Lancet* **ii**:81.
Walton, J. N. (1985) *Brain's Diseases of the Nervous System*, 9th edn. Oxford: Oxford University Press.

5

BEHAVIOUR, MEMORY, INTELLECT, PERSONALITY AND THEIR DISORDERS

INTRODUCTION

The principal difference between the human and the subhuman brain consists in the great development of the cerebral cortex in man. The cortex is, in relation to perception, an end station at which are received nervous impulses derived from the eyes, the ears and other sensory organs. The corresponding regions of the cortex are linked by association paths through which the sensations which form the raw material of perception evoke memories and become enriched with meanings which can be communicated to others by means of speech, writing and gesture (discussed in the earlier chapter on 'human verbal communication' p. 72). The perceptual function of the cerebral cortex, therefore, is primarily discriminative, and its massive development in man compared with that in the lower animals is paralleled by the enhancement of his discriminative faculties. This has occurred in spite of there having been little improvement, and in some cases an actual retrogression, of man's sensory acuity.

By contrast there is far less difference between man and the lower animals with respect to the development of subcortical centres, in particular the thalamus and hypothalamus. These regions of the brain, basal alike in situation and in function, are intimately concerned with the affective element in feeling, with the emotional and instinctive life, with the regulation of the autonomic nervous system, and to some extent with metabolic and endocrine function. The brain, however, works as a whole and there is a constant interplay between cortical and subcortical activity. Perception evokes emotion and, conversely, emotion provides the interest which activates perception.

There is another aspect, however, of this relationship. Discrimination, the function of the cortex, implies inhibition as, if an organism is to react appropriately to a stimulus, inappropriate reactions must be simultaneously inhibited. This is true even at the level of a simple reflex arc. It is far more essential when the range both of potential stimuli and of potential reactions has been so enhanced by the development of the cortex. The cortex, therefore, acquires inhibitory functions as the complement of its discriminative functions.

THE FUNCTION OF THE DIENCEPHALON

The thalamus plays a fundamental role in the organization of animal behaviour. The dorsal thalamus is divided into an external portion and an internal core (Fig. 5.1). Each of these has nuclei that receive impulses from outside the thalamus (extrinsic nuclei) and other nuclei which, as far as is known, do not (intrinsic nuclei). The extrinsic nuclei of the external portion receive the somatic sensory tracts, the optic and auditory pathways; the intrinsic nucleus is the posterior nucleus. The extrinsic nuclei of the internal core receive impulses from the posterior hypothalamus and the central reticular formation; the intrinsic nucleus is the medial. The extrinsic nuclei of the external portion project to the primary sensory cortical areas concerned with somatic sensibility, hearing and vision in the parietal, temporal and occipital lobes, while the intrinsic, posterior nucleus projects to the rest of the parieto-temporo-occipital cortex. The extrinsic nuclei of the internal core project to the limbic areas of the medial aspect of the frontal and parietal lobes and to the anterior rhinencephalon and basal ganglia, and the medial (intrinsic) nucleus projects to the prefrontal cortex. There is an important corticofugal pathway (the medial forebrain bundle) running from the mediobasal part of the frontal lobe to the thalamus and the hypothalamic nuclei, including the corpora mamillaria.

The projections from the extrinsic nuclei of the external part of the dorsal thalamus are the sensory afferent pathways, and interference with them causes sensory loss in the corresponding modalities. Damage to the parts of the cerebral cortex supplied by the projections from the intrinsic nuclei of the external part lead to a failure to differentiate and respond to patterns of sensory stimuli, a condition resembling agnosia (p. 79). These nuclei, their projections, and the corresponding cortical areas therefore provide a higher level perceptual discriminative mechanism.

On the other hand ablations and stimulations of the anatomical systems represented by the nuclei of the internal core of the thalamus (and their projections through the medial and basal telencephalon) affect feeding (eating and drinking), fighting and aggression, fleeing and avoidance, mating, and maternal behaviour. They are therefore concerned with what may in the broadest sense be termed instinctive behaviour. All such activities are linked with emotion to a greater or a lesser extent.

The role of various hypothalamic nuclei in controlling the activity of the autonomic nervous system is now well documented. Emotional disorders and altered autonomic activity are closely interlinked. The hypothalamus, brain-stem reticular system, parts of the thalamus, hippocampus, amygdala, fornix and cingulate gyrus are closely interlinked and play a fundamental integrating role in controlling emotion as well as memory and behaviour. Even though in anatomical terms parts of the hypothalamus and brain-stem reticular substance are not strictly part of the limbic system, functionally they are so closely related that it is reasonable to regard all of these structures as forming the limbic brain (Figs. 5.2 and 5.3).

Some parts of the basal ganglia also possess behavioural functions. Thus the nucleus accumbens, anatomically related to the striatum, seems to act as a 'bridge', bringing limbic influences to bear on motor function. Various neurotransmitters and their respective functions were discussed in chapter 1; however, it is now well known that increased serotonin activity leads to psychomotor retardation, while serotonin antagonist drugs have a stimulant and antidepressant effect. Drugs which reduce catecholamine activity decrease spontaneous locomotion and inhibit conditioned responses and exploratory behaviour, while dopamine agonists can cause stereo-typed behaviour. Both adrenergic and non-adrenergic activity is important in pleasure and reward responses and in hypothalamic activity. The mesolimbic dopamine system seems to be related to motivational arousal and that of the striatum to motor arousal, so that the proper functioning of these systems is needed for the integration of sensory inputs, memory, motivation and motor expression.

In the hypothalamus the anterior and posterior nuclei are concerned with temperature and cardiovascular control and with endocrine activity, and

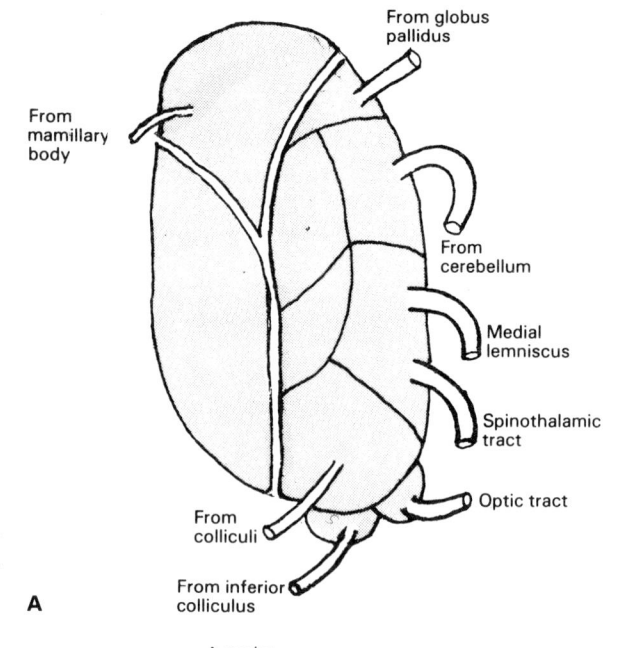

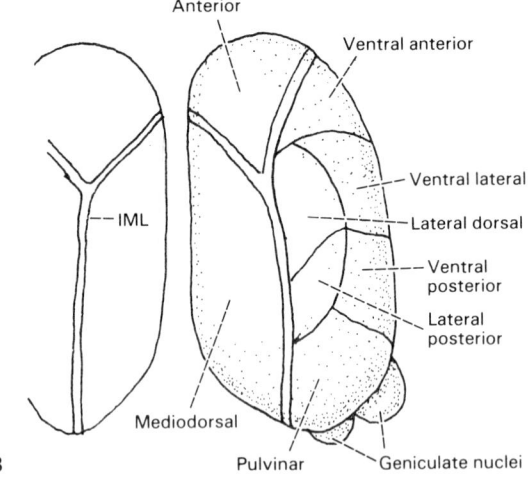

Figure 5.1 A, Thalamus from above, with nuclear subdivisions. IML = internal medullary lamina. B, Diagram indicating sources of input to the specific thalamic nuclei. [Reproduced from Fitzgerald (1985) *Neuroanatomy, Basic and Applied*, by kind permission of the author.]

the supraoptic nucleus produces ADH (p. 114). The perifornical nucleus, if stimulated, causes hunger, increased blood pressure, and sometimes rage; the ventromedial nucleus, satiety, the lateral hypothalamic area, thirst and hunger; and the mammillary body, feeding reflexes (see Guyton, 1981). Many of these functions appear to be mediated through the reticular formation. A series of polypeptides containing between 17 and 21 amino acids, known as endorphins, may play a transmitter role in various parts of the limbic system, thus fulfilling a variety of behavioural functions. Their exact function has yet to be fully defined. Smaller polypeptides known as encephalins seem to act as intrinsic analgesic substances elaborated within the brain itself, as they combine with opiate receptors and are known as endogenous ligands.

THE LIMBIC SYSTEM: BEHAVIOURAL FUNCTIONS

Many hypothalamic and other limbic centres are especially concerned with sensations that have an emotional content and are either pleasant (rewarding) or painful, probably in an emotional rather than a physical sense (punishment or aversion). Centres in the septum, hypothalamic ventromedial nuclei, and medial forebrain bundle may produce such a feeling of reward on stimulation that if an indwelling electrode is inserted and an animal can then apply stimuli himself he will do so repeatedly. By contrast, stimulation of the perifornical nucleus of the hypothalamus and of the mesencephalic central grey matter may give manifestations suggestive of pain, displeasure and punishment, and will outweigh the effects of simultaneous stimulation of a reward centre. Physiologically, both habituation (diminishing response) and reinforcement have been shown with different stimulus patterns. Pharmacologically both reward and punishment can be suppressed by various tranquillizing drugs. It seems probable that much human behaviour is dependent upon the balance of activity in reward and punishment centres.

Intense stimulation of the punishment centres (e.g. the perifornical nucleus) of animals may produce a rage response, whereas stimulation more rostrally gives manifestations of fear and anxiety. By contrast, repeated stimulation of reward centres will result in docility and tranquillity. Stimulation dorsal to the mammillary bodies gives excessive wakefulness and excitement with evidence of sympathetic overactivity, while stimulation in parts of the septum, anterior hypothalamus, or some paths of the thalamic reticular nuclei causes somnolence and sometimes actual sleep (see p. 83).

THE LIMBIC SYSTEM AND EMOTION

Psychophysiologically, emotion involves a number of factors, including (1) some external object which excites it, (2) specific feelings characteristic of particular emotions, and (3) the fact that the emotion tends to find expression in some characteristic action. Accompanying the feelings and the motor activities there are (4) certain other physiological manifestations in which the autonomic nervous system and endocrine activity play an important part. And, finally, there is often (5) a pre-existing physiological state which is necessary if the appetite, or emotional need, is to be fulfilled. This is most obvious in the case of hunger, thirst and the sexual impulse.

The limbic system controls not only the emotions but also memory and much of behaviour. However, the functions of many parts of the limbic system are still poorly understood and what little we know has been largely derived from experiments involving electrical stimulation.

Stimulation of the amygdala can cause changes in heart rate and blood pressure, defaecation and micturition, pupillary dilatation, and an increased output of various anterior pituitary hormones. In other areas involuntary movements (tonic or circling movements, chewing or lip-smacking) may be elicited or, alternatively, an arrest reaction may be produced in which the animal 'freezes' in one posture. Yet other areas, if stimulated, give manifestations of rage, fear, reward or punishment as described above, while elsewhere stimuli produce sexual activity including erection, ejaculation, copulatory movements, ovulation or uterine contraction. Thus, many of the emotional and behavioural manifestations of temporal lobe epilepsy, including fear or hypersexuality, may be reproduced.

The hippocampus distributes many outgoing signals to the hypothalamus and other parts of the limbic system via the fornix. Its other major role appears to relate to memory (see below). Animal experiments suggest that the hippocampus also plays a part in 'goal-directed' behaviour, but its principal function, in consort with the reticular formation and other parts of the limbic system, appears to lie in focusing attention and in acquiring and retaining new information in an orderly manner. Stimulation of other parts of the limbic cortex (the cingulate gyrus and orbitofrontal cortex) can give changes in respiratory and cardiac rate and blood pressure, facilitation of movements induced by cortical stimulation elsewhere, licking, swallowing, changes in gastrointestinal motility and secretion, and various affective reactions (e.g. rage or docility, increased or diminished awareness). Ablation of the cingulate gyri may give tameness in animals and suppression of

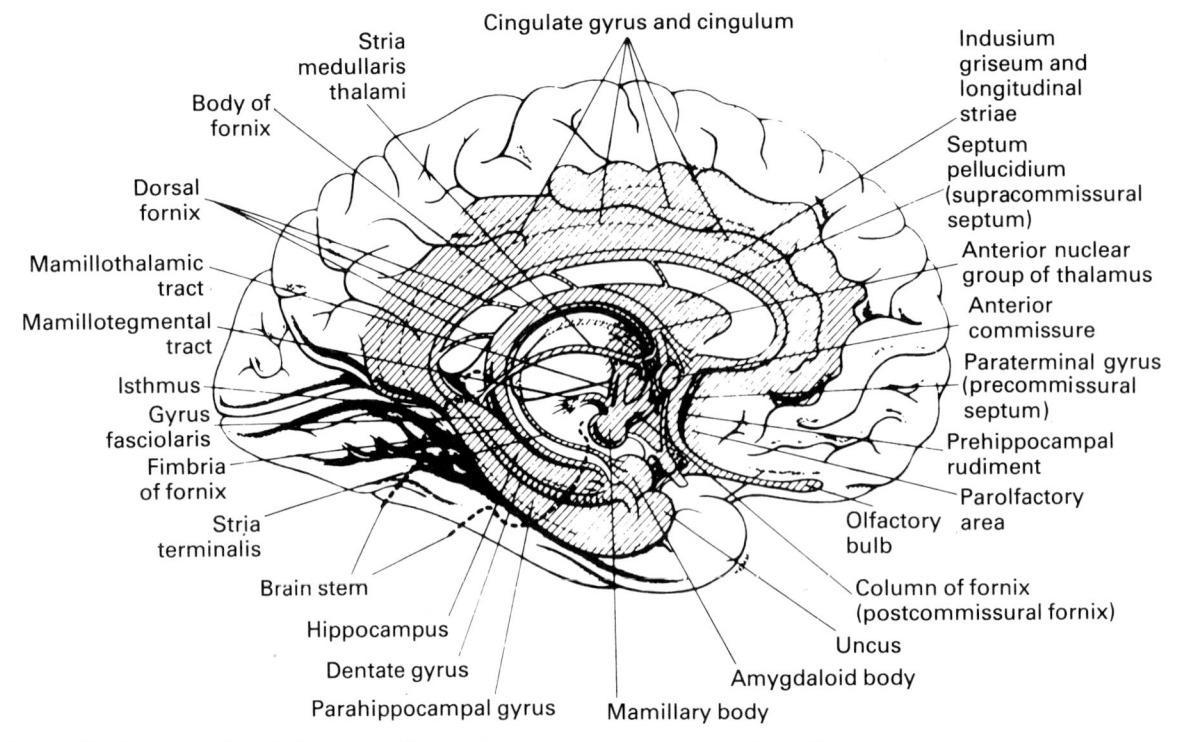

Figure 5.2 Anatomy of the limbic system illustrated by the shaded areas of the figure. [Reproduced from Warwick and Williams (1980) *Gray's Anatomy*, 35th British edn, by kind permission of the authors and publisher.]

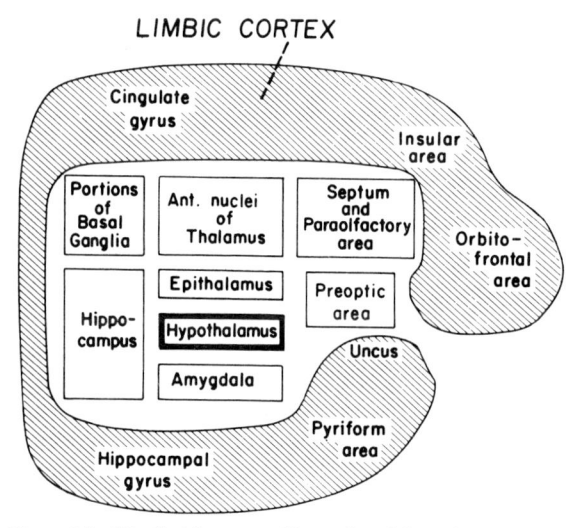

Figure 5.3 The limbic system. [Reproduced from Guyton (1981) *Textbook of Medical Physiology*, 6th edn, by kind permission of the author and publisher.]

previous rage reactions, while bilateral ablations of the orbitofrontal cortex may cause insomnia and motor restlessness. In man, cingulectomy and various other ablations of limbic cortex have been used as psychosurgical procedures for the treatment of obsessional states, hypersexuality and other behaviour disorders.

MEMORY

Types of memory and memory mechanisms

The recording and registration of information is a process known as memorizing. In clinical practice, memory is usually divided into short-term and long-term memory as well as secondary and tertiary varieties (Trimble, 1981). Short-term (or primary) memory is the ability to retain a few facts, words, numbers or letters (such as a telephone number or name and address) for a few seconds or a minute or more at a time. This information can be instantly recalled at will. Long-term memory is the storage in the brain of information which can be recalled minutes, hours, days, months or years later. Secondary memories are those long-term memories which are stored in the form of relatively weak memory traces so that some time may be needed to recall the information or else it can only be recalled for a few days after it has been recorded (recent memory). Tertiary memories, by contrast, are so deeply imprinted that they can be recalled at will throughout life (as in the case of the individual's own name, the letters of the alphabet, prime numerals, etc.).

The mechanism of short-term memory is still uncertain. The recall mechanism has been attributed to (a) activity in precisely defined reverberating neuronal circuits, (b) post-tetanic potentiation in appropriate neurons, and (c) prolonged depolarization of neurons with the production of electrotonic dendritic potentials. Long-term memory is thought to depend upon physical changes in synapses, giving rise to permanent changes in excitability of postsynaptic neurons in appropriate neuronal circuits, thus leading to progressive synaptic facilitation. A role for RNA and for glial cell activity in this process has been postulated but remains unproven. The repetition of information (rehearsal) and the coding of sensory stimuli into different classes of information assist the consolidation of long-term memories and the transfer of short-term into long-term memory. It now appears that while short-term memory involves the modification of pre-existing proteins by second messenger systems, long-term memory requires the expression of additional genes (Goelet et al., 1986).

The pathophysiology of memory

Clinical, behavioural and neuropathological evidence clearly indicates that the recording and registration of information occurs in the hippocampus and its connections, but that the *storage* of the memory trace (engram) plainly involves a considerable part of the limbic system. Severe loss of recent memory with inability to record and retain new impressions occurs as a consequence of lesions of the mammillary bodies in the Wernicke-Korsakov syndrome or after surgery. Remote memory is sometimes impaired in these subjects to a greater extent than is generally realized. Division of the fornix and extensive bilateral frontal lobe damage do not as a rule affect memory, while bilateral anterior cingulectomy produces only transient memory impairment. The effect of bilateral lesions of the thalamic dorsomedial nuclei in animals upon learning tasks may be more profound. In the 'split-brain' animal each hemisphere can be trained to store information so that the corpus callosum is not essential for information processing, storage and retrieval. However, after commissurotomy in man, some defects of memory have been found, suggesting that 'processes mediating the initial encoding of engrams and the retrieval and read-out of contralateral engram elements involve interhemispheric cooperation' (Zaidel and Sperry, 1974). Work carried out in flatworms has suggested that cellular RNA is involved in the memory process and that acquired information can be transferred to a worm that ingests RNA derived from one that has succeeded in learning a task. Much more work upon the transfer of memory by such chemical means has been done, with results which have often been conflicting. As Cooper et al (1982) have pointed out: 'There is evidence that protein and RNA synthesis may occur along with learning but the experiment has yet to be designed which explicitly relates these two events'.

In clinical practice, lesions of the anterior temporal lobe and particularly of the hippocampus have been the ones shown most often to impair memory. Investigations of temporal lobe epilepsy in man, involving electrical stimulation, have shown that memories could be evoked or temporary amnesia induced by hippocampal stimulation. Persistent, profound and generalized loss of recent memory has been reported in cases of bilateral hippocampal excision or infarction, the amnesia being unrelated to any deterioration of the intellect or personality of the subject. Cases of recent memory impairment have also been described after unilateral temporal lobe lesions, but it has been suggested that in such cases the corresponding area on the opposite side must previously have been damaged, and recent neuropathological studies have confirmed this hypothesis. The syndrome of transient global amnesia (see p. 107) is thought to result from bilateral temporal lobe ischaemia due to atherosclerosis or possibly, sometimes, migraine. The use of new and precise techniques of cognitive function, involving dichotic learning tasks and other methods of assessing auditory inattention, have shown that a unilateral defect of 'auditory memory' may follow unilateral anterior temporal lobectomy performed for temporal lobe epilepsy. Hence there is no doubt that bilateral hippocampal lesions are likely to cause permanent and continuing loss of memory for recent events. Such memory loss may be particularly prominent after recovery from herpes simplex encephalitis.

THE FUNCTIONS OF THE FRONTAL LOBE

In animals, experimental damage to the frontal cortex, which derives its thalamic input from the medial nuclear group, affects the ability of the animal to solve problems that depend upon the use of past experience. It has long been believed that the frontal lobes play a particularly important part in the control of intellect, initiative, personality and social consciousness. However, maximum amputation of the right or left frontal lobe produces little change except for some impairment of those processes necessary for planned initiative, sometimes with diminished inhibition of affective responses and a tendency to euphoria, less often with depression. Changes in psychomotor activity may take the form either of restlessness or lack of initiative and interest. The more automatic forms of intelligence are relatively well preserved, together with attention and memory, but the higher forms of reasoning, thinking in symbols and judgement may be impaired, especially after bilateral frontal lesions.

The operation of prefrontal leucotomy or lobotomy threw new light upon the functions of the frontal lobes, which have been summarized as follows:

According to Freeman and Watts, the prefrontal regions in man are concerned with foresight, imagination and the apperception of the self. These psychological functions are invested with emotion by way of the association fibres that link the hippocampus and cingulate gyrus with the thalamus and the hypothalamus. It would seem, then, that the functions of the prefrontal lobes are concerned with the adjustment of the personality as a whole to future contingencies. The imagination, therefore, in the pure sense of the term, may be said to reside in the prefrontal areas. Pure intellection in the sense of analysis, synthesis and selectivity does not appear to require the integrity of the frontal and prefrontal areas to the extent that was previously thought necessary.

Despite the virtual certainty that the frontal lobe is concerned with the storage and maintenance of certain social behaviour patterns, its exact functions are still poorly understood. Disturbances of micturition, including frequency, urgency and incontinence, are well recognized to occur in some patients with bifrontal lesions and less often as a consequence of a unilateral frontal tumour. The frontal lobes presumably possess a regulating function, shaping the development of intellectual resources and the pursuit of long-term goals. The effect upon personality of massive bifrontal lesions was well demonstrated by the celebrated case of Phineas Gage who in 1848 had a crowbar driven through the front of his skull. He was described as 'fitful, irreverent, indulging at times in the greatest profanity... manifesting but little deference for his fellows, impatient of restraint or advice when it conflicts with his desires, at times pertinaciously obstinate, yet capricious and vacillatory'. Thus, a 'frontal lobe syndrome' has come to be recognized. An affected individual previously capable of judgement and sustained application and organization of his life may thus become aimless and improvident, with loss of tact, sensitivity and self-control, and exhibiting impulsiveness and a failure to appreciate the consequences of reckless behaviour.

Destruction of the dorsomedial nuclei of the thalamus has been shown to produce effects similar to those of frontal leucotomy. The syndrome may follow stereotaxic surgery for parkinsonism. Since the efferent frontothalamic pathways are comparatively scanty, it has been suggested that leucotomy works by interrupting the afferent pathways from the dorsomedial nuclei to the frontal cortex and from the anteromedial nuclei to the cingulate gyri. Because the standard prefrontal operation all too often gave relief from stress at the cost of lethargy, social incompetence and other manifestations of the frontal lobe syndrome, it has been replaced by more selective procedures such as undercutting of the orbital cortex, cingulectomy, frontal tractotomy and various stereotaxic techniques which aim at producing relief of emotional tension or behaviour disorder with minimal effects upon intellect and personality.

BRAIN, MIND AND INTELLECT

Although the formulation of thoughts and the correlation and analysis of thought processes are clearly functions of the brain, we still know comparatively little of the ultimate mechanisms by which these important activities are controlled. *Memory*, as discussed earlier, is clearly the ability to record and to recall thoughts and sensorimotor experiences, while *learning* is the ability of the brain to store these memories and to utilize them at will. *Intellect* is the ability to analyse complex sensory information and to formulate abstract thoughts and concepts. This requires (a) the separation of complex sensory inputs into their constituent modalities, which may each be recorded in different areas of the cerebral cortex, (b) the analysis and interpretation of this information in relation to the content of the existing memory store, (c) the establishment of new memory engrams, and (d) the formulation of the appropriate abstract concept or thought, or alternatively of some physical activity which constitutes a response to the information received. These processes may lead to modification of subsequent responses to similar inputs in the light of the past experience. There are many diseases of the brain which involve both intellect and memory, but these two qualities may be disordered independently, or one may be affected more severely than the other, as a consequence of selective and focal cerebral lesions. Subsequent parts of this book will deal with some of the mechanisms and disease processes through which they are disordered.

HALLUCINATIONS AND ALLIED DISORDERS OF PERCEPTION

Hallucinations may be defined as mental impressions of sensory vividness occurring without external stimulus, but appearing to be located or to possess a cause located outside the subject. An *illusion* is defined as a misinterpretation of an external stimulus, but some illusions are closely related to hallucinations and occur as symptoms of hallucinatory states. A *delusion*, by contrast, is an idea or thought (such as a false concept of persecution) which has no substance in fact. In contrast to visual and auditory hallucinations, it is a pure thought process with no sensory content. Hallucinations and delusions may occur together in various toxic/confusional states and in psychotic illnesses such as schizophrenia. Though hallucinations manifest themselves as changes in the content of consciousness, there is considerable evidence that they are often the result of disordered function of the reticulo-hypothalamic and associated pathways concerned with the state of consciousness as a whole.

The principal circumstances in which hallucinations may occur are (1) in dreaming and the hypnagogic state (p. 85), (2) in disorders of sleep, (3) as a result of organic disease of the sense organs or of the central nervous system (including focal epilepsy), (4) in states of intoxication by alcohol and other drugs, and particularly after the administration of substances such as mescaline and lysergic acid or after withdrawal of alcohol, amphetamines, or barbiturates, and (5) in certain psychoses (especially schizophrenia).

Visual hallucinations may occur in patients suffering from severe visual loss as a result of disease of the eyes, such as a detached retina, or may appear as the 'phosphenes' or sparks of light which can result from mechanical distortion of the globe. These are largely illusory, but probably depend upon entrophic images from retinal ganglion cells which exceptionally reach perception. They may also result from lesions in any part of the visual pathways as well as elsewhere in the nervous system. Visual hallucinations have been attributed in the past to lesions of the anterior part of the visual system (including the optic tracts and radiation). While lesions in these areas can cause brief flashes of light, these phenomena are uncommon, and certainly anterior lesions do not cause 'formed' images (see below). When a hemianopia is present, the hallucinations may be seen in the normal half fields or in the blind half fields.

Hallucinations arising in the occipital striate cortex take the form of stars and static lights, those from the parastriate area coloured flashes or rings or, less often, a grey or black 'fog'. Those which arise from visual association areas in the parietal and temporal cortex are more complex and often formed, sometimes involving the evocation of visual memories of people, places or things. Hallucinations arising in the parietal region may be associated with visual agnosia, defective localization of images, perseveration of visual images, and errors in colour-naming or defective colour perception, while those of temporal lobe origin may be associated with auditory hallucinations. The latter, if originating in the primary auditory cortex, are crude and unformed sounds, but lesions of auditory association areas can reproduce auditory memories (music, well-recognized voices, etc.). Temporal lobe lesions not infrequently result in disorders of perception also in that objects look larger or smaller than normal and there may be similar alterations in auditory perception, feelings of unreality of the self and of the surroundings (depersonalization or jamais vu) or conversely feelings of intense familiarity with actual recall of previous experiences (déjà vu). In temporal lobe epilepsy it is often impossible to remember after the attack the actual familiar experience which was recalled. Visual hallucinations of the self have been described in which the individual feels that he is observing his own body from outside his physical self. This unusual phenomenon has some affinities with sensations of intense depersonalization.

Some recent neuropharmacological studies

Hallucinogenic drugs such as lysergic acid diethylamide (LSD) may produce their effects through an action upon the serotonergic system of neurons and especially upon those in the median raphe of the midbrain. The activation of raphe cells by either noradrenaline or serotonin (5-HT) applied electrophoretically in experimental animals can be blocked by LSD, either by inhibiting 5-HT release or by acting at the 5-HT receptor site in the postsynaptic membrane (Fig. 5.4). Monoamine oxidase inhibitors and tryptophan, as well as tricyclic antidepressant agents (imipramine, amitriptyline, and their derivatives), slow down the rate of discharge in median

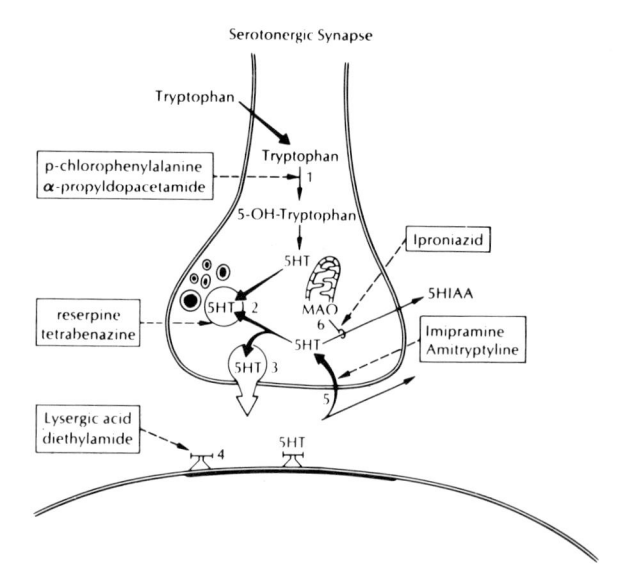

Figure 5.4 Schematic model of a central serotonergic neuron indicating possible sites of drug action.

Site 1: Enzymatic synthesis. Tryptophan is taken up into the serotonin-containing neuron and converted to 5-OH-tryptophan by the enzyme tryptophan hydroxylase. This enzyme can be effectively inhibited by p-chlorophenylalanine and α-propyldopacetamide. The next synthetic step involves the decarboxylation of 5-OH-tryptophan to form serotonin (5-HT).

Site 2: Storage. Reserpine and tetrabenazine interfere with the uptake-storage mechanism of the amine granules, causing a marked depletion of serotonin.

Site 3: Release. At present there is no drug available which selectively blocks the release of serotonin. However, lysergic acid diethylamide, owing to its ability to block or inhibit the firing of serotonin neurons, causes a reduction in the release of serotonin from the nerve terminals.

Site 4: Receptor interaction. Lysergic acid diethylamide acts as a partial agonist at serotonergic synapses in the CNS. A number of compounds have also been suggested to act as receptor-blocking agents at serotonergic synapses, but direct proof of these claims at present is lacking.

Site 5: Reuptake. Considerable evidence now exists which suggests that serotonin may have its action terminated by being taken up into the presynaptic terminal. The tricyclic drugs with a tertiary nitrogen, such as imipramine and amitryptyline, appear to be potent inhibitors of this uptake mechanism.

Site 6: Monoamine oxidase (MAO). Serotonin present in a free state within the presynaptic terminal can be degraded by the enzyme MAO, which appears to be located in the outer membrane of mitochondria. Iproniazid is an effective inhibitor of MAO.

[Reproduced from Cooper et al (1982) *The Biochemical Basis of Neuropharmacology*, 4th edn, by kind permission of the authors and publisher.]

raphe neurons. They may elevate brain 5-HT levels locally through inhibiting its reuptake. Patients with schizophrenia tend to have low monoamine oxidase activity in their platelets. It has been postulated that this may allow the plasma level of tryptamine to rise, thus producing abnormal amounts of dimethyltryptamine, which is known to be a hallucinogenic agent. The possible sequence of events and the actions of various drugs upon a serotonergic synapse are summarized in Fig. 5.4. Recently, evidence has accumulated to suggest that depression is associated with dysfunction of the hypothalamic-pituitary-adrenal axis and with a reduced availability of monoamines, principally noradrenaline and serotonin at several cerebral receptor sites (van Praag, 1982), while many of the physical accompaniments of anxiety are related to neurotransmitter release and can be relieved at least in part by β-adrenergic blockade (Braestrup and Nielsen, 1982). There are further complexities in that various dopaminergic drugs (except bromocriptine) which stimulate dopaminergic neurons have been shown to reproduce many of the symptoms of schizophrenia, in which disease increased numbers of cerebral dopamine receptors and reduced glutamic acid decarboxylase activity have also been reported (Bloom, 1985). The role of hypothalamic endorphins as putative transmitters in the limbic system with their powerful potential influences upon behaviour and memory has already been mentioned.

ABNORMALITIES OF MEMORY, MOOD, INTELLECT AND PERSONALITY

A detailed survey of the classification and differential diagnosis of mental disorders would be inappropriate in a commentary upon neurological pathophysiology. Nevertheless, so many mental symptoms can accompany or imitate organic brain disease that certain general principles must be set down against the background of the anatomical, physiological and pharmacological evidence discussed earlier in this chapter.

Some useful definitions

It was once thought that a neurosis, characterized by anxiety and related symptoms, resulting essentially from psychological causes, was different in both aetiology and prognosis from a psychosis, a term generally implying insanity and typified by a serious derangement of thought processes. It is now evident that the distinction between these two disorders is not absolute and that both neurotic and psychotic reactions can occur in response to organic disease. Amnesia implies loss of memory, while mental retardation or handicap (once called amentia, mental deficiency or oligophrenia) means defective development of intellectual function, and dementia disintegration of previously normal intellect resulting from organic brain disease. Abnormalities of personality and character are more difficult to define but include the shy and introverted or fanatical adherent of outlandish cults who is evidently different in personality from the norm, though not clearly abnormal, and who is often called schizoid, but more particularly the psychopath who, though not insane or mentally retarded, behaves in a socially abnormal manner. The term 'personality disorder' is now generally preferred in modern psychiatric terminology to the more traditional 'psychopathy'.

Affective disorders are characterized by abnormalities of mood or affect of which the most prominent are anxiety and depression. Cyclothymic individuals show excessive mood swings from states of elation verging upon mania to periods of intense depression with psychomotor retardation. The obsessive-compulsive syndrome is a variant of neurosis largely determined by constitutional factors in which insistent thoughts so occupy the patient's mind that they may compel him to perform compulsive acts which he knows are foolish or unnecessary but which he cannot resist. Hypochondriasis, a state of intense introspection in which the patient is preoccupied with his own bodily symptoms, shows many affinities with obsessional neurosis. Hysteria is a common psychiatric reaction in which there are symptoms or signs often mimicking physical disease (loss of voice, blindness, or paralysis) which are not caused by organic pathological change but which are actuated by the desire to obtain real or imagined profit from the symptoms or to escape from stress.

The schizophrenic reaction is often characterized by introversion, severe distortion of thought processes, auditory hallucinations, and paranoid features commonly involving ideas of persecution. The disorder is constitutional and not usually a consequence of exogenous factors.

The assessment of mental changes in cerebral lesions

Many neuropsychological and psychometric tests are available for the assessment of memory, intellect, mood and personality and for the identification of specific defects of speech and perception. Methods of identifying aphasia, apraxia and agnosia have been described previously (see p. 64). The Wechsler intelligence scale for children (WISC) is particularly useful in childhood for identifying, through a discrepancy between verbal and performance intelligence quotients (IQ), defects in the acquisition of motor skills (developmental apraxia), and the measurement of Schonell's 'reading age' is valuable in cases of suspected dyslexia. The Wechsler adult intelligence scale (WAIS) is valuable in identifying early intellectual impairment in cases of presumed dementia and also gives a reasonable assessment of the patient's premorbid IQ. The ability to calculate can be tested by asking the patient to subtract serial 7's from 100.

In examining memory the patient is asked to remember a series of numbers (normally one can recall at least 7 digits forwards and 5 backwards) and recall a name, an address and the name of a flower. These are tests for short-term memory. In testing remote memory the patient is asked for details of his schooling, marriage, children, etc., and for the names of prime ministers or US presidents.

Disorders of personality, emotion and thought processes are more complex. Tests such as the Minnesota Personality Inventory (MMPI) or the Cattell are useful in assessing personality and emotional traits (extraversion, introversion, anxiety, depression, psychopathy). In psychotic states such as schizophrenia the patient sometimes gives concrete interpretations of proverbs, which are intended to be interpreted in an abstract manner. Interpretations of the Rorschach ink-blot test are of greater relevance to psychiatry than to neurology.

Amnesia

Bilateral temporal lobe disease or resection may seriously impair memory. Severe memory loss is characterized particularly by an inability to record, retain and recall recent impressions with comparative sparing of the memory for remote events. Very many metabolic, traumatic, neoplastic, inflammatory and degenerative diseases of the brain may be associated with memory loss. A few of the more specific syndromes are described below.

Transient global amnesia

This syndrome is believed to be due to transient ischaemia in one or both temporal lobes as it is usually of sudden onset in middle-aged or elderly individuals with evidence of cerebral atherosclerosis. Memory loss for recent events develops rapidly. Despite their inability to register new impressions, the patients retain their personal identity, and show no abnormality of behaviour apart from anxiety and no evidence of impaired perception. Recovery is usually complete within a few hours, and retrograde amnesia shrinks rapidly, leaving the patient with no disability other than amnesia for the events occurring in the attack itself.

The Korsakov syndrome

This disorder is sometimes called the 'amnestic syndrome' or the 'Wernicke–Korsakov syndrome' because of its common association with Wernicke's encephalopathy. It is usually due to vitamin B_1 (thiamine) deficiency and is most commonly observed in alcoholic subjects. More rarely the Korsakov syndrome may complicate other metabolic and infective illnesses. Loss of neurons and demyelination with gliosis, capillary proliferation and occasional haemorrhages are found predominantly in the thalamus, mamillary bodies and midbrain. There is characteristically a striking loss of the ability to record and retain new impressions. At one minute the patient appears alert and his conversation is lucid, but within a moment or two he will have forgotten the interview completely. The memory of his remote past may be intact. As a result he becomes disorientated, certainly in time and often in place, and in order to conceal this memory defect he confabulates. For instance, he will describe in detail fantastic activities which he claims to have carried out some few hours or days earlier, though he may never have left his bed. Usually his descriptions have some basis in fact in the remote past, but he is utilizing these previous experiences to fill in the recent period for which his memory is defective.

Hysterical amnesia

Psychological as well as physical causes can seriously impair memory. In hysterical amnesia the patient may have no recollection whatever of his identity, of his address, or of any other details concerning himself despite apparent alertness. The condition is presumably due to some process of psychological inhibition resulting in an inability to reopen voluntarily the pathways where memories are retained. Usually the condition develops acutely as a method of escape from undue stress. Hysterical amnesia may be feigned as a defence against a criminal charge and can then be difficult to distinguish from the genuine disorder.

Disorders of mood

The neural basis of emotion and the integration of the accompanying bodily changes have already been discussed. It is to disorders of this mechanism and of its relationship with higher levels of the nervous system that we must look for the explanation of disorders of mood occurring as a result of organic nervous disease. For more detailed commentaries upon disorders of mood and emotion consequent upon affective and psychotic disorders the reader is referred to textbooks of psychiatry. Such conditions will be mentioned here only in so far as they enter into the differential diagnosis of those mood changes which occur in organic nervous disease.

Emotional instability

Emotional instability or lability is a common symptom of nervous diseases, especially of those in which the lesions are diffuse. The patient is easily moved by almost any form of emotion. He is quickly irritated or angered, easily becomes apprehensive, and is readily depressed or reduced to tears. Less often, he experiences pleasurable emotion with abnormal facility and is readily moved to laughter. Emotional instability of this kind is commonly encountered after head injury, after massive cerebral infarction, and in patients with diffuse cerebral arteriosclerosis. It is frequently present in the early stages of dementia, however produced, and is characteristic of the later stages of multiple sclerosis. This exaggerated emotional activity appears to result from impairment of the control which higher levels of the nervous system normally exercise over the thalamus and hypothalamus.

Impulsive disorders of conduct

The emotional instability described above does not usually lead to disorders of conduct, perhaps because conduct is normally more strongly inhibited than feeling. Exceptionally, however, impairment of higher control releases emotions which pass into action. This most often happens in children or adolescents in whom the control of impulsive action is as yet incomplete. Misdemeanours and acts of violence are sometimes committed by children and adolescents who have suffered disorders causing diffuse brain damage. Similar acts may be committed by aggressive psychopaths, and rarely by epileptics, either before an epileptic attack or in the phase of postepileptic automatism, or even in the intervals between attacks. Such acts of aggression seem most likely to occur in patients with temporal lobe lesions.

Apathy

A general loss of emotional responsiveness without a proportionate intellectual deterioration was once most characteristically seen in association with parkinsonism due to encephalitis lethargica. In view of the known predilection of the virus of this disease for the diencephalic grey matter, it was reasonable to attribute the apathy to injury to the posterior hypothalamus. A similar picture is associated with mental deterioration in the later stages of dementia from any cause. Here it is probable that the apathy is in part, at least, secondary to the deterioration of thought and perception. However, apathy may also be observed in many forms of organic encephalopathy, degenerative brain diseases, and some psychotic disorders, especially severe melancholia and schizophrenia. The apathetic patient loses all his former interests and affects and, lacking the drive of the instinctive life, becomes incapable of effort and sinks into a vegetative existence.

EUPHORIA

Euphoria is the term used to indicate a mood characterized by feelings of cheerfulness and happiness and a sense of mental well-being. Transitory euphoria is induced in many people by the consumption of alcohol. As a prevailing mood it is seen most characteristically in multiple sclerosis. Some sufferers from this disease remain persistently serene and happy in spite of their increasing physical disabilities. Euphoria is also encountered occasionally in patients with intracranial tumours, especially when the tumour is situated in the temporal lobe or, less frequently, in the frontal lobe or corpus callosum. Its psychophysiological basis is little understood.

EXCITEMENT

Excitement is a term somewhat loosely applied to several forms of mental overactivity, which may predominantly involve the intellectual, emotional or psychomotor spheres. All three may be affected together, as in acute mania, characterized by flight of ideas, elation and psychomotor restlessness. Disordered ideas may be linked with excitement in some delirious and confusional states, and in catatonic schizophrenia. Delirium was defined above as confusion with an overlay of excitement. Psychomotor restlessness is associated with anxiety in agitated depression, and the prevailing mood may be one of rage in the outbursts of aggressive psychopaths. There is some evidence that states of excitement can be caused by lesions of the anterior hypothalamus.

DEPRESSION

Depression may be regarded as the converse of euphoria. It is a mood of dejection and gloom for which frequently the patient can offer no explanation. It is encountered in a variety of states. It may be a reaction to an adequate external cause, such as failure or bereavement, or a neurotic reaction to personal difficulties (reactive depression). In sufferers from cyclothymia, depression is liable to occur as a recurrent disorder of mood, sometimes alternating with phases of excitement, though often these are no more than a mild general sense of elation. In cyclothymic individuals the depression is likely to be associated with psychomotor retardation, manifesting itself in a difficulty in concentrating, and with insomnia and loss of appetite. Such patients typically wake early and feel at their worst in the early part of the day. Depression also occurs as the predominant feature of endogenous depression or involutional melancholia, in which it may be associated with agitation. Patients suffering from psychotic depression in a severe form often have delusions of guilt or of a hypochondriacal nature. Individuals with endogenous depression frequently have physical symptoms including headache, fatigue, and facial and/or limb or low back pain. Whereas it was once believed that reactive depression on the one hand and the endogenous disorder on the other were distinct disorders, it is now known that there is considerable overlap between the two, as a depressive illness with all of the features of the endogenous disorder is sometimes precipitated and is certainly accentuated by exogenous factors. Depression is also a mood which is common in patients suffering from organic disease of the brain, sometimes as a natural reaction to their disabilities. It is particularly common in individuals of a cyclothymic temperament in whom the nervous disease may be regarded as having released a pre-existing tendency to depression.

ANXIETY

Fear is the emotional reaction to an imminent danger; anxiety is the reaction to a possible future danger—fear linked with anticipation. Anxiety may be produced in a variety of ways. It can be a normal emotional reaction. It may be the effect of certain toxins which appear to stimulate directly the nervous centres concerned. It can also be induced by drugs which have a stimulating effect upon the sympathetic nervous system, namely adrenaline, noradrenaline, ephedrine, amphetamine, nicotine and thyroxine. Anxiety may be the prevailing mood in patients suffering from organic disease of the brain, as after head injury, and is then probably due in part to diminished control of emotional reactions by higher centres. Fear may be very evident in delirious states, when it appears as a reaction to terrifying hallucinations. It may also be linked with depression in involutional melancholia. In many cases, however, anxiety is neurotic—that is, it is the product of unconscious mental processes.

Mental retardation (handicap)

Mental retardation or handicap implies an intellectual deficit which is present from birth and can be confirmed by psychometric testing, by means of which the intelligence quotient (IQ) and 'mental age' of the patient are assessed. The severely retarded are incapable of guarding themselves against common dangers and must usually be confined in institutions. Moderately retarded individuals are also incapable of managing themselves or their affairs, but are occasionally able to live satisfactorily in a protected domestic environment and may even be able to do work of a simple nature. Patients with mild mental retardation, some of whom have IQs approaching the lower normal limit of 80, are common and mostly live outside institutions. Some can be educated in ordinary schools but others must attend schools for the educationally subnormal. The diagnosis of mild retardation can readily be overlooked and the patient is often regarded as being 'rather stupid', 'incapable of giving a reasonable history' and 'hypochondriacal'. Character or personality defects are common in mentally retarded patients, and many habitual petty criminals, prostitutes, sexual offenders, and murderers fall into this group.

In many severely and moderately retarded individuals there are associated congenital abnormalities involving other organs, and epilepsy or signs of cerebral palsy may co-exist. Mongolism (Down's syndrome) is one of the more common syndromes. Several other conditions causing mental retardation are, like Down's syndrome, associated with chromosomal abnormalities. Sometimes mental retardation is a result of an inborn error of metabolism affecting the nervous system but often it appears to be due to a combination of genetic influences and not to a single factor or to any definable physical or metabolic disease.

Over fifty metabolic disorders, some common and some rare, and many involving amino acid metabolism, have been recognized in association with mental retardation. An example is phenylpyruvic oligophrenia (phenylketonuria). Careful biochemical screening of infants with suspected retardation is paying increasing dividends, although approximately 50% of cases remain unexplained (non-specific mental retardation).

Dementia

Dementia, or progressive disintegration of the intellect, the memory, and the powers of abstract thought, is a disorder of the mind which results from organic disease and generally from physical or metabolic disturbances affecting the brain. The first sign of a dementing process may be an error of judgement incompatible with the patient's previous ability, or a failure to grasp all the facts of a difficult situation. It may simply be said that Mr X is 'losing his grip'. Subsequently, memory, particularly for recent events, becomes impaired so that the patient is forgetful and unable to concentrate, and his attention wanders freely. Increasing emotional lability with inappropriate laughing or crying or with irritability and irrational impulsive acts may follow, and striking changes in mood, taking the form of elation in some cases and apathy in others, often occur. By the time the patient becomes neglectful of his personal appearance and dirty in his habits, the diagnosis is usually obvious, but in the earlier stages it is much more difficult to make. Increasing unpunctuality and neglect of detail are common. Aphasia, apraxia and/or agnosia occur in some cases. It is nevertheless remarkable how often patients with advancing dementia continue to hold responsible jobs, despite increasing so-called 'eccentricity', until some major error of judgement or faux pas brings matters to a head. In the late stages delusions occasionally occur, taking the form of grandiose imaginings ('I am the King of Spain') or ideas of hostility or persecution towards relatives or business associates. Progressive dementing processes must be distinguished from reversible toxic or other confusional states due, for example, to metabolic disorders or subdural haematoma, and from the pseudodementia which may be seen in severe endogenous depression or, rarely, in hysteria. Many forms of organic brain disease give rise to dementia. Most are progressive and incurable, but others (such as those associated with myxoedema, vitamin B_{12} deficiency or neurosyphilis) are eminently treatable and may show no very specific clinical features, so remediable causes should always be borne in mind.

References

Agranoff, B. W. (1975) Biochemical strategies in the study of memory formation. In Tower, D. B. (ed.): Nervous System. Volume 1 in Brady, R. O. (ed.): *The Basic Neurosciences*. New York: Raven Press, 1975.

Andrew, J., and Nathan, P. W. (1964) Lesions of the anterior frontal lobes and disturbances of micturition and defecation. *Brain* **87**: 233.

Barbizet, J. (1963) Defect of memorizing of hippocampal-mammillary origin: a review. *J. Neurol. Neurosurg. Psychiat.* **26**: 127.

Bloom, F. (1985) Neurotransmitter diversity and its functional significance. *J. Roy. Soc. Med.* **78**: 189.

Bond, M. R. (1972) Psychosurgery. In Critchley, M., O'Leary, J. L. and Jennett, W. B. (eds): *Scientific Foundations of Neurology*. London: Heinemann.

Braestrup, C. and Nielsen, Y. (1982) Anxiety. *Lancet* **ii**: 1030.

Brierley, J. B. (1966) The neuropathology of amnesic states. In Whitty, C. W. M., and Zangwill, O. L. (eds.): *Amnesia*. London: Butterworth.

Cooper, J. B., Bloom, F. E. and Roth, R. H. (1982) *The Biochemical Basis of Neuropharmacology*, 4th edn. Oxford: Oxford University Press.

Eadie, M. J. and Tyrer, J. H. (1980) *Anticonvulsant Therapy: Pharmacological Basis and Practice*, 2nd edn. Edinburgh: Churchill Livingstone.

Gellis, S. S. and Feingold, M. (1968) *Atlas of Mental Retardation Syndromes*. Washington, DC: U.S. Department of Health.

Goelet, P., Castelluci, V. S., Schacher, S. and Kandel, E. R. (1986) The long and the short of long-term memory—a molecular framework. *Nature* **322**: 419.

Guyton, A. C. (1981) *Textbook of Medical Physiology*, 6th edn Philadelphia: W. B. Saunders Company.

Humphrey, M. E. (1972) Personality. In Critchley, M., O'Leary, J. L. and Jennett, W. B. (eds) *Scientific Foundations of Neurology*. London: Heinemann.

Isaacson, R. L. (1974) *The Limbic System*. New York: Plenum Press.

Lhermitte, J. (1951) *Les Hallucinations*. Paris: Doin.

Menkes, J. L. (1974) *A Textbook of Child Neurology*. Philadelphia: Lea & Febiger.

Meyer, A. (1974) The frontal lobe syndrome, the aphasias and related conditions—a contribution to the history of cortical localization. *Brain* **97**: 565.

Papez, J. W. (1937) A proposed mechanism of emotion. *Arch. Neurol. Psychiat.* **38**: 725.

Penfield, W. and Mathieson, G. (1974) Memory. Autopsy findings and comments on the role of hippocampus in experiential recall. *Arch. Neurol.* **31**: 145.

Smythies, J. R. (1970) *Brain Mechanisms and Behavior*. New York: Academic Press.

Strub, R. L. and Black, F. W. (1977) *The Mental Status Examination in Neurology*. Philadelphia: F. A. Davis Company.

Trimble, M. R. (1981) *Neuropsychiatry*. Chichester and New York: John Wiley and Sons.

van Praag, H. M. (1982) Depression. *Lancet* **ii**: 1259.

Walton, J. N. (1985) *Brain's Diseases of the Nervous System*, 9th edn. Oxford: Oxford University Press.

Wells, C. E. (ed.) (1977) *Dementia*, 2nd edn (Contemporary Neurology Series, vol. 15). Philadelphia: F. A. Davis Company.

Zaidel, D. and Sperry, R. W. (1974) Memory impairment after commissurotomy in man. *Brain* **97**: 263.

6

THE AUTONOMIC NERVOUS SYSTEM AND HYPOTHALAMUS

INTRODUCTION

The activity of the autonomic nervous system is largely concerned with the control of visceral activity. Its influences are widespread, affecting the cardiac rhythm and output, respiration, blood vessel tone, the behaviour of the hollow viscera of the alimentary and urogenital systems, as well as the secretion of the ducted and ductless (endocrine) glands. Many of these activities are automatic and reflexly controlled, but little influenced by the will. This is fortunate, for many of them are too vital to allow any interference from the capricious behaviour of the mind. The combined activities of the autonomic nerves and of the endocrine glands maintain the constant internal thermal and biochemical environment of the body, a function which Cannon entitled homeostasis. The visceral functions of the autonomic nervous system are diverse in organ distribution and in effect and do not fall exclusively within the domain of any one specialty area of medicine. There are nevertheless many ways in which disease of the central or peripheral nervous system can affect autonomic activity, and accurate interpretation of the abnormalities so produced may be invaluable in diagnosis. A basic knowledge of the distribution of these nerves within the body, and of their function, is necessary for these principles to be rationally applied. The functions of the more peripheral parts of this complex system will be considered before those more centrally placed in the cerebral cortex and hypothalamus.

ANATOMY AND PHYSIOLOGY

The autonomic nervous system can be divided into two principal components: the sympathetic system and the parasympathetic system (Figs. 6.1 and 6.2). These two systems are generally antagonistic, for where one excites the other inhibits.

Activity of the sympathetic system produces dilatation of the pupil and slight protrusion of the eye, increased cardiac output with tachycardia, dilatation of the bronchioles, vasoconstriction of skin vessels but dilatation of the coronary and intramuscular arteries, sweating, inhibition of intestinal movement, closure of vesical and rectal sphincters, and erection of hairs (the pilomotor effect) on the skin. The individual is thus prepared for action in response to an emergency, termed the 'fight or flight' response. Most terminal sympathetic fibres are adrenergic, i.e. (a) they produce their effects upon smooth muscle or other tissues by secreting noradrenaline at their nerve endings, and (b) their effects can be largely reproduced by an increase in the amount of circulating adrenaline or noradrenaline in the blood. There are exceptions to this rule. A few sympathetic fibres, particularly those which innervate the sweat glands (sudomotor fibres), are cholinergic, i.e. they produce their effects by secreting acetylcholine at the effector organ. In skeletal muscle, there are a few adrenergic fibres which cause constriction of intramuscular blood vessels, but many more cholinergic fibres which cause dilatation.

Activity of the parasympathetic system gives constriction of the pupil, slowing of the heart and a diminished cardiac output, constriction of the bronchioles, increased intestinal peristalsis, evacuation of the bladder and bowels, and increased

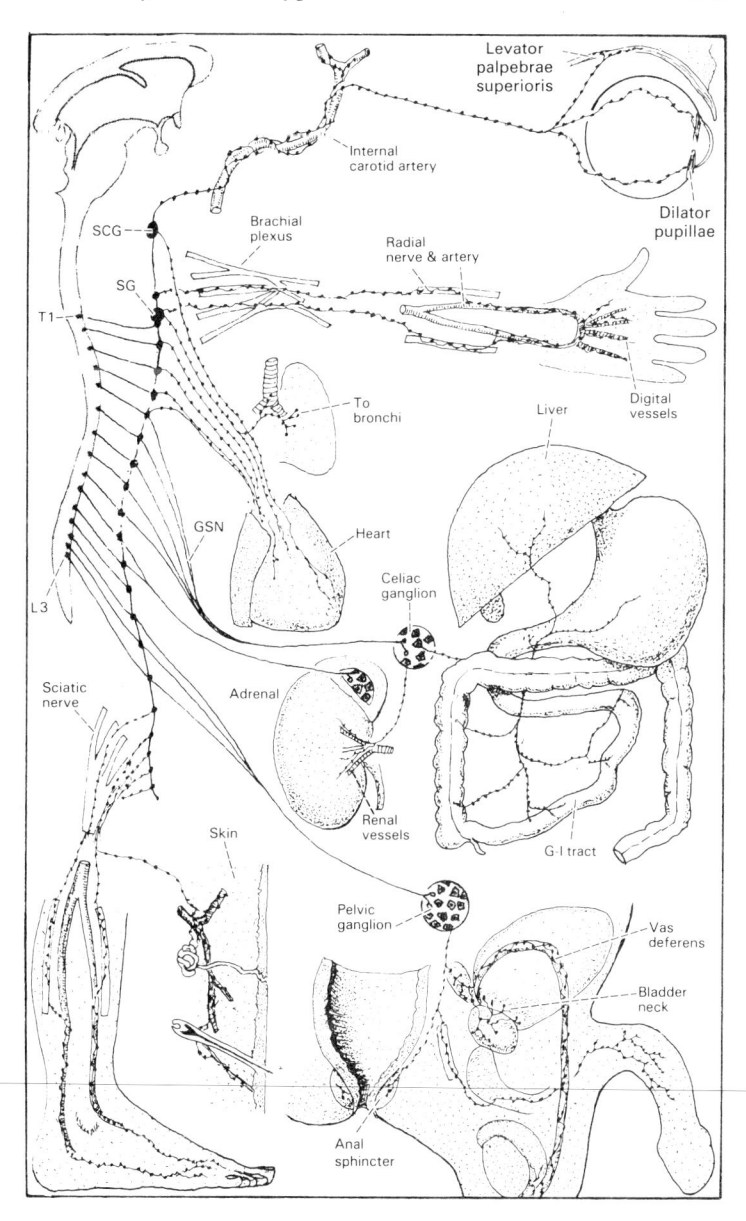

Figure 6.1 Plan of the sympathetic nervous system. GSN, greater splanchnic nerve; SCG, superior cervical ganglion; SG, stellate ganglion.

secretory activity of the salivary and lacrimal glands. The parasympathetic system also plays a principal role in sexual activity, including erection of the penis and probably orgasm in the female. However, ejaculation in the male is controlled by the sympathetic system, and female orgasm is largely a psychological phenomenon with no easily identifiable neurological substrate. Parasympathetic fibres are mainly cholinergic, responding physiologically to the secretion of acetylcholine at the receptor site.

Chemical transmission in the autonomic system

Acetylcholine and noradrenaline are normally released locally at autonomic nerve endings. All preganglionic fibres, both sympathetic and parasympathetic, are cholinergic. In addition, as mentioned, sympathetic activity is influenced by the levels of circulating noradrenaline and adrenaline, much of which is secreted by the adrenal medulla (see p. 12). These biogenic amines, and acetylcholine, produce their effects upon the organs whose activities they influence by combining with receptor sites which lie in close relationship to the nerve endings. Much of the recent progress in our understanding of the autonomic nervous system has been based on studies of the distribution, function and specificity of these receptors.

Acetylcholine receptors are of two types, described by their selective responses to two agents: (a) the so-called *muscarinic receptors*, which are found in all effector cells stimulated by parasympathetic postganglionic neurons (and in cholinergic endings of the sympathetic system), and (b) *nicotinic receptors*, found especially in the neuromuscular junctions of skeletal muscle but also at synapses in the sympathetic and parasympathetic ganglia themselves. Similarly, adrenergic receptors are of two types: (a) alpha receptors, which are stimulated mainly by noradrenaline and which are concerned especially with vasoconstriction, dilatation of the iris, intestinal relaxation, and pilomotor contraction in the skin, and (b) beta receptors, which are stimulated more particularly by adrenaline, and to a lesser extent by noradrenaline and which are responsible for an increased heart rate, vasodilatation of intramuscular blood vessels, intestinal relaxation, uterine relaxation, and bronchodilatation.

The rational use of many therapeutic agents depends upon an understanding of receptor specificity and function in the autonomic nervous system (Tables 1 and 2, pp. 13 and 14). For example, various parasympathomimetic drugs such as pilocarpine and methacholine have a muscarinic effect, whereas others such as neostigmine are essentially nicotinic. Atropine will block the muscarinic effects but not the nicotinic effects of such drugs. Similarly, the activities of sympathomimetic drugs, including adrenaline, ephedrine and methoxamine, depend upon their relative affinities for alpha and beta receptors. Guanethidine may block the release of noradrenaline from sympathetic nerve terminals. Phenoxybenzamine or phentolamine block the alpha receptors, and propranolol blocks beta receptors of the sympathetic nervous system with a high degree of selectivity.

Cerebral control

Parts of the cerebral cortex exercise a controlling influence upon autonomic activity, but the exact areas of the cerebrum concerned and the mechanisms by which they produce their influence in man are not fully defined. Parts of the prefrontal cortex are clearly of importance. In primates, respiratory and vasomotor changes can be evoked by stimulation of Brodmann's area 13 (the posterior insula), and bilateral excision of the posterior parts of area 14 (the arterial insula) causes 'sham rage'. In man, pathways descend to the hypothalamus from the hippocampus, amygdala, prefrontal cortex and cingulate gyrus, all of which are probably concerned with autonomic activity.

Lesions of the cingulate gyrus reduce emotional reactions and are sometimes produced therapeutically in the operation of cingulotomy. Stimulation of the prefrontal cortex may provoke sweating in the opposite arm and leg. The voluntary act of evacuation of the bladder and bowels seems to be initiated in the paracentral lobules of the hemispheres, although the so-called pontine bladder centre also plays a part. Probably, motor impulses from these areas, destined to activate the appropriate parasympathetic nerves, travel downwards with the corticospinal tract. These are but a few examples of cerebral control which future research will almost certainly demonstrate to be much more varied and extensive.

Hypothalamic control

The most important cell stations from which visceral and other autonomic activity are finally controlled lie in the hypothalamus. Nuclei in this area receive fibres from the 'visceral' areas of cerebral cortex mentioned above and in turn give rise to descending pathways which enter the brain stem and spinal cord. The nuclei of the hypothalamus and the functions which they control are shown diagrammatically in Fig. 6.3. The hypothalamic nuclei not only exert important controlling influences upon all autonomic activity but certain nuclei also control secretion from the posterior pituitary, to which, through the infundibulum and tuber cinereum, they are closely related anatomically. They also secrete small polypeptide hormones which control the release of hormones from the anterior pituitary. For example, the cells of the supraoptic nuclei form antidiuretic hormone (ADH) and its precursors, which then travel down the axons into the posterior lobe of the pituitary, being stored there in the form of neurosecretory granules. Similarly, oxytocin, which stimulates contraction of the lactating mammary gland and of the pregnant uterus, is formed in the paraventricular nucleus and is then conveyed to the posterior pituitary. Although the anterior pituitary is not under direct nervous control, humoral substances (mainly polypeptides) secreted by hypothalamic neurons are conveyed to the anterior pituitary through the vessels of the hypophysial venous system, thus exciting gonadotrophic, adrenocorticotrophic, somatotrophic, lactogenic and thyrotrophic hormonal secretion. The posterior lobe (the neurohypophysis), unlike the anterior, receives a direct neural input from the paraventricular nucleus concerned with autonomic activity, and from the supraoptic nucleus, which is primarily involved in the production of ADH or argenine vasopressin. In each of these ways the hypothalamic nuclei exert a powerful influence upon the endocrine system. In general, the anterior nuclei are particularly concerned with parasympathetic activity and with controlling the pituitary gland. The posterior nuclei, by contrast, influence sympathetic

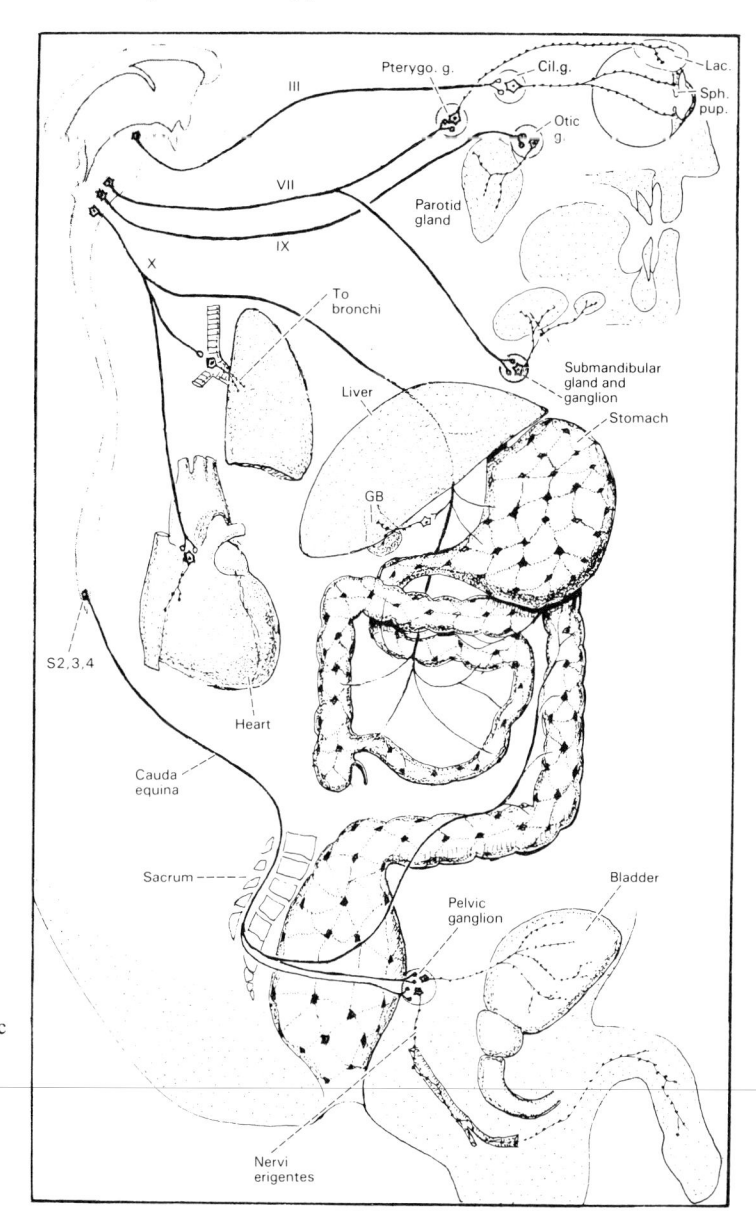

Figure 6.2 Plan of the parasympathetic nervous system. III, oculomotor nerve; VII, facial nerve; IX, glossopharyngeal nerve; X, vagus nerve; Cil. g., ciliary ganglion; Otic g., otic ganglion; Lac., lacrimal gland; Pterygo. g., pterygopalatine ganglion; Sph. pup., sphincter pupillae.

activity; lesions of this area can give rise to emotional disturbances such as 'sham rage' in animals, or conversely to lethargy and hypersomnia. Temperature regulation, control of the emotions, and control of sleep are also mediated through hypothalamic nuclei. The mamillary bodies, which form a part of the hypothalamic system are important in relation to memory function. Lesions in this area may prevent the patient from recording new impressions, a feature typically seen in the Korsakov syndrome.

Pathways descend from the hypothalamus to control sympathetic and parasympathetic activity. Sympathetic fibres are directed to the dorsal portion of the spinal cord to end in relation to cells in the intermediolateral horn of grey matter. The parasympathetic fibres end in the nuclei of the oculomotor, facial, glossopharyngeal and vagus nerves, and in the sacral portion of the spinal cord. No central autonomic fibres travel directly to any viscus. In each case a ganglion which lies outside the central nervous system is interposed. As a result there are always preganglionic fibres arising within the central nervous system and postganglionic fibres originating in the ganglia. The ganglia of the sympathetic nerves lie lateral to the vertebral bodies and with connecting fibres form the sympathetic chain. The postganglionic fibres are therefore long in order to reach effector organs. In contrast, many parasympathetic

POSTERIOR

Posterior hypothalamus
(Increased blood pressure)
(Pupillary dilatation)
(Shivering)
(Corticotrophin)

Dorsomedial nucleus
(GI stimulation)

Perifornical nucleus
(Hunger)
(Increased blood pressure)
(Rage)

Ventromedial nucleus
(Satiety)

Mamillary body
(Feeding reflexes)

Lateral hypothalamic area (not shown)
(Thirst & hunger)

ANTERIOR

Paraventricular nucleus
(Oxytocin release)
(Water conservation)

Medial preoptic area
(Bladder contraction)
(Decreased heart rate)
(Decreased blood pressure)

Supraoptic nucleus
(Water conservation)

Optic chiasm

Infundibulum

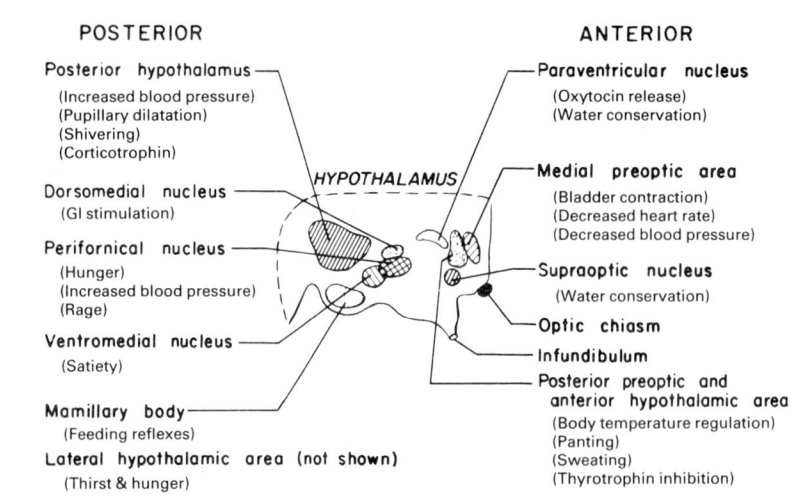

Posterior preoptic and anterior hypothalamic area
(Body temperature regulation)
(Panting)
(Sweating)
(Thyrotrophin inhibition)

Figure 6.3 Autonomic control centres of the hypothalamus. [Reproduced from Guyton (1981) *Textbook of Medical Physiology*, 5th edn., by kind permission of the author and publisher.]

ganglia are situated close to the effector organ, so that the preganglionic fibres are long and the postganglionic short.

The general principles of autonomic innervation are illustrated in Figs. 6.4 and 6.5. The anatomy of the sympathetic pre- and postganglionic fibres is illustrated in more precise detail in Fig. 6.6, and that of the parasympathetic system in Fig. 6.7. The innervation and function of major autonomic effectors are summarized in Table 8.

The sympathetic nervous system

Preganglionic medullated sympathetic fibres (white rami) originate from the intermediolateral horn of grey matter in each segment of the spinal cord from the first thoracic to the second lumbar (Fig. 6.5). [While it has been suggested recently that many (possibly even a half) of all preganglionic fibres are unmyelinated, it is still reasonable to refer to them as 'white rami'.] These fibres then pass laterally to the sympathetic chain (Fig. 6.6), in which there are ganglia corresponding to each of the segments of the cord from which the sympathetic fibres arise. From these ganglia non-medullated postganglionic fibres (grey rami) join the corresponding somatic spinal nerve and are distributed to the blood vessels and skin of the appropriate dermatome. Fibres also extend the chain up to three cervical ganglia [superior, middle, and inferior or stellate (the stellate ganglion is actually constituted by fusion of the inferior cervical and first thoracic ganglia)] and downwards to four lumbar ganglia on each side. There is no direct sympathetic outflow from the spinal cord in either the cervical or lower lumbar region. The thoracic and abdominal viscera receive a sympathetic supply through postganglionic fibres of the thoracic ganglia. These fibres form the splanchnic nerves and the coeliac, mesenteric and hypogastric plexuses. The sympathetic innervation of the hand and neck and of the upper limbs comes from the cervical ganglia. Fibres travelling to the cranium traverse the inferior and middle cervical ganglia to synapse with nerve cells in the superior cervical ganglion. From there, postganglionic fibres enter or overlie the cranium in the coats of the internal and external carotid arteries and

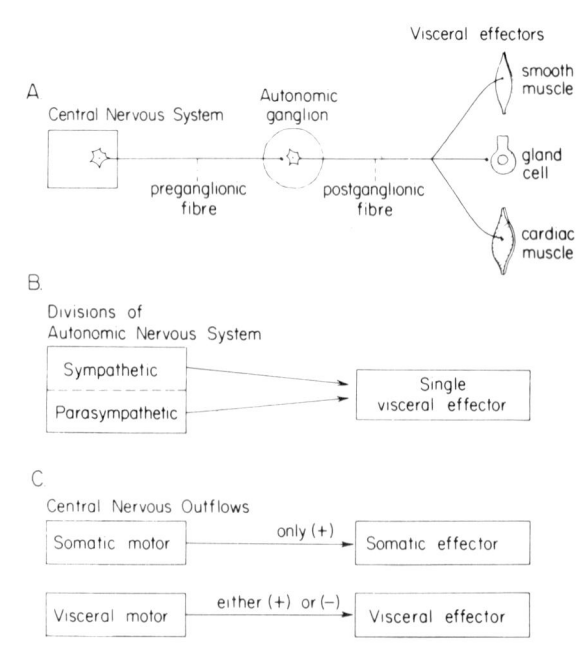

Figure 6.4 General principles of autonomic innervation. A, Overview of the innervation of visceral effectors. B, Dual innervation of visceral effector. C, Contrast between somatic motor outflows and visceral motor outflows. (Reproduced from Patton et al. (1976) *Introduction to Basic Neurology*, by kind permission of the authors and publisher.)

The autonomic nervous system and hypothalamus 117

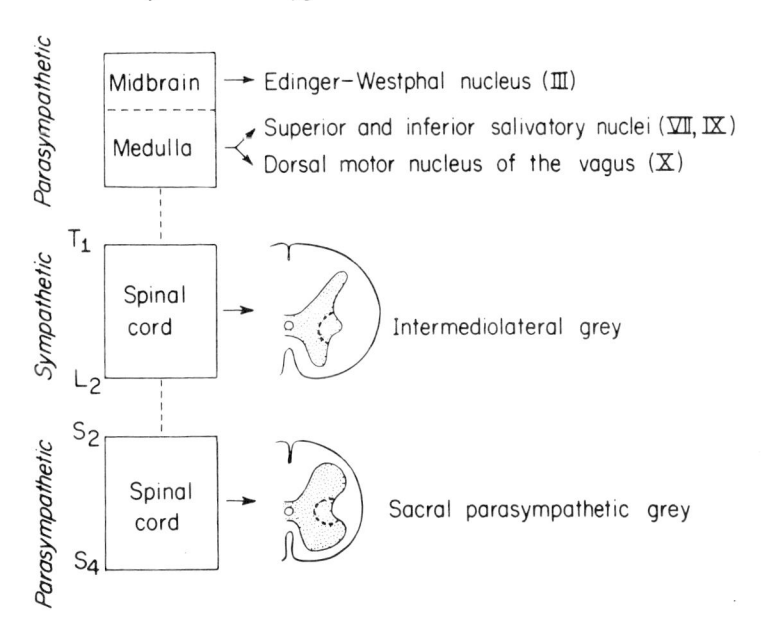

Figure 6.5 The sympathetic and parasympathetic divisions of the autonomic nervous system. The locations of preganglionic cell bodies for the sympathetic and sacral parasympathetic divisions are shown in cross sections of the spinal cord. The nuclei and associated cranial nerves for the cranial parasympathetic division are listed. [Reproduced from Patton et al (1976) *Introduction to Basic Neurology*, by kind permission of the authors and publisher.]

are then distributed to the blood vessels, smooth muscle, and the sweat, lacrimal and salivary glands.

Whether or not there are corresponding afferent sympathetic fibres which are concerned with the transmission of visceral sensation is controversial. Some regard the autonomic nervous system as entirely motor and suggest that afferent fibres accompanying sympathetic efferents are not themselves sympathetic. Whatever their nature, these fibres enter the posterior nerve roots, and visceral sensation is thereafter conveyed centrally along with somatic sensation.

The parasympathetic nervous system

The parasympathetic nervous system (Figs. 6.2 and 6.3) is often called the craniosacral outflow, as its function is motor and its fibres leave the central nervous system only in the cranial nerves and in the sacral region. The cranial outflow is complex. Fibres arising in the oculomotor nucleus (its parasympathetic portion is known as the Edinger-Westphal nucleus) travel with the oculomotor nerve to enter the ciliary ganglion in the orbit, from which short ciliary nerves to the ciliary and pupillary muscles arise. The superior salivatory nucleus in the brain stem gives origin to fibres which travel with the facial nerve, but in the geniculate ganglion some of these leave to form the greater superficial petrosal nerve. This nerve enters the sphenopalatine ganglion from which arise secretomotor fibres to the lacrimal gland. Other fibres from the superior salivatory nucleus are conveyed by the chorda tympani from the facial nerve to the submaxillary ganglion and give rise to fibres which innervate the submaxillary and sublingual glands. The axons of the inferior salivatory nucleus, on the other hand, travel with the glossopharyngeal nerve. They form the lesser petrosal nerve and enter the otic ganglion, and postganglionic fibres promote secretion by the parotid gland. Finally, the preganglionic fibres which arise in the dorsal nucleus of the vagus nerve end in a great

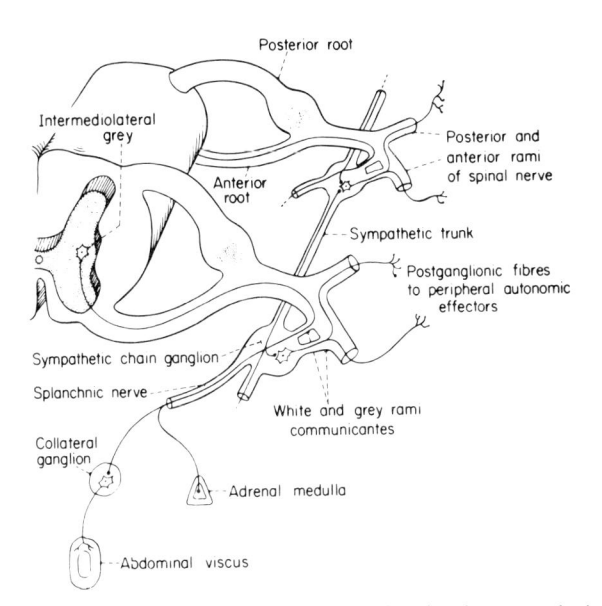

Figure 6.6 The origin of the routes taken by the sympathetic preganglionic and postganglionic fibres. [Reproduced from Patton et al (1976) *Introduction to Basic Neurology*, by kind permission of the authors and publisher.]

TABLE 8. Summary of the innervation and function of major autonomic effectors*

	PREGANGLIONIC NEURON	POSTGANGLIONIC NEURON	FUNCTION
Head Structures			
Eye: pupillary and ciliary muscles			
Sympathetic	Cord segments T1 to T2	Superior cervical ganglion	Pupillary dilatation (mydriasis); accommodation for far vision
Parasympathetic	Edinger–Westphal nucleus (oculomotor nerve—III)	Ciliary ganglion	Pupillary constriction (miosis); accommodation for near vision
Lacrimal gland			
Sympathetic	Cord segments T1 to T2	Superior cervical ganglion	Vasoconstriction
Parasympathetic	Lacrimal part of superior salivatory nucleus (facial nerve—VII)	Sphenopalatine ganglion	Tear secretion and vasodilatation
Parotid, submandibular, and sublingual salivary glands			
Sympathetic	Upper thoracic cord segments	Superior cervical ganglion	Salivary secretion (mucus, low enzyme, vasoconstriction)
Parasympathetic			
Parotid gland	Inferior salivatory nucleus (glossopharyngeal nerve—IX)	Otic ganglion	Salivary secretion (water, high enzyme, vasodilatation)
Submandibular and sublingual glands	Superior salivatory nucleus (facial nerve—VII)	Submandibular ganglion	Same as above
Thoracic Viscera			
Heart			
Sympathetic	Cord segments T1 to T4	Upper thoracic to superior cervical chain ganglia	Acceleration of heart rate and force of contraction; coronary vasodilatation
Parasympathetic	Dorsal motor nucleus (vagus nerve—X)	Cardiac plexus	Deceleration of heart rate and force of contraction; coronary vasoconstriction
Oesophagus			
Sympathetic	Thoracic cord segments	Thoracic and cervical chain ganglia	Vasoconstriction
Parasympathetic	Dorsal motor nucleus (vagus nerve—X)	Intramural plexuses	Peristalsis and secretion
Lungs			
Sympathetic	Cord segments T2 to T6	Thoracic chain ganglia	Bronchial dilatation
Parasympathetic	Dorsal motor nucleus (vagus nerve—X)	Pulmonary plexus	Bronchial constriction
Abdominal Viscera			
Stomach and intestine			
Sympathetic	Cord segments T5 to T12 (thoracic splanchnic nerves)	Coeliac and superior mesenteric ganglia	Inhibition of peristalsis and secretion; sphincter contraction
Parasympathetic	Dorsal motor nucleus (vagus nerve—X)	Intramural plexuses	Peristalsis and secretion
Adrenal medulla			
Sympathetic	Cord segments T8 to T11 (thoracic splanchnic nerves)	The adrenomedullary cells are derived from neural crests but have no dendrites or axons. They are endocrine cells	Secretion of adrenaline and noradrenaline directly into the blood
Parasympathetic (none)			
Descending colon			
Sympathetic	Cord segments T12 to L2 (lumbar splanchnic nerves)	Inferior mesenteric ganglion	Inhibition of peristalsis and secretion; vasoconstriction
Parasympathetic	Cord segments S2 to S4 (pelvic splanchnic nerves)	Intramural plexuses	Peristalsis and secretion
Pelvic Viscera			
Sigmoid colon, rectum and anus, bladder, gonads and associated ducts and organs, and erectile tissue			
Sympathetic	Cord segments T12 to L2 (lumbar splanchnic nerves)	Inferior mesenteric ganglion (hypogastric nerves)	Inhibition of peristalsis and secretion; anal and bladder sphincter contraction; vasoconstriction; ejaculation
Parasympathetic	Cord segments S2 to S4 (pelvic splanchnic nerves)	Intramural or specific organ plexuses	Peristalsis and secretion; bladder detrusor muscle contraction; penile and clitoral erection

*Reproduced from Patton et al (1976) *Introduction to Basic Neurology*, by kind permission of the authors and publisher.

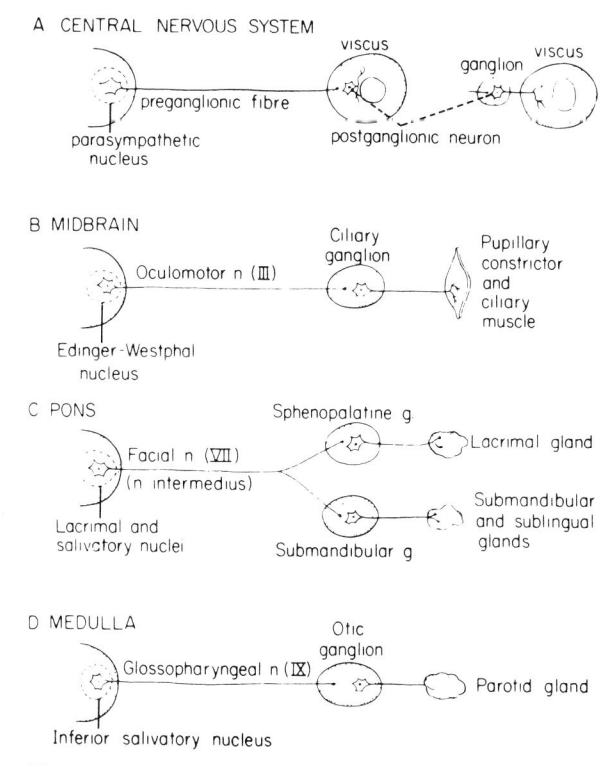

Figure 6.7 Parasympathetic innervation. A, General plan (most appropriate for vagal and sacral outflows). B, Oculomotor nerve. C, Facial nerve. D, Glossopharyngeal nerve. [Reproduced from Patton et al (1976) *Introduction to Basic Neurology*, by kind permission of the authors and publisher.]

many ganglia lying in the walls of the numerous thoracic and abdominal viscera which this nerve innervates.

The sacral outflow of the parasympathetic system leaves the spinal cord in the second, third and fourth sacral nerves, the so-called nervi erigentes. These preganglionic fibres pass to the vesical plexus and to numerous ganglia in the walls of the bladder, rectum and other pelvic organs, and from these ganglia postganglionic fibres emerge in order to fulfil specific functions.

The bladder and bowel

The wall of the bladder consists of smooth muscle, which forms the detrusor. The detrusor and the internal sphincter are both supplied by parasympathetic nerves arising from the nervi erigentes. Stimulation of these parasympathetic fibres causes contraction of the detrusor and relaxation of the internal sphincter. Evacuation of the bladder cannot, however, occur until there is relaxation of the external sphincter, which consists of striped muscle supplied by the pudendal nerve and is therefore under voluntary control. Normally the tone of the detrusor keeps the bladder contracted upon its contents, but when the intravesical pressure rises to a certain level, rhythmical contractions of the bladder wall develop followed by reflex relaxation of the internal sphincter. Evacuation can then be resisted only by voluntary contraction of the external sphincter. When the sphincter is relaxed and micturition occurs, the abdominal muscles also contract.

Sympathetic fibres from the hypogastric nerves also supply the bladder wall and may inhibit contraction. In fact, however, section of these nerves has little practical effect upon bladder function. Some of the afferent fibres concerned in the vesical reflexes travel with these fibres but others travel with the pelvic nerves.

The physiological stimulus for bladder evacuation is an increase in the intravesical pressure, which gives rise to the desire to micturate. If this desire is unfulfilled, repeated contractions eventually follow. As previously mentioned, there are also higher centres in the paracentral lobules of the cerebral cortex and also in the pons which exercise some control over micturition. From these centres fibres descend close to the spinal grey matter. Hence disease of the spinal cord, as we shall see below, can profoundly influence bladder function. Disordered function is often assessed by measuring with a manometer the changes in intravesical pressure that follow the introduction of a standard volume of fluid into the bladder via a catheter. Normally this cystometrogram reveals a sudden rise in pressure as the fluid is introduced, followed by a gradual fall, and thereafter by rhythmical contractions of the bladder wall. If the bladder is hypotonic as a result of nervous disease, these reflex contractions fail to occur.

The innervation of the rectum is similar in many respects to that of the bladder. Stimulation of the parasympathetic nerves gives contraction of the rectal musculature but relaxation of the internal sphincter. The striated external sphincter of the anus, however, is supplied by the pudendal nerve which enables evacuation to be resisted voluntarily. As with the bladder, distension with faeces gives reflex contraction of the rectum and the desire to defecate.

Sexual activity

Sexual function in the male requires (a) desire or libido, which is essentially an emotional function, (b) erection of the penis due to tumescence of the corpora cavernosa, and (c) emission and ejaculation of semen. The second and third functions are mediated through the activity of parasympathetic nerves, while closure of the internal bladder sphincter through sympathetic action is also necessary during emission and ejaculation. Emission, which begins with contraction of the epididymis, the vas deferens and the ampulla, expels sperm into the internal urethra and this is followed by contraction of the seminal vesicles which then propels forward the sperm, mixed with prostatic fluid and mucus from bullo-urethral fluid. Ejaculation results from rhythmical nerve impulses which stimulate erectile tissue at the base of the penis, expelling the semen from the urethra in a series of spurts. Loss of libido may be of emotional or endocrine origin, while impotence (retention of desire but inability to achieve an effective penile erection) can also be psychologically based. Impotence can also be caused by disease of the spinal cord or cauda equina, due to a lesion of the parasympathetic motor pathway or of the afferent sensory pathways. In such a case the ability to ejaculate is also absent. The sexual act is a function which, once initiated, is largely controlled reflexly; therefore erection and ejaculation can occur despite a severe transverse lesion of the cord. Indeed, in some cases of severe spinal cord injury, persistent erection of the penis (priapism) may occur. Premature ejaculation is due to sympathetic overactivity, which inhibits penile erection but which causes contraction of the seminal vesicles, and is usually due to anxiety.

Disorders of sexual function in the female are less well understood. Lack of desire (frigidity) is common in otherwise normal females and is usually psychogenic. Disease of the cauda equina or of the lower spinal cord may abolish the ability to achieve orgasm, but the effects of nervous disease upon female sexuality are much less apparent than in the male.

Precocious sexual development is generally the result of overactivity of the adrenals or ovaries, but can occasionally be seen in patients with neoplasms in the hypothalamus or midbrain or in the region of the pineal. Excessive sexuality is a constitutional disorder, which is of psychic rather than physical origin, and usually shows some affinities with psychopathy.

Some autonomic and related sensory reflexes

Certain cutaneous reflexes which depend upon autonomic pathways may help in neurological diagnosis. Thus, local warming of a limb will initially give rise to vasodilatation and flushing of the skin, followed by sweating in the part that is warmed. Subsequently, general vasodilatation and sweating occur in other parts of the body. This occurs even when all nervous connections between the stimulated limb and the remainder of the body have been divided and must therefore depend upon stimulation of the hypothalamus by the warm blood. The converse effects (vasoconstriction, a pilomotor response or 'gooseflesh') follow cooling of a limb. Sweating and pilomotor activity may, however, be lost in a part of the body which has lost its sympathetic nerve supply, whether it be the postganglionic or preganglionic fibres which are at fault. The absence of sweating in a localized area of skin can be demonstrated by dusting the skin with either quinizarin powder or a starch and iodine mixture. Sweat turns quinizarin purple, and starch and iodine blue. Similarly, autonomic denervation of the vessels supplying an area of skin can give rise to local flushing and a rise in skin temperature which may, however, require sophisticated thermometry for its detection.

The 'flare' reaction is another important reflex which occurs independently of the central nervous system. It is an axon reflex; in other words the afferent stimulus travels centrally along a fibre, spreads to other branches of the same fibre, and then travels peripherally to produce an effect. The CNS is not included in this circuit. If the skin is scratched firmly there is temporary blanching along the scratchline due to local injury to capillaries, but this is soon followed by a spreading vasodilatation or 'flare', resulting from the axon reflex. A central weal will also occur as a result of local histamine release, but the flare, and the pilomotor response which may also occur in the same area, are reflexly determined. Since this axon reflex does not traverse the spinal cord, it remains intact in spinal cord lesions and in lesions lying central to the posterior root ganglia. The reflex is impaired only when the afferent sensory fibres or the ganglia themselves are diseased. Hence an absence of the flare can be a valuable physical sign of a lesion of the somatic sensory nerves. The cold vasodilatation response is another useful test. If normal fingers are immersed in water at 5°C they cool rapidly, but 5 or 10 minutes later there is vasodilatation. This does not happen if the finger is denervated. Like the flare, this is not strictly an autonomic reflex, since it is dependent upon the integrity of sensory axons. In disease of the efferent sympathetic pathways, whether preganglionic or postganglionic, reflex vasodilatation (flushing of the skin) and sweating are abolished but a flare will develop. When the sensory nerves from an area of skin are diseased, sweating may occur, but the flare and cold vasodilatation are abolished.

Tests involving the accurate measurement of arterial blood pressure and its response to various stresses are of considerable value in determining whether or not there is widespread reflex vasomotor paralysis. Blood pressure normally rises when one assumes an erect posture; in a patient with central sympathetic denervation it may fall (postural hypotension). Valsalva's manoeuvre (a deep inspiration followed by attempted forcible expiration against a closed glottis) normally produces a fall in heart rate and a rise in blood pressure, but when there is central autonomic denervation the blood pressure falls. The integrity of vagal function may also be tested by pressure upon the eyeball or upon the carotid sinus, both of which may cause reflex slowing of the heart. These tests must be used with caution, as cardiac asystole and even arrest may occur if the carotid sinus is unusually sensitive.

SOME COMMON DISORDERS OF THE AUTONOMIC NERVOUS SYSTEM

Horner's syndrome

A lesion of the cervical sympathetic chain or ganglia results in a number of ipsilateral abnormalities of the eye: (a) constriction of the pupil on the same side due to unopposed action of the parasympathetic, (b) drooping of the eyelid, due to paralysis of that part of the levator palpebrae which is composed of smooth muscle and innervated by sympathetic nerves, (c) slight retraction of the globe of the eye because of paralysis of smooth orbital muscle which is similarly innervated, and (d) loss of sweating on the affected side of the head and neck. These are the features of Horner's syndrome: miosis, ptosis, enophthalmos, and anhidrosis of head and neck, all on the same side as the lesion. A lesion of the cervical sympathetic ganglia may be due to disease or operation. Rarely, the syndrome is congenital or can result from a lesion of the cervical and upper dorsal spinal cord (such as syringomyelia), which destroys the intermediolateral horn of grey matter. A lesion destroying the sympathetic fibres which ascend into the cranium in the coat of the internal carotid artery (e.g. aneurysm or carotid thrombosis) may rarely give all of the ocular features of a Horner's syndrome, but facial sweating is normal, since the relevant fibres travel in the unaffected external carotid and its branches. As the lesion responsible may be in the neighbourhood of the trigeminal ganglion (in which case there may be signs of dysfunction of the fifth and other adjacent cranial nerves), this condition is often called Raeder's paratrigeminal syndrome.

Cranial nerve syndromes

A lesion of one oculomotor nerve usually gives a fixed dilated pupil on the affected side, owing to paralysis of parasympathetic fibres and unopposed action of the sympathetic fibres. Lesions of the glossopharyngeal and vagus nerves rarely produce any obvious evidence of autonomic disturbance. After a facial palsy, misdirection of regenerating parasympathetic fibres can result in fibres intended for the salivary glands reaching the lacrimal gland so that lacrimation occurs when the patient eats (the syndrome of crocodile tears). Facial sweating during meals (gustatory sweating) is another reflex phenomenon which is occasionally seen in apparently normal individuals and can often be controlled by atropine and related drugs.

The *Holmes–Adie syndrome* (the myotonic pupil) results from a lesion of the ciliary ganglion, almost always of unknown cause. It is much more common in young women than in men and usually causes unilateral pupillary dilatation, often of relatively sudden onset with consequent blurring of vision. The affected pupil either fails to constrict in response to light or does so very slowly and through a small range. The reaction on accommodation/convergence is either lost or, again, occurs very slowly, though constriction may ultimately be full. Many patients also have absent deep tendon reflexes in the limbs and there is depression of the monospinal reflex arc, confirmed by recording the H-reflex. The condition is entirely benign but frequently persists unchanged for many years.

Lesions of the cauda equina and spinal cord

A severe lesion of the cauda equina profoundly affects bladder and bowel function as a result of damage to the sacral parasympathetic outflow. The bladder becomes toneless and reflex contraction can no longer occur as it distends, so that retention of urine develops. As distension increases, the elasticity of the bladder wall forces urine into the urethra. As the external sphincter is generally paralysed as well, dribbling incontinence or retention with overflow occurs. If the lesion of the cauda equina is permanent, reflex bladder activity cannot be re-established, and owing to enforced catheterization and urinary stasis, severe urinary infections may supervene. In some such cases permanent suprapubic drainage of the bladder is necessary, but eventually in many cases evacuation by manual compression is achieved. Similarly, retention of faeces occurs, sometimes with incontinence, and regular enemas may be required to empty the bowel.

The initial effects of an acute transverse lesion of the spinal cord are similar. There is retention of urine with overflow and also faecal retention. As spinal shock wears off, reflex bladder and bowel evacuation are gradually established, occurring solely in response to increasing intravesical and intrarectal pressure and independently of the will. Thus, automatic bladder and bowel activity develop; micturition and defecation can be evoked by anything which increases intravesical pressure, including pressure upon the abdomen, or straining. They can also occur as a result of stimuli applied to the lower limbs, as part of the 'mass reflex' which includes flexor withdrawal of the limbs. The patient with a total transverse lesion of the cord may become aware that his bladder is full through sensations of headache, sweating or abdominal fullness, and will then be able to initiate micturition by pressure upon the abdomen.

Retention of urine can also result from parasagittal lesions affecting both paracentral lobules of the cerebral hemispheres (the 'cortical bladder centres'). Incomplete lesions of the spinal cord affecting the corticospinal tracts, in close association with which the descending fibres controlling micturition are believed to travel, can also affect bladder function. Sometimes, in such a case, there is delay in the ability to initiate micturition and even incomplete retention with overflow. More often, in the patient with a spastic paraparesis, there is heightened reflex activity of the bladder, and precipitancy or urgency of micturition results. The patient cannot resist the desire to micturate, and precipitate evacuation of the bladder occurs.

Apart from their effects upon bladder and bowel function, lesions of the spinal cord can influence other autonomic activities. Thus, following an acute transverse lesion, and during the stage of spinal shock, the skin of the body below the level of the lesion is dry, pale and cool, but subsequently, when reflex activity is established, profuse sweating in the affected area is common and can be provoked by many cutaneous and other stimuli. Local disease of the thoracic segments of the spinal cord may also damage the intermediolateral horn of grey matter, giving sympathetic denervation of the affected segments with physical signs corresponding to those produced by division of preganglionic fibres.

Referred pain

The afferent pathway for visceral sensation is initially along afferent fibres which accompany autonomic nerves, and particularly along the sympathetic. These fibres enter posterior nerve roots and travel centrally with somatic afferents. Pain of visceral origin can be felt in skin areas which are not at first sight anatomically related to the viscus concerned. As an example, cardiac pain may be referred to the substernal region, but also to the left arm, to both arms, or to the jaw. The mechanism of referred pain is discussed on p. 207.

Afferent fibres concerned in autonomic reflexes may possibly provide an alternative path for painful sensation from areas deprived of their somatic sensory nerves. Certainly pain sensation can be carried by somatic afferents which accompany the autonomic nerves that supply the blood vessels. This probably explains pain associated with intra- and extracranial arterial dilatation in disorders such as migraine. A similar mechanism may possibly account for the pain of causalgia (see below).

Degenerative disorders of the autonomic system

In *idiopathic orthostatic hypotension* (the Shy–Drager syndrome) attacks of fainting may occur whenever the patient assumes the upright posture. Anhidrosis, impotence, dysuria and disorders of bowel function are also common, and the normal autonomic reflexes are generally abolished. Cells of the intermediolateral column of the spinal cord degenerate for unknown reasons. The patient often shows features of parkinsonism, cerebellar ataxia or corticospinal tract dysfunction (so-called progressive multisystem degeneration) and occasionally dementia. The term *progressive autonomic failure* is now generally preferred to that of idiopathic orthostatic hypertension (Bannister, 1983) and it is clear that in many cases the syndrome develops gradually and the patient does not go on to develop manifestations of parkinsonism or multiple system atrophy. If signs of neurological dysfunction other than those of involvement of the autonomic nervous system do not appear within 5 years, they are unlikely to do so. On the other hand, autonomic failure is sometimes seen in association with rare familial degenerative nervous disorders such as olivopontocerebellar degeneration and striatonigral degeneration.

Familial dysautonomia (the Riley–Day syndrome) is a rare disorder of autosomal recessive inheritance, usually seen in Jews, in which defective lacrimation, hyperhidrosis, epilepsy, and episodic hyperpyrexia generally occur. Most patients have no sense of taste and are relatively insensitive to pain. They usually die in childhood from respiratory infection. The condition appears to be accompanied by an as yet unidentified inborn error of catecholamine metabolism, and there is marked reduction in the number of unmyelinated nerve fibres in the peripheral nerves.

Acute autonomic neuropathy is a rare condition presenting in childhood or adult life with the rapid onset of postural hypotension, paralysis of ocular accommodation, anhidrosis and urinary and faecal retention. Spontaneous recovery usually occurs within a few months, hence the alternative title of 'pure pan-dysautonomia with recovery'. The cause is unknown.

Peripheral nerve lesions

A lesion of the lower motor neuron usually produces no recognizable autonomic effects. As a result of disuse, the skin of the affected part may become smooth, shiny and inelastic, while subcutaneous tissue, denervated muscle and even bone will atrophy. Owing to loss of the 'pumping' action of the muscles upon the veins, the affected part, especially a hand or foot, often becomes cyanotic and oedematous. These so-called trophic changes are due to disuse and not to a lesion of autonomic nerves. The autonomic reflexes are intact.

The sequelae of a sensory nerve lesion are often more serious, particularly if pain fibres are involved, as injury to the insensitive skin and joints will readily occur, giving indolent or perforating ulcers and gross joint disorganization (Charcot's arthropathy). Section of a sensory nerve peripheral to its posterior root ganglion usually abolishes the flare response in the anaesthetic area. Other trophic changes, such as loss of sweating and of the pilomotor response, only follow a lesion of preganglionic or postganglionic sympathetic efferents and do not always result therefore from lesions of peripheral somatic nerves unless these contain sympathetic fibres.

After an incomplete lesion of a peripheral nerve, particularly in the region of the forearm and wrist, a curiously unpleasant type of pain may develop in the affected hand, with excessive sweating and excessive sensitivity to touch and pain. This syndrome is called causalgia, and it seems that the afferent stimuli responsible for the pain are carried with autonomic nerves, as block or division of somatic sensory nerves may fail to relieve the pain, while sympathectomy does. The pathogenesis of causalgia is not fully understood. Similarly, the mechanism by which painful swelling of the hand, often leading to atrophy of muscles and even of bone (Sudeck's atrophy), develops in some cases of pericapsulitis of the shoulder joint or 'frozen' shoulder (the 'shoulder-hand' syndrome or algodystrophy) is obscure, but this condition too is often relieved by cervical sympathectomy.

Hyperhidrosis

Excessive sweating, particularly of the hands and feet, can be due to emotional disturbances or to endocrine disorders such as thyrotoxicosis, acromegaly or phaeochromocytoma. It may also be congenital and, if intolerable, it can be alleviated by sympathectomy. Hyperhidrosis occasionally occurs in Parkinson's disease. Localized cutaneous areas of increased sweating sometimes occur following peripheral nerve lesions, as in causalgia. Similarly, any peripheral stimulus may produce excessive perspiration, a pilomotor response, and an increased skin temperature below the level of a transverse lesion of the spinal cord once spinal shock has passed.

Hypothalamic syndromes

Disorders of sleep, taking the form of either hypersomnia or wakefulness with reversal of the sleep rhythm, can result from hypothalamic lesions (see p. 84). Excessive appetite can also occur. Conversely, some hypothalamic lesions, especially gliomas, can produce anorexia leading to extreme cachexia. A syndrome of this nature may also result from a hypothalamic lesion in infancy and early childhood. The affected children show rapid longitudinal growth with almost total loss of subcutaneous fat despite adequate food intake and no evidence of malabsorption. They are alert and often hyperactive. In most cases a diencephalic or optic nerve glioma is eventually found but in a few cases no cause is demonstrable.

Disorders of memory, and Korsakov's syndrome in particular, can result from lesions of the corpora mamillaria. Actual visual hallucinations (so-called peduncular hallucinations) can also be produced by lesions in this area, while many emotional and personality disorders, including excessive anger and irritability on the one hand and apathy leading to akinetic stupor on the other, have been attributed to hypothalamic lesions. The region clearly plays a major part in regulation of the body temperature, and irritation of anterior hypothalamic nuclei may give rise to hyperpyrexia. A similar mechanism involving posterior nuclei or the tuber cinereum probably accounts for the hyperglycaemia and glycosuria, albuminuria, and acute gastric ulceration with haemorrhage that sometimes occur in patients with brain disease. Basal neoplasms and subarachnoid haemorrhage are particularly liable to produce these effects.

Diabetes insipidus, a condition in which the patient passes very large quantities of dilute urine and consequently has polydipsia and excessive thirst, may also be the result of a hypothalamic lesion or one involving the tuber cinereum or posterior pituitary, impairing the production of anti-diuretic hormone (ADH).

Obesity and sexual underdevelopment are other signs which are sometimes due to disease of the hypothalamus or pituitary or both. There are also several hypothalamic disorders of early life whose cause is unknown. In idiopathic adiposogenital dystrophy (Fröhlich's syndrome) the obesity is present from birth and is greatest around the shoulders and hips, and there is genital hypoplasia and immaturity. The condition is more common in males, but when females are affected sexual function is more often normal.

CONCLUSIONS

Disease or dysfunction of the hypothalamus, which is in essence the control centre from which autonomic activities are regulated, can give rise to many different clinical manifestations. From an understanding of the simple principles which govern the behaviour of this part of the nervous system, it may be possible to interpret the significance of these important symptoms and physical signs. Similarly, a knowledge of the structure and function of the more peripheral components of the autonomic nervous system is necessary in order to interpret the consequences of autonomic dysfunction, and particularly those of abnormal bladder and bowel activity which may occur in patients with nervous disease.

References

Appenzeller, O. (1976) *The Autonomic Nervous System*. 2nd edn. Amsterdam: North-Holland.

Bain, H. W., Darte, J. M. M., Keith, W. S. and Kruyff, E. (1966). The diencephalic syndrome of early infancy due to silent brain tumor: with special reference to treatment. *Pediatrics* **38:**473.

Bannister, R. (1983) *Autonomic Failure*. London: Oxford University Press.

Bannister, R. and Oppenheimer, D. R. (1972) Degenerative diseases of the nervous system associated with autonomic failure. *Brain* **95:**457.

Bannister, R., Davies, B., Holly, E., Rosenthal, T. and Sever, P. (1979) Defective cardiovascular reflexes and supersensitivity to sympathomimetic drugs in autonomic failure. *Brain* **102:**163.

Blackwell, R. E. and Guillemin, R. (1973) Hypothalamic control of adenohypophyseal secretions. *Ann. Rev. Physiol.* **35:** 357.

Dancis, J. and Smith, A. A. (1966) Familial dysautonomia. *N. Engl. J. Med.* **274:**207.

Guyton, A. C. (1981) *Textbook of Medical Physiology*, 6th edn. Philadelphia: W. B. Saunders Company.

Hayward, J. N. (1975) Neural control of the posterior pituitary. *Ann. Rev. Physiol.* **37:**191.

Johnson, R. H. and Spalding, J. M. K. (1974) *Disorders of the Autonomic Nervous System*. Oxford: Blackwell Scientific Publications.

Johnson, R. H., Lambie, D. G. and Spalding, J. M. K. (1984) *Neurocardiology* (Major Problems in Neurology, vol. 13). Philadelphia: W. B. Saunders Company.

Johnson, R. H., Smith, A. C. and Spalding, J. M. K. (1969) Blood pressure response to standing and to Valsalva's manoeuvre: independence of the two mechanisms in neurological diseases including cervical cord lesions. *Clin. Sci.* **36:**77.

Patton, H. D., Sundsten, J. W., Crill, W. E. and Swanson, P. D. (1976) *Introduction to Basic Neurology*. Philadelphia: W. B. Saunders Company.

Smith, A. A., Taylor, T. and Wortis, S. B. (1963) Abnormal catecholamine metabolism in familial dysautonomia. *N. Engl. J. Med.* **268:**705.

Tolis, G., Labrie, F., Martin, J. B. and Naftolin, F. (eds) (1979) *Clinical Neuroendocrinology: A Pathophysiological Approach*. New York: Raven Press.

Walton, J. N. (1985) *Brain's Disease of the Nervous System*, 9th edn. chap. 20. Oxford: Oxford University Press.

Young, R. R., Asbury, A. K., Corbett, J. L. and Adams, R. D. (1975) Pure pan-dysautonomia with recovery—description and discussion of diagnostic criteria. *Brain* **98:**613.

7

THE SPECIAL SENSES

INTRODUCTION

The special senses include the faculties of smell, vision, hearing and taste. Closely related to hearing, at least in an anatomical sense, is the maintenance of equilibrium (vestibular function). These functions are mediated through those cranial nerves which convey the sensory impulses concerned in the appreciation of these sensations to the appropriate areas of the cerebral cortex. Thus, the first or olfactory nerve contains the peripheral pathway for the sense of smell, while the second or optic nerve carries visual impulses. The ability to see is closely related to mechanisms subserving binocular vision and ocular movement, so that in considering visual processes we must also discuss the functions of the third (oculomotor), fourth (trochlear) and sixth (abducens) cranial nerves, which control external ocular movement. The third nerve, along with sympathetic fibres derived from the autonomic nervous system, also influences those intrinsic ocular muscles controlling the size of the pupils as well as the process of accommodation–convergence. Hearing and the control of bodily equilibrium are respectively mediated through the cochlear and labyrinthine divisions of the eighth or auditory nerve. Taste sensations from the anterior two-thirds of the tongue travel in the chorda tympani along with the seventh or facial nerve, and those from the posterior one-third are conveyed by the ninth or glossopharyngeal nerve. Disorders of function of the special senses may be produced by lesions of the primary sensory receptors, of the cranial nerves concerned, or of their central connections. They are common in patients with neurological disease, and an adequate understanding of the means by which these lesions produce their clinical effects is essential for accurate diagnosis. It may be useful at this point to formulate certain unifying physiological principles which are of general relevance to sensory physiology, applying equally to the special senses and to somatic sensation (chapter 9). The Weber–Fechner law formulated in the last century said that the intensity of the sensation experienced by a subject is proportional to the logarithm of the strength of the stimulus:

$$I = K \log \frac{S}{S_0}$$

when I is the intensity of the subjective experience, S_0 is the threshold, S the suprathreshold stimulus used in the estimation of stimulus magnitude, and K is a constant. In the 1950s it was shown that the subjective experience is proportional not to the logarithm but to the nth power of the suprathreshold stimulus. This power function has been shown to be more accurate over an extended range for describing the sensation-stimulus intensity relationship. In general terms there is also evidence that the rate of firing of afferent fibres is related to stimulus intensity, so that this firing rate is also related to the perceived magnitude of the sensation experienced (Kandel and Schwartz, 1985).

SMELL

The olfactory receptors are a series of bipolar nerve cells situated in the upper part of the mucous membrane on either side of the nasal cavity. Inhaled gases given off by all odorous materials become dissolved in the nasal secretions which continually bathe the surface of these sensitive cells. Impulses so produced are conveyed by nerve fibres through the cribriform plate of the ethmoid bone into the cranial cavity to join the olfactory bulb which lies on the undersurface of the ipsilateral frontal lobe. From there, impulses travel posteriorly in the olfactory tracts to reach the prepyriform cortex and uncus in the rostral part of the parahippocampal gyrus of the temporal lobe, which can be regarded as the primary rhinencephalic (olfactory) area of the cerebral cortex. The anterior commissure unites the olfactory cortical regions of the two hemispheres and carries fibres from each olfactory tract to the opposite side; nevertheless, olfaction is not a crossed sensation (i.e. olfactory impulses from one side are recorded and recognized on the same side of the brain).

There is a strong relationship between the faculties of smell and taste, which combined give the sensation of flavour. If either faculty is impaired, so too may be the ability to appreciate flavours. In such a patient it is not sufficient to test taste sensation alone, as an inability to perceive olfactory sensations may be the primary abnormality. While the human brain can probably distinguish about 3000 different odours, in clinical practice the most useful test substances are coffee, oil of peppermint, camphor and (possibly) oil of cloves. Disease of the nasal mucosa such as rhinitis, a severe coryza, or even excessive smoking can so impair the sensitivity of the olfactory nerve cells that the sensation of smell is lost or greatly impaired (anosmia). Bilateral loss is thus not always significant neurologically. Unilateral impairment of the sense of smell is, however, an important physical sign. In the absence of a primary nasal abnormality it may indicate compression of one olfactory bulb or tract, possibly by a tumour underlying the ipsilateral frontal lobe. Total anosmia can also be hysterical or feigned; these cases are detected by the fact that the patient will deny that he can appreciate concentrated ammonia, which stimulates trigeminal rather than olfactory nerve endings. Olfactory hallucinations may be a manifestation of schizophrenia but can also occur in patients with lesions in one or other temporal lobe, as in some cases of temporal lobe epilepsy (uncinate seizures) that result from abnormal discharges arising in the anterior temporal cortex. Parosmia is an abnormal or perverted sense of smell occasionally due to organic lesions but more often occurring in mental illness (e.g. severe depression).

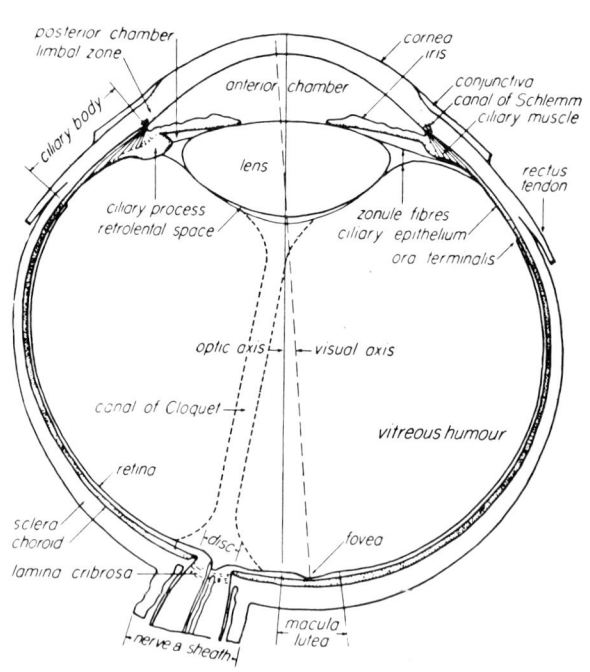

Figure 7.1 A horizontal section through the equator of the right eye. [Reproduced from Patton et al (1976) *Introduction to Basic Neurology*, and previously published in Ruch and Patton (eds) *Physiology and Biophysics*, by kind permission of the authors and publishers.]

TASTE

Taste receptors (taste buds) are situated on the dorsal surface of the tongue and occupy the vallate, fungiform and foliate papillae. There are also a few taste buds on the hard and soft palate and the epiglottis. Each consists of a cluster of about 50 receptor cells the tips of which project on the surface, forming a gustatory pore that is stimulated by substances, dissolved in the saliva, that give rise to taste. A single axon may innervate about eight taste cells; the afferent nerve fibre leaving the taste bud is myelinated. A generator potential arising from a single taste cell can be recorded with a microelectrode. Such studies have shown that different taste receptors vary considerably in their sensitivity to different tastes, and recent studies have shown that the zinc ion plays an important role in taste sensation.

Taste fibres from the anterior two-thirds of the tongue travel through the lingual nerve to the chorda tympani, joining the facial nerve at the geniculate ganglion and proceeding to the pons in the nervus intermedius, which lies alongside the facial nerve. Taste sensations from the posterior one-third of the tongue are conveyed by the glossopharyngeal nerve. In the pons, the fibres of these nerves enter the tractus solitarius, relay across the midline, and proceed in the gustatory fillet or lemniscus to the optic thalamus, from which they are conveyed to the lower end of the postcentral gyrus.

Loss of taste (ageusia) on the anterior two-thirds of the tongue can result from lesions of the geniculate ganglion. A facial paralysis due to a lesion at or proximal to this point is usually associated, therefore, with unilateral loss of taste, whereas a paralysis resulting from a more distally situated lesion is not. A lesion of the glossopharyngeal nerve will result in loss of taste on the posterior third of the tongue on the same side, but taste sensation is so difficult to test in this region with even a reasonable degree of accuracy that disorders of taste in this region are of little value in clinical neurological diagnosis. Bilateral loss of taste sensation can sometimes follow head injury. Much more often, the head-injured patient who complains of loss of taste sensation is found to be suffering from anosmia with resultant impairment of sense of flavour, but on testing, the primary taste sensations (sweet, salt, bitter and sour) are found to be intact. Hallucinations of taste may occur in association with those of smell as a result of lesions in the neighbourhood of the uncus. Lesions here may also cause parageusia, a perversion of taste in which many substances possess the same unpleasant flavour. This symptom occasionally develops without apparent cause in elderly subjects, causing anorexia and showing little if any response to treatment.

VISION

General considerations

In the so-called special senses, physical stimuli are extensively modified or transduced as they are transmitted through non-neural tissue before reaching the neural sensory receptor specifically designed to record them. Thus the eye (Fig. 7.1) can be likened superficially to a camera in that light rays pass through an aperture which can be varied at will, then through a lens of variable focus, being eventually recorded upon a light-sensitive receptor surface (the retina). The neural process of visual perception is, however, much more complex than the simple recording of a single visual image upon a light-sensitive film.

A detailed consideration of physiological optics would be beyond the scope of this volume, and for such information the reader is referred to texts on ophthalmology. The process by means of which the lens focuses images upon the retina is known as refraction. The human eye focuses upon near objects by increasing the refractive power of the lens through the process of accommodation. As a light source moves closer to the eye, contraction of both the circular and longitudinal fibres of the ciliary muscle allows the lens to bulge passively and to become more nearly spherical. The degree of change is proportional to the strength of ciliary muscle contraction. This change in shape of the lens shortens its focal length, thus bringing the near object into focus. It is accompanied by convergence of the two eyes, a reflex action due to contraction of the medial recti which ensures that the images recorded by each eye are focused on the macular area of each retina at the fovea centralis. This process is also accompanied by reflex pupillary constriction or miosis (see p. 136), which blots out light rays that would otherwise fall upon the periphery of the lens, and thus prevents distortion of images due to chromatic and spherical aberration (which would otherwise give visual blurring as the lens approaches a more nearly spherical shape).

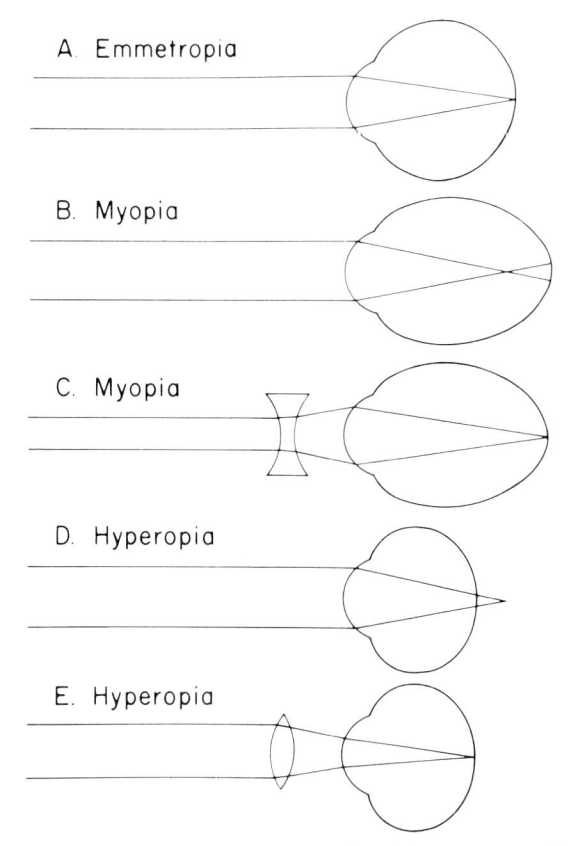

Figure 7.2 Normal vision (A) and optical defects uncorrected (B and D) and corrected by appropriate lenses (C and E). [Reproduced from Patton et al (1976) *Introduction to Basic Neurology*, by kind permission of the authors and publisher.]

Among the disorders of visual refraction commonly seen in clinical practice are (a) *myopia*, which is short sight due to abnormal length of the globe of the eye and which is usually constitutional or developmental, requiring concave lenses for its correction, and (b) *hypermetropia* or *hyperopia*, which is long sight due to abnormal shortness of the globe and which is somewhat less common. Longsightedness commonly develops with increasing age (*presbyopia*) at the rate of about one-quarter of a diopter per year after the age of about 25 years, and can be corrected by the use of convex lenses. Presbyopia is due to increasing impairment of the accommodation process resulting from progressive lack of elasticity of the lens (Fig. 7.2). Astigmatism, a more complex defect, is due to asymmetry in the curvature or shape of the lens.

The retina

STRUCTURE

The retina contains two types of receptors, the rods and the cones, which have entirely different properties and which account for the so-called duplicity theory of retinal function (Table 9). The cones are found throughout the retina but are most heavily concentrated in the fovea or macular region, which subserves central vision. They have a high stimulus threshold, function mainly in daylight or conditions of high illumination, and are responsible for detailed high-acuity vision and colour vision. The rods, by contrast, are absent from the fovea, have very low thresholds of stimulation, are insensitive to colour and to visual detail, and subserve vision in conditions of poor illumination (night vision).

The retina lines the inside of the globe of the eye as far forwards as the ciliary body. Posteriorly it is interrupted by the optic nerve head or disc, where the axons of the retinal ganglion cells come together to form the optic nerve.

The retina is strikingly laminated in cross-section (Fig. 7.3). Its outer pigment layer, loosely bound posteriorly to the choroid and anteriorly to the receptor layer, is the point at which retinal detachment often occurs, especially in myopic individuals. It contains a single layer of epithelial cells with finger-like processes penetrating between the outer segments connected by an eccentric waist-like constriction (Fig. 7.4). It is the shape of their outer segments which distinguishes the two. Each outer segment contains free-floating discs to which are attached the light-sensitive pigments which are rhodopsin or visual purple in the rods, and three pigments not yet fully characterized in the cones, of which one may be iodopsin. In the rods, new discs are constantly being formed at the base of the outer segment, while others at the tip bud off and are ingested by pigment cells. A similar process may occur in the cones, but this is not yet finally established and the cone discs certainly have a longer life than those of the rods. Studies on animal models of the disease retinitis pigmentosa, which causes progressive visual failure and pigmentary degeneration of the retina, have indicated that the phagocytic activity of the epithelial cells is impaired so that cellular debris accumulates between them and the tips of the photoreceptors (Kandel and Schwartz, 1985).

The inner segments of these receptors contain many mitochondria and also expand to contain nuclei that are larger in the cones than in the rods which, in light micrographs (Fig. 7.3), constitute the outer nuclear layer of the retina. Beyond the nuclei, the inner segments continue through the outer plexiform layer, terminating in expansions that make synaptic contacts with the dendrites of the bipolar cells, which in turn constitute the inner nuclear layer. In this layer there are flat bipolar cells, each of which receives connections from about seven cones, midget bipolar cells (especially in the foveal region) connecting with a single cone, and rod bipolar cells which receive impulses from rods exclusively. There are also retinal interneurons, the horizontal cells which connect rods and cones, and amacrine cells (neurons without identifiable axons), which form connections between bipolar terminals and dendrites of ganglion cells. The ganglion cells form the innermost cell layer of the retina, and their dendrites form synapses with axons of the bipolar cells in the inner plexiform layer (Fig. 7.5). The axons of the ganglion cells traverse the retina to enter the optic nerve. The photosensitive receptors lie deepest in the retina so that light must traverse several retinal layers to excite them. In the foveal (macular) region, however, there is a cup-shaped shallow depression in the retina where the ganglion and bipolar cells are pushed aside, thus exposing the receptors. This area is concerned with central vision and with maximal acuity, clarity and discrimination of visual images.

Ganglion cell responses to diffuse retinal illumination include 'on' responses, 'off' responses, and 'on–off' responses. 'On' cells discharge with increasing frequency during illumination, 'off' cells do so when light stimulation ends, and 'on–off' cells discharge at the beginning and end of photic stimulation. Stimulation of the retina with minute light spots has shown that many ganglion cells have receptive fields with 'on-centre, off-surround' characteristics, while others show the reverse arrangement. Receptive fields for foveal cells are very small and may correspond to the on response of a single cone, the 'off-surround' being mediated by interneurons. The latter cells (the horizontal and amacrine neurons) appear to be responsible for lateral inhibitory responses which enhance the contrast generated by visual images.

There are two pathways by which information is transferred from the receptors to the ganglion cells. The on-line pathway is the simplest, representing a direct receptor-bipolar-ganglion cell route. The off-

The special senses

TABLE 9.   Comparison of rods and cones*

	Cones	**Rods**
Threshold	Relatively high	Exquisitely low
Distribution	Ubiquitous, concentrated at fovea	Non-foveal, peripheral retina only
Convergence	Limited in fovea	Extensive
Illumination	Photopic (daylight)	Scotopic (twilight)
Function	Central vision	Peripheral vision
	Colour vision	Achromatic vision
	Detail vision	Poor detail vision

* Reproduced from Patton et al (1976) *Introduction to Basic Neurology*, by kind permission of the authors and publisher.

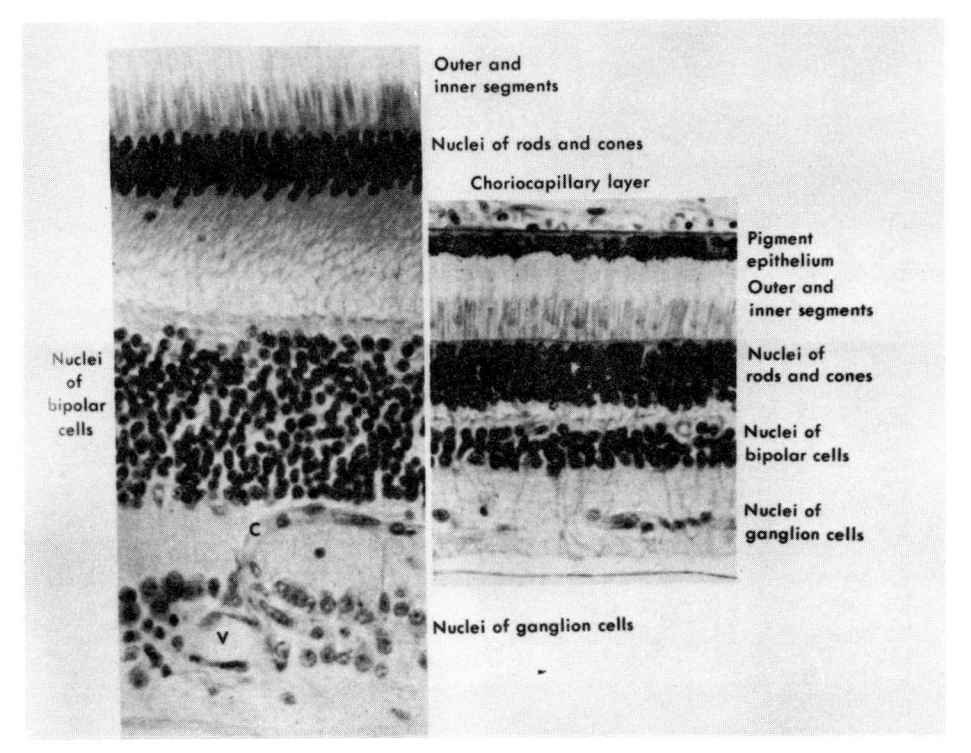

Figure 7.3   Photomicrographs of a human retina, both at the same magnification (about × 525). Right, section from the periphery of the retina. Note the scarcity of ganglion cells. The external limiting membrane (not labelled) is visible as a thin, dark line immediately above the nuclei of the rods and cones. The internal limiting membrane (not labelled) is a thin, dark line that forms the inner surface of the retina. Left, section near the fovea, where cones predominate (the pigment epithelium separated during processing for microscopic sectioning). Note the thickness of the bipolar and ganglion cell layers, evidence of a much greater tendency to a one-to-one ratio from photoreceptors to ganglion cell in the cone-dominated portions. The layer labelled 'Nuclei of bipolar cells' also contains nuclei of glial cells and interneurons. V = venule; C = capillary. [Reproduced from Gardner (1972) *Fundamentals of Neurology*, 6th edn, by kind permission of the author and publisher.]

line pathway involves a receptor-horizontal-bipolar-ganglion cell circuit through which horizontal and amacrine cells (laterally orientated interneurons) help to integrate and transfer information from distant receptors to the bipolar-ganglion cell circuits (see Kandel and Schwartz, 1985). Synaptic chemical transmitters in the retina have not yet been fully characterized, although acetylcholine, dopamine and GABA are all known to be present.

FUNCTION

Photochemical and electrophysiological mechanisms
Retinal photoreceptors are sensitive to light with wavelengths from 400 to 700 nm, that is from blue through green to red. Light stimuli falling upon such receptors ultimately lead to firing in ganglion cells, as mentioned earlier. From stores in the liver, vitamin A is released intermittently into the bloodstream, to be taken up by retinal epithelial cells.

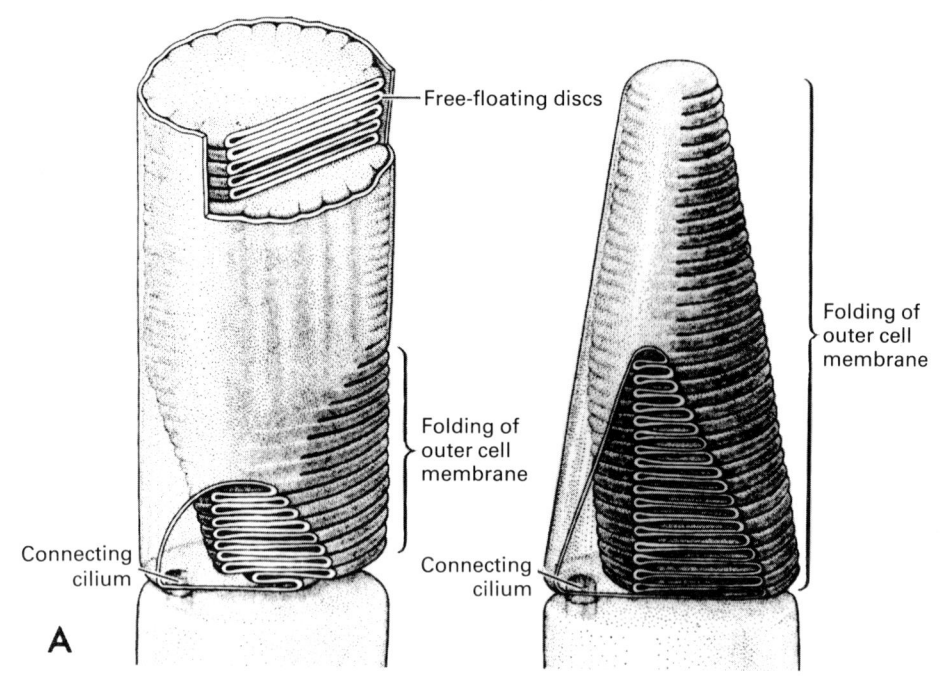

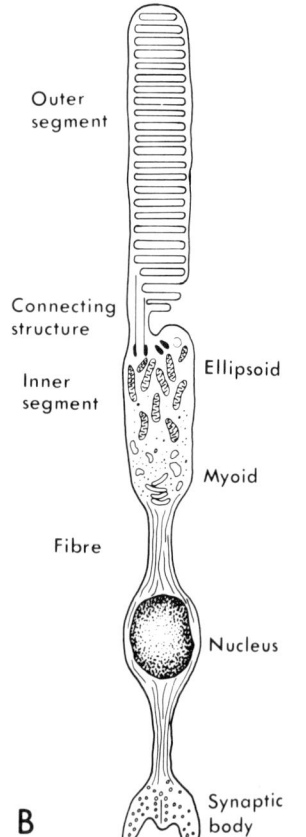

Figure 7.4 A, Outer segments of rod (left) and cone (right). In both receptors discs are formed by infolding of plasma membrane. In rods the folds pinch off so that discs become free-floating within the outer segment. Cone discs persist as folds; the disc space communicates with extracellular space. [Reproduced from Patton et al (1976) *Introduction to Basic Neurology*, and previously published in 'Visual Cells', by Richard W. Young, Scientific American Inc., 1970, by kind permission of the authors and publishers.]

B, Schematic representation of the essential features of a vertebrate photoreceptor. The outer segment contains membrane discs on which the photosensitive pigment molecules are concentrated. The inner segment consists of two zones: an ellipsoid, which is a dense aggregation of mitochondria, and a myoid, containing the Golgi complex and granular endoplasmic reticulum. The organelles give way to a fibre, which is succeeded by the nucleus, and the cell ends as a complex synaptic body. [Reproduced from Gardner (1975) *Fundamentals of Neurology*, 6th edn, by kind permission of the author and publisher; based on Young, R. W., in Straatsma, B. R., et al (eds) *The Retina*. Berkeley, University of California Press, 1969.]

In the eye, vitamin A (retinol) is converted into retinene by dehydrogenation in the following reaction:

$$C_{19}H_{27}CH_2OH + NAD^+ \underset{}{\overset{\text{alcohol dehydrogenase}}{\rightleftharpoons}} C_{12}H_{27}CHO + DPNH + H^+$$
Vitamin A \hspace{3cm} Retinene

The equilibrium of this reaction favours vitamin A so that in the retina the vitamin A concentration is normally greater than that of free retinene. The carotenoid pigment retinene combines with the protein scotopsin to form rhodopsin, which is then stored in the outer segments of the rods. Rhodopsin has a characteristic absorption maximum for light with a wavelength of 497 nm. When light falls upon these outer segments some rhodopsin is bleached, the amount being dependent upon the intensity of the light. A single photon of light when absorbed by a single rhodopsin molecule initiates structural change in that molecule. When the stimulus ceases, the rhodopsin is resynthesized. Vitamin A, therefore, is essential for rod function, and dietary deficiency of this vitamin causes night blindness. A similar process of bleaching of pigment followed by resynthesis is presumed to occur with respect to the poorly characterized cone pigments, which have three different absorption spectra.

The conformational changes resulting from the breakdown of rhodopsin result in a decrease of Na^+ conductance in the plasma membrane of the outer segments. It is uncertain as yet as to whether this results from the fact that cGMP is believed to achieve signal amplification enzymatically and that rhodopsin, when split by light, initiates the breakdown of cGMP with resultant dephosphorylation of channel proteins and closing of the Na^+ channels. An alternative hypothesis suggests that Ca^{2+} is sequestered in outer segment discs of dark-adapted rods and that light releases these Ca^{2+} ions which flow through rhodopsin-formed Ca^{2+} channels, subsequently combining with Na^+ channels and blocking them (Kandel and Schwartz, 1985).

These photochemical changes are succeeded by the generation of graded responses in bipolar cells, which in turn excite action potentials in ganglion cells. In the 1960s the first successful intracellular voltage recordings were made from vertebrate photoreceptors (which resembled in many respects auditory and vestibular hair cells). It was found that they failed to display the conventional 'all-or-none' action potentials but produced graded potentials related to light intensity. It was also found that the polarity of response was different from that found in many other sensory receptors, in that stimulation (by light) gave a negative voltage signal. More recently new techniques have been developed which enable the current (rather than the voltage) to be recorded from a single photoreceptor. It has thus become possible to record the electrical responses of rods to individual photons of light and to show that single photon signals are reliably detectable (Lamb, 1984). These signals are then conveyed by axons in the optic nerve to the lateral geniculate body. The accompanying electrical changes can be recorded in the electroretinogram (ERG) through an electrode applied to the globe of the eye.

DARK AND LIGHT ADAPTATION

In complete darkness the sensitivity of the eye to light is increased almost a thousandfold. This sensitivity is almost wholly in the green portion of the light spectrum where the greatest absorption by rhodopsin occurs. Stimulation with light of other wavelengths reveals reduced sensitivity, and a scotopic luminosity curve can be charted (Fig. 7.6). (The term 'scotopic' refers to vision in dim light, which is dependent on the rods, while the term 'photopic' refers to vision in daylight, which is dependent on the cones.) Some of the decreased sensitivity at the violet end of the spectrum is due to absorption of light of shorter wavelength by the lens, so that patients whose lenses have been removed for cataract (aphakia) can sometimes see objects in the ultraviolet spectral range which are invisible to others. By contrast, the dark-adapted eye is totally insensitive to light of longer wavelength (i.e. red). Thus, dark adaptation can be achieved at least in part by wearing dark red goggles in daylight.

By contrast, if an eye is exposed to daylight or strong artificial light (phototopic luminosity), it becomes light-adapted, and the greatest sensitivity is then at about 557 nm (Fig. 7.6), representing a shift to the yellow–red end of the spectrum (the Purkinje shift).

VISUAL SENSITIVITY AND ACUITY

The rods are therefore primarily concerned with visual sensitivity in conditions of dark adaptation, the cones with visual acuity in the light-adapted eye and with colour vision. The distinction is not absolute as the rods also function in daylight, and nocturnal animals, for instance, can see during the day.

Visual acuity is defined by the ability to see minute objects in sharp outline. In clinical practice this is determined by asking the patient to read letters of diminishing size at a standard distance from the eye (distance vision) or to read lines of print held at reading distance (reading acuity). It may be tested alternatively by measuring the eye's resolving power, that is the smallest visual angle, say between two

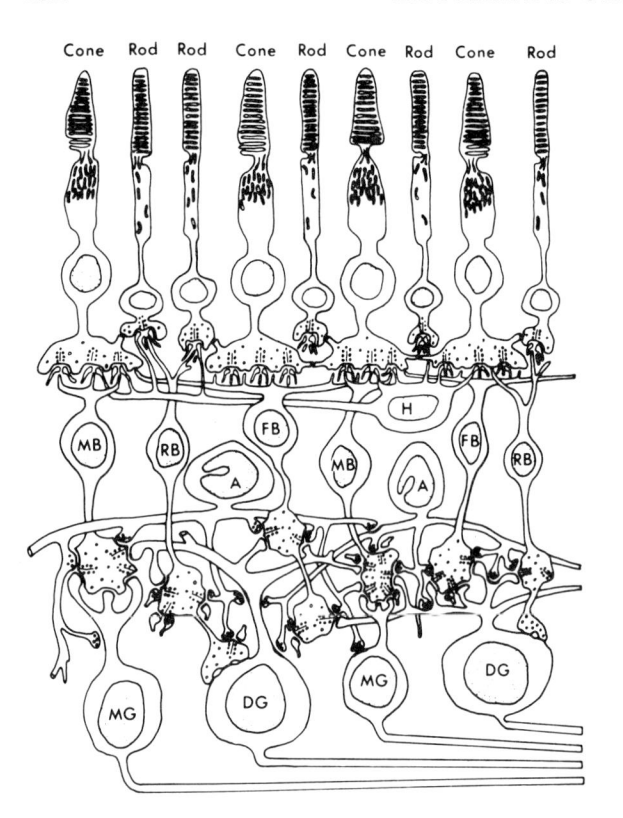

Figure 7.5 A summary diagram illustrating the organization of the primate retina. MB, midget bipolar, RB, rod bipolar, FB, flat bipolar. H, horizontal cell. A, amacrine cell. MG, midget ganglion cell. DG, diffuse ganglion cell. The direction followed by light falling upon the retina is from below upwards (see p. 128). [Reproduced from Gardner (1975) *Fundamentals of Neurology*, 6th edn, and previously published by Dowling, J. E. and Boycott, B. B. (1966) *Proc. R. Soc. Lond.* B, **166**:80–111, by kind permission of the authors and publishers.]

determined at which point the flashes can no longer be distinguished and a single continuous image is perceived. Motion pictures and television make use of this faculty in that the frequency of the visual images is so great that there is no sensation of 'flicker'.

COLOUR VISION

The eyes are sensitive to light of wavelengths varying from 400 to 700 nm, from violet through green to red (Fig. 7.6). Coloured objects absorb light of varying wavelength, the colour or hue being a function of wavelength. Brightness or brilliance of a colour is a function of stimulus intensity, and purity or saturation of a colour depends upon the extent to which it is diluted by the admixture of white light. The three primary colours of the visual spectrum are red, green and blue, intervening hues or shades being due to mixtures of the primary colours. It is now known that the genes for red and green vision are X-linked, while that for blue vision is autosomal. In the Young–Helmholtz theory of colour vision, three different types of cones are postulated, each responsive to one of the primary colours. The fact that there are known to be three cone pigments which absorb light of three different wavelengths supports this concept. Colour perception is affected by the point or area of the retina upon which the stimulus falls. A stimulus falling upon the fovea, for instance, may be perceived as different in a colour sense from the same stimulus striking a more peripheral part of the retina. The interpretation of colour is probably not a simple all-or-none phenomenon due to the direct transmission

vertical lines, at which their separation can be clearly recognized. This is determined, at least in part, by the grain of the retina, i.e. the density of its photoreceptors. If these were to lie far apart, then light from either of the vertical lines or from the contrasting areas between them could fall upon an insensitive part of the retina, preventing clear resolution of the two lines. Acuity also involves a process of intensity discrimination, which is a function of the cerebral cortex rather than of the cone receptors themselves. For example, if the two vertical lines are dark on a white background, the white area between them gives stimuli of greater intensity than the dark lines themselves.

Frequency of stimulation is another important variable in visual acuity. A single flash of light evokes a burst of electrical impulses in the optic nerve and visual cortex. If such flashes are applied with increasing frequency, a critical fusion frequency can be

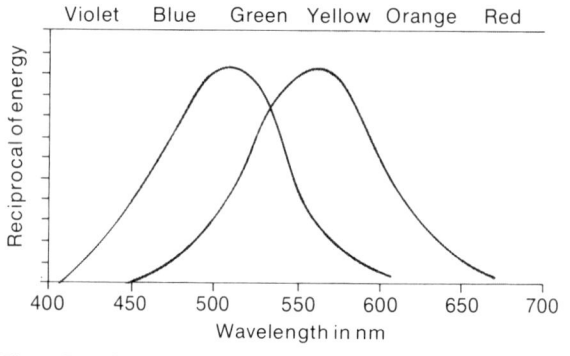

Figure 7.6 Scotopic and photopic luminosity curves, illustrating the Purkinje shift. The scotopic curve shows that the maximum sensitivity of the dark-adapted eye (achromatic vision) is 505 nm. The photopic curve shows that the maximum sensitivity of the light-adapted eye (chromatic vision) is about 560 nm. The two curves, for convenience, are plotted in the same units of sensitivity, although the scotopic eye is much more sensitive. [Reproduced from Gardner (1975) *Fundamentals of Neurology*, 6th edn, by kind permission of the author and publisher.]

of impulses from colour-sensitive cones to the visual cortex. It is affected by patterns of firing from colour-coded receptors but also by the integration of excitatory and inhibitory signals from populations of cones with different spectral sensitivities, both in the ganglion cell layer of the retina and at subsequent cellular relay stations on the way to the cortex.

The visual pathways

Visual impulses recorded upon the retina are conveyed by the optic nerves through the optic chiasm. In the chiasm, fibres from the nasal half of each retina decussate, whereas temporal fibres do not. Hence each optic tract carries fibres from the temporal half of the ipsilateral retina and from the nasal half of the contralateral one (Fig. 7.7). This means that impulses from the right half-field of both eyes are carried in the left optic tract and vice versa. The tract continues to the lateral geniculate body where the axons synapse with nerve cells which give origin to the optic radiation. The optic radiation then travels backwards through the temporal lobe, hooking around the tip of the temporal horn of the lateral ventricle in the process, and onwards to that part of the cerebral cortex which lies in the lips and in the depth of the calcarine fissure of the occipital lobe. This primary visual receptive area (the striate cortex) has profuse connections with the surrounding association areas in which visual sensations are recognized and interpreted.

Afferent fibres from the retina and from the muscles of accommodation also travel in the optic nerve. These fibres synapse in the lateral geniculate body and in the superior corpora quadrigemina of the upper midbrain, from which fibres arise which travel to the third, fourth and sixth nerve nuclei and to a sympathetic centre in the hypothalamus nearby. These pathways are responsible for constriction of the pupil in response to light fixation on near objects, and dilatation when the visual field is darkened or when distant objects are being observed. A similar reflex pathway, controlled by visual impulses from the retina, influences the ocular movements necessary for ocular convergence and fixation and for following objects with the eyes.

VISUAL ACUITY (CLINICAL ASPECTS)

The visual acuity in each eye can be measured independently by means of test types of the Snellen and Jaeger variety. The acuity is essentially a measurement of the efficiency of macular or central vision, as it depends very largely upon normal functioning of this part of the retina and its nervous connections, provided the mechanism for focusing light upon the retina is intact. Peripheral retinal lesions rarely influence acuity, but a small lesion of the macula or of the fibres of the optic nerve which come from the macular area may seriously affect the ability to read or to distinguish small objects. Visual acuity can also be seriously impaired by disorders of refraction, and primary abnormalities of the eye which influence the passage of light to the retina, as well as by disorders which damage retinal sensitivity.

COLOUR BLINDNESS

Colour blindness is an inherited defect which occurs in 8% of the male population and in less than 0.5% of females. It is generally inherited as a sex-linked (X-linked) recessive character. Although it occurs in many forms, the commonest variety is red–green blindness, either partial or complete, in which the affected individual finds it difficult to distinguish reds from greens. Many complex defects of colour vision have been described. Thus, trichromats (three-colour vision) include normal individuals but also some with weak red vision or weak green vision. Dichromats are those who are unable to perceive red or green; blue–violet colour blindness (autosomal) is extremely rare. Monochromats (with total colour blindness) are also very rare and some also show severe photophobia. Many patients are unaware of their colour blindness as they recognize 'colours' by their brightness, but the diagnosis can be confirmed with the Ishihara charts. The defect is of no serious significance except in those occupations where the recognition of coloured lights or signals is important. In patients with minimal lesions of the visual pathways, however, field defects for coloured objects (red is commonly used) can often be demonstrated at a time when the field for white objects is full. The field for red is normally smaller than that for white.

THE VISUAL FIELDS

The demonstration of defects of the peripheral visual fields or of the central fields may be of great value in neurological diagnosis (Fig. 7.7). From a knowledge of the anatomy of the visual pathways it is generally possible to localize with considerable accuracy the site of the lesion which is responsible. Circumscribed defects of the central fields are referred to as scotomas. In each central field there is a normal 'scotoma', medial to the fixation point. This is the 'blind spot', corresponding to the optic nerve head or disc in which there are no visual receptors. A scotoma that surrounds the fixation point or macular area is known as a central scotoma, and generally results in severe impairment of visual acuity. It is most commonly seen as a sequel of retrobulbar neur-

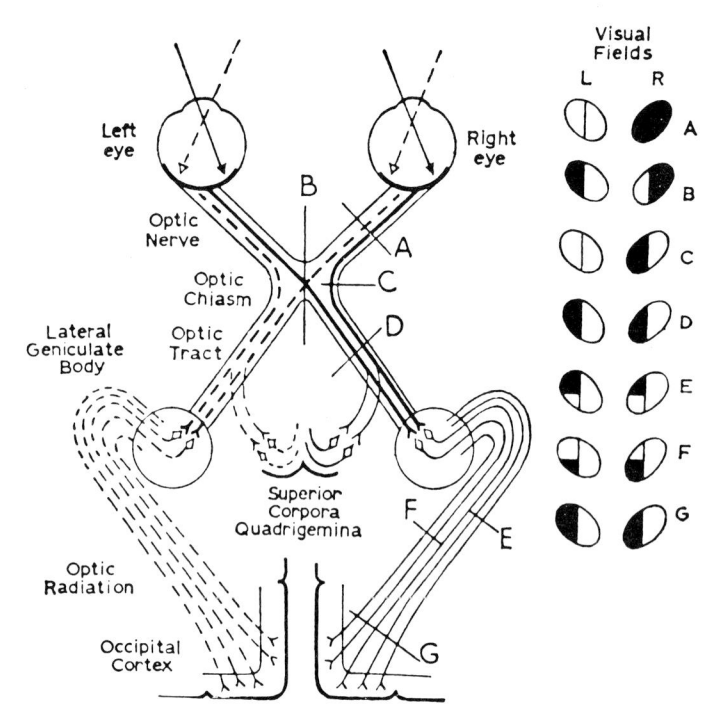

Figure 7.7 A diagram of the visual pathways. On the right are examples of visual field defects produced by lesions interrupting these pathways at the points signified by the letters A to G. [Reproduced from Walton (1982) *Essentials of Neurology*, 5th edn, by kind permission of the publisher.]

itis, an inflammatory lesion of the optic nerve which is frequently a manifestation of multiple sclerosis. Rarely, a central scotoma may result from compression of one optic nerve by a retro-orbital tumour, presumably because macular nerve fibres may be the most sensitive to pressure ischaemia. Central scotomas may also be observed in vitamin B_{12} deficiency and various nutritional deficiencies, in neuromyelitis optica, or in retrobulbar neuritis due to a variety of toxic and metabolic causes, of which methyl alcohol poisoning is a good example. Tobacco is a cause of progressive visual failure in smokers of certain brands of pipe tobacco, possibly related to the effect of cyanide in the tobacco upon vitamin B_{12} utilization. It usually gives a centrocaecal scotoma, joining the fixation point to the blind spot. Many authorities deny that tobacco alone is responsible (tobacco amblyopia) and suggest that heavy alcohol consumption and possibly multiple B group vitamin deficiency may also be needed to produce the syndrome (tobacco–alcohol amblyopia).

A severe lesion of one optic nerve gives complete blindness of the ipsilateral eye, while the peripheral field of the other eye is full. Lesions of the optic chiasm can give many types of field defect, depending upon the character and situation of the causal lesion. Although atherosclerotic ischaemia of the chiasm is occasionally responsible, chiasmal field defects most frequently are secondary to external compression by parasellar neoplasms and aneurysms. Tumours of the pituitary gland, as they protrude from the sella turcica, will first compress the decussating fibres from the lower nasal portions of the retinas, producing defects in the upper temporal fields of both eyes, and eventually a bitemporal hemianopia. A lesion which compresses the chiasm asymmetrically from above, such as a suprasellar meningioma, a craniopharyngioma or a suprasellar aneurysm, may produce first a defect in the nasal field of one eye, progressing to complete unilateral blindness, and then a defect in the temporal field of the other eye. Other possible variations can readily be deduced on anatomical grounds.

A complete lesion of one optic tract gives rise to a contralateral homonymous hemianopia, that is complete loss of the nasal field of the ipsilateral eye and of the temporal field of the contralateral eye. In a lesion of the left optic tract, the right half-field of both eyes is lost. Since optic tract compression is frequently asymmetrical, the defect is often initially larger in one half-field than in the other until the hemianopia is complete. When homonymous defects in the two fields are unequal in size and shape they are said to be incongruous.

Lesions of one optic radiation, whether in the internal capsule, temporal lobe or occipital lobe, also give rise to homonymous defects. A large lesion gives a complete homonymous hemianopia, but a smaller lesion affecting the lower fibres of the radiation may give a contralateral upper quadrantic homonymous defect. Since the nerve fibres coming from the retina are closely intermixed in the radiation, so that fibres from homologous portions of the two retinas lie alongside one another, field defects due to radiation lesions are almost always congruous, i.e. they are the same in both eyes. In a homonymous hemianopia resulting from an occipital lobe lesion, the macular area of the blind half-field is split. Visual acuity remains unimpaired in a patient with a complete homonymous hemianopia, but reading is difficult, since in the normal reading process words are read in groups of two or three. In a patient with a hemianopia, ability to see only half the words in the group can cause great difficulty, so that he must learn again to read word by word.

Abnormalities of the visual fields may result from local ocular conditions such as glaucoma and retinal detachment, but these disorders are generally apparent on examination of the eye and rarely give rise to diagnostic difficulty. Some concentric diminution of the fields with enlargement of the blind spot is seen in severe papilloedema and less often in optic atrophy, due to syphilis or constriction of the optic nerve due to arachnoiditis. Complete loss of the peripheral field with retention of only a small central area (tubular vision) is usually a hysterical phenomenon.

The optic fundus and its abnormalities

Ophthalmoscopic examination of the optic nerve head or disc, of the retinal vessels, and of the retina itself is an essential and often revealing part of a neurological examination. The optic disc is normally slightly pink in colour, but its temporal half is generally somewhat paler than the nasal, while some lack of definition of its nasal margin is common. In the centre of the disc, or slightly more towards its temporal margin, is the physiological cup into which the vessels dip. This cup is frequently much paler than the remainder of the disc, and its appearance must not be confused with that of optic atrophy. Excessive cupping of the disc is seen in glaucoma. Not uncommonly a leash of pale fibres is seen spreading for a short distance across the retina, in fanlike manner, from one part to the edge of the disc. These medullated nerve fibres are a common abnormality and have no pathological significance.

The two most frequent abnormalities of the optic disc are swelling (papilloedema) and excessive pallor (optic atrophy).

Papilloedema generally results from some obstruction to the venous return from the retina, so that the first sign may be a distension of the retinal veins. This is followed by obliteration of the physiological cup, and later the centre of the optic disc becomes raised above the level of the surrounding retina, while its margins become progressively more blurred and indistinct. When swelling is severe, haemorrhages and sometimes patches of white exudate develop around the disc margins in a radial manner. A star-shaped patch of white exudate (a 'macular star') may also develop in the macular area, which is normally a relatively avascular area of the retina, lying about two disc-breadths lateral to the disc. The two principal causes of papilloedema are increased intracranial pressure and retrobulbar or optic neuritis (or neuropathy). The latter is an 'inflammatory' neuritis (or neuropathy) of the optic nerve, due most often to a demyelinating lesion of multiple sclerosis or the related neuromyelitis optica, but rarely resulting from syphilis or from toxic, nutritional or metabolic disorders. Disc swelling due to retrobulbar neuritis can generally be distinguished from that due to increased intracranial pressure by the fact that visual acuity is seriously impaired at an early stage in retrobulbar neuritis. Furthermore, the oedema is rarely as great in retrobulbar neuritis as it is in true papilloedema, while haemorrhages and exudates are uncommon in such cases. The optic disc may look surprisingly normal even in the acute stage of optic neuritis when the visual acuity is severely impaired. The typical history of this condition is one of progressive failure of vision in one eye, often associated with local pain, and usually leading to partial or total monocular blindness within a few hours or days. There is often complete recovery from this condition after several weeks or months, although a central scotoma may remain. The condition must be presumed to be due to multiple sclerosis unless some other cause is clearly apparent. It may be many months or years before other neurological manifestations of multiple sclerosis develop, and in some cases they never do so. By contrast, severe papilloedema due to increased intracranial pressure is often present without loss of visual acuity. There may be some concentric diminution of the fields with enlargement of the blind spot, and the patient sees flashes of light or 'haloes' around lights, symptoms which may presage impending visual failure. These symptoms indicate that measures to reduce the intracranial pressure should be undertaken urgently, since visual loss as a result of papilloedema is due to compression of the central retinal artery and is often complete and irreversible. Transient episodes of visual loss in patients with papilloedema, provoked often by stooping, are due to retinal ischaemia and give warning of impending arterial occlusion. Papilloedema can also result from severe arterial disease, as in chronic nephritis and malignant hypertension, from local lesions giving venous obstruction in the orbit or elsewhere, or from polycythaemia vera.

Occasionally, congenital hyaline bodies ('drusen') lying on or in relation to the optic disc can give sufficient blurring of the disc margins (pseudopapilloedema) to make diagnosis from true papilloedema difficult. Fluorescein retinal angiography may then be diagnostic.

The optic disc in patients with optic atrophy is chalky-white or grey in colour, its pallor being in striking contrast to the surrounding retina. The edges of the disc are clear-cut and often somewhat irregular. The form of optic atrophy which typically follows an attack of retrobulbar neuritis in multiple sclerosis affects the temporal half of the disc much more than the nasal, as the fibres from the macular area of the retina enter this part of the disc. This so-called temporal pallor, which is sometimes difficult to distinguish from the normal comparative pallor of the temporal part of the disc, is almost diagnostic of multiple sclerosis. Optic atrophy may also be inherited. It is a feature of cerebral lipidosis of the Tay–Sachs type (cerebromacular degeneration) and of some of the other neuronal storage disorders, of diseases in the hereditary ataxia group, and of retinitis pigmentosa. Other causes of optic atrophy include neurosyphilis, compression of the optic nerve (tumour, arachnoiditis or aneurysm), occlusion of the central retinal artery, and various metabolic, toxic and nutritional disorders.

Changes in the retinal vessels also have considerable diagnostic value. The venous engorgement which occurs in papilloedema has already been mentioned. In subarachnoid haemorrhage, the rapid inflow of blood into the optic nerve sheath can give such severe venous obstruction that a large brick-red haemorrhage, known as a subhyaloid haemorrhage, is to be seen extending from the edge of the optic disc. Early changes of atherosclerosis and hypertension may take the form of slight 'silver-wiring' of the retinal arteries (Grade I retinopathy) with subsequent narrowing of the veins where the arteries cross them (Grade II). When the changes are more severe, flame-shaped haemorrhages and patches of hard white exudate appear in the retina (Grade III), and eventually papilloedema develops (Grade IV). In diabetic patients, small microaneurysms are sometimes found on peripheral retinal arteries. These can be very difficult to visualize with the ophthalmoscope but are well demonstrated by fluorescein retinal angiography. Occlusion of the central artery of the retina may give sudden unilateral blindness. The arteries are seen to be greatly reduced in calibre, and optic atrophy follows. While this syndrome can result from atherosclerosis, in elderly patients it is often due to cranial (temporal or giant cell) arteritis. Transient unilateral blindness (amaurosis fugax) is often due to embolism of the central retinal artery, and occurs most commonly in patients with internal carotid artery stenosis. Emboli of platelets or cholesterol may be seen in retinal arteries during attacks.

Among other abnormalities of the retina which are of diagnostic value are retinal angiomas (tangles of abnormal blood vessels) found in patients with haemangioblastoma of the cerebellum (von Hippel–Lindau disease), retinal tubercles (yellowish nodules, often about half the size of the optic disc) which help to confirm a diagnosis of tuberculous meningitis or miliary tuberculosis, and flat yellow plaques or phakomas, which may be seen in tuberous sclerosis or neurofibromatosis.

The pupils

The parasympathetic nerve fibres which innervate the constrictor of the pupil travel in the trunk of the third cranial (oculomotor) nerve, while the sympathetic fibres responsible for pupillary dilatation arise in the hypothalamus and travel through the tegmentum of the brain stem and the cervical cord to the lateral horn of grey matter in the eighth cervical and first and second dorsal segments. They leave the spinal cord in the anterior roots and reach the superior cervical ganglion, from which postganglionic fibres arise and enter the skull in the plexus in the wall of the internal carotid artery. Some then pass to the ophthalmic division of the fifth (trigeminal) nerve and enter the orbit with its branches, while others go from the carotid plexus directly to the ciliary ganglion in the orbit, giving rise to the short ciliary nerves.

Both pupils normally constrict when a light is shone upon one retina. The reaction in the illuminated eye is called the direct reaction, that in the opposite eye the consensual one. The afferent pathway for the light reflex travels in the optic nerve to the lateral geniculate body and superior colliculus and from there to the third nerve nucleus from which efferent constrictor fibres arise. Hence a lesion on the afferent side of the pathway (e.g. optic atrophy) impairs both the direct and the consensual reaction to light, while a lesion in the efferent pathway (e.g. third-nerve paralysis) to the eye that is being stimulated will affect the direct but not the consensual reaction. In unilateral retrobulbar neuritis if a light is shone into the affected eye, both the direct and consensual reactions are sluggish or absent, but on light stimulation of the normal eye both reactions are brisk (the retrobulbar pupil reaction). Constriction of the pupil also occurs when vision is focused upon a near object, a procedure which involves both accommodation (through contraction of the ciliary muscle) and convergence, and which is subserved by a complicated series of reflexes involving the oculomotor nuclei. Both the light and accommodation reactions are impaired by a lesion of the third nerve. Paralysis of the pupillary reaction to accommodation with preservation of the light reflex is a very rare finding, though it can occur occasionally in lesions of the midbrain and may seem to be present when ocular convergence is impaired, as may rarely occur with ageing or in postencephalitic parkinsonism. Loss of the light reflex with retention of that to accommodation is, however, one feature of the *Argyll Robertson pupil* of tabes dorsalis and sometimes of general paresis. Additional features are that the pupils are small, irregular and unequal, with atrophy of the iris, and loss of the ciliospinal reflex (pupillary dilatation on pinching the skin of the neck). There is some controversy about the location of the lesion responsible for the Argyll Robertson pupil. Some believe it to be in the periaqueductal region of the midbrain, while others have inferred that it is in the ciliary ganglion; the former view has more adherents. In congenital syphilis, the light reflex may be lost, but in such cases the pupils are usually large and are not therefore of the typical Argyll Robertson type. Pupils with most, if not all, of the features of the Argyll Robertson pupil are sometimes seen in patients with diabetes (diabetic pseudotabes) and other autonomic neuropathies and in patients with hereditary motor and sensory neuropathy of the Charcot–Marie–Tooth variety.

A lesion of the third-nerve nucleus or of the nerve in its intracranial course can give paralysis of the pupilloconstrictor muscles, so that the pupil becomes dilated and fixed. Since the parasympathetic fibres lie relatively superficially in the nerve, along with those innervating the levator palpebrae superioris, this pupillary change may be the first sign of a third-nerve lesion, being followed by ptosis and later by external ophthalmoplegia. Pressure upon the nerve trunk by an aneurysm or pituitary neoplasm, and ischaemia or infarction of the nerve in diabetes mellitus, are common causes of a unilateral third-nerve palsy. A similar effect can result from herniation of the temporal lobe through the tentorial hiatus, so that a unilateral fixed dilated pupil may be an early sign of a space-occupying lesion in or overlying one cerebral hemisphere (such as an extradural or subdural haematoma). Histological studies have shown that in transverse sections of the trunk of the third nerve, the pupilloconstrictor fibres lie most superficially with motor fibres to the levator palpebrae superioris just beneath them. This is why, when the nerve is compressed from above, pupillary dilatation is the first physical sign followed by ptosis, and paresis of other external ocular muscles comes later.

A lesion of the sympathetic pathway gives rise to a constricted pupil (miosis) and is generally accompanied by the other features of *Horner's syndrome* (miosis, ptosis, enophthalmos and loss of sweating on the affected side of the face) as described earlier. The lesion responsible may lie in the descending pathway in the brain stem, in the cervical sympathetic ganglia, or in the internal carotid artery, damaging sympathetic fibres which run in the wall of the vessel. Sympathetic overactivity, due for instance to fright or sympathomimetic drugs, dilates the pupils. Lesions in the brain stem commonly affect the size and reactivity of the pupils. Changes of localizing value in comatose patients and in identifying the site of brain-stem lesions have been described under 'Consciousness and its disorders' (p. 82).

Drugs have a profound influence upon pupillary size and activity. Miotics, which cause pupillary constriction, include morphine, pilocarpine, neostigmine and eserine, whereas mydriatics (dilators) include the long-acting atropine, homatropine, which is used to dilate the pupil for ophthalmoscopy, and cocaine. Local ocular conditions can influence pupillary shape and size. Iridocyclitis, for instance, often gives irregularities of the iris and adhesions to the lens (synechiae), which may restrict the range of pupillary movement. Hippus is a phenomenon of intermittent rhythmical pupillary contraction and dilatation; it has no diagnostic value.

The myotonic pupil is another interesting pupillary abnormality. When this pupillary abnormality is associated with sluggishness or absence of the tendon reflexes, the condition is referred to as *Adie's syndrome*. Characteristically the syndrome occurs in young women, though it is occasionally seen in males. The patient may notice the sudden onset of slight blurring of vision in one eye or alternatively she observes on looking into the mirror that one pupil is dilated. On examination the pupil is widely dilated and shows a sluggish, delayed reaction to light. The reaction to accommodation is usually better, but this too may be impaired and indeed it is occasionally impossible to produce pupillary constriction with either stimulus. The condition is benign, but its aetiology is unknown and it is uninfluenced by treatment. The lesion responsible is a loss of cells (of unknown aetiology) in the ciliary ganglion.

The eyelids and orbital muscles

The part of the levator palpebrae superioris which consists of voluntary muscle is innervated by the third cranial nerve, but there is also a smooth muscle component (Muller's muscle) innervated by the sympathetic. Hence a paresis of the third nerve or of the sympathetic can give rise to ptosis. However, that due to sympathetic paralysis is relatively slight, in that the lower margin of the upper eyelid usually covers only the upper third of the cornea, while that due to a third nerve lesion may be complete, with the lid covering the entire globe. Ptosis can also be congenital and either unilateral or bilateral. It is also seen in myasthenia gravis, in which case it characteristically worsens as the day wears on.

Lid retraction, or a failure of the upper lid to follow the globe in downward movement of the eye, is typically seen in thyrotoxicosis in which condition exophthalmos, or protrusion of the eye, is also common. The term proptosis is sometimes used to identify a unilateral exophthalmos, particularly when it is asymmetrical. In some patients with thyrotoxicosis there may be considerable swelling of the external ocular muscles and orbital tissues, and ophthalmoplegia is common (ophthalmic Graves' disease). This ocular syndrome, known to be of autoimmune origin, is now more often called thyroid ophthalmopathy. Other conditions which may give rise to exophthalmos include orbital tumour, 'pseudotumour' and other inflammatory lesions in the orbit or paranasal sinuses, retro-orbital intracranial tumours (meningiomas in particular) and thrombosis of, or arteriovenous aneurysm in, the cavernous sinus. In patients with a carotico-cavernous fistula (rupture or leakage of the carotid artery within the cavernous sinus, whether due to trauma or aneurysmal rupture) the exophthalmos usually pulsates and there is a loud bruit over the globe of the eye.

External ocular movement and its abnormalities

THE NATURE AND CONTROL OF OCULAR MOVEMENTS

The ocular movements include horizontal movement outwards (abduction), horizontal movement inwards (adduction), vertical movement upwards (elevation), and vertical movement downwards (depression). The eye is capable of diagonal movements at any intermediate angle. The term 'rotation' should be reserved for wheel-like movements around an imaginary pivot passing from before backwards through the centre of the pupil. Such movements of rotation do not normally occur, but are observed only as a result of the unbalanced action of certain muscles. Inward rotation is a movement similar to that of a wheel rolling towards the nose, and outward rotation is the opposite rotatory movement. Normally the movements of the two eyes are harmoniously symmetrical, constituting conjugate ocular movement or deviation, which is described as horizontal or lateral, upwards and downwards. Conjugate adduction of the two eyes is known as convergence. Other varieties of ocular movement will be considered below.

The nuclei of the ocular muscles
The lower motor neurons which innervate the ocular muscles originate in the nuclei of the third, fourth and sixth cranial nerves. The first two lie in the midbrain just anterior to the cerebral aqueduct at the level of the superior and inferior colliculi. The nuclei of the sixth nerve lie in the pons beneath the floor of the upper part of the fourth ventricle and are partly encircled by the fibres of the seventh nerve (Fig. 7.8).

The precise representation of muscles in the nucleus of the third nerve is still somewhat uncertain, but Figure 7.9 shows the probable arrangement. The median, unpaired nucleus of Perlia is the centre for convergence and accommodation, while the lateral, paired nucleus of Edinger-Westphal innervates the parasympathetic constrictor of the pupil. The remainder of the nucleus is the paired, lateral nucleus in which the muscles are represented from above downwards as follows: levator palpebrae, superior rectus, inferior oblique, medial rectus, inferior rectus. Decussating fibres unite the lower parts of the nuclei. Immediately below the third-nerve nucleus lies that of the fourth nerve, which innervates the opposite superior oblique. This nucleus and the adjacent lowest part of the third-nerve nucleus innervate the two muscles concerned in depression of the eye, and the two elevating muscles are innervated by mutually adjacent portions of the upper half of the third-nerve nucleus.

The extrinsic ocular muscles
The extrinsic ocular muscles are the four recti (superior and inferior, lateral and medial) and the two obliques, superior and inferior. The action of each of these muscles is shown in Fig. 7.10. Only the lateral and medial recti act in a single plane. The other muscles always act in concert in such a way that their conflicting tendencies cancel and a harmonious resultant is produced. When the two obliques aid the lateral rectus in abduction, their vertical and rotatory forces cancel out. When the superior rectus and inferior oblique contract together in elevating the eye, their horizontal and rotatory components also cancel.

Owing to the planes in which the superior and inferior recti and the obliques are placed, their actions are influenced by the position of the eye in the orbit. When it is rotated outwards 23 degrees, the superior rectus is a pure elevator and the inferior rectus a pure depressor. The more the eye is turned inwards, the more the muscles act as internal and external rotators. The converse is true of the obliques. In conjugate deviation there is a harmonious contraction of the appropriate muscles of the two eyes. In lateral conjugate deviation the lateral rectus of one eye and the medial rectus of the other are associ-

The special senses 139

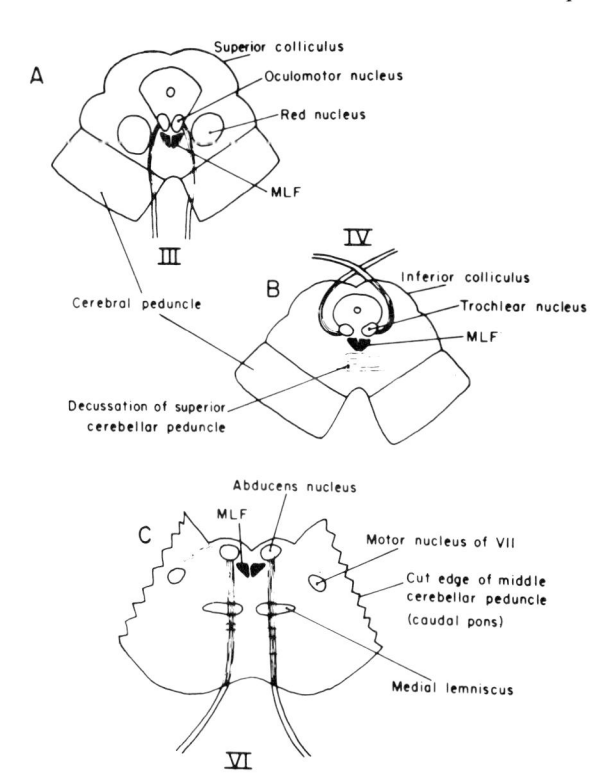

Figure 7.8 Diagrammatic cross sections at the levels of the nuclei for the (A) oculomotor nerve (III); (B) trochlear nerve (IV); and (C) abducens nerve (VI), MLF locates the medial longitudinal fasciculus. [Reproduced from Patton et al (1976) *Introduction to Basic Neurology*, by kind permission of the authors and publisher.]

Squint
Squint, or strabismus, is the term applied to a failure of the normal coordination of the ocular axes. It is necessary to distinguish paralytic squint from concomitant squint. Paralytic squint may be present when the eyes are at rest, in which case it is due to the unbalanced action of the normal antagonist of the paralysed muscle. For example, the affected eye may be slightly adducted when the lateral rectus is paralysed. More often it is apparent only when the eyes are deviated in the direction in which the eye should be pulled by the paralysed muscle, or, if squint is present at rest, it is increased by such a movement. Concomitant squint, however, is present at rest and is equal for all positions of the eyes, and, if the fixing eye is covered, the movements of the squinting eye are found to be full. Concomitant squint is not usually associated with diplopia; paralytic squint, at least in the early stages, usually is. However, when there is long-standing ocular muscle imbalance (latent concomitant squint or heterophoria) the patient may be able for many years to contract the ocular muscles so as to fuse the images from the two eyes. As he becomes older the effort may no longer be possible

ated; in conjugate deviation upwards and downwards, the elevators and depressors of the two eyes respectively are associated; and in convergence, the medial recti are associated. Graded contraction and relaxation of their antagonists play an important part in orderly movement.

Paralysis of individual ocular muscles
The more important results of paralysis of an ocular muscle are (1) defective ocular movement, (2) squint, (3) erroneous projection of the visual field, and (4) diplopia.

Defective ocular movement
Defective ocular movement is demonstrated by asking the patient to fix his gaze on an object, such as the observer's finger, which is then moved upwards and downwards and to either side, convergence being tested by bringing it towards the patient. The movement is defective in the direction in which the eye is normally moved by the muscle which is paralysed. Slight weakness of a muscle, especially of one of the elevators or depressors, may not lead to any defect of ocular movement evident to the observer.

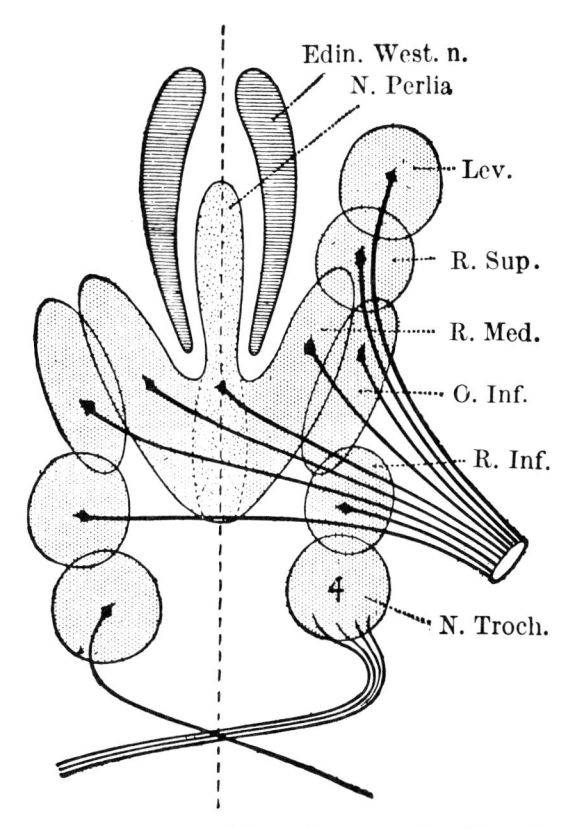

Figure 7.9 Diagram of the oculomotor nucleus. [Reproduced from Walton (1985) *Brain's Diseases of the Nervous System*, 9th edn, by kind permission of the publisher.]

Erroneous projection of the visual field

If we look at a light straight in front of us and then, turning the eyes but not the head, look at one placed to one side, in each case the image of the light falls upon the macula. When the right lateral rectus is paralysed, on conjugate deviation to the right the left eye moves normally but the right eye remains directed forward. The image of the object regarded falls in the left eye upon the macula, and in the right eye upon the nasal half of the retina. The patient is accustomed to regard an object, the image of which falls upon the nasal half of the right retina, as situated to the right of one of which the image falls upon the macula. Consequently he sees two images and projects the false image perceived by his affected eye to the right of the true image perceived by his normal eye. If now his normal eye is covered and he is asked to touch the object, he will direct his finger to the right of its true position. The erroneous projection is always in the normal direction of action of the affected muscle. When it produces sufficient spatial disorientation, subjective giddiness may result.

Diplopia

Erroneous projection of the visual field of the affected eye is responsible for double vision. When both eyes are used, two images are seen, one correctly and one erroneously projected—the true and the false images.

To take one example, in paralysis of the right lateral rectus the right eye is not abducted. If the patient attempts to deviate his eyes horizontally to the right, the image of a small object falls in the left eye upon the macula. In the right eye, which is not displaced, it falls upon the nasal half of the retina; hence it is seen in (or projected into) the temporal field of the right eye. The false image is thus parallel with and to the right of the true image. The further the test object is moved to the right, the further into the nasal half of the right retina its image moves, and the further the false image appears to move to the right. From these facts two simple rules about diplopia can be deduced:

1. The separation of the images increases the further the eyes are moved in the normal direction of pull of the paralysed muscle.
2. The false image is displaced in the direction of the plane of action of the paralysed muscle.

When the gaze is so directed that the separation of the images is greatest, the more peripherally situated image is the false one, derived from the affected eye, which can thus be ascertained. The simplest method is to cover one eye with a red glass and the other with a green glass. The patient is then made to look at a light source. This is moved until the maximal separation of the images is obtained, and they are then distinguishable by their colour. If coloured glass is

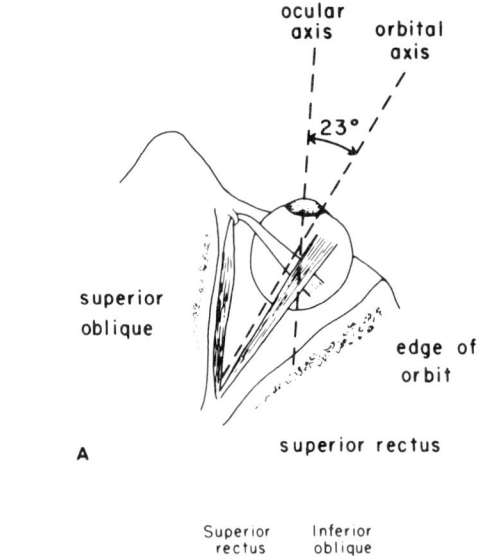

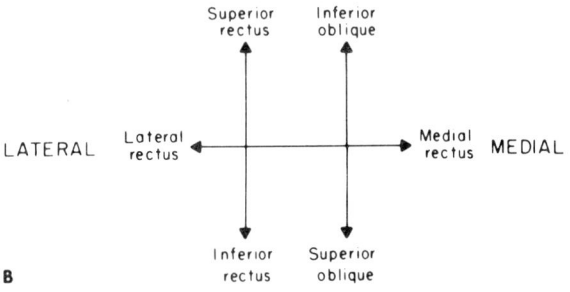

Figure 7.10 A, Dorsal view of the orbit, globe, superior rectus muscle, and superior oblique muscle. Note the relationship of the ocular axis to the orbital axis with regard to insertion of each muscle. B, Primary directon of pull by each of the six extraocular muscles. [Reproduced from Patton et al (1976) *Introduction to Basic Neurology*, by kind permission of the authors and publisher.]

so that the latent squint breaks down and diplopia may result. Similarly, in long-standing paralytic squint, one image may ultimately be suppressed so that diplopia disappears. Suppression of this type often results in one eye becoming amblyopic as a result of untreated concomitant squint in early childhood.

When the lateral rectus is paralysed, the ocular axes converge and the squint is said to be convergent. Paralysis of the medial rectus causes divergent squint. The deviation of the axis of the affected eye from parallelism with that of the normal eye is called the 'primary deviation'. If the patient is made to fix an object in a direction requiring the action of the affected muscle and at the same time is prevented from seeing it with his normal eye, the latter is found to deviate too far in the required direction. This is called 'secondary deviation', and is due to the increased effort evoked by his attempt to move the affected eye.

not available, an intelligent and cooperative patient is usually able to distinguish the images by noticing which disappears when each eye is covered separately.

When the affected eye has been discovered, the paralysed muscle can be determined. It is the muscle which normally displaces the eye in the direction of displacement of the false image. The positions of false images which result from paralysis of the various ocular muscles are described below for the right eye. The description will apply to the left eye if right be substituted for left and vice versa. The diplopia is said to be simple, or uncrossed, when the false image lies on the same side of the true image as the affected eye, and crossed when it lies on the opposite side.

Position of false image in paralysis of the ocular muscles of the right eye
Lateral rectus. The diplopia is uncrossed and the maximal separation of the images occurs on abduction when the false image is level with, and parallel with, the true image.
Medial rectus. The diplopia is crossed and the maximal separation of the images occurs on adduction, when the false image is level with, and parallel with, the true image.
Superior rectus. The false image is above and to the left of the true image and tilted away from it. Vertical separation of the images is greatest on abduction, and tilting is greatest on adduction. The diplopia is crossed.
Inferior rectus. The false image is below and to the left of the true image and tilted towards it. Vertical separation of the images is greatest on abduction, and tilting on adduction. The diplopia is crossed.
Inferior oblique. The false image is above and to the right of the true image and tilted away from it. The diplopia is uncrossed. Vertical separation of the images is greatest on adduction, and tilting on abduction.
Superior oblique. The false image is below and to the right of the true image and tilted towards it. The diplopia is uncrossed. Vertical separation of the images is greatest on adduction, and tilting on abduction. Since the diplopia occurs on looking downwards it is particularly troublesome to the patient when walking downstairs.

A patient suffering from diplopia usually rotates or tilts the head into the position in which the least demand is made upon the paralysed muscle.

The pathophysiology of nuclear and infranuclear lesions affecting ocular movement
Having confirmed which muscle or muscles are affected and hence which nerve is diseased, it is then necessary to decide the nature of the lesion responsible. Rarely, an isolated paralysis of abduction of one eye simulating a sixth nerve lesion is congenital (and often familial) and is due to fibrosis of the lateral rectus muscle (Duane's syndrome). A great many traumatic, inflammatory, neoplastic and degenerative disorders arising in the brain stem or in the basal cisterns or orbital foramina can give rise to paralysis of one or more of the oculomotor nerves. Thus, sphenoidal ridge meningioma can cause multiple ocular palsies, while orbital periostitis due to a granulomatous process involving the apex of the orbit and the margins of the superior orbital fissure, or granulomatous vasculitis in the cavernous sinus (the Tolosa–Hunt syndrome) are among the causes of painful ophthalmoplegia. A painful sixth nerve palsy may be due to petrous apicitis (Gradenigo's syndrome). Painless ophthalmoplegias can result from cranial polyneuritis (in the Guillain–Barré syndrome), from infarction of the nerve trunk (as in diabetes mellitus), or from infiltration by carcinomatous deposits involving the skull base and/or the meninges (as, for example, in nasopharyngeal carcinoma). Progressive supranuclear degeneration (the Steele–Richardson–Olszewski syndrome) is a rare degenerative disorder causing ophthalmoplegia, especially involving vertical gaze and associated with parkinsonian features and, sometimes, dementia.

The third nerve in particular is vulnerable in patients with basal arterial aneurysms or pituitary tumours, and it can be paralysed as a result of a cerebral hemisphere lesion, giving tentorial herniation. When complete third, fourth and sixth nerve palsies develop and are associated with sensory loss in the upper face, then an aneurysm in the cavernous sinus, compressing also the first and second divisions of the trigeminal nerve (which accompany these nerves within the sinus), is possible.

Lesions of the myoneural junction and of the ocular muscles themselves can give rise to ptosis, strabismus and diplopia. In myasthenia gravis, for instance, drooping of the eyelids towards the end of the day and intermittent strabismus and diplopia are common. An uncommon condition in which there is slowly progressive bilateral ptosis, with eventual impairment of ocular movement in all directions, is ocular myopathy. The process responsible is only occasionally nuclear and is more often a progressive dystrophy of the external ocular muscles.

The supranuclear and internuclear control of ocular movement

TYPES OF OCULAR MOVEMENT

During conjugate movements of the eyes the visual axes remain parallel, whereas during disconjugate movements the axes intersect. Conjugate movements are of two types: saccadic movement, in which the eyes jump rapidly and successively from one point of fixation to another, and smooth-pursuit movement, in which the eyes follow a moving object smoothly.

Saccadic movements are fast in that the eyes can move 40° in 100 ms. All voluntary eye movements, except when the subject is viewing a moving object, are saccadic. In reading a line of print the eyes read one to four words in the course of a single fixation and then jump to the next series of words. Speed and efficiency of reading depend upon the number of words read during each fixation. Saccadic movements can be recorded by an eye movement camera. The latency of successive movements is 200 to 500 ms. During each movement visual acuity is reflexly suppressed via a pathway which appears to involve the lateral geniculate body. Physiological studies in animals have demonstrated bursts of 400 to 600 spike discharges per second in the oculomotor, trochlear and abducens nuclei immediately prior to the onset and throughout each saccadic movement, with steady firing at a slower rate during the intervening periods of fixation. Saccadic movements are little influenced by drugs but are selectively impaired in some diseases such as Huntington's chorea and progressive supranuclear palsy.

Smooth pursuit movements, used to track moving targets, are slower, having a maximum velocity of about 50° per second. During such movements, visual acuity is unimpaired. Such movements cannot be performed at will without the stimulus of a moving target. The pursuit movement follows displacement of the target after a latency of about 13 ms. Drugs such as barbiturates and anticonvulsants depress this type of movement, breaking it down into saccadic movements.

In contrast to saccadic and smooth pursuit movements, which involve conjugate deviation of the eyes, vergence movements track approaching (convergence) or receding (divergence) objects. During vergence movements the eyes move in opposite directions. The vestibular system plays a part in the control of ocular movement in reflexly maintaining ocular fixation upon a visual target during head movement. Lesions of the labyrinth or vestibular nerve or nucleus may result in impaired ocular fixation and consequent blurred vision when the head is moved.

Supranuclear and internuclear pathways
The supranuclear pathway concerned with voluntary conjugate eye movement in a lateral direction originates in the frontal eye field in the contralateral middle frontal gyrus. The pathway from the cortical area descends through the corona radiata, internal capsule and cerebral peduncle, subsequently decussating in the midbrain and descending in the pons to join the medial longitudinal fasciculus at about the level of the sixth nerve nucleus. Thus, stimulation in the pons, below the decussation of this pathway, causes conjugate deviation of the eyes towards the lesion or point of stimulation, while a unilateral lesion of the pontomesencephalic reticular formation may cause paralysis of conjugate gaze towards the affected side. There is also evidence that visual input into the superior colliculus has a powerful controlling influence upon this fronto-mesencephalic-pontine (supranuclear) pathway, as bursts of spikes can be recorded from collicular neurons during saccades.

Another important cortical centre concerned with ocular movements lies in or near the visual cortex in the occipital lobe. The occipitomesencephalic pathways appear to be concerned especially with smooth pursuit movements and occipitopretectal pathways with vergence.

Less is known about supranuclear pathways controlling vertical conjugate deviation. Probably they also originate in the middle frontal gyrus, but bilateral activation may be needed to evoke vertical movements. As a result, defective vertical conjugate gaze of cerebral origin as a rule occurs only as a result of massive bifrontal lesions. Lesions in the neighbourhood of the posterior commissure may also paralyse vertical gaze.

Because coordination of the movement of the two eyes is essential to binocular vision, the nuclei of the individual third, fourth and sixth cranial nerves are linked together in the medial longitudinal fasciculus, which is the principal internuclear pathway controlling ocular movement. The fasciculus also receives an extensive input from vestibular, cerebellar and other nuclei and pathways concerned with reflex ocular movement, as well as from the supranuclear pathways described above. Cerebellar lesions often cause over- or undershoot of saccadic movements and/or the breaking down of smooth-pursuit into saccadic movements.

Reflex ocular movement
In voluntary conjugate deviation of the eyes the patient turns his eyes spontaneously or on command. Other ocular movements are reflexly induced. Visual stimuli usually result in movement of the head (or, if the head is held fixed in one position, of the eyes) in order to keep the image of the stimulus upon the macula. Continuous movement of a series of objects or lines in one direction evokes optokinetic nystagmus (see below). Similarly, auditory stimulation may give deviation of the eyes towards the origin of the sound, while caloric or electrical excitation of

one labyrinth evokes conjugate ocular deviation and nystagmus (see below). If the patient is asked to fix his gaze upon an object and the head is then flexed, rotated or extended at the neck, reflex ocular deviation occurs in an attempt to keep the image of the object upon the macula. This so-called oculocephalic reflex (the doll's head manoeuvre) is dependent upon the integrity of the medial longitudinal fasciculus and of its connections with the vestibular system, and is thus valuable clinically in determining whether pontine vestibulo-ocular connections are intact in patients in coma. Very exceptionally, the reflex can be severely impaired or even lost in patients with supratentorial lesions receiving therapeutic doses of anticonvulsant drugs.

Supranuclear and internuclear lesions
Spasmodic conjugate lateral movements of the eyes may occur in focal attacks of epilepsy due to lesions involving the contralateral frontal eye field and, less often, involving the contralateral occipital cortex. It can also be an occasional consequence of a deep contralateral intracerebral haemorrhage involving the thalamus and basal ganglia.

Paralysis of conjugate lateral movement may occur as the result of a lesion at any point in the supranuclear pathway described above, but this effect is always transient in lesions situated above the pons. A lesion involving the decussation of the pathways at the pontomesencephalic junction can give paralysis of conjugate gaze to both sides. A unilateral pontine lesion may give long-lasting paralysis of both voluntary and reflex conjugate gaze to the affected side. This may result from encephalomyelitis or Wernicke's disease, but is more often due to brain-stem infarction.

Dissociation of conjugate lateral movement is usually a consequence of a lesion of the medial longitudinal fasciculus (an internuclear lesion). Much the commonest effect is the so-called anterior internuclear ophthalmoplegia (Harris's sign, or 'ataxic nystagmus') in which there is phasic nystagmus confined to the abducting eye, associated with failure of medial movement of the adducting eye. While rarely this sign can be a consequence of brain-stem tumour or infarction, it is much more often due to multiple sclerosis and can be unilateral or bilateral. Very rarely, a posterior internuclear ophthalmoplegia resulting from a lesion (usually an infarct) of the fasciculus just rostral to the abducens nucleus may occur, giving paralysis of abduction of one eye with normal adduction of the other, and with nystagmus, thus differentiating this sign from the effects of a sixth nerve lesion. Another rare manifestation of an acute brain-stem lesion involving the paramedian pontine recitular formation and the medial longitudinal fasciculus is paralytic pontine exotropia in which there is external deviation of the contralateral eye with total horizontal immobility of the ipsilateral eye.

Skew deviation of the eyes, in which one eye is deviated upwards and outwards, and the other downwards and outwards, is a rare consequence of an acute brain-stem lesion, usually in the pons on the side of the lower eye, less often in the midbrain, medulla or cerebellum, and usually resulting from infarction.

Spasmodic conjugate vertical movement of the eyes upwards is a rare phenomenon, occasionally occurring in an attack of epilepsy, especially petit mal, but it is also characteristic of the oculogyric crises of postencephalitic parkinsonism.

Paralysis of conjugate vertical deviation in an upward direction is not uncommon, but paralysis of downward movement is excessively rare. In lesions of the upper midbrain in the region of the superior colliculus, voluntary vertical deviation can be lost even though the movement can still be excited reflexly in eliciting the oculocephalic reflexes. The term 'Parinaud's syndrome' is often applied to isolated defects of upward conjugate gaze. Rarely, the defect is congenital, but in the fully developed syndrome due to lesions of the midbrain tectum there is often loss of the pupillary light reflexes and paralysis of convergence in addition. This may result from encephalitis, from tumours of the third ventricle, midbrain or pineal body, from Wernicke's disease, or from infarction.

Paralysis of convergence is occasionally seen in postencephalitic parkinsonism as a result of head injury or midbrain infarction, and rarely results from ageing. Loss of convergence is occasionally hysterical, and spasm of convergence invariably hysterical.

Ocular motor apraxia is an inability to move the eyes voluntarily in a desired direction when random and reflex eye movements are intact. The condition is usually congenital. The patients show increased latencies and decreased amplitudes of voluntary saccadic eye movements in the horizontal plane, especially when the head is fixed, but when the head is free to move they make conspicuous, thrusting, compensatory head movements in the direction in which they wish to look. Rarely a similar syndrome develops in patients with an acquired lesion of the prefrontal motor cortex.

Nystagmus
Nystagmus refers to an oscillatory movement of the eyes which is often rhythmic and repetitive. It is sometimes present with the eyes at rest, but it may appear only when they are moved conjugately. If present at rest, it may be accentuated by ocular movement. It can be rotary in type (occurring in more

than one plane) or it may occur only in a lateral or vertical direction. Occasionally both phases of the to-and-fro oscillation are of equal duration, but more often there is a quick phase in one direction succeeded by a slower recoil (phasic nystagmus). In this case the nystagmus is said to be occurring in the direction of the quick phase. Nystagmus is described as first degree when present on lateral gaze to one side only, second degree when present on looking ahead but accentuated when looking to one side, and third degree when present on fixation and on looking to both sides and when it is much more striking on looking to one side. Acquired forms of nystagmus sometimes cause apparent movement of objects seen by the patient (oscillopsia). Nystagmus can be recorded by electronystagmography. This phenomenon is essentially a disorder of the posture of the eyes and can be produced by disease of the reflex pathways which influence ocular posture. Stimuli from the retina and labyrinths play an important role in the maintenance of posture of the eyes as of other parts of the body, and cerebellar activity is also of importance, so that lesions of any of these structures can give rise to nystagmus.

Nystagmus of labyrinthine origin can be evoked by caloric stimulation of the semicircular canals. If only the horizontal canals are stimulated it is lateral in type, but involvement of the vertical canals gives a rotary type which is therefore more common in disease of the internal ear. The quick phase of the nystagmus takes place in a direction away from the affected ear. In acute labyrinthine vertigo the amplitude of the nystagmus is increased on looking to the side away from the lesion. Sometimes nystagmus is produced only by sudden movement of the head in a particular direction (positional nystagmus). This occurs in a disorder of the internal ear known as benign positional nystagmus, but it is occasionally seen in lesions of the brain stem or in patients with neoplasms in the neighbourhood of the fourth ventricle.

Phasic nystagmus on lateral gaze may not infrequently be due to many drugs, including alcohol, barbiturates, anticonvulsants and many more (toxic nystagmus). The commonest causes of nystagmus in neurological practice are lesions of the cerebellum or of cerebellar and vestibular connections in the brain stem. In a unilateral cerebellar lesion the nystagmus is increased on lateral deviation of the eyes towards the side of the lesion. So profuse are the structures in the brain stem which are concerned with cerebellar, vestibular and oculomotor function (the medial longitudinal fasciculus is one of the most important) that virtually any lesion in this location, whether inflammatory, neoplastic, degenerative or metabolic, gives rise to this physical sign. It is almost impossible to attribute any specific localizing or diagnostic value to the nystagmus under these circumstances, except in the case of the ataxic nystagmus or internuclear ophthalmoplegia mentioned above. Often the nystagmus resulting from a brain-stem lesion occurs particularly on lateral movement of the eyes, the quick phase occurring towards the direction of gaze. Many other varieties occur and vertical nystagmus is particularly common in cases of the Chiari malformation or in other disorders at or near the foramen magnum. Statistically, multiple sclerosis is the commonest cause of nystagmus, but encephalitis, vascular lesions, syringobulbia, Wernicke's encephalopathy and tumours can also produce this sign. There is no convincing evidence that lesions at any level lower than the medulla oblongata and cerebellar tonsils ever produce nystagmus.

HEARING

General considerations

Sound waves are mechanically induced by vibrations which spread as pressure waves throughout the surrounding medium, whether this is gaseous, liquid or solid. They are perceived by the ear, which is a specialized mechanoreceptor. Vibrations so recorded are modified in the conduction system (external auditory canal, tympanic membrane, ossicular system and cochlear perilymph and endolymph) before reaching the auditory receptors, the hair cells of the organ of Corti. These hair cells are exquisitely sensitive, being responsive at frequencies of maximal sensitivity to displacements of as little as 10^{-10} cm.

The conduction system transmits some frequencies more efficiently than others. Sound waves travel in air with a velocity of 344 m/s at 20°C. A simple sinusoidal wave gives rise to a pure tone and its frequency (in cycles/s or Hz) determines its pitch, which is higher the greater the frequency. Similarly there is a correlation between amplitude and loudness. Musical sounds produced by various instruments produce complex tones consisting of a basic pure tone admixed with various harmonics which help to confer quality or timbre upon the sound, allowing one to recognize the distinctive sounds made by different instruments playing the same note. In addition, human experience is full of sounds producing multiple and very complex wave forms simply called noises.

The intensity of sound, which is closely correlated with but not identical to loudness, is measured on a logarithmic scale in units known as bels (B), but for convenience the decibel (dB) is much more often

The special senses 145

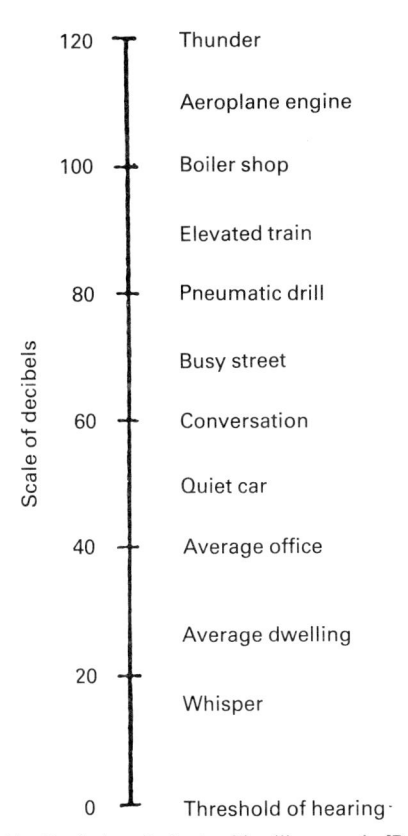

Figure 7.11 Decibel equivalents of familiar sounds. [Reproduced from Patton et al, (1976) *Introduction to Basic Neurology*, and previously published in Stevens and Davis *Hearing. Its Psychology and Physiology* (New York: John Wiley & Sons, 1938), by kind permission of the authors and publishers.]

used. Ten decibels implies a tenfold increase, 20 dB a hundredfold increase in intensity, and so on. Fig. 7.11 gives some indication of the relative intensities of some everyday sounds.

Structure and function

STRUCTURE

The outer, middle and internal ear are illustrated in Fig. 7.12. Sound passing via the pinna or auricle into the external auditory canal impinges on the tympanic membrane, which communicates the vibrations into the middle ear. The middle ear is an air-filled bony cavity which communicates with the nasopharynx via the eustachian tube in order to maintain it at atmospheric pressure. The chain of auditory ossicles (malleus, incus and stapes) transmits the sound vibrations across the cavity of the middle ear to the oval window of the cochlea where they are conveyed to the cochlear endolymph. This process is affected by two small muscles, the tensor tympani and the stapedius, which together tend to increase tension in the ossicular chain, thereby reducing energy transmission and protecting the ear reflexly against sound of exceptional intensity. In Bell's palsy, when muscles innervated by the facial nerve are paralysed, hyperacusis is sometimes noted as the result of paralysis of the stapedius.

The structure of the inner ear is exceptionally complex (Fig. 7.13). The bony labyrinth contains fluid (perilymph), within which is the membranous labyrinth filled with endolymph. Two parts of the labyrinth are concerned with balance and equilibrium: the semicircular canals, containing the semicircular ducts, and the vestibule, containing the utricle and saccule. The cochlear portion, containing the cochlear duct, is concerned solely with hearing. The cochlea makes two and a half turns around its central pillar from which a bony shelf projects into the canal. Attached to the free edge of this shelf is the basilar membrane, joined to the lateral wall of the spiral ligament. Below this membrane is the scala tympani filled with perilymph; above it is the cochlear duct containing endolymph. The delicate upper wall of the cochlear duct (Reissner's membrane) separates its endolymph from the perilymph of the scala vestibuli, which is continuous with that of the vestibule. The columnar cells which line the lateral wall of the cochlear duct control the composition of the endolymph. At the apex of the cochlea, the scala tympani and scala vestibuli communicate through a tiny opening. The scala tympani ends below at the round window, closed by a membrane which separates it from the middle ear.

The organ of Corti (Fig. 7.13), the final sensory receptor organ of the cochlea, lies on the dorsal surface of the basilar membrane. The rods or pillars of Corti form a triangular arch enclosing the tunnel of Corti, flanked by columns consisting of phalangeal (Deiters') cells and hair cells. Projections from the phalangeal cells extend upwards between the hair cells and fuse to form the reticular lamina or articular plate forming the roof of the organ. Above this is the tectorial membrane, a stiff, fibrogelatinous plate to which the stereocilia of the hair cells are attached and which therefore bend to and fro as the basilar membrane vibrates. Soft columnar cells of Hensen and Claudius cover the basilar membrane on either side of the hair cells. Up to 80 hairs or stereocilia join the tips of each hair cell to the tectorial membrane. The to-and-fro movement of these hairs is thought to generate potentials stimulating the cells of the spiral ganglion, which are the primary auditory neurons. Two types of nerve terminals can be ident-

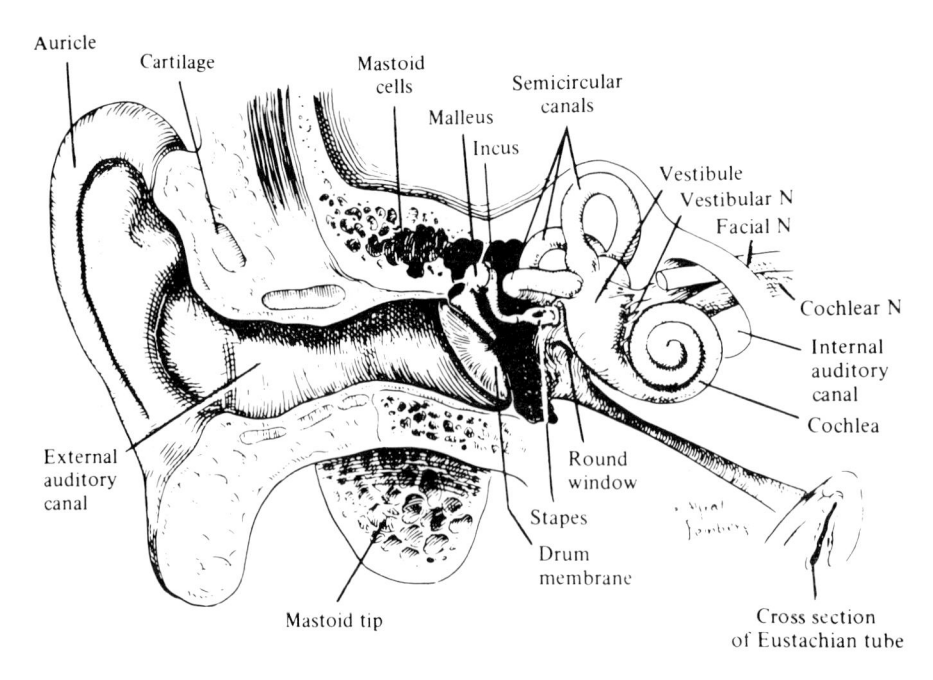

Figure 7.12 The peripheral auditory apparatus. The cochlea is turned slightly to show its coils. The Eustachian tube runs forwards as well as downwards and inwards. [Reproduced from Patton et al (1976) *Introduction to Basic Neurology*, and previously published in Davis and Silverman *Hearing and Deafness* (New York: Holt, Rinehart and Winston, 1970), by kind permission of the authors and publishers.]

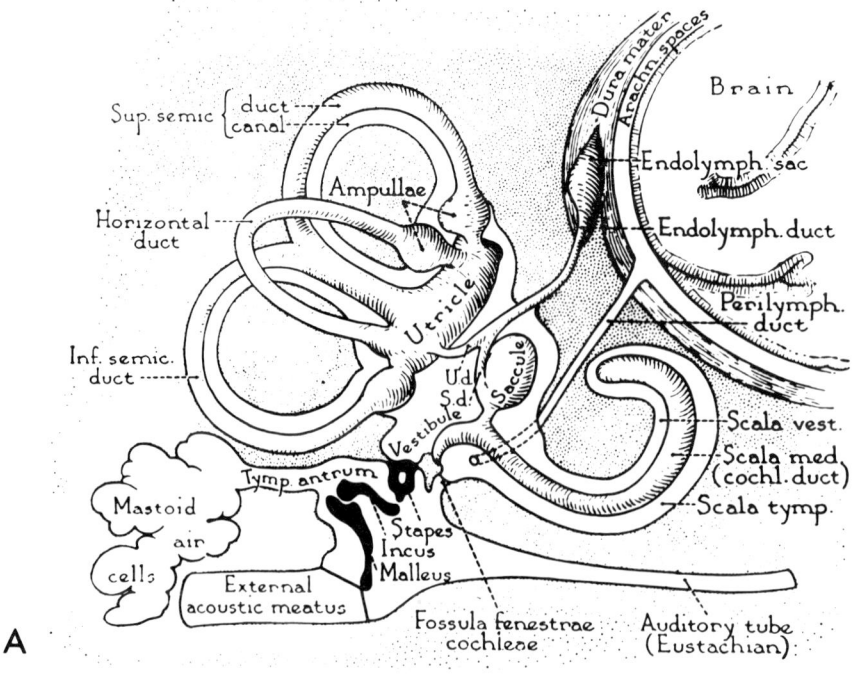

Figure 7.13 A, The relationship of the osseous and membranous labyrinths. The former is filled with perilymph and at the vestibule communicates with the subarachnoid space via the perilymphatic duct. The membranous labyrinth floats in the perilymph and contains endolymph. Only part of the coiled cochlea is shown. Note that the cochlear duct (scala media) is part of the membranous system. It ends blindly at the cochlear apex and contains endolymph. The perilymph-filled scala vestibula communicates with the vestibule and through the helicotrema, with the scala tympani, which ends at the round window. [Reproduced from Patton et al (1976) *Introduction to Basic Neurology*, and previously published in Bast and Anson *The Temporal Bone and the Ear* (Springfield, Ill., Charles C. Thomas, 1949) by kind permission of the authors and publishers.]

Illustration continued on the opposite page

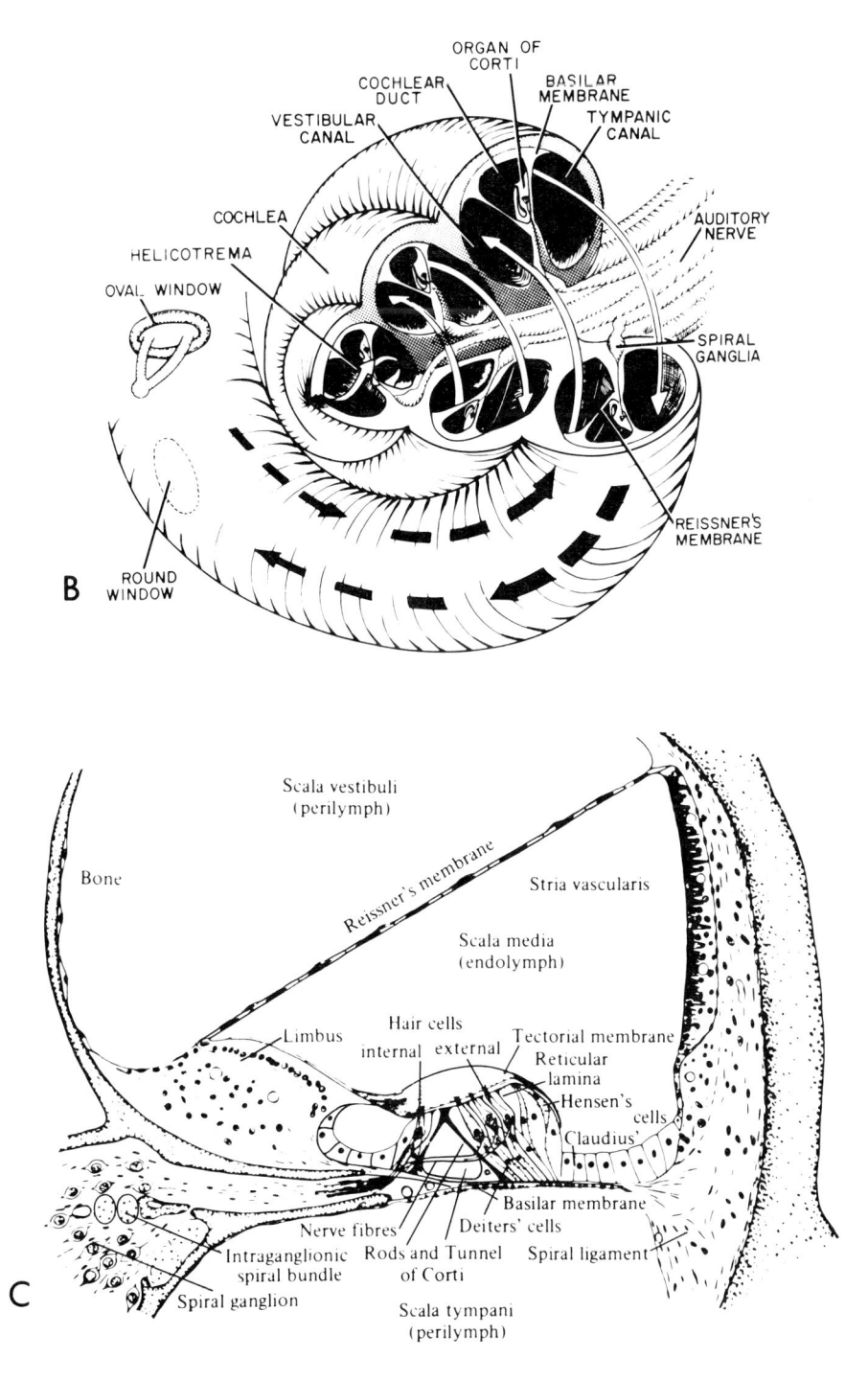

Figure 7.13 *(continued)* B, The cochlea and the organ of Corti. Diagram of cochlea cut through to show the partition of the cavity by the basilar membrane and cochlear duct (scala media). Arrows show the pathway of transmission of pressure waves originating at the oval window. (Reproduced from Patton et al: *Introduction to Basic Neurology*, and previously published in Curtis, Jacobson, and Marcus: *An Introduction to the Neurosciences* [Philadelphia, W. B. Saunders Co., 1972]; by kind permission of the authors and publishers.)

C, The cochlear partition and the organ of Corti. (Reproduced from Patton et al: *Introduction to Basic Neurology*, and previously published in Davis and Silverman, *Hearing and Deafness* [New York, Holt, Rinehart and Winston, 1970]; by kind permission of the authors and publishers.)

ified in the base of the hair cells: (a) clear endings, which are afferent and convey the auditory impulse into the spiral ganglion, and (b) granular terminals, which are efferent, originating in the superior olivary nucleus and subserving the function of depressing hair-cell excitability.

FUNCTION

Conduction
The external auditory canal acts in some respects like an organ pipe in adding resonance to the sound which enters it. The ossicular system, through a rocking action which gives a piston-like effect to the stapes in the oval window, efficiently transmits pressure waves from a gaseous medium (air in the external canal and middle ear) to a liquid medium, the perilymph. The resonance of the external canal and the mechanical properties of the ossicular chain determine that sensitivity will be most acute in the middle range of frequencies, which predominate in human speech (400–3000 Hz). In addition to transmission through the ossicular chain, air conduction can also occur through the round window of the scala tympani, and the perilymph can be made to vibrate by oscillations conducted through the bony skull (bone conduction). Bone conduction is much less sensitive than air conduction, a fact made use of in certain tuning fork tests. Nevertheless bone conduction is utilized in various hearing aids.

Sound-induced pressure waves in the perilymph of the scala vestibuli impinge on the basilar membrane, causing a shearing displacement of the stereocilia of the hair cells. At the same time, pressure alters in the perilymph of the scala tympani with consequent bulging of the round window in and out of the middle ear. Outward movement of the stapes causes the organ of Corti to move upwards and the hairs to bend laterally, with consequent neuronal discharge which is then turned off by movement in the opposite direction.

Cochlear mechanisms
The auditory nerve fibres derived from the hair cells have an upper frequency response of 1000 Hz, whereas the upper limit of the range of auditory perception and discrimination is about 20 000 Hz. This discrepancy was explained by Helmholtz in the place theory of pitch perception, which concluded that the basilar membrane, as a consequence of its variable structure and the variable tension upon its fibres, is differentially tuned at different points. This would allow different parts of the membrane to respond to pressure waves of varying frequency. Subsequently, Bekesy showed that such waves in the perilymph produce propagated waves in the basilar membrane proceeding from the base towards the apex of the cochlea, and that the amplitude of these waves at different points varied with the frequency of the sound wave. High-frequency waves reach maximal amplitude in the basal portion and die out before reaching the apex, whereas low-frequency waves produce minimal displacement at the base and much more displacement towards the apex. Recent work has shown that the mechanical response of the basilar membrane is tuned very sharply indeed (Pickles, 1985), and there is believed to be a physiologically active process which restores mechanical energy in the membrane, particularly after low-intensity or high-frequency stimulation. Thus, each frequency in the audible range has a point of maximal displacement of the membrane (mechanical processing) at which the relevant hair cells produce maximal rates of action potential discharge through which the pitch of the sound is ultimately recognized.

Cochlear microphonics are non-propagated hair cell potentials generated by movement of the organ of Corti. These are best recorded from the round window but in man they can be picked up by electrodes applied behind the pinna just above the mastoid process. The amplitude of the microphonic is proportional to the intensity of the sound and can be accepted as giving an accurate indication of hair-cell displacement. The membrane potential of the hair cells also produces a current which passes through the scala media and ultimately leaves the base of the hair cell to release a transmitter (as yet unidentified) which excites afferent neuronal endings. Movement of the membrane and consequently of the stereocilia of the hair cells causes variations in this leakage current, which are responsible for the cochlear microphonic, the receptor potential of the ear. The hair cell is not truly an excitable cell; rather it acts as a variable resistor sensitive to mechanical distortion of its hairs. It is now known that deflection of the stereocilia in one direction decreases membrane resistance and produces intracellular depolarization, while deflection in the opposite direction increases resistance and causes hyperpolarization (Pickles, 1985). These changes are associated with the pressure flow of ions through ionically non-specific channels. It seems likely that the changes in membrane resistance produce the receptor potential while alterations in intracellular polarization release transmitter and activate auditory neurons.

Auditory nerve
The central processes of bipolar cells in the spiral ganglion of the cochlea form the cochlear nerve. The distal processes emerge and lose their myelin sheaths medial to the inner pillar of the organ of Corti. About 95% of them innervate the inner hair cells, 20 fibres

The special senses

from fibres supplying different groups of hair cells at various points on the basilar membrane.

An individual nerve fibre can respond to a range of frequencies as a substantial area of the basilar membrane moves in response to a single frequency of sound even at moderate intensity. However, each fibre's tuning curve shows one frequency region of great sensitivity (the 'tip' region) and the tip frequency is called the characteristic frequency. This is directly related to the region of the basilar membrane innervated by the fibre, those areas near the oval window having high characteristic frequencies, while low frequencies are typical of those parts of the membrane near the apex. Some fibres with low characteristic frequencies can phase-lock to a pure tone stimulus. If stimulus intensity is varied for a tone of any one frequency, there is a sigmoidal relationship between firing rate and stimulus intensity. The intensity range from threshold to the maximum or saturation rate is 30–50 dB for most fibres. In addition, one auditory stimulus can often reduce the responsiveness of the cochlea to other stimuli (suppression). Thus, inhibitory interaction is probably related to the non-linearity of the transduction process, including the basilar membrane mechanics. It is not true neural inhibition (Pickles, 1985).

Most of the granular, vesicle-containing efferent nerve endings (Fig. 7.14) are the terminations of neurons lying in the contralateral superior olivary nucleus in the brain stem. The relevant fibres traverse the auditory nerve and spiral ganglion without synapsing, to terminate either on the base of inner hair cells alongside the afferent terminals or else on the afferent fibres themselves which innervate the outer cells. In addition, 20–25% of efferent fibres arise from the ipsilateral olive and are largely distributed to the inner hair cells. Both ipsilateral and contralateral fibres branch extensively and have many terminal knobs. Like afferent fibres they show tuned behaviour, each having a best frequency of response. They respond to auditory stimuli, having a threshold of about 40 dB. Stimulation of these efferent fibres either blocks or reduces the neural response to auditory stimuli, but the cochlear microphonic is not reduced and is sometimes increased. It therefore seems likely that this efferent system diminishes the masking effect of background noise, thus improving the signal-to-noise ratio.

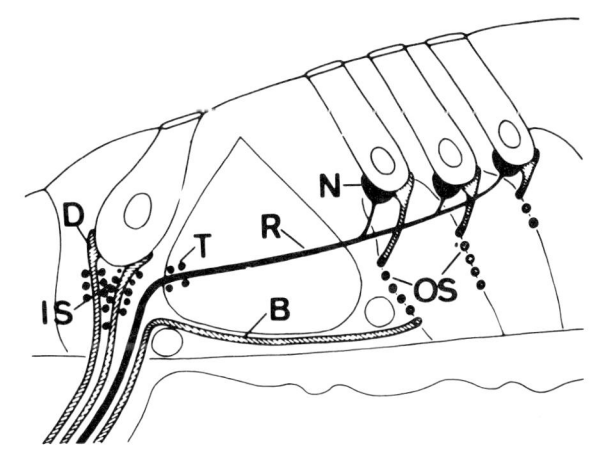

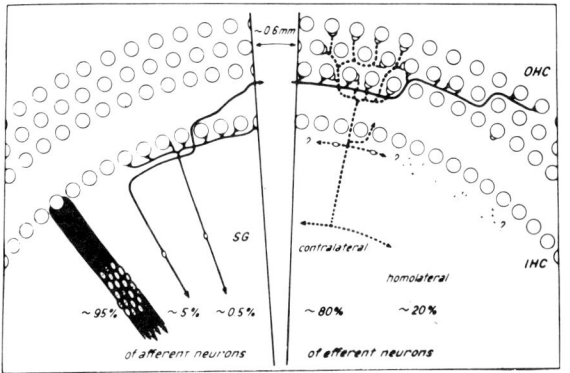

Figure 7.14 Distribution of afferent and efferent fibres to inner and outer hair cells.
Upper diagram: Afferent fibres are cross-hatched; efferent fibres, solid. D, direct afferent fibres to inner hair cells, IS, inner spiral efferent fibres. T, tunnel spiral efferent fibres. R, upper tunnel efferent fibres to outer hair cells (N). B, basal fibres (afferent). OS, outer spiral afferent fibres.
Lower diagram: Quantitative distribution of afferent (left) and efferent (right) fibres to inner and outer hair cells.
[Reproduced from Patton et al (1976) *Introduction to Basic Neurology*; upper diagram previously published by Spoendlin in Møller (ed.) *Basic Mechanisms in Hearing* (New York: Academic Press, 1973); lower diagram previously published by Spoendlin (1971) *Arch. klin. exp. Ohr-Nas-Kehlkoptheilkunde* **200**:275–291, by kind permission of the authors and publishers.]

to a cell, while the remaining 5% cross under the tunnel and branch repeatedly, each innervating about 10 outer hair cells (Fig. 7.14). Afferent neurons in the auditory nerve show random spontaneous resting discharges (about 100 spikes per second), even in conditions of absolute silence. These are possibly due to the leakage current from the hair cells mentioned above. When pure tones are applied to the ear, single fibres derived from different parts of the organ of Corti each respond to a specific band of frequencies. There is one 'best or characteristic frequency', so that V-shaped 'tuning curves' for each fibre can be plotted, and it is assumed that different curves are derived

Central auditory pathways

The afferent fibres of the auditory nerve synapse with secondary auditory neurons in the cochlear nuclei which lie dorsolaterally in the medulla just below the inferior cerebellar peduncle. In each there is one dorsal and two ventral nuclei, and the projection is organized tonotopically so that high frequencies are

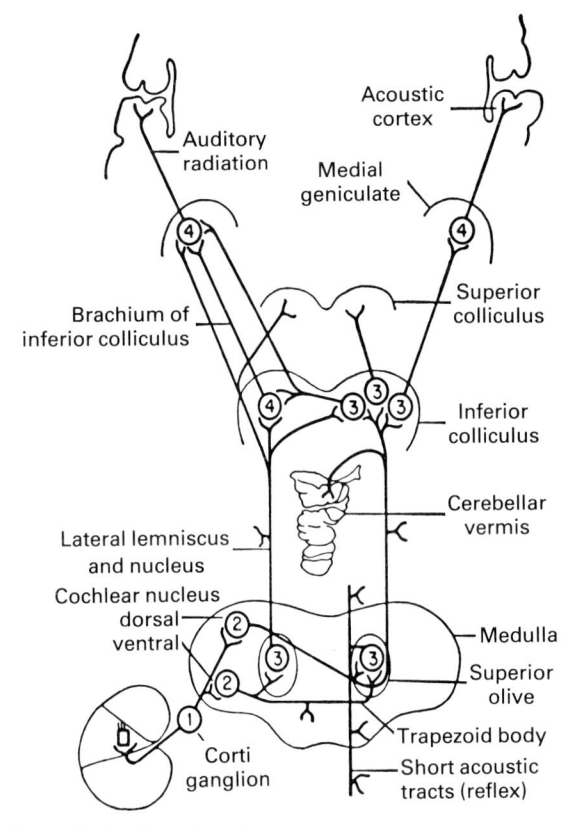

Figure 7.15 Central auditory pathways. Numbers label first-, second-, third-, and fourth-order neurons. [Reproduced from Patton et al (1976) *Introduction to Basic Neurology*, and previously published by Davis in Stevens (ed.) (1951) *Handbook of Experimental Psychology* (New York: John Wiley & Sons); by kind permission of the authors and publishers.]

recorded dorsally, and low frequencies are recorded ventrally. Pathways projecting centrally from these nuclei are exceptionally complex (Fig. 7.15). All fibres synapse in the inferior colliculus and again in the medial geniculate body, but their pathways are diverse. The fibres of the principal crossed pathway decussate in the trapezoid body and then enter the lateral lemniscus, with or without synapsing in the superior olive, while uncrossed fibres follow a similar route without crossing the midline. Most cells of the inferior colliculus project to the ipsilateral medial geniculate body, but some projections cross between the inferior colliculi to reach the contralateral medial geniculate. The final common path for auditory stimuli from the cells of the medial geniculate body is to the auditory (acoustic) cortex in the superior temporal gyrus. Multiple and complex tonotopic representation of the cochlea has been demonstrated in the lateral lemniscus, superior olive, inferior colliculus, medial geniculate body, and especially in the auditory cortex. This complex organization with multiple decussations and bilateral representation explains why clinically overt disturbances of hearing only rarely result from discrete lesions of the brain stem or auditory cortex, unless the lesions are bilateral.

There is good evidence that in the lateral part of the superior olive most cells are excited by ipsilateral stimuli and inhibited by contralateral ones. This mechanism is clearly closely related to the ability to localize a sound in space, and is related to *intensity* differences recognized by each of the two ears. Such differences are greatest for high frequencies. In the medial superior olive, however, most cells are excited by stimuli applied to either ear but they are able to localize sound sources on the basis of differences in the *timing* of stimuli reaching each ear independently. These mechanisms, combined with that of frequency-representation made possible by phase-locking of individual neurons, are fundamental in relation to sound localization, and in recognition of both musical notes and the quality of musical sounds.

TESTS OF AUDITORY FUNCTION

Damage to hair cells of the organ of Corti causes sensorineural deafness, while lesions of the auditory nerve produce nerve deafness. Lesions of the conducting mechanism in the middle ear give conductive deafness. Various tests are available to distinguish these clinically.

Weber's test
A vibrating tuning fork (C-256) is applied to the forehead or vertex in the midline and the patient is asked whether the sound is heard in the midline or is localized in one ear. In normal individuals the sound appears to be in the midline. In conductive deafness it is usually localized in the affected ear; in nerve deafness it is usually localized in the normal ear. This is due to the fact that in sensorineural or nerve deafness bone conduction is reduced as well as air conduction, whereas in conductive deafness air conduction is reduced but bone conduction is relatively enhanced.

Rinne's test
A vibrating tuning fork is applied to the patient's mastoid process, the ear being closed by the observer's finger. The patient is asked to say when he ceases to hear the sound, and the fork is then held at the external meatus. In conductive deafness the sound cannot be heard by air conduction after bone conduction has ceased to transmit it. In nerve deafness, as in normal individuals, the reverse is the case. It is important also to occlude the opposite ear during the performance of the test. Even so, the results of

Rinne's test may be misleading in unilateral sensorineural or nerve deafness when the sound of the tuning fork applied to the mastoid process of the deaf ear is heard in the opposite normal ear.

In nerve deafness loss of hearing is most marked for high-pitched tones; in conductive deafness it is most marked for low-pitched tones.

Audiometry and other quantitative methods

Pure tone audiometry, a quantitative method of testing hearing, should now be a routine procedure in all patients suspected of having hearing loss. The threshold in decibels for the perception of pure tones of different frequencies is measured in each ear using both air and bone conduction, with the other ear masked. Characteristic patterns are then obtained for nerve deafness (of high and low frequencies or both), for conductive deafness, and for mixed types of deafness. Various special techniques have been devised for the examination of young children.

Loudness recruitment is a technique of particular value in detecting unilateral sensorineural deafness (due to cochlear end-organ disease, as in Ménière's syndrome). A pure tone of constant frequency is applied with increasing intensity (in decibels) to each ear alternately. In conductive deafness and in nerve deafness due to disease of the cochlear nerve central to the sensory end-organs in the cochlea, the ratio between the intensities required to produce sounds of equal loudness in the two ears remains constant. In sensorineural deafness, however, with increasing loudness the sound eventually seems equally loud in the two ears.

The greatest social disability of the deaf is inability to hear and understand the spoken word; hence free-field speech audiometry is useful in the distinction between conductive, cochlear and retrocochlear hearing loss and in helping to correct cochlear deafness with hearing aids. The measurement of auditory-evoked potentials is being used increasingly in diagnosis. When a click is delivered to the external auditory meatus, neurons in the internal ear, the brain stem and the auditory and association areas of the cortex are activated sequentially, and the electrical activity so generated can be recorded by means of sophisticated averaging techniques through electrodes placed over the mastoid process and vertex. At least seven components of the auditory-evoked response have been identified of which five, occurring in the first 8 ms, are believed to originate from the auditory nerve and brain stem. These short-latency components, known as the brain stem auditory-evoked potentials (BAEP), measurement of their interwave intervals, amplitude ratios, and responses to changing stimulus rates are being used increasingly as aids in the localization and identification of brain-stem lesions in adults and children. Intermediate-latency (8–50 ms) and long-latency responses (over 50 ms) probably reflect activity in the auditory cortex and association areas but are as yet of much less diagnostic value.

LESIONS RESPONSIBLE FOR DEAFNESS

The commonest causes of conductive deafness include simple remediable lesions such as wax in the ear or blockage of the eustachian tube, inflammatory processes such as acute or chronic otitis media, and otosclerosis, a disorder in which abnormal bone growth immobilizes the stapes in the oval window. The latter condition may require stapedectomy or the surgical provision of a new window (fenestration). Nerve deafness may result from lesions of the hair cells of the organ of Corti or of the auditory nerve or its terminals. The commonest causes are sensorineural deafness due to Ménière's disease, trauma, damage by drugs, spread of acute or chronic infection from the middle ear, virus infection causing so-called acute labyrinthitis, ageing (presbyacusis), and occlusion of the internal auditory artery due to atherosclerosis. Streptomycin and its analogues cause deafness by damaging the cochlear end-organ. Other causes include congenital syphilis, otosclerosis, many causes of hereditary deafness, and acoustic neuroma. Other lesions or processes which may damage one or both auditory nerves in the subarachnoid space include meningitis, especially when granulomatous in type (e.g. tuberculosis, meningovascular syphilis, sarcoidosis). Rare causes include avitaminosis, mumps and polyneuritis cranialis. Deafness is a rare symptom of lesions within the central nervous system, though unilateral deafness may rarely be caused by a vascular lesion of the pons, or by multiple sclerosis, and total bilateral deafness and loss of vestibular function may be associated with other signs of brain-stem damage in a case of head injury. Clinical deafness does not occur as a result of lesions of the temporal lobe unless the lesions are bilateral and very extensive, but unilateral temporal lesions can disrupt the discrimination of patterned sequences of tonal stimuli. Central deafness in childhood may be due to birth injury, perinatal anoxia, maternal rubella, or kernicterus.

Tinnitus

Tinnitus, or noise in the ears, is an important symptom of disease of the auditory nerve, though it can result from wax or from eustachian catarrh or middle-ear disease. Characteristically it is a hissing or machinery-like noise which may be unilateral or bilateral, and continuous or intermittent. It is often severe in elderly people and can be so distressing as to interfere continuously with sleep and hearing. In such cases it may be due to atherosclerotic ischaemia of the inner ear, though it is sometimes a manifestation of severe depression. Degeneration of Corti's organ, of unknown cause, is the commonest cause in the elderly. Drugs such as quinine, salicylates and streptomycin may also produce tinnitus. When unilateral, it may be an important symptom of disease of the labyrinth (e.g. Ménière's disease) or the auditory nerve (e.g. acoustic neuroma).

THE VESTIBULAR SYSTEM

The vestibular portion of the eighth cranial nerve conveys impulses from the receptors of the vestibular labyrinth concerned with spatial orientation of the body into the central nervous system. There the information so derived is correlated with visual and proprioceptive inputs in order to control and modulate posture, balance and other motor activity.

Each vestibular labyrinth (Fig. 7.13) includes the three semicircular canals and the utricle and saccule, and each contains a sensory epithelium containing receptor hair cells and supporting structures. At one end of each semicircular canal there is a dilatation or ampulla containing the receptor organ or crista ampullaris. A gelatinous cupula covers the hair cells of this organ, each of which have numerous short stereocilia and a single longer kinocilium (Fig. 7.16). Movement of endolymph in the membranous labyrinth bends the cupula towards or away from the utricle. Such a deflection bends the stereocilia towards the kinocilium and evokes increased discharge in afferent vestibular nerve fibres, while a deflection in the opposite direction reduces such neuronal firing. The extent of the angular deflection of the cupula determines the frequency of firing in the vestibular neuron. The relative position of the three semicircular canals in relation to one another is so disposed that any movement of the head in space evokes a neuronal discharge which can be shown to be proportional to the velocity of movement. In fact the three canals are arranged approximately at right angles to one another (Fig. 7.13A) so that when the head is inclined 30° forwards from the erect position, the lateral canal is horizontal; this fact is used in the performance of caloric tests (see below). The polarization of the stereocilia in relation to the kinocilia of respective groups of hair cells is such that vestibular nerve fibres derived from receptors in the horizontal canal are excited when endolymph moves towards the ampulla, whereas in the vertical canals excitation is induced by movement away from the ampulla.

In the utricle and saccule the sensory epithelium,

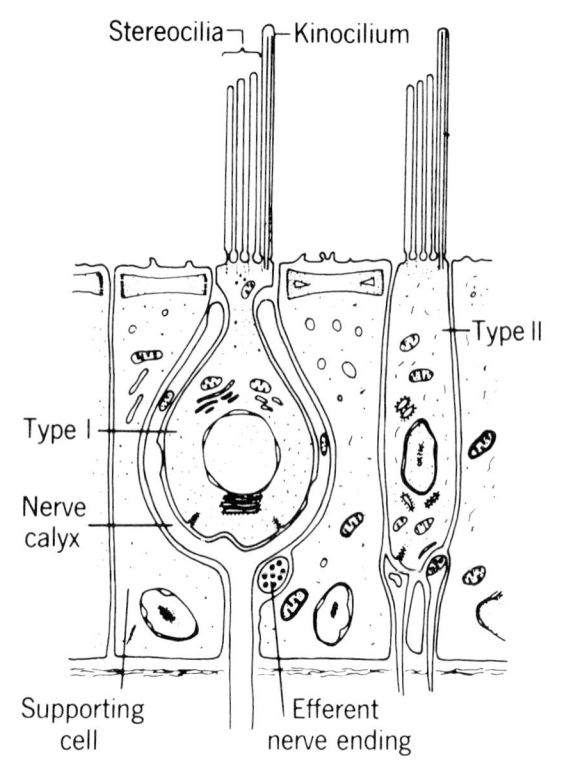

Figure 7.16 Schematic drawing of vestibular epithelium (from electron micrographs), showing two types of hair cells. [Reproduced from Patton et al (1976) *Introduction to Basic Neurology*, and previously published in Brodal (1969) *Neurological Anatomy in Relation to Clinical Medicine* (New York: Oxford University Press), by kind permission of the authors and publishers.]

called the macula, contains hair cells like those of the crista ampullaris. In addition, crystals of calcium carbonate (otoliths) lie in the gelatinous material overlying other hair cells. Because these organs lie horizontally, movement of the upright head produces little deflection of the hair cell cilia, but tilting of the head means that the effect of gravity upon the otoliths causes such deflections. These organs, static vestibular receptors, are not affected, as are the semicircular canals, by velocity of head movement but by change of the position of the head in relation to gravity.

The cell bodies of the neurons of the vestibular nerve lie in Scarpa's ganglion in the internal auditory canal. Most of their axons travel to the vestibular nuclei in the lateral pons and medulla, but a few pass through the nuclei without synapsing to enter the cerebellar flocculonodular lobe. The vestibular nuclear groups are connected with the spinal cord via the vestibulospinal tracts with the third, fourth and sixth cranial nerve nuclei and proprioceptive pathways from the neck muscles via the medial longitudinal fasciculus, and with the cerebellum via the inferior cerebellar peduncle. Thus, ocular deviation to the opposite side with nystagmus induced by stimulation of one horizontal semicircular canal is mediated via the medial longitudinal fasciculus as in the oculocephalic or vestibulo-ocular reflexes previously discussed.

The function of the vestibular system is to assist the motor system in maintaining equilibrium by providing a continuing inflow of information into the nervous system relating to the effects of movement and of gravitational forces upon the body. If there is excessive output from the system, as after rapid rotation, or differing input from the two sides because of pathological processes, an illusion of movement or vertigo (see below) results. Such vertigo is nearly always accentuated by closing the eyes, and lessened by opening them.

Examination of vestibular function

Tonic vestibular input on one side causes deviation of the eyes to the opposite side which is, however, quickly overcome by cerebral cortical mechanisms concerned with saccadic eye movements, so that there is a rapid recoil. A vestibular lesion may cause spontaneous nystagmus with a slow phase towards the opposite side and a rapid recoil. While the tonic vestibular component of the nystagmus is the slow phase, it is customary in clinical practice to describe the direction of nystagmus as being that of the quick phase, which is normally therefore towards the affected labyrinth. Unlike the nystagmus which results from central brain stem lesions, that of labyrinthine origin is not altered by the direction of voluntary gaze.

INDUCED MANIFESTATIONS OF VESTIBULAR DYSFUNCTION

Induced manifestations are shown by various clinical tests of vestibular function. Caloric tests and tests for positional and optokinetic nystagmus may be necessary for diagnosis. Electronystagmography makes it possible to record details of the nystagmus.

Caloric tests
Caloric tests are a means of demonstrating dysfunction of the canal and tonus elements of the vestibular system. The results remain remarkably constant regardless of repetition.

A moderate but effective thermal stimulus is applied to each labyrinth separately. The stimulus used is water at 7°C below and 7°C above body temperature. This produces equal and opposite horizontal nystagmus lasting for approximately 2 minutes in the normal individual.

During the test the patient lies supine on a couch with his head raised 30 degrees from the horizontal. In this position the lateral semicircular canals are vertical, the position of maximal thermal sensitivity. The patient is asked to look at a suitable spot so that a fixed gaze is maintained. Water at 30°C is run into one ear continuously for 40 seconds, not less than 250 ml being used. In the normal subject second-degree nystagmus away from the stimulated labyrinth occurs. The time is recorded in seconds from the beginning of irrigation to the point when nystagmus can no longer be seen. Irrigation at 30°C is repeated in the other ear. Water at 44°C is then used in each ear in turn, when the induced nystagmus is towards the irrigated side. Accuracy of temperature and duration of irrigation are essential. Experience in observation of the end point and in interpretation of the caloric patterns is necessary for reaching a correct diagnosis.

The caloric tests are of great value in the diagnosis of organic lesions at all levels of the vestibular system. They may show suppression of activity on one side, canal paresis, or a directional preponderance of nystagmus, which means that nystagmus in one direction, from whichever canal it is obtained, is stronger and lasts longer than in the other direction. Combined responses showing directional preponderance and canal paresis frequently occur (Fig. 7.17).

In cerebral lesions involving the posterior temporal lobe, marked directional preponderance of caloric nystagmus towards the side of the lesion is found.

In brain-stem lesions directional preponderance away from the lesion is found more frequently than canal paresis, which occurs when the lesion is at or above the level of the entry of the eighth nerve. Combined responses sometimes occur. Simple stimulation of one ear with a small quantity of ice-cold water in an attempt to induce nystagmus is a useful rapid test of the responsiveness of pontine vestibular nuclei in comatose patients. Absence of any response implies a severe disturbance of brain-stem function.

In peripheral lesions the commonest abnormality found is canal paresis, due to a lesion of the lateral semicircular canal or its peripheral neurons. Canal paresis is found in a high proportion of patients with Ménière's disease, vestibular neuronitis and acoustic neuroma. Combined lesions indicating a change in the utricle or its peripheral neurons as well as in the lateral canal occur in approximately 20% of cases of Ménière's disease. Directional preponderance of caloric nystagmus alone is found less commonly in peripheral labyrinthine disease.

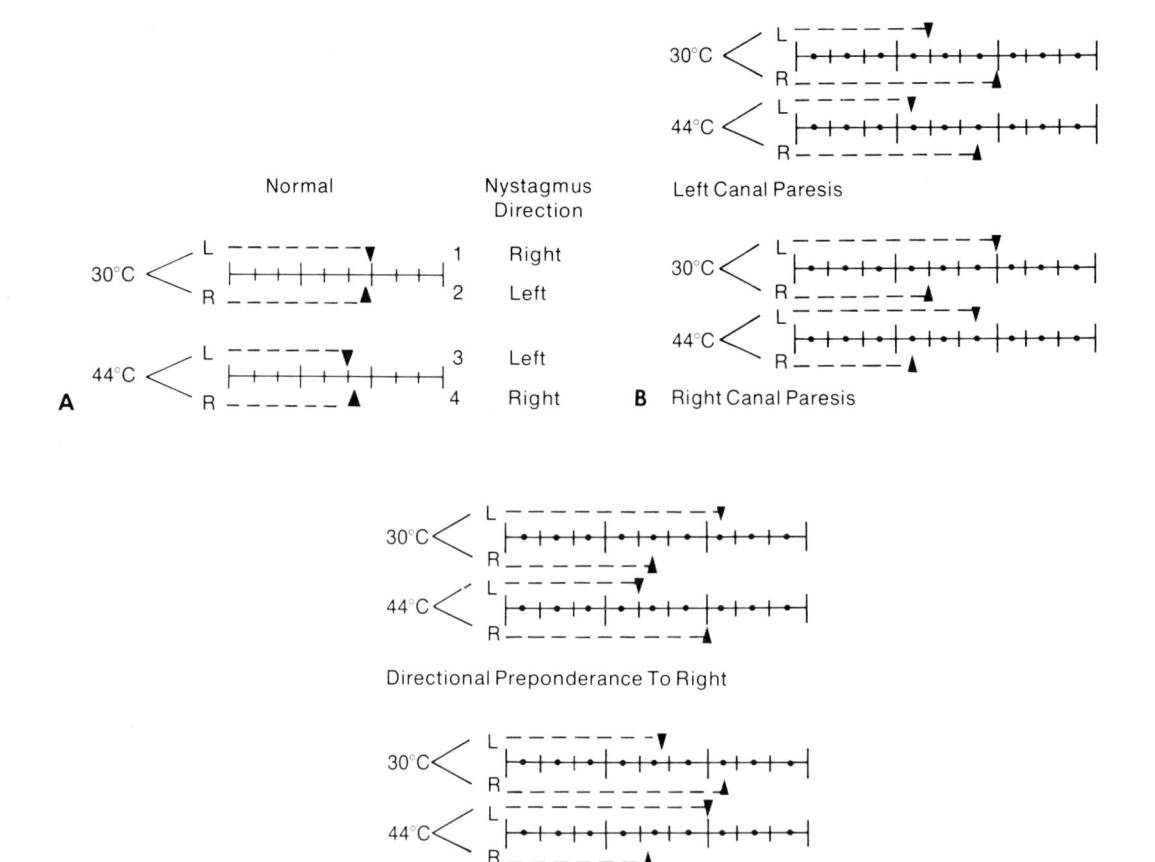

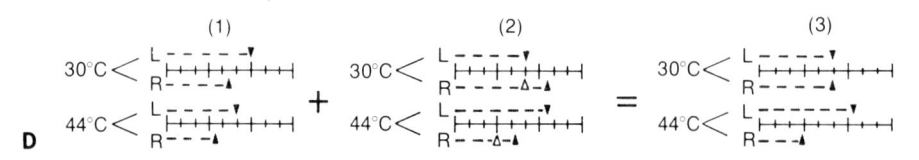

Figure 7.17 Caloric responses: A, Normal. B, Canal paresis. C, Directional preponderance. D, From a case of Ménière's disease of the right labyrinth. Combination of right canal paresis (1) and directional preponderance to the left (2). [Reproduced from Walton (1985) *Brain's Diseases of the Nervous System*, 9th edn, A, B, and C previously published by Fitzgerald, G. and Hallpike, C. S. (1942) *Brain* **65**:115, D by Hallpike, C. S. (1965) *Proc. R. Soc. Med.* **58**:185, by kind permission of the authors and publishers.]

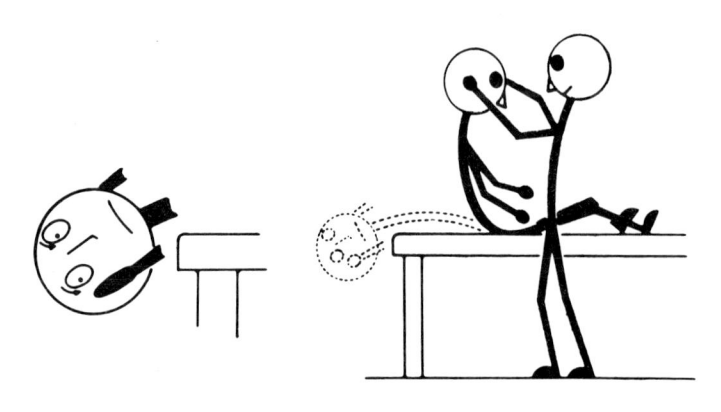

Figure 7.18 The method of eliciting positional nystagmus. [Reproduced from Walton (1985) *Brain's Diseases of the Nervous System*, 9th edn, and previously published by Hallpike, C. S. (1955) *Postgrad. Med. J.* **31**:330, by kind permission of the author and publishers.]

Positional tests

Nystagmus on sudden movement of the head in certain directions is produced by changes in the otolith organ of the utricle.

Tests for otolith function cannot be confined to one ear, but there is a useful and easily performed test to elicit positional nystagmus. The patient is seated on a couch. His head is held and he is briskly laid back so that his head becomes 30 degrees below the horizontal and rotated 30–40 degrees towards the observer (Fig. 7.18). In the normal subject no nystagmus or vertigo occur. In benign paroxysmal positional nystagmus, after a short, characteristic latent period, severe vertigo and rotary nystagmus towards the lowermost ear (the affected one) occur and last for several seconds. If the critical position is maintained, the nystagmus and vertigo gradually stop. On the subject's returning to a sitting position a similar, though usually less severe, episode occurs. If the test is then repeated the phenomenon may not be observed, as adaptation occurs rapidly.

Positional nystagmus is sometimes seen in patients with posterior fossa lesions and especially in patients with ependymomas or metastases in the fourth ventricle or in others with brain-stem lesions of multiple sclerosis. In contrast to those with the benign syndrome, in these individuals nystagmus develops without a latent period, neither adapts nor fatigues, and is variable in direction depending upon how the head is moved. There is less severe subjective vertigo or even none at all.

Vertigo

Vertigo is a disorder of equilibrium characterized by a sensation of rotation of the self or of one's surroundings. Often the objects around the patient appear to be moving, either continuously in one direction or in a to-and-fro manner. Sometimes the patient feels that he himself is twisting or spinning or falling. Commonly, vertigo is accompanied by staggering or even by actual falling, with clumsiness of the limbs, vomiting, depression and pallor. Nystagmus is generally present and in severe cases the vision is blurred or momentarily lost. Rarely, transient loss of consciousness may occur. It is important to distinguish true vertigo from mild 'giddiness' or 'swimming in the head', which are commonly psychogenic, or else may be due to syncope or presyncope.

Disorders of many different nervous pathways concerned in the normal maintenance of posture may cause vertigo. Visual impulses from the retina and from proprioceptive receptors in the external ocular muscles convey information concerning the relationship between the individual and his surroundings.

Transient vertigo may result from looking down from heights or when observing a rapidly moving object. The proprioceptive impulses derived from the neck muscles are closely related to labyrinthine function, while similar stimuli from the muscles of the trunk and limbs give information concerning the position of the body. Lesions of these proprioceptive pathways do not usually produce vertigo, but it can result from disorders of the central coordinating mechanisms in the brain stem and of the cerebellum. Lesions of the cerebral cortex rarely cause vertigo, although this symptom has been described as the aura of an epileptic fit and can occasionally result from tumours of the temporal lobe. Even though the cerebellum is of such importance in the control of posture, it is comparatively uncommon for cerebellar hemisphere lesions, however massive, to give rise to vertigo. An exception is primary intracerebellar haemorrhage in which intense vertigo and vomiting often occur at the outset. Brain-stem lesions involving central cerebellar connections, however, often give severe vertigo. The two most common brain-stem causes are multiple sclerosis and infarction or transient ischaemia. Occasionally the first symptom of multiple sclerosis is a sudden severe attack of vertigo, often lasting for hours or days, and associated with severe nystagmus and perhaps with other signs of a brain-stem lesion. The lateral medullary infarct produced by posterior inferior cerebellar or vertebral artery thrombosis characteristically produces sudden vertigo, vomiting and prostration as an initial manifestation, while less severe attacks can occur as a feature of the recurrent ischaemic episodes of vertebrobasilar insufficiency. Drugs such as alcohol, anticonvulsants (e.g. phenytoin) and barbiturates, if taken in excess, produce vertigo, drowsiness and ataxia through an action on central vestibular and cerebellar connections, and a similar mechanism probably accounts for vertigo resulting from metabolic disorders such as hypoglycaemia. Lesions of the vestibular nerve (such as acoustic neuroma) sometimes cause giddiness and nystagmus along with deafness and tinnitus due to involvement of the cochlear nerve, but severe vertigo is uncommon in such cases.

Lesions of the labyrinth are the most frequent cause of vertigo. Sudden vertigo may result from an extension of a middle-ear infection to the labyrinth, but an 'acute vestibular neuronitis', often erroneously called 'labyrinthitis', can occur without a preceding middle-ear infection. In such a case vertigo develops suddenly and is generally associated with severe vomiting and prostration, some ataxia of the ipsilateral limbs, and a rotary nystagmus to the opposite side. The patient is often febrile and the illness may last for several hours, days or weeks. The condition can occur in epidemic form. As diplopia and a lymphocytic pleocytosis in the cerebrospinal fluid occasionally occur, some believe this condition to be an acute virus infection of the brain stem, involving vestibular nuclei rather than a labyrinthitis. Hence the title 'epidemic vertigo' is often preferred, even for sporadic cases. A similar clinical picture, which can generally be identified by the accompanying unilateral deafness, can result from atherosclerotic occlusion of the internal auditory artery. The distinction between epidemic vertigo and a first episode of multiple sclerosis due to a plaque of demyelination in the brain stem can be difficult and often depends solely upon the subsequent course as acute vestibular neuronitis generally recovers completely, whereas in multiple sclerosis subsequent manifestations of neurological disease are to be expected. Furthermore, other signs of brain-stem dysfunction (e.g. diplopia) may accompany the vertiginous presentation of multiple sclerosis. Even in the benign labyrinthine disorder, however, one or more relapses may occur within the first few months.

Ménière's syndrome (recurrent aural vertigo) is a condition characterized by recurrent attacks of vertigo, often with vomiting and prostration, and accompanied by unilateral tinnitus and progressive sensorineural deafness. The condition occurs at any age, but is rare in young children. It is commonest in middle life and is somewhat more frequent in males. Ménière's syndrome appears to be due to a hydrops of the membranous labyrinth, of unknown aetiology, resulting in dilatation of the endolymph system with consequent pressure atrophy of the hair cells of the organ of Corti. Sometimes the deafness and tinnitus have been present for some time before the attacks of vertigo develop, but more often the latter are the presenting feature. Attacks may initially be mild and brief, increasing in severity and frequency, but the manifestations are extremely variable. Typically a sudden attack of vertigo occurs with unsteadiness, vomiting and prostration and can be so violent that the patient is literally thrown to the ground. Pallor, perspiration, depression and tachycardia are common accompaniments, and rotary nystagmus is present. Occasionally, transient loss of consciousness due to syncope occurs in a severe attack. The attack may last for only a few minutes or several hours, but the patient is sometimes lethargic, unsteady and depressed for several days afterwards. The episodes can occur at intervals of a few days, weeks or even months, but tend to become increasingly less frequent and eventually to disappear completely when deafness is complete in the affected ear. Unfortunately the contralateral ear is occasionally affected, sometimes concurrently but more often subsequently. A benign form of paroxysmal vertigo of childhood giving recurrent vertiginous attacks occurring for only a few months or years and a similar syndrome of benign recurrent vertigo of adult life have been described, in neither of which are deafness or tinnitus a feature.

A somewhat similar condition which gives rise to episodic attacks of vertigo is the so-called benign positional nystagmus, which results from a degenerative lesion, again of unknown aetiology, in the otoliths of the utricle and saccule. In this condition, however, the attacks of vertigo occur only on certain specific movements of the head (e.g. stooping or lying down on one side) and can be reproduced at will by carrying out such movements. Most patients learn to avoid the offending position that evokes the attacks, and in many cases the condition improves spontaneously after months or years. Transient vertigo evoked by head movement and presumed to be due to damage to the utricle is a common sequel of closed head injury (Cartlidge and Shaw, 1981).

Motion sickness is another closely related disorder, and is due to the stereotyped repetitive stimulation of the semicircular canals produced by movement of a motor car, ship, train or aeroplane. There is a wide variation in individual susceptibility. Commonly lassitude, vague depression and drowsiness are the earliest manifestations and are followed by vomiting and vertigo, though the vertigo is not usually severe. A considerable degree of adaptation usually occurs in the habitual traveller.

References

Barany, R. (1921) Diagnose von Krankheitserscheinungen im Bereiche des Otolithen-apparates. *Acta Oto-Lar* **2**:434.

Carmichael, E. A., Dix, M. R. and Hallpike, C. S. (1965) Observations upon the neurological mechanism of directional preponderance of caloric nystagmus resulting from vascular lesions of the brain-stem. *Brain* **88**:51.

Cartlidge, N. E. F. and Shaw, D. A. (1981) *Head Injury*. Philadelphia: W. B. Saunders Company.

Cawthorne, T., Dix, M. R., Hood, J. D. and Harrison, M. S. (1969) Vestibular syndromes and vertigo. In Vinken, P. J. and Bruyn, G. W. (eds) *Handbook of Clinical Neurology*, vol. 2. Amsterdam: North-Holland.

Cogan, D. G. (1970) *Neurology of the Visual System*. Springfield, Ill.: Charles C. Thomas.

Cogan, D. G. and Adams, R. D. (1953) A type of paralysis of conjugate gaze (ocular motor apraxia). *Arch. Ophthalmol.* **50**:434.

Cogan, D. G. and Wray, S. H. (1970) Internuclear ophthalmoplegia as an early sign of brainstem tumors. *Neurology* **20**:629.

Davis, H. and Silverman, S. R. (1970) *Hearing and Deafness*, 3rd edn. New York: Holt Rinehart & Winston.

de Jong, R. N. (1979) *The Neurologic Examination*, 4th edn. Hagerstown, Md.: Harper and Row.

Dix, M. R. (1969) Modern tests of vestibular function, with special reference to their value in clinical practice. *Br. Med. J.* **3**:317.

Dix, M. R. and Hood, J. D. (eds) (1984) *Vertigo*. Chichester: John Wiley.

Doig, J. A. (1972) Auditory and vestibular function and dys-

function. In Critchley, M., O'Leary, J. L. and Jennett, W. B. (eds) *Scientific Foundations of Neurology*. London: Heinemann.
Fitzgerald, M. J. T. (1985) *Neuroanatomy, Basic and Applied*. Eastbourne: Baillière Tindall.
Gardner, E. (1975) *Fundamentals of Neurology*, 6th edn. Philadelphia: W. B. Saunders Company.
Gay, A. J. and Newman, N. M. (1972) Eye movements and their disorders. In Critchley, M., O'Leary, J. L. and Jennett, W. B. (eds) *Scientific Foundations of Neurology*. London: Heinemann.
Hallpike, C. S. (1965) Clinical otoneurology and its contributions to theory and practice. *Proc. R. Soc. Med.* **58**:185.
Hood, J. D. and Poole, J. P. (1971) Speech audiometry in conductive and sensorineural hearing loss. *Sound* **5**:30.
Hood, J. D. and Korres. S. (1979) Vestibular suppression in peripheral and central vestibular disorders. *Brain* **102**:785.
Kandel, E. R. and Schwartz, J. H. (1985) *Principles of Neuroscience*, 2nd edn. London: Edward Arnold.
Lamb, T. D. (1984) Electrical response of photoreceptors. *Recent Advances in Physiology*, 10th edn, chap. 2. Edinburgh: Churchill Livingstone.
Leigh, R. J. and Zee, D. S. (1983) *The Neurology of Eye Movements*. Philadelphia: F. A. Davis.
Mayo Clinic, Section of Neurology (1981) The cranial nerves, and neuroophthalmology. In *Clinical Examinations in Neurology*, 5th edn. Philadelphia: W. B. Saunders Company.
Nylén, C. O. (1939) The otoneurological diagnosis of tumours of the brain. *Acta Otolaryngol.*, Suppl. 33.
Patton, H. D., Sundsten, J. W., Crill, W. E. and Swanson, P. D. (1976) *Introduction to Basic Neurology*. Philadelphia: W. B. Saunders Company.
Pickles, J. O. (1985) Hearing and listening. In Swash, M. and Kennard, C. (eds) *Scientific Basis of Clinical Neurology*. Edinburgh: Churchill Livingstone.
Steele, J. C., Richardson, J. C. and Olszewski, J. (1964) Progressive supranuclear palsy: a heterogeneous degeneration involving the brain stem, basal ganglia and cerebellum with vertical gaze and pseudobulbar palsy, nuchal dystonia and dementia. *Arch. Neurol.* **10**:333.
Sumner, D. (1964) Post-traumatic anosmia. *Brain* **87**:107.
Sumner, D. (1967) Post-traumatic ageusia. *Brain* **90**:187.
Victor, M. and Adams, R. D. (1974) Dizziness, vertigo and disorders of gait, and common disturbances of vision, ocular movement and hearing. In Wintrobe, M. M. et al (eds) *Harrison's Principles of Internal Medicine*, 7th edn. New York: McGraw-Hill Book Company.
Walton, J. N. (1982) *Essentials of Neurology*, 5th edn. London: Pitman.
Walton, J. N. (1985) *Brain's Diseases of the Nervous System*, 9th edn. Oxford: Oxford University Press.
Zeki, S. (1985) Looking and seeing. In Swash, M. and Kennard, C. (eds) *Scientific Basis of Clinical Neurology*. Edinburgh: Churchill Livingstone.

8

THE MOTOR SYSTEM

INTRODUCTION

Disorders of movement produce some of the commonest symptoms professed by patients with disease or disordered function of the nervous system. Sometimes the ability to move a part in response to the will is impaired (weakness or paresis) and sometimes it is lost completely (paralysis). On other occasions, willed movements are clumsy, ill-directed or uncontrolled (ataxia or incoordination), or else the part moves spontaneously or independently of the will (involuntary movements). The examiner may be able to confirm the presence of these abnormalities and may also discover abnormalities of tone in which normal response to passive stretching of a muscle is altered. Tone can be reduced (hypotonia) or increased in one of two ways: spasticity or rigidity. Abnormalities of this type, and particularly weakness or paralysis, are sometimes emotionally determined (hysteria). Alternatively they can be apraxic, resulting from a cortical lesion which has impaired the ability to recall acquired motor skills.

Disorders of movement are most often due to a disturbance in function of the motor pathway which begins in the motor area of the cerebral cortex and ends in the voluntary musculature. There are a number of important physical signs which assist in the localization of lesions within this motor apparatus, but for a full appreciation of their significance a working knowledge of the organization of movement is essential.

THE ORGANIZATION OF MOVEMENT

General considerations

The motor system of man consists of (a) the descending pathways derived from the cerebral cortex and brain stem which are concerned with the suprasegmental control of movement, (b) the basal ganglia and cerebellum, (c) the continuation of these pathways within the spinal cord, and (d) the neuromuscular system, which is made up of the nuclei of the motor cranial nerves and the muscles which they innervate, as well as the anterior horn cells of the spinal cord together with the segmentally organized voluntary musculature of the trunk and limbs. Major afferent pathways project to these motor structures both at the higher and at the segmental levels, providing an input of information about the relative positions of different parts of the body and about muscle length, which fulfils an important role in the control of movement. The basal ganglia and cerebellum do not project directly to the segmental motor structures of the brain stem and spinal cord but process information from other parts of the nervous system and project backwards on to the cortical and brain-stem structures from which the suprasegmental pathways arise. A schematic outline of the motor system is given in Fig. 8.1.

The components of the motor system

THE CORTICOSPINAL AND CORTICOBULBAR (PYRAMIDAL) SYSTEM

Strictly speaking, the pyramidal tract is that bundle of descending motor nerve fibres which traverses the

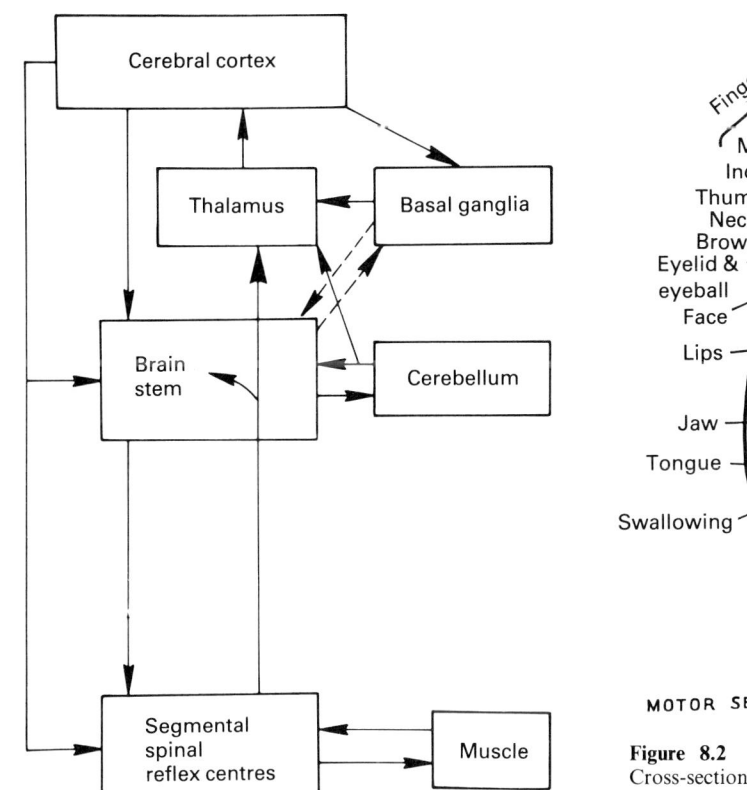

Figure 8.1 A highly schematic flow diagram of the motor system. The arrows should not be taken to represent direct monosynaptic connections. [Reproduced from Patton et al (1976) *Introduction to Basic Neurology*, by kind permission of the authors and publisher.]

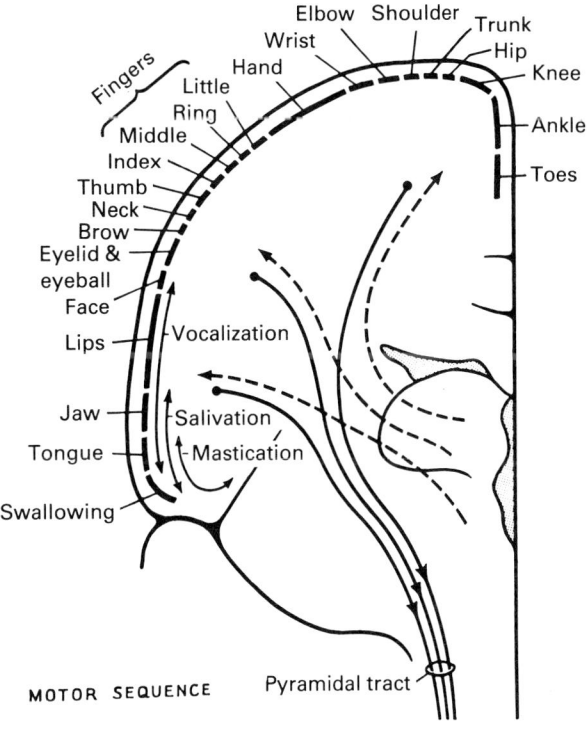

Figure 8.2 Corticospinal motor pathway (pyramidal tract). Cross-section through right hemisphere along the plane of the precentral gyrus. The sequence of responses to electrical stimulation of the surface of the cortex (from above down, along the motor strip from toes through arm and face to swallowing) is unvaried from one individual to another. The broken arrows represent afferent thalamocortical pathways. [Reproduced from Walton (1985) *Brain's Diseases of the Nervous System*, 9th edn, by kind permission of the publisher.]

medullary pyramid to enter the spinal cord and thus contains both corticospinal fibres and others derived from brain-stem structures. It has been conventional, if slightly inaccurate, to regard the terms corticospinal and pyramidal as being synonymous in referring to descending motor pathways.

Structure
The upper motor neurons arise in part from nerve cells in the motor cortex of the cerebrum. This area of cortex lies anterior to the rolandic fissure, in the precentral convolution. Some of these neurons arise from the giant Betz cells which are common in this area, but many of the other upper motor neurons arise from nerve cells in or near this area which are not structurally distinctive. In man, the pyramidal tract contains about 1 000 000 fibres, of which 94% are myelinated. A few of the fibres of this tract are small demyelinated fibres that arise from neurons lying around the central or rolandic sulcus.

Activation of cells in the lower end of the precentral gyrus causes bilateral movement of the pharynx and larynx, while stimulation of others just above the gyrus gives rise to movement of the contralateral half of the tongue (Fig. 8.2). Facial movement can be elicited at a point slightly higher still with bilateral movement of the upper face but unilateral movement only of the lower face. Movement of the contralateral hand, arm, trunk, leg and foot will then be produced in turn as one ascends the gyrus, and in each case 'representation' is strictly unilateral. The leg and foot 'area' lies partly on the medial surface of the hemisphere and partly on its superior aspect. Nerve fibres arising from the cells in this cortical area come together in the corona radiata and converge upon the internal capsule, which lies deep in the hemisphere between the thalamus and caudate nucleus medially and the lenticular nucleus laterally (Fig. 1.25C, p. 35). From the internal capsule the tract passes down to enter the midbrain. In the pons it is broken into bundles by transverse pontine fibres, but in the medulla it again becomes a compact tract, the pyramid, which forms an anterior prominence.

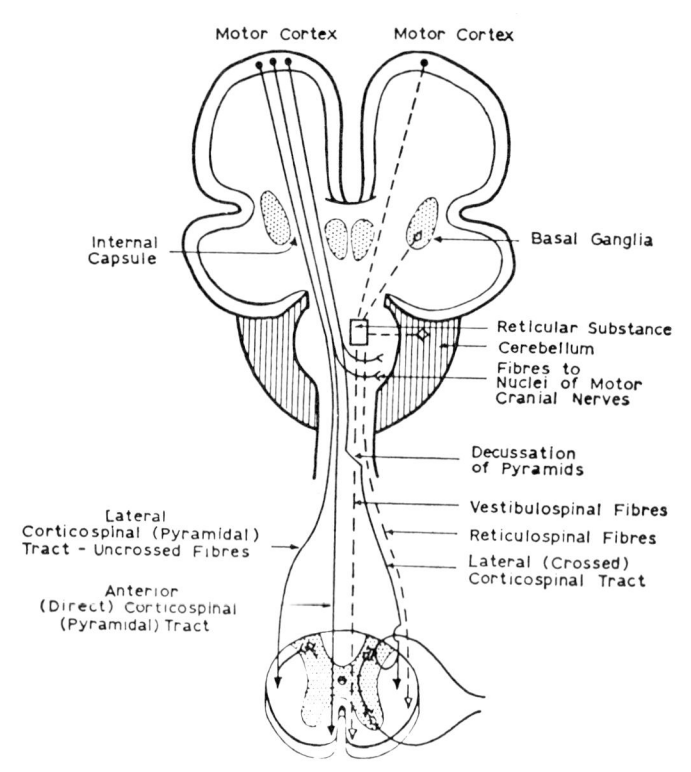

Figure 8.3 A diagram of the principal pathways of the motor system. The continuous lines represent pathways of the pyramidal system, and the interrupted lines those of the extrapyramidal system. The nuclear masses of the basal ganglia, the brain-stem reticular substance, and the dentate nucleus of the cerebellum, which are some of the most important relay stations in the extrapyramidal system, are represented diagrammatically.
[Reproduced from Walton (1982) *Essentials of Neurology*, 5th edn, and redrawn from Gardner (1975) *Fundamentals of Neurology*, 4th edn, by kind permission of the author and publisher.]

Throughout the brain stem the tract gives off corticobulbar fibres which travel to the contralateral motor nuclei of the cranial nerves. In the lower part of the medulla, most of the fibres in the pyramidal tract decussate to form the crossed pyramidal tract, which travels down in the lateral column of the spinal cord on the opposite side, but a small proportion do not do so and continue downwards in the anterior column of the cord, forming the direct or uncrossed pyramidal tract (Fig. 8.3). As a rule, fibres of the pyramidal tract do not synapse directly with the anterior horn cells from which the lower motor neurons arise. Rather, they synapse with internuncial (propriospinal) neurons in the grey matter of the spinal cord, which in turn pass on to synapse in the anterior horns.

The lower motor neurons (alpha neurons) transmit impulses from the motor nuclei of the cranial nerves and from anterior horn cells of the spinal cord to the voluntary muscles. They constitute the final common path of motor activity. All nervous mechanisms that influence muscular activity must produce their final effects through impulses which travel along these fibres. Their structure and function and that of the motor unit will be considered below.

Other small motor neurons (gamma neurons) innervate only the intrafusal fibres of the muscle spindle and form part of the reflex mechanism concerned with the control of muscle tone.

Function

The organization of movement is very much more complex than the preceding simple schema of the basic functional units would suggest. For instance, no single cell in the motor area of the cerebral cortex can be said to innervate any single muscle. It is not single muscle twitches, but organized movements, which are initiated in the motor cortex. These movements involve several muscles or muscle groups, of which only some act as prime movers or agonists. Other muscles, the antagonists, must relax smoothly as the agonists contract. Still others are required to fix a limb proximally, say, in order to allow a movement which is occurring distally to be efficient. Other muscles or synergists may also be brought into play in order to counteract unwanted effects which would be produced by the unmodified action of the agonists. In general, stimulation of pyramidal tract neurons excites those muscles which fulfil physiologically a flexor role, and inhibits the antigravity or extensor muscles. Those portions of the tract primarily involved with voluntary movement excite the agonists concerned with fine or precise movements while inhibiting the antagonists, many of which are concerned with segmental postural mechanisms. The descending fibres of the tract also exercise an effect upon gamma motor neurons as well as alpha motor neurons. The profusion of internuncial neurons in the spinal cord, which receive impulses from many pyramidal axons and may influence many anterior horn cells, are clearly important in this organization. Incoming sensory impulses from stretch receptors (muscle spindles) in the muscles themselves, as well as other proprioceptive sensations, continually inform the individual of the position of the part which is being moved. These impulses can also modify motor activity through a series of spinal reflexes. Additional modifying influences are exerted through sensory impulses from the eyes and labyrinths, which enter the brain stem and initiate activity in the vestibulospinal tracts.

Within the last 20 years these concepts have been illuminated by a number of neurophysiological studies. Stimulation with microelectrodes in the depths of the motor cortex in experimental animals produces contractions of individual flexor or extensor muscles as well as restricted muscle groups. By contrast, stimuli applied to the cortical surface result in contraction of several muscles or groups of muscles. The points where stimulation with lowest current densities elicit contraction of any given muscle are grouped in relation to columns of cells orientated perpendicularly to the cortical surface. These columnar arrays, reminiscent of the columns in the somatosensory and visual cortex, are called cortical efferent zones (Kandel and Schwartz, 1985). It has also been found that a specific relationship exists between the target muscle on the one hand and peripheral receptor fields (in the muscles and/or skin) which excite neurons within each efferent zone on the other. For example, neurons within the efferent zone which control flexor muscles of the digits may be activated by stretching these muscles (proprioceptive input) or by cutaneous stimuli applied to the flexor surfaces of the digits. These relationships enable the cortex to function as a positive feedback system which provides servo assistance when the moving limb segment encounters an unexpected obstacle.

Recent work has also shown that axons from the thalamus and other areas synapse with distant dendrites of pyramidal tract neurons and on interneurons in the superficial layers of the motor cortex. The interneurons form a cascade through which impulses spread down the cortical columns to pyramidal neurons. As the axons of pyramidal tract neurons vary considerably in diameter, their conduction velocities also vary. The giant Betz cells thus tend to fire in short, high-frequency bursts followed by rapid adaptation, much more rapid than that of the small, more slowly conducting pyramidal tract neurons. There is now increasing evidence to show that single neurons in the system code for the intended force of voluntary movements, but that such intention also requires a preparatory 'set'.

Other important effects are exerted by the so-called extrapyramidal motor system and by the cerebellum, which will be considered below. These structures exercise their effects through a series of independent descending pathways which may profoundly influence the activity of the pyramidal tract.

THE RUBROSPINAL, VESTIBULOSPINAL AND RETICULOSPINAL TRACTS

Axons arising from the red nucleus, which lies in the tegmentum of the midbrain, cross the midline immediately and then descend through the lateral brain stem and lateral column of the spinal cord. They are closely related to fibres of the pyramidal tract and synapse with internuncial neurons in the lateral part of the ventral grey matter. Excitation of these fibres gives facilitation of both alpha and gamma neurons supplying distal limb muscles. The red nucleus itself receives an input from the cerebral cortex, largely through corticospinal tract collaterals, and also from the cerebellum. As in the motor cortex, the red nucleus shows clear-cut somatotopic organization; the topographical relationships between input and output which hold for the stretch reflex also hold for the efferent zones of the red nucleus and motor cortex (Kandel and Schwartz, 1985). In primates, division of the rubrospinal tract causes paresis of distal limb muscles, but in man this tract is vestigial and clinically insignificant; certainly there is no clinical syndrome recognized as being due to interruption of this pathway.

The principal or lateral vestibulospinal tract originates in neurons of the lateral vestibular (Deiters') nucleus of the pons, which receives an input from vestibular neurons and from cerebellar Purkinje cells as well as midline cerebellar nuclei. The fibres of this tract synapse with alpha and gamma neurons and with internuncial neurons in the ipsilateral anterior horns of the cord, and especially with those which supply axial and proximal limb muscles. Stimulation of this tract excites the neurons that innervate extensor or postural muscles and inhibits those which fulfil a flexor role. The shorter medial vestibulospinal tract arising from the medial vestibular nuclei extends downwards only as far as the mid-dorsal level and appears to subserve a similar function in relation to neck and paraspinal muscles.

Descending reticulospinal tracts originating respectively in the pontine and medullary reticular systems excite both alpha and gamma neurons; pontine reticulospinal fibres mainly supply extensor muscles, while fibres from the medulla mostly travel to flexor ones.

Conclusions

A particular movement is presumed to initiate when the idea of the movement is first invoked in the association areas of the cortex in which acquired motor skills (praxis) are stored. The appropriate motor cells of the precentral cortex are then activated and impulses travel down the pyramidal tracts in order to activate the appropriate anterior horn cells and their motor units. Simultaneously the movement is influenced and controlled by the activity of the cerebellum and of the components of the extrapyramidal motor system. At the same time as the agonists are being stimulated to contract, the synergists to assist, and the fixators to fix, an inhibitory mechanism must be invoked to produce controlled relaxation of the antagonists. Once the movement has begun it will then be subject to continued modification depending upon sensory impulses arriving from the proprioceptors, or from the eyes and labyrinths. Clearly, therefore, in view of its complexity, movement can be disorganized by lesions of many different nervous pathways. Some of the principles which aid in deciding which pathway or pathways are diseased will be considered later.

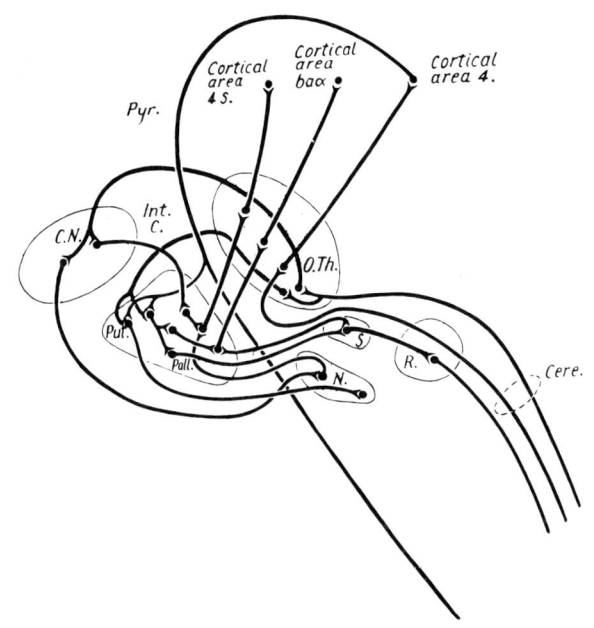

Figure 8.4 Diagram of the principal connections of the basal ganglia. Pyr., corticospinal tract. Int. C., internal capsule. C.N., caudate nucleus. Put., putamen. Pall., globus pallidus. O. Th., optic thalamus. S., subthalamic nucleus. N., substantia nigra. R., red nucleus. Cere., ascending cerebellar pathways. [Reproduced from Walton (1985) *Brain's Diseases of the Nervous System*, 8th edn, by kind permission of the publisher.]

THE BASAL GANGLIA

Structure

The basal ganglia are a group of nuclei situated deep within the substance of the cerebral hemispheres and brain stem (see Fig. 1.25, p. 35). They include the caudate nucleus, the putamen, the globus pallidus or pallidum, the claustrum, the subthalamic nucleus and the substantia nigra. The putamen and pallidum together form the lentiform nucleus, while the streaky appearance of the caudate, putamen, pallidum and claustrum in myelin-stained sections has resulted in those nuclei being referred to collectively as the corpus striatum. The thalamus, in addition to its important sensory functions, plays a crucial part in the control of movement. In particular, thalamic nuclei mediate the connections of the basal ganglia to the motor cortex. Phylogenetically the pallidum (paleostriatum) is older than the caudate nucleus and putamen (neostriatum). Some of the principal interconnections of the basal ganglia are shown in Fig. 8.4.

The principal connections of the basal ganglia, organized topographically, are from the cerebral cortex to the striatum, to the pallidum and onwards to the thalamus, with further projections rostrally from the nucleus ventralis anterior (VA) and nucleus ventralis lateralis (VL) back to the motor areas of the cortex. Efferent pathways also connect the striatum and pallidum with the subthalamic nucleus and substantia nigra. Recent work has also demonstrated an important reverse pathway (not shown in Fig. 8.4) from the substantia nigra to the striatum. The basal ganglia influence movement largely through the thalamic relays which project to the motor cortex, by integrating their output with cerebellar input to the ventralis lateralis nucleus, and by descending impulses conveyed by the rubrospinal and reticulospinal tracts.

Function

The function of the basal ganglia is complex and much remains to be elucidated. The corpus striatum plays an important role in the regulation of posture. The globus pallidus is the final efferent cell station of the basal ganglia, its activity being influenced by inputs from the cortex, striatum, substantia nigra and subthalamic nucleus. Its efferent pathway passes rostrally via the VL nucleus of the thalamus and caudally via the subthalamic and red nuclei. It plays a vital role in the initiation of movement so that lesions of this nucleus can give severe akinesia (inability to initiate movement) or bradykinesia (excessively slow movement).

Recording from single neurons in various parts of the basal ganglia in monkeys has shown first that there are many cells which change their activity during movement of a single part of the body. Such neurons are often clustered in a type of somatotopic representation. For example, in the pallidum, neurons whose activity relates to movements of the arms lie ventral to those concerned with leg movement. Changes in activity of some such neurons occur before movement of the body part and before firing of motor cortical and cerebellar neurons, confirming the role of the pallidum in the initiation of movement.

The basal ganglia also exert a controlling influence upon the balance of alpha and gamma motor neuron activity. When disease causes imbalance of these activities, abnormalities of muscle tone or tremor may result. The concerted activity of the basal ganglia results in the smooth coordination of voluntary movement depending upon a delicate physiological balance. Certain lesions of individual components of the system distort this balance, allowing the release, due to removal of inhibitory mechanisms, of characteristic involuntary movements (chorea, athetosis, dystonia, hemiballismus) which will be considered later.

In parkinsonism the concentration of dopamine in certain nuclei of the basal ganglia is reduced. Many of the neurons of the substantia nigra, and especially those of the nigrostriatal pathway, are dopaminergic, while striatonigral neurons, by contrast, appear to employ GABA as their transmitter. Reserpine and some phenothiazine drugs may deplete dopamine stores and give rise to drug-induced parkinsonism, while phenothiazines may also produce facial dyskinetic movements (tardive dyskinesia) or dystonic phenomena. Levodopa, a dopamine precursor, restores dopamine stores and ameliorates parkinsonism, but can produce movements resembling athetosis as a troublesome side-effect. Many neurons in the striatum are cholinergic, and cholinergic activation can enhance the manifestations of parkinsonism. The clinical features of disease or dysfunction of the basal ganglia may often be due to an imbalance in the relative activities of cholinergic and dopaminergic neurons and their receptors.

THE CEREBELLUM

Structure
The gross morphology and the cellular organization of the cerebellum have been described and illustrated in chapter 1 ('The structure and function of the nervous system').

Function
The archicerebellum, consisting of the flocculonodular lobe and uvula, receives afferent fibres from the vestibular neurons directly and also via the vestibular nuclei. In turn, efferent fibres from Purkinje cells in this lobe travel via the fastigial nucleus and the inferior cerebellar peduncle to the vestibular nuclei. This area is concerned with the control of eye movements and with postural reflexes involving the neck and axial muscles. Its major role, however, is the control of equilibrium. Lesions in the midline give dysequilibrium without vertigo (truncal ataxia) and often positional nystagmus.

The paleocerebellum consists of the vermis and of contiguous portions of the cerebellar hemispheres. The spinocerebellar and cuneocerebellar tracts end in mossy fibres which enter this structure. The dorsal spinocerebellar tract originates in Clarke's column of cells near the lateral horn area of spinal grey matter in segments T1 through L2, which receive afferents from the muscle spindles and Golgi tendon organs. The fibres of this tract enter the cerebellum through the inferior cerebellar peduncle and project to the paleocerebellar cortex, carrying especially information conveyed by ipsilateral muscle spindle afferents concerned with the control of muscle tone. The cuneocerebellar tract conveys similar information from the head and neck musculature. The ventral (from the legs and trunk) and rostral (from the arms) spinocerebellar tracts project similarly to the paleocerebellum but enter via the superior cerebellar peduncles and carry incoming information from the spindle afferents and from cutaneous sensory receptors. There is also an efferent pathway from the paleocerebellum via the fastigial nucleus to the vestibular and reticulospinal tracts. These pathways exercise a modulating effect upon muscle spindle activity and integrate many afferent signals relating to the length of muscle fibres, providing a kind of positive servomechanism. Clinical lesions of this part of the cerebellum may increase decerebrate rigidity, causing a shift from a gamma to an alpha type of rigidity (see below) and, like some lesions of the archicerebellum, selective damage to this area may cause truncal ataxia with a broad-based unsteady gait.

The remainder of the cerebellum, constituting the major part of the cerebellar hemispheres, is known as the neocerebellum. It receives collateral branches from pyramidal neurons and mossy pontocerebellar fibres originating in contralateral pontine nuclei. Efferent fibres from the deep nuclei of the cerebellar hemispheres leave the cerebellum through the superior peduncles, cross the midline, and then project to the VL nucleus of the thalamus. This part of the cerebellum is especially concerned with the regulation and smooth coordination of limb movements, fulfilling a graduating and harmonizing role and also playing a part in the control of posture. Striking differences in firing rates (some increasing, some decreasing) occur in the Purkinje cells and in the neurons of cerebellar nuclei during voluntary movement. The clinical effects of dysfunction of the neocerebellum will be considered later.

In summary, then, it is now believed that the intention to carry out a movement involves first activation of association areas of the motor cortex. These areas act with the lateral portions of the cerebellar hemispheres and dentate nuclei during the early phases of planning a movement, ultimately leading to a 'command to move' (Kandel and Schwartz, 1985). These areas of the neocerebellum thus receive an input from the frontal association cortex and send their output back to the motor cortex via the thalamus. The motor cortex is then the executive which conveys the final command, via pathways described above, to the appropriate muscle group. The intermediate parts of the cerebellar hemisphere are kept informed of this cortical command by pyramidal tract fibre collaterals so that the evolving movement can be controlled and modified by the inhibitory effect of Purkinje cells on the cells of the cerebellar nuclei. The latter in turn, via efferents to the red nuclei and on to the motor cortex, exert yet another coordinating and modifying influence.

THE NEUROMUSCULAR SYSTEM

The lower motor neurons
The cell bodies of the lower motor neurons are situated in the motor nuclei of the brain stem and in the anterior horns of grey matter of the spinal cord. The cell bodies or perikarya of the alpha neurons which innervate voluntary muscle are remarkably consistent in total number and distribution throughout the various segments of the spinal cord. Various groups of cells lying in specific locations constantly supply certain muscle groups and even individual muscles. The gamma neurons supply the intrafusal fibres of the muscle spindles. Each motor neuron is influenced by impulses concerned with both excitation and inhibition. Spinal interneurons constitute an important set of networks for processing both peripheral sensory inputs (feedback) and commands descending from centres in the brain. The properties of these networks ultimately determine the pattern and sequence of impulses distributed to different motor neuron pools. These networks can transform an input at steady frequency into rhythmical patterns of impulses conveyed to different muscle groups and thus play a fundamental role in the organization of smooth movement. The generation of graded forces of muscular contraction requires both recruitment (recruiting large numbers of motor neurons to increase muscle tension) and rate coding (tension increase resulting from an increased rate of firing in a single neuron). The axons of the motor neurons leave the central nervous system via the cranial nerves or the spinal ventral roots. From the latter the axons enter the peripheral nerves, those destined for the limbs being organized into brachial and lumbosacral plexuses.

The structure and function of voluntary muscle
A voluntary muscle is composed of muscle fibres, each of which is a multinucleate cell, consisting of myofibrils, sarcoplasm and a number of discrete intracellular organelles including mitochondria, ribosomes and the sarcotubular system. Each fibre is enclosed within a sarcolemmal sheath (with an outer basement membrane and an inner plasma membrane), deep to which the muscle nuclei are situated, and each has a motor endplate in which the nerve fibre terminates. Under normal conditions muscle fibres never contract singly. The functional unit of muscle activity is known as the motor unit, being that group of muscle fibres supplied by a single alpha neuron and its axon. Discharge of such a single anterior horn cell results in the simultaneous contraction of all of the muscle fibres which it innervates. In most human limb muscles each motor unit contains between 500 and 2000 muscle fibres.

The motor unit
The fibres of a single motor unit are usually widely scattered throughout a muscle rather than being gathered into groups or fasciculi. Only after denervation and subsequent reinnervation by regenerating neurons are fibres innervated by a single anterior horn cell gathered together into groups. Contraction of the muscle fibres which make up a motor unit is preceded by electrical excitation of the fibre membranes. The appearance of this electrical activity in the electromyogram depends on physical factors such as the dimensions of the electrode used, as well as on the muscle chosen for examination. For example, in the biceps brachii of a healthy young adult, the electrical activity of a single motor unit usually appears as a di- or triphasic wave with a duration of 5–10 ms and an amplitude of 250–500 μV. The variation in form, amplitude and duration of the motor unit action potential is considerable, however.

Neuromuscular transmission
The release of acetylcholine (ACh) is responsible for transmission of the nerve impulse at the neuromuscular or myoneural junction (Fig. 8.5). The synaptic vesicles in the motor nerve terminal are actually packets of ACh. Single packets of ACh are continually being released spontaneously and give rise to small depolarizations (miniature end-plate potentials) which can be recorded electrically with a micro-

The motor system 165

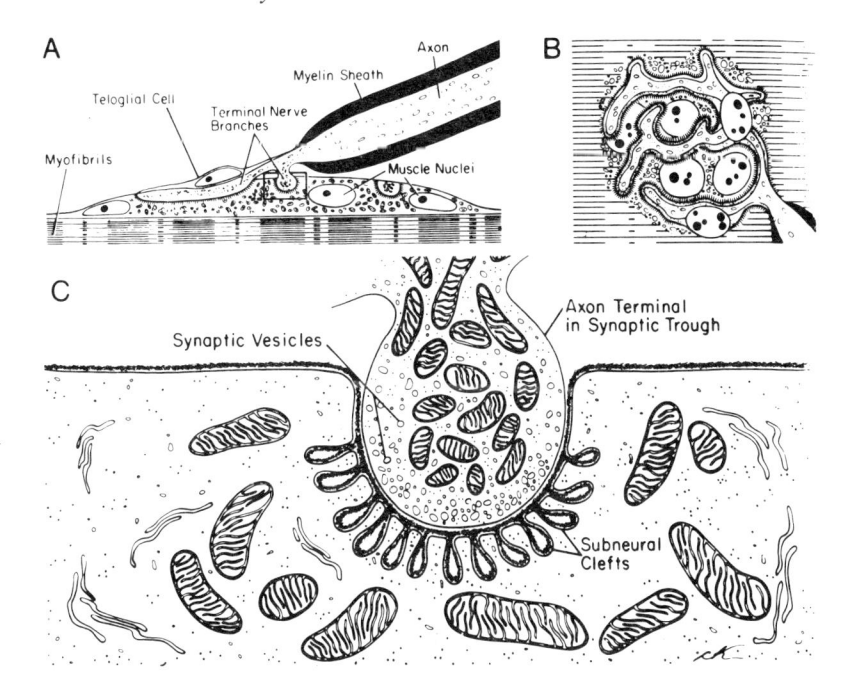

Figure 8.5 Schematic drawings of motor end-plates. A and B, Views from the side and from above, respectively. C, Enlarged view (as seen in electron micrographs) of the region outlined by the rectangle in A. [Reproduced from Patton et al (1976) *Introduction to Basic Neurology*, and previously published in Bloom and Fawcett (1970) *A Textbook of Histology* (Philadelphia, W. B. Saunders Co.), by kind permission of the authors and publishers.]

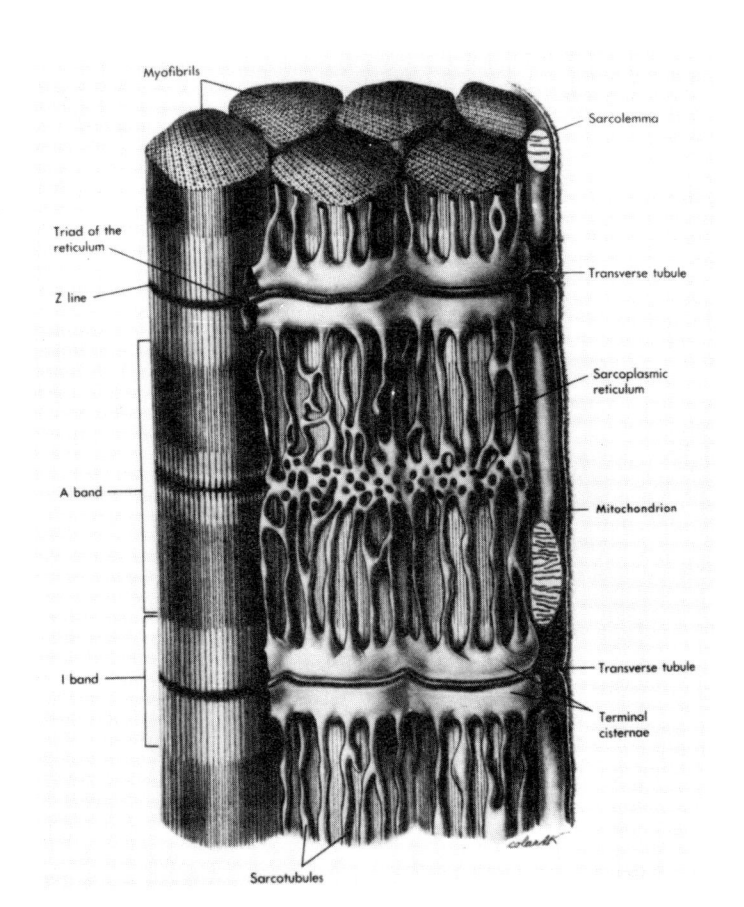

Figure 8.6 Muscle structure, showing relation of endoplasmic reticulum and of transverse tubular system to fibrils. [Reproduced from Patton et al (1976) *Introduction to Basic Neurology*, and previously published in Bloom and Fawcett (1970) *A Textbook of Histology* [Philadelphia, W. B. Saunders Co.; by kind permission of the authors and publishers.]

electrode in the region of the end-plate. ACh so released combines with specific ACh receptors (AChR) on the postjunctional membrane. The arrival of a nerve impulse at the motor end-plate results in the synchronous release of many packets or quanta of ACh, which produces a localized depolarization of the muscle fibre membrane in the region of the end-plate. This is the end-plate potential. When the end-plate potential reaches a certain critical size it triggers off an excitatory wave, the action potential, which then travels away from the end-plate along the surface membrane of the fibre. Under normal circumstances ACh receptors are confined to the area of the end-plate. After denervation, extrajunctional receptors may be identified on other parts of the sarcolemmal membrane. This is accompanied by a hundredfold increase in sensitivity of the muscle fibre to ACh (denervation hypersensitivity). At rest the inside of the fibre membrane is some 80 mV negative with respect to the outside. During the action potential the polarization of the membrane momentarily reverses, so that for about 1 ms the inside of the fibre becomes positive. This reversal of electrical polarity is caused by increased sodium permeability of the fibre membrane. There is evidence that the wave of excitation spreads inwards into the substance of the muscle fibre along the transverse system of tubules—the 'T' system (Fig. 8.6)—and that the consequent mobilization of calcium ions in the sarcoplasmic reticulum initiates contraction of the myofibrils. Among the many biochemical reactions which follow, creatine phosphate, in the presence of calcium, is broken down into creatine and phosphate, and adenosine triphosphate (ATP) to adenosine diphosphate (ADP), also releasing phosphate. This release of high-energy phosphate bonds provides much of the energy required for muscular contraction.

Muscle ultrastructure
The unit of structure of the individual myofibril of skeletal muscle is the sarcomere (Fig. 8.7) extending from one Z-line (situated in the midst of the I-band) to the next. Attached to each Z-line are a series of thin filaments of the protein actin. There is also a second type of filament which is rather thicker and is composed of myosin. These filaments correspond to the dark (birefringent) A-bands of the myofibrils. Each filament of myosin is surrounded by a hexagonal array of actin filaments; in addition, molecular cross-bridges reach out from the myosin to the actin filaments. During contraction, the cross-bridges repeatedly disengage and re-engage at successive sites on the actin filaments. The propulsion imparted to the actin filaments causes them to slide over the myosin filaments so as to interdigitate more fully with the latter. In this way the whole myofibril, and consequently its parent fibre, shortens. The energy metabolism of muscle contraction was described above.

Types of muscle fibre
Skeletal muscles are not homogeneous. In man they contain at least two main types of muscle fibre which are morphologically and histochemically distinct. The so-called type I fibre tends to be somewhat small and contains myofibrils which are generally somewhat slender. This type of fibre has a high concentration of mitochondria and enzymes such as succinic dehydrogenase and NADH diaphorase which are concerned with aerobic metabolism. The larger type II fibres have more coarse and more widely dispersed myofibrils. They contain fewer mitochondria but a higher concentration of glycogen and enzymes such as phosphorylase and myofibrillar adenosine triphosphatase, which are concerned with anaerobic metabolism. In man, all skeletal muscles contain an admixture of type I and type II fibres so that in transverse sections stained histochemically, a characteristic checker-board pattern is observed. These fibres are functionally different, and refinements of histochemical technique have shown that the type II fibres can be further subdivided into subtypes IIa and IIb. In mammals other than man there are certain muscles (such as the soleus) which are made up predominantly of type I fibres (so-called red muscles). These muscles are considered to be concerned largely with the maintenance of posture, and upon stimulation are found to contract and relax relatively slowly (slow 'twitch' muscles). By contrast, other muscles concerned more directly with phasic motor activity, such as the flexor digitorum longus, are made up predominantly of type II fibres (white muscle) and contract more rapidly (fast 'twitch' muscles). The motor nerve not only appears to control the physiological behaviour but also largely determines the histochemical structure of the muscle fibres. Transposition of the motor nerve supply from a fast muscle to a slow muscle, and vice versa, may almost completely alter the physiological and histochemical characteristics of the muscle fibres. The neurons seem to control the behaviour of the muscle fibres which make up their motor units, so that one can speak of type I and type II alpha neurons. When a group of muscle fibres which have lost their nerve supply are reinnervated by a sprouting neuron they become of uniform histochemical type (so-called 'type grouping').

The effect of drugs
A number of drugs may act upon the neuromuscular junction. When ACh is released at the neuromuscular

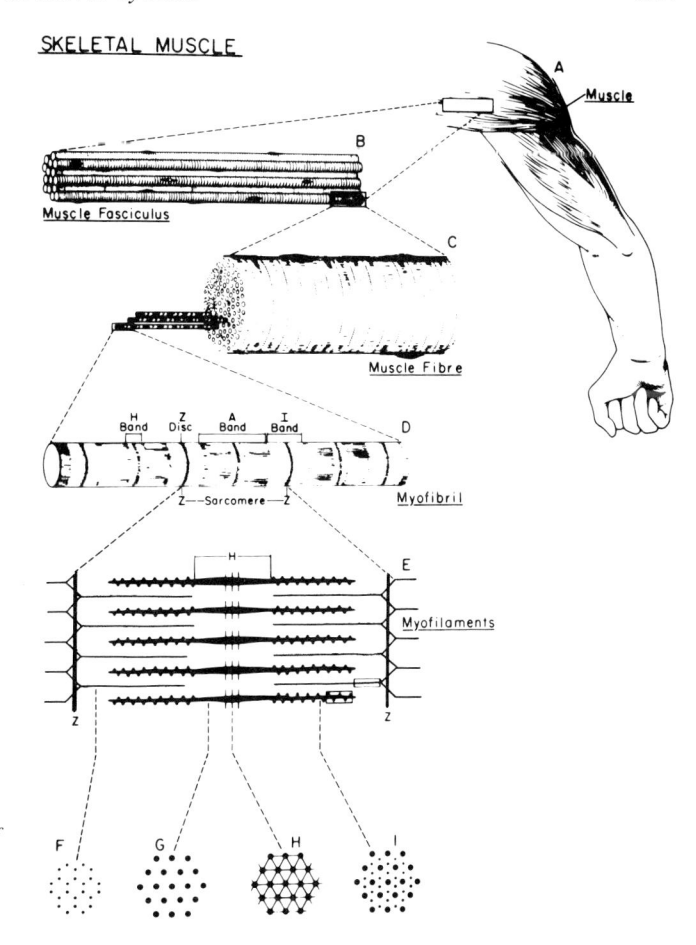

Figure 8.7 Histological and molecular structure of skeletal muscle. [Reproduced from Patton et al (1976) *Introduction to Basic Neurology*, and modified from Bloom and Fawcett (1970) *A Textbook of Histology* (Philadelphia: W. B. Saunders Co.) by kind permission of the authors and publishers.]

junction, it is broken down by cholinesterase, which is normally present in the subneural apparatus. Curare acts on the postjunctional membrane, where it reduces or prevents the depolarizing effect of the transmitter excited by the nerve impulse. Botulinum toxin blocks ACh release. Drugs such as physostigmine and neostigmine inhibit cholinesterase and allow ACh liberated at the myoneural junction to accumulate. Guanidine hydrochloride increases the output of ACh at the nerve endings and may thus be helpful in botulism. If ACh accumulates in excess, as in overdosage with neostigmine or guanidine, depolarization of the muscle fibre membrane persists and may result in blockage of the muscle action potential (depolarization block). Tubocurarine and gallamine compete with ACh for the end-plate chemical receptors and are therefore competitive inhibitors. Decamethonium and suxamethonium first produce muscle paralysis as a result of depolarization block but subsequently also produce competitive block, so that they are said to have a 'dual' action. In myasthenia gravis ACh receptors become coated with circulating anti-AChR antibodies, preventing ACh from having its full normal effect.

The muscle spindles (the fusimotor system) and other muscle and tendon receptors

The stretch detectors of muscle and tendon are the Golgi tendon organs and the muscle spindles. Strictly, the Golgi organs are tension receptors, and the muscle spindles are length detectors. The Golgi neurotendinous endings lie most often on tendons and are thus excited by stretch, as in tension applied to the tendon during muscular contraction. These stimuli produce a tonic generator potential and repetitive spike discharge in the afferent fibres. The effect of such discharge is to activate inhibitory motor neurons which inhibit alpha neuron activity.

The muscle spindles (Figs 8.8 and 8.9) are present in all voluntary muscles and contain on the average seven or eight muscle fibres, called intrafusal because they are enclosed in a fluid-containing connective tissue capsule. These fibres are of two types: nuclear-bag fibres, which are few, relatively large in diameter, and show a collection of nuclei at their equator, and the narrower and often more numerous nuclear chain fibres, each of which contains a single row of nuclei. Axons of gamma (effector) neurons enter the striated poles of these fibres. At the equatorial region of the

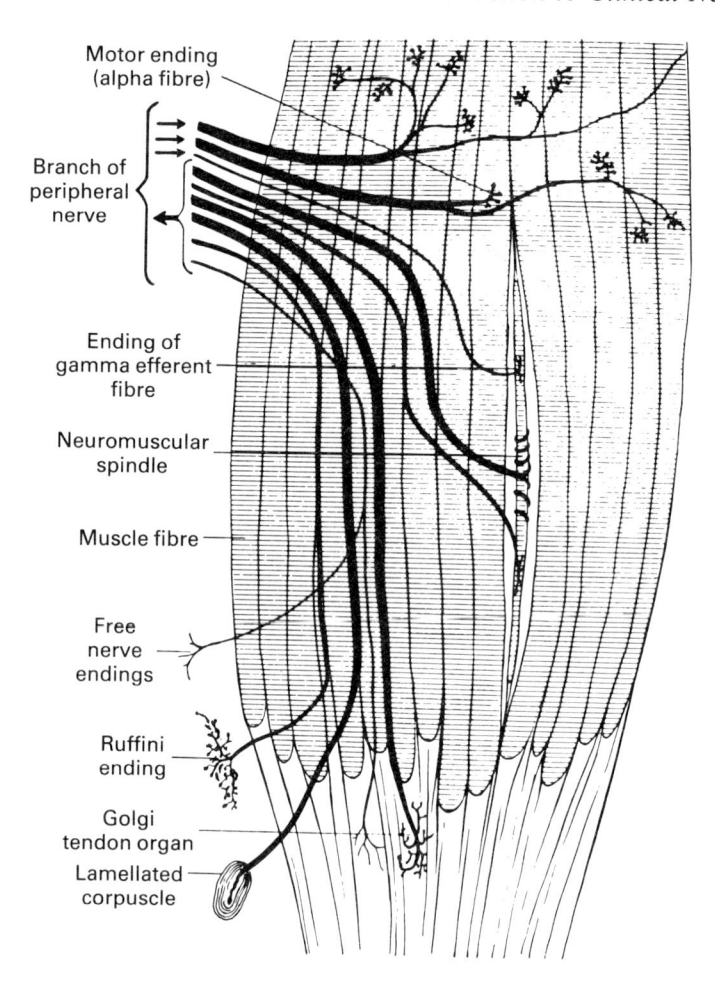

Figure 8.8 Schematic representation of a muscle and its nerve supply. Arrows indicate direction of conduction. Each muscle fibre has a motor ending from a large myelinated (alpha) fibre. The muscle fibres within a spindle have motor endings from small myelinated (gamma) fibres. Muscle nerves contain many sensory fibres. Some are large myelinated fibres from primary (annulospiral) endings in spindles, from neurotendinous spindles (Golgi tendon organs), and from pacinian corpuscles in the connective tissue within and external to the muscle. Smaller myelinated and non-myelinated fibres arise from Ruffini endings in the connective tissue in and around muscle, and in joints. Finally there are small myelinated and non-myelinated fibres that form free endings in the connective tissue in and around muscle. [Reproduced from Gardner (1975) *Fundamentals of Neurology*, 6th edn, by kind permission of the author and publisher.]

fibres there are two types of sensory endings: (a) annulospiral endings giving rise to group I myelinated axons, and (b) secondary or flower-spray endings, which give origin to group II myelinated axons. Both types of receptors are tonic receptors which are depolarized by stretch. The tendinous ends of the intrafusal muscle fibres project beyond the capsule at each end of the spindle and are attached either to the tendon of the muscle or to the perimysium of nearby extrafusal fibres, so that stretching of the extrafusal fibres applies tension to the intrafusal ones, whereas contraction of the muscle causes them to relax.

Sensory endings in the spindle are arranged in parallel with the extrafusal muscle fibres, while tendon endings are in series. The group I afferent fibres from these two receptors are thus conventionally divided into IA afferents (from the annulospiral spindle endings) and IB afferents (from the tendon endings). The respective arrangement of these receptors determines the fact that during muscular contraction IA afferents are silent (owing to relaxation of intrafusal fibres), while IB afferents discharge. These afferent fibres play a crucial role in the control of monosynaptic spinal reflexes, while the group II afferents from the flower-spray endings of the spindle are more concerned with polysynaptic reflex activity. Gamma-neuron discharge increases the sensitivity of the muscle to tension through contraction of the intrafusal fibres and stretching of the sensory receptors in the equatorial region. The fusimotor fibres are of two types: dynamic fibres which respond to afferent stimuli concerned with the velocity of stretch, and static fibres concerned with changes solely in length.

Passive stretching of a muscle gives rise to afferent impulses which reach the spinal cord, stimulating the alpha neurons which then discharge, causing the muscle to contract and regain its former length. This process is responsible for monosynaptic spinal reflex activity as in the tendon jerks (see below). Sensory impulses from the spindles also reach the brain stem, cerebellum and cerebral cortex by a number of ascending pathways. In turn the descending path-

groups IA and IB and group II afferents from all of the receptors in the muscle, eliciting stretch reflexes which are more complex, often polysynaptic, and which are modulated by activity in the many descending pathways concerned in the control of posture and of muscle tone. Essentially the response consists of tonic or continuous muscle contraction (the tonic stretch reflex).

Segmental and peripheral organization of the neuromuscular system

The motor nuclei of the cranial nerves are derived from branchial columns of cells in the brain stem which innervate structures derived from the branchial arches. In the adult the anatomical organization of these nuclei in the brain stem retains some semblance of segmental organization, but this is much less clear than is the segmental arrangement of the spinal cord. Corresponding to each spinal segment is one pair of spinal nerves composed of the ventral and dorsal roots derived from that segment. The sensory neurons in the dorsal root ganglia are completely separated in each segment from those of the contiguous segments. The organization of the alpha motor neurons is less clearly segmental in that their cell bodies are arranged in longitudinal columns and those innervating a single muscle often extend over more than one segment. Several muscles may be represented in one segment. A lesion of the anterior horn of a single segment gives weakness of all muscles innervated by that segment but paralyses completely only those which have no nerve supply from adjacent segments.

The motor cranial nerves

The pathophysiology of the third, fourth and sixth cranial nerves, which innervate the external ocular muscles, has been detailed earlier (p. 138). The motor root of the fifth or trigeminal nerve leaves the lateral aspect of the inferior surface of the pons, passes forward beneath the gasserian ganglion, leaves the skull via the foramen ovale, and unites with the third sensory division to form a single trunk in the infratentorial fossa. Its branches then innervate the temporalis, masseter and pterygoid muscles as well as the anterior belly of the digastric, the mylohyoid muscle, the tensor tympani and the tensor palatini. Lesions of this root therefore give weakness of the masticatory muscles, and when the mouth is opened the mandible deviates to the side opposite to the lesion.

The seventh or facial nerve is primarily motor, but it also contains fibres which excite salivary secretion and others which convey taste impulses from the anterior two-thirds of the tongue. The nerve emerges

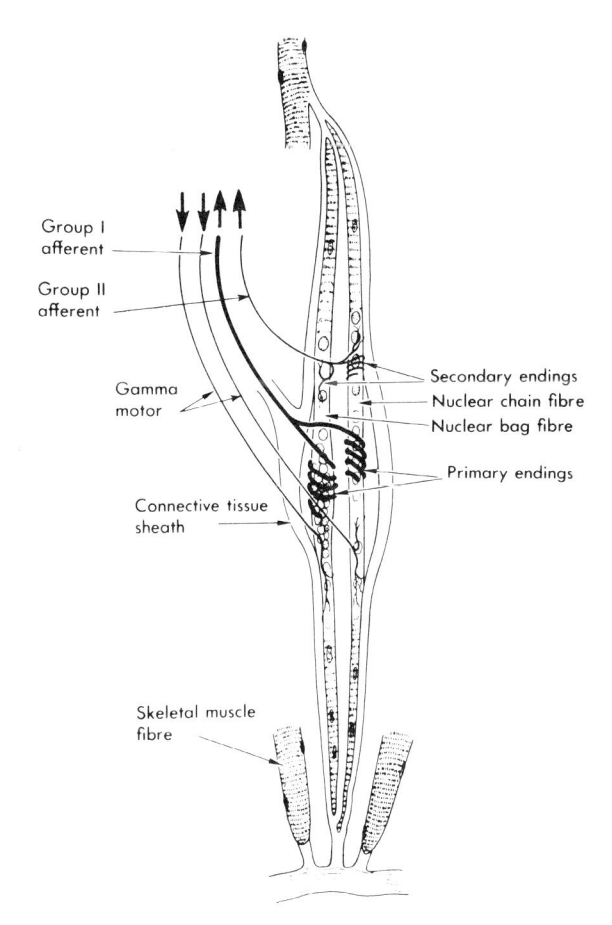

Figure 8.9 Schematic representation of a neuromuscular spindle. Parts of three skeletal muscle fibres are shown (cross-striated, nuclei at edge). Inside the connective tissue sheath of the spindle are three muscle fibres (thinner than regular skeletal muscle fibres, with central nuclei, and striations minimal or absent in region of sensory endings). Sensory nerve fibres form primary (annulospiral) and secondary (flower-spray) endings, the primary arising from the large fibres. (The form of primary and secondary endings varies according to species. In some, such as rabbit and man, the primary endings of the large fibre may be flower-spray in type, not winding around the muscle fibre.) Small nerve fibres (gamma efferents) form motor endings at each end of the spindle muscle fibres. Motor discharges over gamma efferents cause the muscle spindle fibres to contract at each end, thus stretching the intervening, noncontractile sensory region and activating the sensory endings. Arrows indicate direction of conduction. [Reproduced from Gardner (1975) *Fundamentals of Neurology*, 6th edn, by kind permission of the author and publisher, and based on Barker, D. (1948) *Quart. J. Micr. Sci.* **89**:143–186, Boyd, I. A. (1962) *Phil. Trans. Roy. Soc. Lond. Ser. B.* **245**:81–136, and Matthews, P. B. C. (1964) *Physiol. Rev.* **44**:219–288.]

ways from these structures influence the excitability of gamma neurons, thus exercising important controlling influences over muscle tone. Sudden and transient stretching of a muscle, as in the tendon jerks, causes selective discharge in Group IA afferents thus eliciting a monosynaptic reflex. Steady stretch or vibration applied to the muscle, by contrast, excites

from the lateral aspect of the pons, enters the internal auditory meatus with the eighth nerve, and then travels through the middle ear in the facial canal (Fig. 8.10) to emerge from the skull via the stylomastoid foramen. In the middle ear it gives a branch which innervates the stapedius. After leaving the skull it gives branches to the stylohyoid muscle, the posterior belly of the digastric, and the posterior part of the occipitofrontalis before entering the parotid gland, where it divides into a number of branches which then innervate the facial musculature or muscles of expression, including the frontalis, orbicularis oculi, orbicularis oris, buccinator and platysma.

Facial weakness due to supranuclear lesions of the contralateral corticospinal tract affect movements of the lower part of the face much more severely than those of the upper part. Voluntary retraction of the corner of the mouth is impaired, whereas eye closure remains relatively normal, as do emotional movements of the face as in smiling. Such emotional movements may, however, be reduced (mimetic paralysis) as a result of lesions of the opposite frontal lobe anterior to the precentral gyrus, or less often as a result of lesions in the region of the thalamus where there may be a centre for emotional expression. Lesions of the facial nerve itself may involve the nucleus in the pons, as in pontine tumour or infarction, for example. The nerve can also be involved in its intracranial course in the posterior fossa (e.g. by acoustic neuroma), or within the petrous temporal bone (e.g. by otitis media or cholesteatoma). Herpes zoster of the geniculate ganglion (the Ramsay Hunt syndrome) often gives facial paralysis and loss of taste on the anterior two-thirds of the tongue, sometimes with ipsilateral deafness and facial sensory loss due to involvement of the fifth and eighth nerves. Vesicles are usually seen in the external auditory meatus and on the soft palate. Perineural and interstitial oedema of undetermined cause of the nerve in its canal above the stylomastoid foramen appears to be the mechanism usually responsible for idiopathic facial paralysis (Bell's palsy). Fibrosis and irritation of the nerve in a similar location has been thought to be the usual cause of clonic facial spasm (hemifacial spasm), a benign but embarrassing condition which gives rise to irregular intermittent twitching or spasm of the muscles of one side of the face, but it has become apparent that compression of the intracranial trunk of the nerve in the subarachnoid space, caused by an aberrant trunk (a condition readily relieved by surgery), is a much commoner cause. Aberrant reinnervation of regenerating facial nerve fibres after facial paralysis can result in various patterns of paradoxical facial movement and/or in gustatory sweating (facial sweating during meals). After leaving the skull the fibres of the nerve may also be damaged in the parotid gland. Facial muscle weakness is seen in various forms of myopathy but here it is the muscles themselves rather than the facial nerve which are affected.

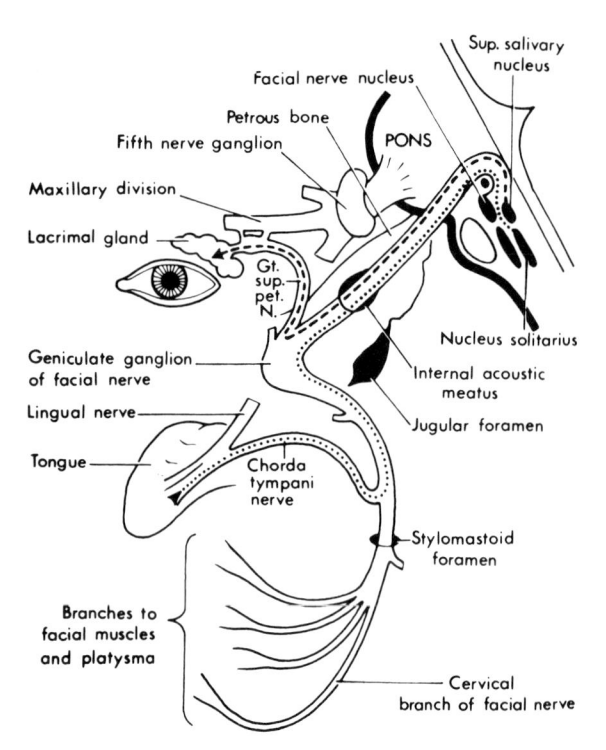

Figure 8.10 The facial nerve.

Lesions involving the facial nerve trunk above the geniculate ganglion will cause loss of lacrimation (greater petrosal nerve), and loss of taste in the anterior two-thirds of the tongue (chorda tympani nerve), as well as paralysis of both upper and lower facial muscles.

Lesions between the geniculate ganglion and the point where the chorda tympani nerve leaves the facial nerve (6 mm above the stylomastoid foramen) will cause loss of taste sensation in the anterior two thirds of the tongue, as well as paralysis of the facial muscles, but lacrimation will still be present.

Lesions below the point where the chorda tympani leaves the facial nerve will cause paralysis of the facial muscles, but both taste and lacrimation will be present.

[Reproduced from Walton (1985) *Brain's Diseases of the Nervous System*, 9th edn, by kind permission of the publisher, and redrawn from an original drawing by Charles Keogh.]

The ninth or glossopharyngeal nerve is principally sensory, carrying taste from the posterior one-third of the tongue. Its fewer motor fibres, arising from the nucleus ambiguus, supply the stylopharyngeus muscle. The motor function of this nerve can for practical purposes be ignored in clinical neurology.

The motor fibres of the tenth or vagus nerve originate in the nucleus ambiguus and leave the medulla oblongata in a series of radicles at the anterior margin of the inferior cerebellar peduncle in line with the roots of the glossopharyngeal nerve above and the accessory below. These radicles combine into a single trunk which leaves the skull through the jugular foramen with the accessory nerve and then comes to lie in the carotid sheath behind the carotid arteries and the internal jugular vein. In the thorax the course of the two vagus nerves differs on the two sides. That on the right passes downwards behind the trachea and superior vena cava to reach the right lung root, while that on the left passes between the left common carotid and subclavian arteries and then crosses the aortic arch to reach the root of the left lung. In the posterior mediastinum both nerves contribute parasympathetic fibres to the pulmonary and oesophageal plexuses and enter the abdomen at the oesophageal opening in the diaphragm, the left in front, the right behind the oesophagus, going on in a purely parasympathetic capacity to supply the stomach and other abdominal organs. The principal motor branches of the vagus are (a) the pharyngeal branch, which leaves the inferior ganglion of the nerve just below the jugular foramen and which innervates the muscles of the soft palate, (b) the external laryngeal division of the superior laryngeal branch, which innervates the cricothyroid muscle (the remainder of the superior laryngeal nerve is sensory), and (c) the recurrent laryngeal branch, which innervates most of the intrinsic muscles of the larynx as well as the cricopharyngeus, which is the principal muscle of the inferior pharyngeal sphincter. The right recurrent laryngeal nerve arises in the root of the neck and loops backwards and upwards behind the subclavian artery. The left nerve loops similarly around the arch of the aorta, where it is especially vulnerable to damage by aortic aneurysm but more particularly by other lesions in the mediastinum such as metastases in lymph nodes.

A unilateral lesion of the vagus gives ipsilateral paralysis of the muscles of the soft palate, the three pharyngeal constrictors, the intrinsic and extrinsic laryngeal muscles, and the lower pharyngeal sphincter. This results in difficulty in swallowing food and saliva, hoarseness of the voice, and sometimes a nasal intonation as well as impaired coughing. With unilateral palatal paralysis there may be few if any symptoms, but when the patient opens his mouth and says 'ah' the soft palate and uvula deviate to the opposite side. Bilateral palatal paralysis gives a nasal quality to the voice, mouth breathing, and loud snoring and regurgitation of ingested fluids through the nose. Palatal myoclonus is a rare rhythmical and repetitive movement of the soft palate due to a degenerative lesion of unknown cause in the inferior olivary nucleus.

Unilateral pharyngeal paralysis causes delay in pharyngeal emptying with the accumulation of mucus overflowing into the larynx. On attempting to swallow there is a 'curtain' movement of the posterior pharyngeal wall towards the normal side. In bilateral lesions dysphagia is more complete.

In the normal larynx the cricothyroid muscles (external laryngeal nerve) tense the vocal cords, while the abductors and adductors of the cord are supplied by the recurrent laryngeal. Abduction of the cords occurs during inspiration, and the cords are adducted during phonation and coughing. A unilateral lesion of one vocal cord and of the cricopharyngeus muscle on the same side (Fig. 8.11) results in hoarseness of the voice (dysphonia) and some accumulation of mucus with dysphagia. If the external laryngeal nerve is also damaged or if the lesion affects the vagus between the nucleus ambiguus and its inferior ganglion, these symptoms are more severe. In the latter instance, the palate and pharynx are paralysed on the same side. Bilateral paralysis of the larynx usually gives inspiratory stridor and a weak but clear voice, a very poor cough, and difficulty in expelling mucus from the larynx.

The eleventh or accessory nerve arises in part from the most caudal portion of the nucleus ambiguus and in part from the anterior horn cells of the first to the fifth cervical segments of the spinal cord. At the jugular foramen the medullary fibres join the vagus; the spinal fibres form a single trunk which lies between the internal carotid artery and the internal jugular vein, descending to supply the sternomastoid muscles and the upper part of the trapezius in conjunction with branches of the second, third and fourth cervical nerves. A unilateral lesion of this nerve gives paralysis of the sternomastoid, which results in difficulty in rotating the head to the opposite side and (owing to weakness of the trapezius) in elevating the shoulder on the same side, while the affected shoulder also droops at rest. Lesions damaging this nerve are much the same as those which damage the vagus except that isolated lesions of this nerve rarely result from inflammation (in cervical lymph nodes) or from penetrating injuries or surgical operations on the neck.

The twelfth or hypoglossal nerve originates in the hypoglossal nucleus of the medulla, this nucleus being an upward extension of the anterior horn of the cervical cord. It emerges from the medulla between the inferior olive and the pyramid and leaves the skull via the hypoglossal canal. Near the hyoid bone it turns medially over the two carotid arteries and between the mylohyoid and hyoglossus muscles to reach the tongue, where it innervates all the intrinsic tongue muscles. Other branches supply the infrahyoid and thyrohyoid muscles. Lesions of this nerve cause weakness and wasting of the affected half of the tongue in which fasciculation can often be seen. The tongue deviates to the paralysed side when pro-

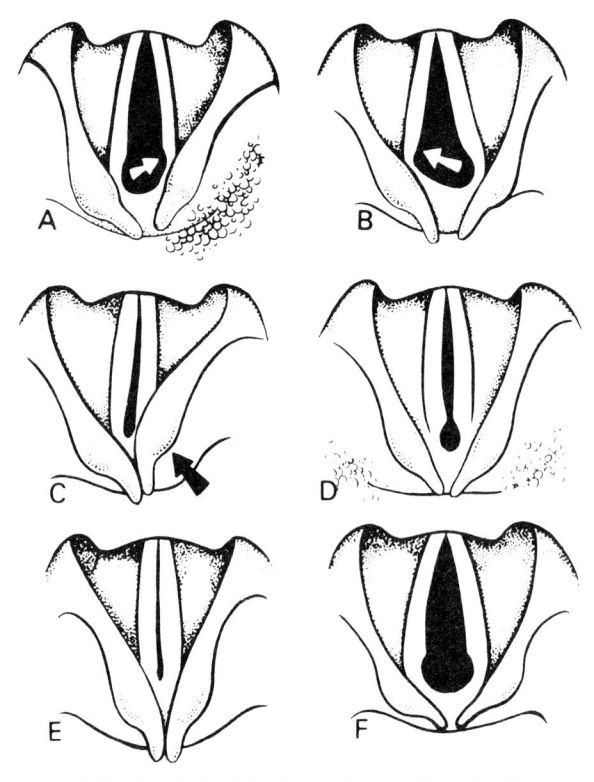

Figure 8.11 Paralysis of the larynx (as seen through a laryngoscope).

A, Paralysis of the left recurrent laryngeal nerve (neurofibroma). The paralysed arytenoid always lies slightly in front of the non-paralysed right arytenoid. Froth tends to collect around the opening of the oesophagus, owing to paralysis of the left cricopharyngeus muscle (lower sphincter of the pharynx, supplied by the same recurrent laryngeal nerve). On adduction, the non-paralysed right vocal cord moves across to meet the paralysed left cord.

B, Paralysis of the right recurrent laryngeal nerve (thyroidectomy). There is no collected froth at the opening of the oesophagus, because compensation is so good by the intact left paired cricopharyngeus muscle that it has been able to overcome the delay due to the paralysis of the right cricopharyngeus muscle.

C, The same case as B, showing closure of the larynx on adduction. The left non-paralysed cord now moves up to the paralysed cord, and the non-paralysed arytenoid now lies in front of the paralysed arytenoid.

D, Paralysis of both vocal cords at the same time (thyroidectomy). The cords are held in adduction because their muscles are all paralysed except for the chief tensors of the cords, the cricothyroid muscles (supplied by the external branch of the superior laryngeal nerve).

E, Normal closure of the vocal cords as seen in a laryngeal mirror.

F, Normal abduction of the vocal cords as seen in a laryngeal mirror.

[Reproduced from Walton (1985) *Brain's Diseases of the Nervous System*, 9th edn, by kind permission of the publisher, and redrawn from an original drawing by Charles Keogh.]

truded. Unilateral lesions do not cause impairment of articulation (dysarthria), but when paralysis is bilateral (as in advanced progressive bulbar palsy—motor neuron disease), speech is markedly impaired. Spasticity of the tongue giving dysarthria without atrophy can result from bilateral corticospinal tract lesions in the cerebral hemispheres or upper brain stem, as in progressive bulbar palsy (motor neuron disease), pseudobulbar palsy due to bilateral infarction, and brain-stem tumour.

The innervation and organization of the voluntary muscles of the trunk and limbs

The axons derived from the alpha and gamma motor neurons in each spinal cord segment leave that segment in the anterior or ventral root which joins with the posterior root in the spinal nerve of that segment. After leaving the spinal column via the intervertebral foramina, each spinal nerve divides into dorsal and ventral rami. The dorsal rami largely supply the muscles of the trunk, the larger ventral rami those of the limbs. But in the brachial and lumbosacral plexuses the axons are redistributed and enter into new groupings in the peripheral nerves. Hence the fibres from a single spinal segment may reach several peripheral nerves, and conversely a single peripheral nerve often receives fibres from several spinal segments. In addition many peripheral nerves divide into several branches, each supplying one or more voluntary muscles. In clinical neurology a working knowledge of anatomy of the peripheral neuromuscular system is necessary in order to be able to distinguish between lesions involving (a) a spinal cord segment or anterior horn or one ventral root, (b) a spinal nerve, in which case somatic sensory afferent fibres are also involved, (c) one or more components (e.g. cords) of the brachial or lumbosacral plexus, (d) a single peripheral nerve or one of its branches, and (e) the voluntary muscles themselves. To assist the reader in this differential diagnostic process, the brachial plexus is illustrated in Fig. 8.12 and the distribution to the musculature of various peripheral nerves in Fig. 8.13; the root and nerve supply of the muscles commonly examined in clinical practice are listed in Table 10. The principles governing the examination of the individual skeletal muscles have been described earlier.

WEAKNESS AND PARALYSIS

Weakness (paresis) of a group of muscles implies that the power produced on voluntary contraction of the affected muscles is reduced, whereas complete paralysis indicates that the power to move the part con-

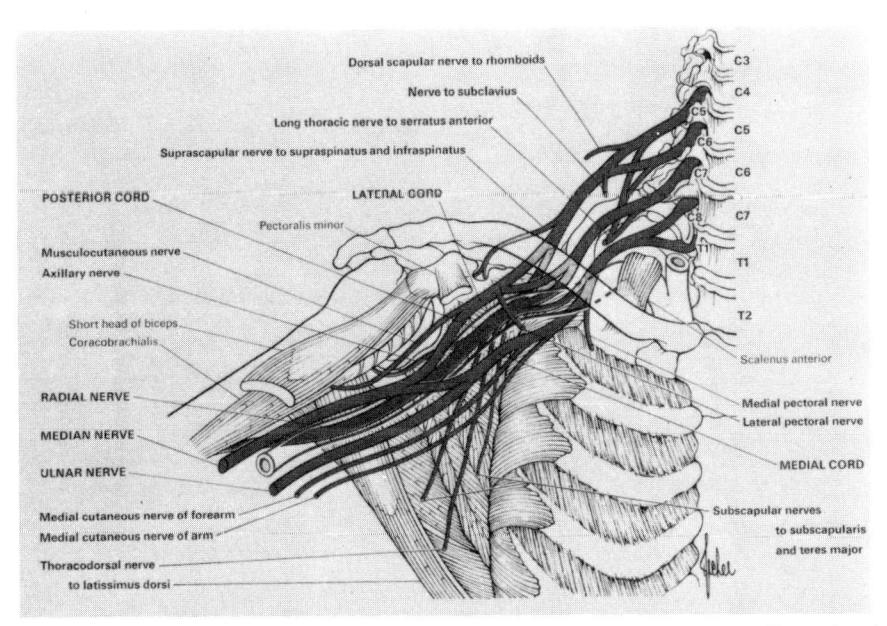

Figure 8.12 Diagram of the brachial plexus, its branches, and the muscles which they supply. [Reproduced from *Aids to the Examination of the Peripheral Nervous System*. Medical Research Council Memorandum No. 45, by kind permission of the authors and publisher.]

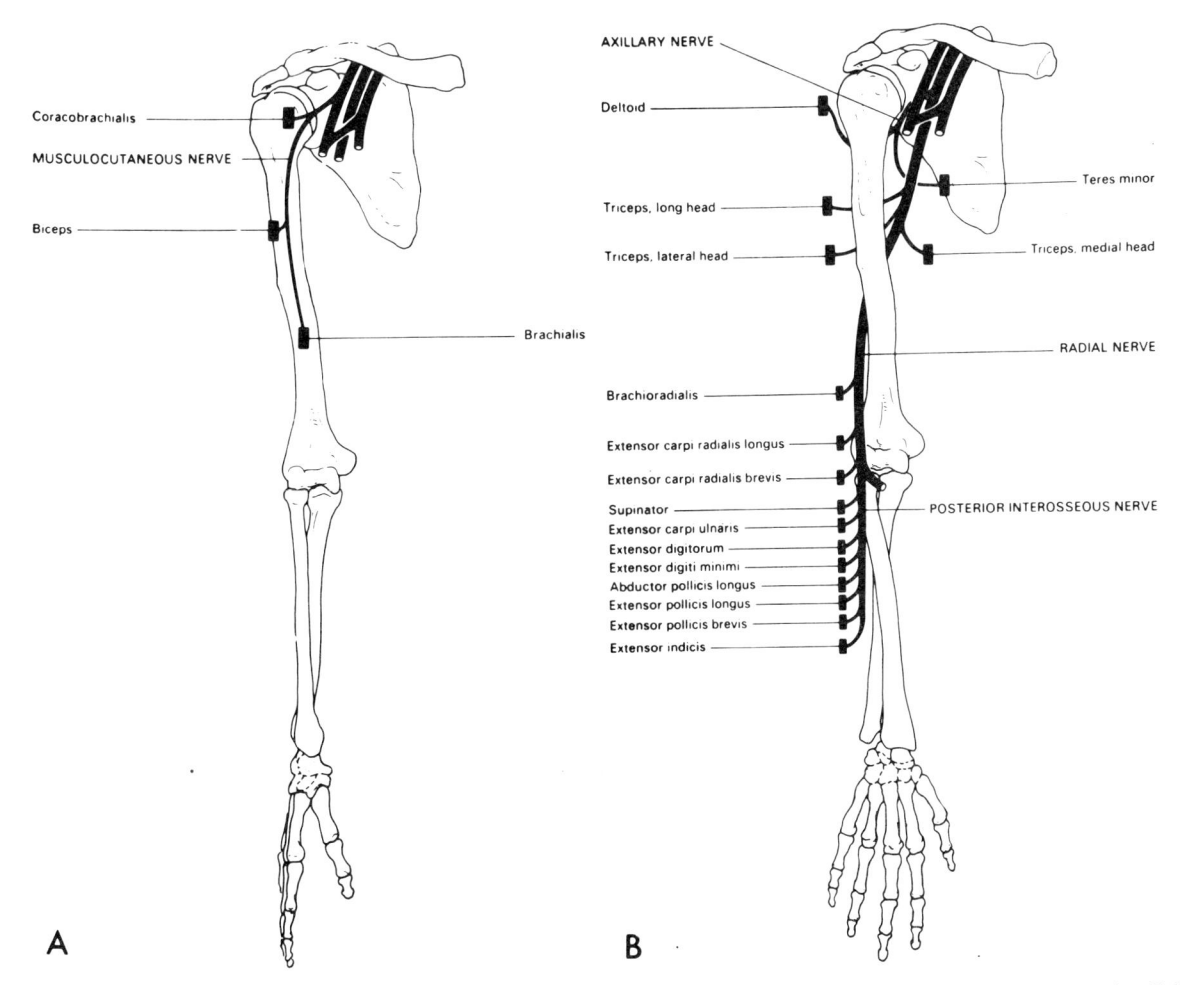

Figure 8.13 A, Diagram of the musculocutaneous nerve and the muscles which it supplies. B, Diagram of the axillary and radial nerves and the muscles which they supply.

Illustration continued on the following pages

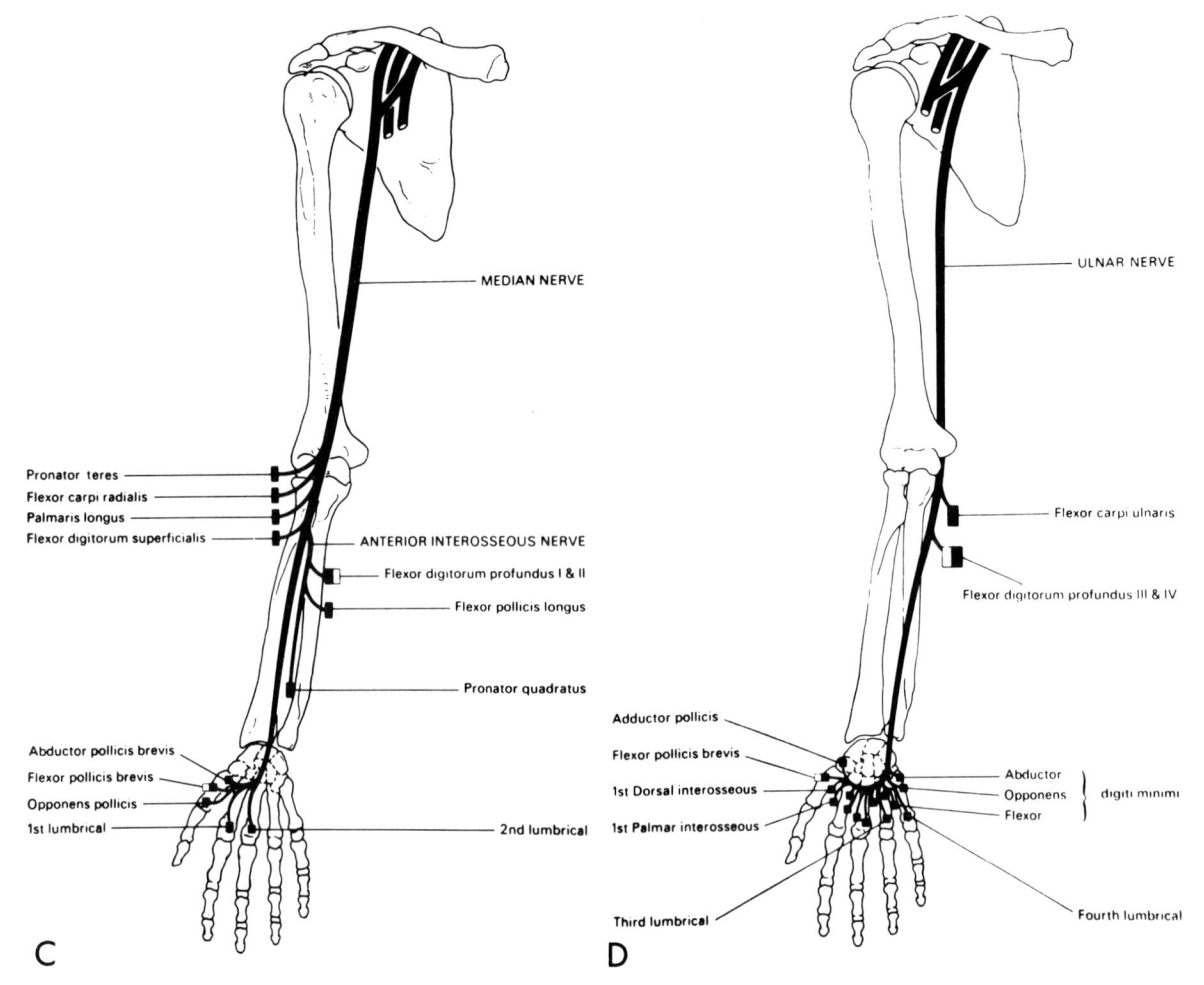

Figure 8.13 (*continued*) C, Diagram of the median nerve and the muscles which it supplies. Note: the white rectangle signifies that the muscle indicated receives a part of its nerve supply from another peripheral nerve (see D, E, and F). D, Diagram of the ulnar nerve and the muscles which it supplies.

Illustration continued on the facing page

cerned is totally lost. Weakness of one limb is referred to as a monoparesis, while total paralysis of a limb is called a monoplegia. Hemiplegia is the term used to identify paralysis which afflicts one side of the body, and particularly the arm and leg, while paraplegia signifies a paralysis of both lower limbs. When all four limbs are paralysed, the terms quadriplegia or tetraplegia are used. A symmetrical weakness of all four limbs, affecting the lower limbs more markedly than the upper limbs, and occurring in children with cerebral palsy, is often called a diplegia. The term 'palsy' can be used interchangeably with 'paralysis', but is more often used in modern neurological practice to identify the paralysis of individual muscles or muscle groups that results from peripheral nerve lesions.

Paralysis may result from a lesion of either the upper or lower motor neuron; under certain circumstances it can be due to a defect in conduction at the neuromuscular junction or to a biochemical or structural abnormality of the muscle fibres themselves. Some principles governing the differentiation of these causes of paralysis will be discussed below.

MUSCLE 'TONE' AND ITS DISORDERS

General considerations

The tone of a muscle can be regarded as the response it shows to passive stretching. Contrary to the views once held, a completely relaxed and resting muscle is not in a state of continuous partial contraction and is silent electrically. It has elasticity, but not tone. Tone can be assessed only when the muscle is moved or when it is concerned with maintaining a posture

The motor system 175

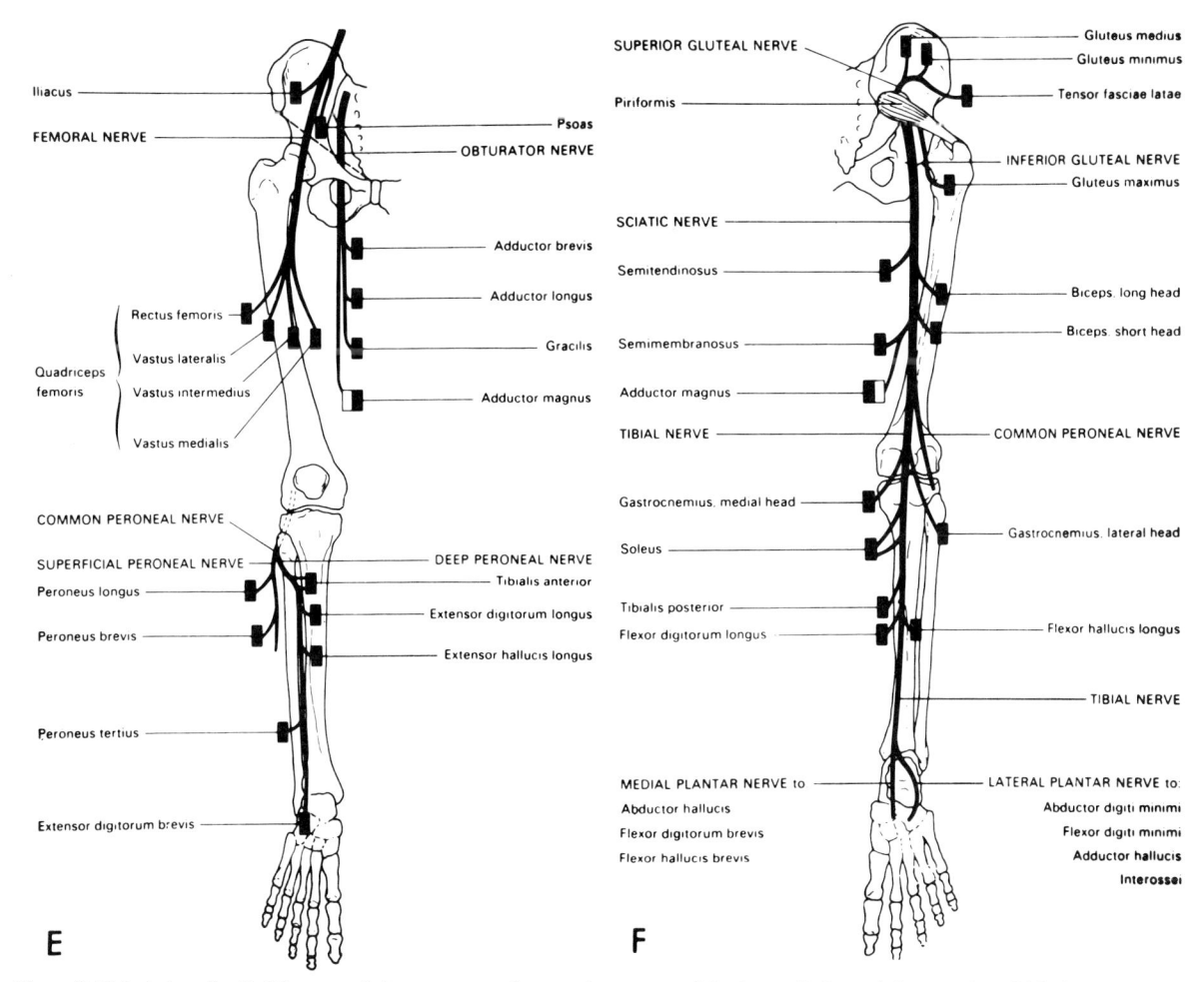

Figure 8.13 (*continued*) E, Diagram of the nerves on the anterior aspect of the lower limb, and the muscles which they supply. F, Diagram of the nerves on the posterior aspect of the lower limb, and the muscles which they supply. [Reproduced from *Aids to the Examination of the Peripheral Nervous System*, Medical Research Council Memorandum No. 45, by kind permission of the authors and publisher, and modified from Pitres and Testut (1925) *Les nerfs en Schémas*. Doin, Paris.]

against an applied force such as that of gravity. Postural tone is that state of partial contraction of certain muscles which is needed to maintain the posture of the parts of the body. The muscles involved and the force of muscular contraction required will depend upon the position of the parts concerned at any one time.

Tone is usually assessed by moving a limb or some other part passively and by observing the reaction which occurs in the muscles which are being stretched. The moment this stretching begins, stretch receptors in the muscle concerned, and particularly in the muscle spindles, give out afferent stimuli, and reflex partial contraction of the muscle results. The responses to momentary and to more prolonged stretching are different, the former being responsible, for instance, for the tendon jerks, the latter eliciting more complex responses, often in the form of tonic contraction. Variations in the degree of sensitivity of these reflexes account for the alterations in tone which occur as a result of nervous disease. Forceful continued contraction of a group of muscles (e.g. clenching one hand or pulling firmly with the flexed fingers of both hands opposed to one another) temporarily causes an increased flow of afferent impulses in the sensory fibres from the spindles. While this appears to increase slightly the rate of discharge in gamma neurons, causing a slightly increased sensitivity of the spindles to stretch, and it was once believed that in consequence the 'set' of the spindles (the state of contraction of their intrafusal fibres) was altered, it is now known that the exaggeration of the tendon reflexes which results is principally due to increased alpha (as distinct from gamma) neuronal discharge. This phenomenon, known as reinforcement or Jendrassik's manoeuvre, is often used clin-

TABLE 10. Nerve and main root supply of muscles†

(The list given below does not include all the muscles innervated by these nerves, but only those more commonly tested, either clinically or electrically, and shows the order of innervation.)

UPPER LIMB	Spinal Roots
Spinal Accessory Nerve	
Trapezius	C3, C4
Brachial Plexus	
Rhomboids	C4, C5
Serratus anterior	C5, C6, C7
Pectoralis major	
Clavicular	**C5**, C6
Sternal	C6, **C7**, C8
Supraspinatus	**C5**, C6
Infraspinatus	**C5**, C6
Latissimus dorsi	C6, **C7**, C8
Teres major	C5, **C6**, C7
Axillary Nerve	
Deltoid	**C5**, C6
Musculocutaneous Nerve	
Biceps	C5, C6
Brachialis	C5, C6
Radial Nerve	
Triceps (Long head, Lateral head, Medial head)	C6, **C7**, C8
Brachioradialis	C5, **C6**
Extensor carpi radialis longus	C5, **C6**
Posterior Interosseous Nerve	
Supinator	C6, C7
Extensor carpi ulnaris	**C7**, C8
Extensor digitorum	**C7**, C8
Abductor pollicis longus	**C7**, C8
Extensor pollicis longus	**C7**, C8
Extensor pollicis brevis	**C7**, C8
Extensor indicis	**C7**, C8
Median Nerve	
Pronator teres	C6, C7
Flexor carpi radialis	C6, C7
Flexor digitorum superficialis	C7, **C8**, T1
Abductor pollicis brevis	**C8, T1**
Flexor pollicis brevis*	**C8, T1**
Opponens pollicis	**C8, T1**
Lumbricals I & II	**C8, T1**
Anterior Interosseous Nerve	
Flexor digitorum profundus I & II	C7, **C8**
Flexor pollicis longus	C7, **C8**

	Spinal Roots
Ulnar Nerve	
Flexor carpi ulnaris	C7, **C8**, T1
Flexor digitorum profundus III & IV	C7, **C8**
Hypothenar muscles	**C8, T1**
Adductor pollicis	**C8, T1**
Flexor pollicis brevis	**C8, T1**
Palmar interossei	**C8, T1**
Dorsal interossei	**C8, T1**
Lumbricals III & IV	**C8, T1**
LOWER LIMB	Spinal Roots
Femoral Nerve	
Iliopsoas	L1, **L2**, L3
Rectus femoris, Vastus lateralis, Vastus intermedius, Vastus medialis (Quadriceps femoris)	L2, **L3, L4**
Obturator Nerve	
Adductor longus, Adductor magnus	L2, **L3, L4**
Superior Gluteal Nerve	
Gluteus medius and minimus	
Tensor fasciae latae	L4, **L5**, S1
Inferior Gluteal Nerve	
Gluteus maximus	L5, **S1**, S2
Sciatic and Tibial Nerves	
Semitendinosus	L5, **S1**, S2
Biceps	L5, **S1**, S2
Semimembranosus	L5, **S1**, S2
Gastrocnemius and soleus	S1, S2
Tibialis posterior	L4, L5
Flexor digitorum longus	L5, **S1**, S2
Flexor hallucis longus	L5, **S1**, S2
Abductor hallucis, Abductor digiti minimi, Interossei (Small muscles of foot)	S1, S2
Sciatic and Common Peroneal Nerves	
Tibialis anterior	**L4**, L5
Extensor digitorum longus	**L5**, S1
Extensor hallucis longus	**L5**, S1
Extensor digitorum brevis	**L5**, S1
Peroneus longus	**L5**, S1
Peroneus brevis	**L5**, S1

* Flexor pollicis brevis is often supplied wholly or partially by the ulnar nerve.
† Reproduced from Medical Research Council *Aids to the Examination of the Peripheral Nervous System*, by kind permission of the authors and publisher.

---

ically to bring out tendon reflexes which at first seem to be absent. In spasticity and extrapyramidal rigidity, however (see below), the 'set' of the spindles is continuously abnormal.

On stretching, the tone of the muscle may be increased (spasticity or rigidity, or hypertonia) or it may be reduced (flaccidity or hypotonia); these alterations are of great value in neurological diagnosis. Both spasticity and rigidity can cause a subjective sense of stiffness in the muscles and this is sometimes severe.

Muscle tone is normally regulated by reticulospinal fibres which accompany the pyramidal tract through its course in the spinal cord and which have an inhibitory effect upon the stretch reflex. This inhibition balances the background facilitatory impulses conveyed by the pontine reticulospinal and lateral vestibulospinal pathways. These influences are in turn influenced by multisynaptic reflex arcs traversing the cerebellum, basal ganglia and brain stem. Dorsal reticulospinal fibres appear specifically to inhibit flexor lower limb reflexes. When lesions of the pyramidal and reticulospinal tracts release stretch reflexes from inhibition, the increased tone which results is initially associated with hyperactivity of dynamic fusimotor neurons. If such increased tone persists (spasticity), increased alpha neuron discharge develops so that spasticity in man at different stages may be associated with both increased gamma (dynamic fusimotor) and alpha neuron activity. The role of the basal ganglia appears to be of particular importance in balancing alpha and gamma neuron activity.

Spasticity

Spasticity is one form of increased tone or hypertonia resulting from lesions of the pyramidal pathways and often of the reticulospinal pathways. Released from descending inhibitory influences, the stretch reflexes become hyperactive as a consequence of increased excitability of dynamic fusimotor neurons and alpha neurons, as mentioned above. If the dorsal reticulospinal system is also damaged, there is disinhibition of afferent flexor reflex pathways. Release of such flexor reflexes may give flexor spasms in the lower limbs in response to stimulation of the legs, bladder or bowels. The 'extensor' plantar or Babinski reflex is one component of the primitive flexor withdrawal reflex similarly released. In spasticity the affected limb or limbs usually show an increase in resistance to passive stretching. This resistance is particularly severe initially, but then tends to 'give' suddenly as the movement is continued. This sign is known as 'clasp-knife' rigidity. It is seen particularly well in the legs of a patient with a spastic paraplegia due to bilateral pyramidal tract disease. In individuals with spastic weakness, movement is impaired owing to defective conduction of motor impulses by the pyramidal tracts, while there is also 'clasp-knife' rigidity on passive movement. Hyperactivity of tendon reflexes is often accompanied by clonus, a phenomenon in which sustained stretch of a muscle evokes repetitive contraction and relaxation owing to reverberating activity in the hyperexcitable fusimotor system.

Extrapyramidal hypertonia

Rigidity of extrapyramidal type occurring in patients with disease of the basal ganglia or substantia nigra is different from spasticity. The rigidity is either uniform in degree throughout the entire range of passive movement, in which case it is known as 'plastic' or 'lead-pipe' rigidity, or else it intermittently 'gives' and returns throughout the movement, being then referred to as 'cogwheel' in type. In contrast to spasticity, alpha neuron discharge predominates over gamma neuron discharge in extrapyramidal rigidity. There is usually increased activity as well in static fusimotor fibres, although not in the dynamic ones which are involved in spasticity. In dystonia there is simultaneous contraction of agonists, antagonists and synergists, so that reciprocal inhibition of antagonists is seriously deranged and there is greatly increased alpha neuron discharge. As a result parts of the body become virtually fixed in an abnormal posture.

Decerebrate rigidity

A transverse lesion across the midbrain at about the level of the superior colliculus or red nucleus releases the brain stem, cerebellum and spinal cord from cerebral control. This results in strong continuous contraction in extensor groups of muscles so that the animal placed upright with support will remain standing, or if pushed over cannot rise. Excitatory mechanisms controlling posture or extensor muscles predominate, and inhibitory mechanisms as well as those excitatory to the flexor muscles are suppressed. These mechanisms are clearly mediated by the reticulospinal and vestibulospinal pathways, and a further lesion induced at the level of the vestibular nuclei, as Sherrington showed, abolishes this rigidity. In this decerebrate state tonic rather than phasic stretch reflexes are increased and there is increased gamma efferent discharge to extensor muscles, especially involving static fusimotor fibres. In man, a somewhat similar state may accompany severe midbrain lesions, which almost invariably cause loss of consciousness. In such a case all four limbs are rigidly extended, the back is arched, and there may be neck retraction, so that the patient, if lying supine, is virtually supported by the back of the neck and the heels—a posture known as *opisthotonos*. The arching of the back can be increased by any sensory stimulus, and there is striking resistance to any attempt to flex the limbs passively. Tonic neck reflexes may often be elicited; thus, turning the head to one side gives extension of the limbs on that side and flexion on the other.

Hypotonia

Flaccidity, or hypotonia, is a reduction in tone. It may be due to cerebral or spinal shock, a phenomenon which may result from acute and extensive lesions of the brain or spinal cord which have the effect of suppressing transiently all motor reflex activity. It is a common manifestation of cerebellar disease, being then associated with diminished gamma efferent activity. It also occurs whenever a lesion of the afferent or efferent pathway interrupts the spinal reflex arc. In patients with total flaccid paralysis, all resistance to passive stretch is lost and the limbs are limp and flail-like. Lesser degrees of hypotonia in the upper limbs, for instance, can be elicited by asking the patient to hold out his arms horizontally in front of him. The forearms are then tapped briskly. When tone is increased (spasticity) the recoil is sharp, immediate and exaggerated. When one limb is hypotonic the recoil is slower and the arm swings through a wider range. If the patient is asked to contract the biceps brachii against resistance by bending an arm towards his face, and the examiner's restraining hand is suddenly removed, the patient's hand may strike his face if the limb is hypotonic. If the tone is normal he will be able to stop the movement before it does so. Furthermore, if the subject is asked to raise his arms above his head with the palms facing forward, the palm of a hypotonic limb will be seen to be externally rotated and facing more laterally than the other. In the lower limbs it is useful to place one's hands beneath the knee and lift the leg from the bed, and then to allow it to fall back quickly. With experience it will soon be possible to judge whether tone is increased or reduced from the degree of resistance the limb shows to this movement.

ATAXIA AND INCOORDINATION

General considerations

Ataxia is clumsiness of motor activity, resulting from an inability to control accurately the range and precision of movement. It can result from a defect in the sensory pathways responsible for the transmission of proprioceptive information from sensory receptors in the periphery. When this occurs the appreciation of the position of the parts of the body in space is impaired. Controlled movement requires continuous and accurate information of this nature for its performance and therefore may be seriously deranged, resulting in sensory ataxia (to be considered later). In such a case, the cause of the unsteadiness will become apparent on sensory examination. Similarly, sensory stimuli from the labyrinths are of great importance in the maintenance of posture. Disease of the labyrinths, or of the vestibular nerves or their central connections, may result in distorted information concerning the position of the head. The patient's gait may become grossly unsteady and the movements of his limbs clumsy and poorly controlled. Ataxia as a result of labyrinthine dysfunction is much less common than that due to cerebellar dysfunction.

Cerebellar dysfunction

The controlling activity of the cerebellum upon the motor system is concerned particularly with the fine coordination of movement and with the judgement of distance. It is these faculties which are selectively impaired as a result of cerebellar disease. Central cerebellar structures (the paleocerebellum) have predominantly vestibular connections and are concerned particularly with equilibration. Lesions in this location produce an ataxia which involves central structures of the body, particularly apparent when the patient walks. The patient is unsteady and staggers in a drunken manner. He walks on a wide base and has considerable difficulty in stopping suddenly or in turning. Lesser degrees of ataxia can be revealed by asking the patient to walk 'heel to toe'. Even in mildly ataxic individuals this is usually impossible. There may also occasionally be a rhythmical nodding or 'titubating' tremor of the head. The tests of cerebellar function described earlier (p. 69) which are concerned with the demonstration of ataxia in lateral structures such as the limbs, may be singularly uninformative. Because these tests are negative, it is a common pitfall to regard such patients as being hysterical, particularly if the doctor fails to recognize that a cerebellar lesion that is centrally located gives this particular type of so-called truncal or central ataxia.

Lesions of the lateral cerebellar hemispheres (the neocerebellum) produce a number of physical signs which are more readily identifiable. If the lesion is predominantly unilateral, then these signs are apparent in the limbs on the same side as the lesion. There may also be ocular signs. Nystagmus is common, being of greatest amplitude on looking to the side of the lesion. Occasionally the head is tilted to the affected side. Hypotonia is often present in the ipsilateral limbs, and ataxia is evidenced by a striking clumsiness and incoordination of movement. The patient is unable to button his clothes, and his handwriting is scrawling and illegible. Judgement of distance is grossly impaired, a phenomenon known as dysmetria. The hand performing a movement may wildly overshoot the mark (past-pointing). Tremor of the limbs may be apparent at rest but is sometimes greatly accentuated by movement, especially in disease of the cerebellar connections in the brain stem, in which it may be much worse towards the end of an action (intention tremor). These signs are particularly apparent on carrying out the 'finger–nose' and 'heel–knee' tests. Rapid alternating movements of the limbs, such as pronation and supination of the forearms, are poorly and jerkily performed (dysdiadochokinesis). The patient with a unilateral cerebellar lesion also tends to stagger and to deviate towards the affected side when walking. A minimal cerebellar lesion on one side can sometimes be identified most easily by asking the patient to walk a few paces with his eyes closed, in which case he will deviate to the affected side. Alternatively, if the patient is asked to walk in a circle around the examiner, first clockwise and then counterclockwise, the deviation away from the examiner in one direction and towards him in the other will be apparent.

THE REFLEXES

The simplest form of a reflex arc consists of an afferent or sensory neuron and an efferent or motor neuron with whose parent cell the terminal fibres of the afferent neuron synapse. Stimulation of the sensory neuron will then produce a motor response mediated by the motor neuron. Only a few reflexes are as simple as this. Examples are the monosynaptic spinal reflex arc, exemplified by the tendon jerks. Withdrawal of a limb in response to a painful stimulus is a polysynaptic reflex. In many pathways concerned with reflex activity, however, the sensory and motor neurons are separated by connecting interneurons, once called internuncial neurons, most of which lie in the grey matter of the cord. These interneurons receive impulses from ascending and descending fibre pathways which exercise important controlling influences upon reflex activity. Unquestionably there are some very long reflex pathways which run a course involving brain-stem as well as spinal structures, while some traverse the cerebral cortex. There are many reflexes concerned with autonomic and visceromotor activity, and even endocrine secretion. Clinical neurology is largely concerned with the simpler reflexes which, when activated, result in somatic motor activity. Various oculocephalic and labyrinthine reflexes were considered in the preceding chapter on 'The special senses'.

Reflex activity will be lost or impaired if a lesion is present at any point in the reflex arc. A break in the afferent or efferent pathway will mean that a particular form of reflex activity can no longer be elicited. For instance, the corneal reflex (the contraction of the orbicularis oculi which follows stimulation of the cornea) may be lost if the cornea is anaesthetic as a result of a lesion of the trigeminal nerve or if the face is paralysed due to a lesion of the seventh nerve. The reflexes which are most informative in the physical examination of patients with nervous disease are the stretch and cutaneous reflexes.

The jaw jerk is a stretch reflex elicited by means of a sharp downward tap on the chin with the mouth held partly open. A positive response consists in contraction of the masseters with elevation of the lower jaw. If this reflex is exaggerated it usually indicates a bilateral pyramidal tract lesion in or above the upper brain stem.

The stretch reflexes normally utilized on examination of the limbs are so-called tendon reflexes. These consist in a reflex contraction of the muscle concerned, produced in practice by a sharp blow upon the tendon of the muscle near its point of insertion. In the upper limb those commonly elicited are the biceps and radial jerks, which obtain their motor innervation from the fifth and sixth cervical roots, the triceps jerk, which is mainly innervated by the seventh root, and the finger jerk, which receives its supply from the seventh and eighth roots. In the lower limbs the knee jerk is innervated by the second, third and fourth lumbar roots, the ankle jerk by the first and second sacral roots. Any of the tendon reflexes can be diminished or lost if there is a lesion of the sensory pathway carrying afferent impulses from the muscle to the spinal cord, if there is a lesion of the lower motor neurons supplying the muscle concerned at any point along its course, or even if a primary disorder of the muscle itself—a myopathy—has impaired its ability to contract. These reflexes are also lost temporarily during the stage of so-called 'shock' which follows an acute and severe lesion of the brain or spinal cord, even if there is no break in the reflex arc. All of the tendon reflexes may be symmetrically exaggerated by tension and anxiety or by increased neuromuscular excitability arising from toxic (e.g. drugs), metabolic or other causes. The tendon reflexes are most strikingly increased when there is a lesion of the pyramidal tract. A unilateral lesion is particularly easy to identify as the reflexes are exaggerated on one side of the body and not on the other. The finger jerk, for instance, is normally present in some patients and not in others, but it is of real significance only if it is present unilaterally. The phenomenon of clonus as described earlier consists of an intermittent muscular contraction and relaxation evoked by sustained stretching of a muscle. Clonus can occur apparently spontaneously in spastic limbs, but it is best elicited as a physical sign in the lower limbs by sudden pressure applied in a distal direction to the upper margin of the patella (patellar clonus) or by a sharp dorsiflexion of the foot carried out with the leg extended (ankle clonus).

Inversion of upper limb reflexes may be an important physical sign of spinal cord disease. Thus if there is a lesion of the C5–C6 segments of the spinal cord, this will break the reflex arc for reflexes innervated by these segments, namely the biceps and radial jerks, which are therefore lost or diminished. If, however, the same lesion is compressing the spinal cord and giving pyramidal tract dysfunction, reflexes innervated by lower segments of the cord (triceps, finger jerks) are exaggerated and can be obtained by stimuli applied over a wide field. Thus, tapping the biceps tendon may cause contraction of the triceps, while an attempt to elicit the radial jerk may produce finger flexion but no radial jerk. This so-called inversion of either of these reflexes is diagnostic of a cervical cord lesion.

The cutaneous or superficial reflexes commonly used in neurological diagnosis are the abdominal reflexes, the cremasteric reflex, the anal reflex and the plantar reflex. The abdominal reflexes are elicited by stroking the skin of the abdomen (the point of a pin is a suitable instrument), which should produce movement of the umbilicus towards the stimulus. The level of a segmental lesion in the dorsal portion of the spinal cord can sometimes be identified by loss of the lower abdominal reflexes and preservation of the upper abdominal reflexes. The abdominal reflexes are unilaterally diminished in amplitude or lost (or they may simply fatigue rapidly on repetitive stimulation) when there is a lesion of the pyramidal tract on the same side of the body. There are certain conditions (e.g. multiple sclerosis) in which the abdominal reflexes may be lost at a comparatively early stage of the disease, whereas in others (e.g. motor neuron disease), in which there is also evidence of pyramidal tract disease, they often survive to a relatively late stage. Total absence of the abdominal reflexes is usually a finding of definite pathological significance, except in the very obese, in multipara with lax abdominal muscles, and in the elderly. The cremasteric reflex (contraction of the cremaster on stroking the medial side of the thigh) is also impaired or lost as a result of a pyramidal tract lesion. The anal reflex (contraction of the external sphincter on scratching the perianal skin) is particularly likely to be lost when there is a lesion of the cauda equina involving the fourth and fifth sacral roots.

One of the most important reflexes in clinical neurology is the plantar response. On stroking the lateral aspect of the sole of the foot from the heel towards the fifth toe, there is normally plantar-flexion of all five toes (the flexor response). The abnormal response, which consists of a dorsiflexion of the great toe and a simultaneous downward and 'fanning-out' movement of the remaining toes, is known as an extensor response or the *Babinski response*. The Babinski response refers only to the abnormal or extensor type of reflex movement, and it is semantically inaccurate to say that the Babinski is 'negative' or 'positive'. It is far better to avoid the eponymous term and to refer to the plantar response as being 'flexor' or 'extensor'. An extensor plantar reflex is virtually diagnostic of a lesion or dysfunction of the pyramidal tract at any point on its course from the contralateral motor cortex down through the brain stem and the ipsilateral lateral column of the spinal cord. It is essentially part of a primitive flexor withdrawal response 'uncovered' or 'released' by a pyramidal tract lesion. The word dysfunction is deliberately used above since while an extensor plantar response usually implies that there is a definable pathological process involving the pyramidal pathways, there are many circumstances when, as, for example, in severe fatigue or transient biochemical disorders (such as hypoglycaemia), the response becomes extensor only temporarily, with reversion to the normal response after recovery. Often, along with the extensor plantar response, there is contraction of the hamstrings. If the spinal cord lesion is severe and complete, stroking the sole will also evoke flexion at the hip and knee and even evacuation of the bladder and bowels (a 'mass' reflex). In such a case the extensor plantar response is readily elicited by a variety of stimuli applied over a wide area (e.g. pressure upon the shin bone, pricking the leg with a pin, etc.)

In decerebrate patients, as in neonates, the tonic neck reflexes may be greatly exaggerated so that on forcibly turning the head to one side the limbs on that side extend while the contralateral limbs flex. Persistence of this reflex response after the first 3 months of life, and of the Moro reflex (flexion of all four limbs on sharply tapping the bed upon which the baby lies) indicates a serious disorder of cerebral development. The activity of the frontal lobes in man is sufficient after the first year or two of life to inhibit the reflex grasping and groping which result from stroking the palm of the hand. This grasp reflex may return unilaterally as the result of a lesion of the contralateral frontal lobe.

THE CLINICAL FEATURES OF UPPER AND LOWER MOTOR NEURON LESIONS

An example of the effects of an upper motor neuron lesion is the hemiplegia produced by an extensive lesion of the contralateral motor area of the cerebral cortex, or of the internal capsule. If the lesion is an acute one, the paralysed limbs are at first limp and flaccid, immobile, and without tone, owing to the phenomenon of so-called 'shock'. A sudden and extensive lesion may produce an abrupt depression of reflexes subserved by relatively remote areas of the nervous system, even though the reflex arc or arcs concerned remain intact. At this stage, all reflexes on the affected side are absent. Gradually over the course of a few days or weeks the flaccidity lessens and the affected limbs become spastic, though rarely the hemiplegia may remain permanently flaccid, particularly if there is also an extensive parietal lobe lesion. Whereas the affected arm and leg are completely paralysed, those parts of the body which are bilaterally 'represented' in the cerebral cortex can still be moved voluntarily, even on the paralysed side. Thus, facial weakness affects mainly the lower part of the face and the upper part slightly or not at all, while no defect in palatal movement will be apparent. Furthermore, since emotional movement of the face, as in smiling, appears to be controlled not by the cerebral cortex but by more deeply situated structures, a patient who is completely unable to move the lower half of one side of the face at will may yet smile symmetrically.

As flaccidity passes off in the paralysed limbs and spasticity makes its appearance, the tendon reflexes return, become greatly exaggerated, and may be accompanied by clonus. The abdominal and cremasteric reflexes on the affected side remain absent and the plantar response is clearly extensor. Spasticity is often greatest in the flexor muscles of the upper limbs and in the extensor muscles of the lower, so that in a patient with a long-standing hemiplegia the arm is flexed at the elbow and at the wrist and fingers, while the leg remains fully extended. In hemiplegic spasticity, dynamic fusimotor drive (gamma discharge) predominates, though alpha neuron hyperexcitability may develop later in long-standing cases.

Sometimes the lesion of the pyramidal tract is not sufficiently severe to cause total paralysis, but produces only a relatively minor degree of weakness. In such a case the finer and more skilful movements, those most recently acquired by man in the process of evolution, are the ones most severely impaired. Independent finger and toe movements are very poor, though the strength of movement at proximal joints such as the elbow and knee remains good. A useful way to detect early pyramidal tract dysfunction is to observe the patient with his hands and arms outstretched in front of him and his eyes closed. A downward 'drift' of the arms may be an early sign of upper motor neuron weakness. While difficulty in opposing the thumb and individual fingers may be an early sign, objective testing of muscle power often shows that 'pyramidal' weakness is first apparent on abduction of the shoulder and in the hand grip in the upper limbs, and in hip flexion and foot dorsiflexion in the lower limbs. During the process of recovery from a pyramidal tract lesion, movement usually returns first at the proximal joints. It is the cruder movements which are first regained, while the more delicate activity of the fingers and toes is the last to return. A patient who is recovering from a hemiplegia may be able to use his hand to grip or to lift objects, but will often be quite unable to write or to fasten buttons or shoelaces. He walks with his arm flexed across the front of his chest and with stiffness, dragging and circumduction of the affected leg.

Similar physical signs are apparent in patients with bilateral pyramidal tract lesions giving rise to spastic paraplegia. If the lesion responsible is in the brain stem or spinal cord, however, concomitant involvement of reticulospinal and other descending pathways modifies the nature of the spasticity. Increased alpha-neuron excitability as well as dynamic fusimotor drive often appear earlier, and the primitive flexor withdrawal reflex may be released from inhibition. If the lesion responsible is an acute transverse lesion of the cord, there is a total flaccid paralysis of the limbs below the affected segment during the initial stage of spinal shock. Subsequently spasticity, increased tendon reflexes, and extensor plantar responses appear. As the lower motor neuron and the spinal reflex arc are intact, severe wasting of muscle does not occur, although when paralysis has been present for some time, some degree of disuse atrophy appears, affecting all muscles of the limb or limbs. When the spinal cord lesion is incomplete and affects principally the pyramidal tracts, the tone of the spastic lower limbs is particularly increased in the extensor muscles (paraplegia-in-extension). When both pyramidal tracts are severely diseased and there are also lesions of other descending spinal pathways as mentioned above, the legs become progressively more flexed at the knees and hips, and stimulation provokes painful flexor spasms (paraplegia-in-flexion).

The rate of development of an upper neuron lesion affects its manifestations. An acute lesion will give a total flaccid paralysis initially, with spasticity slowly evolving over the subsequent days or weeks. A chronic or slowly progressive lesion such as a tumour may give little more initially than a slight impairment of fine finger movement in one hand, or simply a minimal increase in tendon reflexes in the affected arm. Subsequently, however, a spastic monoparesis or hemiparesis slowly develops.

A lesion of lower motor neurons interrupts the final common path of all forms of motor activity. The muscle or muscle groups involved become paralysed and flaccid, and remain so. Any reflex movement for which the paralysed muscles are necessary will be lost. Another invariable feature is that all muscles deprived of their motor nerve supply undergo rapid atrophy. They may shrink to half the normal size within about 6 weeks and will eventually disappear almost completely, being virtually replaced by fibrous connective tissue. Before this stage of total atrophy is reached, and particularly if the lesion responsible lies in the anterior horn cells of the spinal cord (as in motor neuron disease, for example), fasciculation is commonly seen. Individual muscle fasciculi contract spontaneously, and an irregular but recurrent flickering of these fibre bundles can be seen through the intact skin to be occurring in a muscle which is apparently completely at rest. Although most often seen in patients with motor neuron disease, fasciculation is not diagnostic of this condition as it may occur following old poliomyelitis, and is also observed occasionally in polyneuropathy and as a result of other lesions of the peripheral nerves. It can also be a benign phenomenon not due to an identifiable lesion.

Fibrillation, or spontaneous contraction of individual muscle fibres, also occurs following a lesion of the lower motor neuron. It cannot be seen through the skin, though it can be recorded electromyographically. The clinical features of an acute lower motor neuron lesion are total flaccid paralysis with absence of all reflexes, and rapid atrophy of the affected muscle or group of muscles. In a slowly progressive lesion, by contrast, weakness and atrophy increase gradually and only eventually are the reflexes lost. In such a case it can be difficult to decide whether the lesion involves a single peripheral nerve, several peripheral nerves, a group of spinal anterior roots, or the anterior horn cells of the cord. Knowledge of the anatomy and innervation of muscles is all-important in making this distinction. If more muscles are affected than could be supplied by a single peripheral nerve, lesions of one or a group of spinal roots could be responsible, in which case there may also be some associated evidence of spinal cord disease or dysfunction. If the muscular weakness and wasting is more widespread still, and particularly if it occurs symmetrically in the peripheral muscles of limbs, the two most likely diagnoses are polyneuropathy (polyneuritis) and motor neuron disease (progressive muscular atrophy). However, motor neuron disease more often begins in one limb, and the weakness and wasting is commonly asymmetrical in distribution and severity for many months or years. Symmetrical involvement of all four limbs may be more suggestive of an inherited spinal muscular atrophy (see below). Sensory loss, particularly if present symmetrically in the periphery of the limbs, will support a diagnosis of polyneuropathy, while if there is profuse fasciculation, no sensory loss, and some evidence of pyramidal tract disease, motor neuron disease can be diagnosed with reasonable confidence.

Muscular weakness and wasting which can mimic that due to a lower motor neuron lesion may result from a primary disease of the muscles themselves, a myopathy. Here too there is flaccid weakness with atrophy and absence of tendon reflexes. Even in disorders of conduction at the motor end-plate, such as myasthenia gravis, the muscles may be weak and hypotonic, though atrophy is uncommon. In general, myopathic as distinct from neuropathic disorders tend to affect the proximal rather than the distal muscles of the limbs. Fasciculation does not occur. Some comments upon the pathophysiology of neuromuscular disease are given below.

INVOLUNTARY MOVEMENTS

Movements of parts of the body which do not occur in response to the will and are thus involuntary can be of the greatest importance in neurological diagnosis.

Tic or *habit spasm* is a term which covers a variety of twitching or jerking movements which occur irregularly and which tend particularly to involve the muscles around the eyes, the remainder of the face, and the shoulders. The subject is well aware of the movement, and in fact it is voluntarily performed, as from it the patient obtains relief from tension which would otherwise become almost intolerable. This affliction is clearly related to anxiety. Though initially under the control of the will, the movements often become so habitual as to be almost involuntary.

The *epileptic fit* or *convulsion*, whether focal or general, is clearly involuntary, and was discussed in detail on p. 193. The closely related phenomenon of *myoclonus* (see p. 194) is a sudden shock-like muscular contraction which can involve a small group of muscles, several muscle groups, or even the greater part of the voluntary musculature, either simultaneously or successively. Myoclonic jerks may occur while falling asleep and are not then pathological, though when they occur repeatedly throughout the night the condition is in all probability an epileptic manifestation and many such persons also have occasional major seizures. Repetitive and sometimes rhythmical twitching of one half of the face should not be confused with either habit spasm or myoclonus, for this condition—*hemifacial* or *clonic facial spasm*—is due to an irritative lesion of the seventh nerve.

Tremor is a rapid, rhythmically repetitive movement which tends to be consistent in pattern, amplitude and frequency, and usually consists of intermittent contraction of a muscle group and then of its antagonists. A physiological tremor with a frequency of 8–9 Hz may be seen in normal individuals with the hands outstretched, but usually disappears at rest and may not be perceptible at all in many individuals. Tremor may be static (present at rest), action (present throughout the entire range of movement) or intention (accentuated towards the end of movement) in type. A static tremor of the head and hands, rapid in frequency and small in range, and not generally abolished by movement, constitutes the so-called senile tremor which is seen in a proportion of elderly patients. A more coarse rhythmical nodding of the head is seen in some patients with cerebellar disease. The most typical form of static tremor, however, is the rhythmical 'pill-rolling' movement of the fingers and hands, often affecting also the arms and legs and sometimes the lips and tongue, which is seen in patients with parkinsonism. Though accentuated by embarrassment and attention, this tremor is generally abolished by movement, though occasionally in this disease an action tremor is present as well. The principal lesion responsible for this tremor appears to be in the substantia nigra of the midbrain. Rarely, a similar tremor (often called, perhaps erroneously, 'striatal' tremor) is seen in other degenerative diseases of the nervous system (e.g. olivopontocerebellar degeneration).

Many different forms of disease can give rise to action tremors, which are observed particularly well in the actions of writing, in taking hold of an object, or in holding the arms outstretched. This is essentially an accentuation of physiological tremor. Fatigue and anxiety are common causes. The fine tremor of the outstretched hands seen in patients with thyrotoxicosis is usually easy to recognize. Much coarser movements occur in individuals with a variety of toxic and metabolic disorders, including delirium tremens (alcoholism), various forms of drug intoxication, mercury poisoning and chronic liver disease. In the latter condition there may be a remarkable 'flapping' movement of the outstretched hands, often like the beating of wings (*asterixis*). In Wilson's disease (hepatolenticular degeneration), this type of movement of the hands will be seen if the liver disease is sufficiently advanced, but facial grimacing, rigidity and tremor of the limbs are also present as a result of the pathological changes that occur in the lenticular nuclei. The condition of so-called benign familial or essential tremor is also accentuated by movement. It is remarkable that this form of tremor, though sometimes gross, does not often interfere much with fine movements such as threading a needle, which would appear, at first sight, to be impossible.

Intention tremor is virtually diagnostic of disease of the cerebellum or more often of its brain-stem connections. When unilateral it may indicate a lesion of the ipsilateral cerebellar hemisphere or of the dentato-vestibular pathway and/or other central pontine projections from the cerebellar hemisphere on the same side. If the tremor is severe, there may be some degree of static and action tremor as well, but this invariably becomes very much worse towards the end of movement. Movements cannot be accurately controlled, and such activities as writing and feeding are grossly disorganized. The patient may spill a cup whenever he brings it close to his mouth.

Many types of involuntary movement can result from lesions of the extrapyramidal system, in addition to the parkinsonism tremor already described. The movements of *chorea*, for instance, though involuntary, may appear at first to be semi-purposive and to show a high degree of organization. Facial grimacing, raising of the eyebrows and rolling of the eyes, curling of the lips, and protrusion and withdrawal of the tongue are common. In the limbs the movements are very largely peripheral, with intermittent wriggling or squirming of the fingers and toes. Often, too, there is striking hypotonia of the limbs, and the reflexes may be pendular in type, in that a single blow on the quadriceps tendon causes the dependent leg to swing forwards and backwards several times like a pendulum. The limb movements cease during sleep. The lesions causing the movements involve principally the caudate and lenticular nuclei. The condition occurs in two main forms, namely rheumatic or Sydenham's chorea of children or young adults, and Huntington's chorea, an inherited degenerative cerebral disease of late adult life in which progressive dementia also occurs. Much less often chorea is symptomatic. Thus, it can occur unilaterally as a consequence of a cerebral vascular lesion, occasionally complicates systemic lupus erythematosus of the nervous system, may follow oral contraceptive medication, and is a rare consequence of liver disease.

Athetosis tends to involve the more proximal limb muscles to give movements which are writhing in character, slower in their execution, and of greater amplitude than those of chorea. Often choreiform and athetotic movements are combined in the same patient, in which case the condition is referred to as choreoathetosis. Athetosis can be bilateral and of congenital origin, resulting from degenerative changes in the corpus striatum. Lesions of the corpus striatum can also result in another type of involuntary movement in which the trunk muscles are predominantly involved, termed *dystonia musculorum deformans* or *torsion spasm*. In this condition there is a striking increase in tone with frequent irregular spasmodic contraction of the muscles of the neck, back and abdomen, and also of the limbs, giving rise to bizarre alterations in posture. These postural changes are often constant over long periods, with superimposed painful spasms, and the affected muscles often show a striking degree of hypertrophy. *Spasmodic torticollis* is a condition of frequent spasm of the sternomastoid and of other neck muscles, which results in a spasmodic turning of the head and neck to one side. Some consider it to be a fractional variety of dystonia.

Long-continued use of drugs of the phenothiazine group can cause irreversible *facial dyskinesias* (involuntary grimacing and protrusion of the tongue), while athetosis, foot-tapping and paddling movements are among the many side-effects of treatment of parkinsonism with levodopa.

Hemiballismus is a wild, purposeless, 'flinging' movement of one arm and leg which may occur in elderly patients as a result of a lesion, generally an infarct, that involves particularly the subthalamic nucleus of Luys on the opposite side. The movements can be so violent and distressing that if untreated they result in death from exhaustion. The condition resembles in many respects a very violent form of unilateral chorea.

Among the many other uncommon involuntary movements sometimes seen in clinical practice is *blepharospasm–oromandibular dystonia* (Meige's or Brueghel's syndrome) due to a degenerative process, rarely familial, of unknown cause. It is characterized by severe and almost continuous blepharospasm and by repetitive spasms of facial, mandibular and lingual musculature. *Palatal myoclonus*, in which rhythmical movements of the soft palate occur 60–180 times a minute, often develops insidiously, again for no evident cause, and seems to be due to a dysfunction of the olivocerebellar modulatory projection on to the rostral brain stem. Even less common is the *Gilles de la Tourette's syndrome*, characterized by persistent multiple tics and coprolalia (recurrent compulsive verbal utterances, often of an obscene nature).

THE PATHOPHYSIOLOGY OF NEUROMUSCULAR DISEASE

General considerations

Disease processes involving the neuromuscular apparatus may affect the motor nuclei of the cranial nerves or anterior horn cells of the spinal cord, the ventral roots, the spinal nerves, the plexuses, the peripheral nerves, the neuromuscular junctions, or the muscles themselves. Those disorders which involve the lower motor neurons at some point within their course are conventionally classified as neuropathic, while those involving the neuromuscular junctions or muscles are generally called myopathic. The neuromuscular diseases embrace both categories. Focal lesions and/or diffuse pathological processes of the spinal cord may involve the anterior horns, giving rise to muscular weakness and wasting, but there are usually other accompanying features indicating associated dysfunction of ascending and descending tracts. However, there is a group of degenerative disorders known as the spinal muscular atrophies in which there is selective involvement of the motor cranial nerve nuclei and of the anterior horn cells, often giving fasciculation, progressive weakness, and atrophy of the muscles. In adult sporadic motor neuron disease there is associated degeneration of the pyramidal tracts without evidence of sensory involvement, and three clinical syndromes (progressive bulbar palsy, progressive muscular atrophy and amyotrophic lateral sclerosis) have been described, depending upon whether the motor cranial nerve nuclei, the anterior horn cells of the cord, or the pyramidal tracts are predominantly affected in the early stages. In the autosomal recessive spinal muscular atrophies of early infancy and childhood, by contrast, the pyramidal tracts are usually spared.

Differentiation between lesions involving roots of spinal nerves, plexuses and peripheral nerves depends upon a careful analysis of the distribution of the weakness, wasting, reflex change and sensory loss and upon a thorough knowledge of the anatomical organization described in detail above. There also is a group of disorders known as the polyneuropathies or neuropathies which, through a variety of metabolic, inflammatory and other processes, cause diffuse dysfunction of peripheral nerves. There is generally symmetrical muscular weakness and sensory loss involving especially the distal muscles of the limbs and abolition of the tendon reflexes. On occasion motor nerve fibres are predominantly involved (motor neuropathy), less often the sensory nerve fibres (sensory neuropathy), and occasionally the proximal rather than the distal muscles are affected first. Sometimes individual peripheral nerves are picked out serially by the process (mononeuropathy), but generally a diffuse and symmetrical distal sensorimotor neuropathy is the commonest variety. In these conditions both the myelin sheaths and the axons of the nerves are usually involved by the process, but there are some conditions in which the process primarily attacks the myelin sheaths, at first in the region of the internodes (demyelinating neuropathies), while still others mainly involve axonal degeneration (axonal neuropathies). Measurement of nerve conduction velocity is very helpful in distinguishing these subvarieties, and the information so derived may be of considerable diagnostic value.

In myasthenia gravis, impaired conduction at the neuromuscular junction is the principal abnormality. A specific antibody coats the acetylcholine receptors upon the postjunctional muscle fibre membrane and blocks its interaction with acetylcholine. Fatigability is the predominant symptom. Weakness increases with repetitive muscular contraction, and the muscles involved become much weaker as the day goes on. Drugs which inhibit cholinesterase (e.g. pyridostigmine) partially reverse the process, while corticosteroids or removal of the thymus gland may suppress or modify the disordered autoimmune processes now known to be responsible for the condition. By contrast, in the myasthenic–myopathic (Eaton–Lambert) syndrome which may complicate bronchial carcinoma and which rarely occurs in the absence of malignant disease, there is a paradoxical increase in strength with repeated contraction. In this condition, as in botulism, there is diminished release of acetylcholine from motor nerve terminals, a defect which may be partially corrected by the administration of guanidine hydrochloride.

Myotonia results from an ill-defined and poorly understood abnormality of the muscle fibre membrane, associated with changes in its chloride conductance. There is an electrical after-discharge in the affected muscles after voluntary excitation of their motor nerves has ceased, giving an appearance of impaired relaxation. For example, on attempting to relax after gripping an object the fingers uncurl abnormally slowly. On percussing a muscle a dimple forms and slowly disappears. Myotonia may occur diffusely throughout the skeletal musculature from birth in dominantly inherited myotonia congenita (Thomsen's disease), and is similar to the recessively inherited form, but often of slightly later onset. It is made worse by cold and improved by exercise. In the commoner myotonic dystrophy (dystrophia myotonica), myotonia is accompanied by facial myopathy, weakness of sternomastoids, cataracts, a distal myopathy in the limb muscles, and various systemic and endocrine manifestations. This is a progressive disease causing increasing disability, usually in middle life. While myotonia may be relieved by drugs such as quinine, procaine amide and phenytoin, the accompanying dystrophic (myopathic) process in dystrophia myotonica is uninfluenced by treatment.

The term *myopathy* is most often used to identify any disease or syndrome in which the patient's symptoms and/or physical signs can be attributed to pathological, biochemical or electrophysiological changes involving the muscle fibres or the interstitial tissues of the muscle, and in which there is no evidence that the symptoms are secondary to disordered function of the central or peripheral nervous system. This group of diseases includes many which are genetically determined, progressive and of unknown aetiology (such as the muscular dystrophies), others which are primarily of biochemical origin (a large group of metabolic and endocrine myopathies), and yet others in which the process is primarily inflammatory and often due to disordered immunity (e.g. polymyositis).

Some important principles in clinical nosology

Pain, muscular weakness and fatigability are the most important symptoms of muscle disease. Muscle cramps commonly occur in the elderly, particularly in bed at night, and may be relieved by a nocturnal dose of quinine or phenytoin. In younger individuals cramp may follow unaccustomed exertion but can on occasion be a manifestation of metabolic muscle disease. Spontaneous muscle pain at rest usually occurs in inflammatory disorders of muscle. Pain experienced on exertion generally implies either muscle ischaemia or a metabolic disorder such as hypothyroidism or phosphorylase deficiency, although some cases of severe and long-standing exercise-induced muscle pain remain unexplained. Muscle weakness is the predominant symptom of most varieties of myopathy. It is important to judge its distribution and tempo of development. Thus, proximal muscle weakness in the upper limbs gives difficulty in lifting the arms above the head, while weakness in the lower limbs gives difficulty in climbing stairs and in rising from a low chair. In most of the genetically determined disorders of muscle, weakness develops gradually over a period of many months or years. A more rapid onset of muscular weakness suggests that the patient is more probably suffering from an inflammatory or metabolic myopathy. Periodic attacks of weakness with complete recovery in between the episodes strongly suggest that the patient may be suffering from one of the group of periodic paralyses. When weakness is accompanied by sensory symptoms such as numbness or other paraesthesiae, this strongly suggests a diagnosis of polyneuropathy. Fatigability is characteristic of myasthenia gravis and myasthenic syndromes.

The importance of a general physical examination must be stressed, as there may be changes in the eyes, skin, lymph nodes or viscera indicating that the muscular weakness of which the patient complains is but one manifestation of a systemic multisystem disease. On examining the muscular system itself, the presence of atrophy, hypertrophy, contractures or fasciculation of muscle may be of diagnostic value. Myotonia and myoedema were described previously. Physiological contracture differs from the pathological contracture resulting from permanent shortening of muscles and tendons due to fibrosis in chronic muscle disease in that it is a reversible shortening of muscle lasting for some minutes after exercise. It may be seen particularly in muscle phosphorylase deficiency (McArdle's disease) and in other related enzymatic defects which impair glycogen breakdown, such as phosphofructokinase deficiency. Direct myotatic irritability is the reflex contraction which occurs in the belly of a muscle when it is percussed or stimulated directly by mechanical means. As with the tendon reflexes, this direct reflex response may be accentuated by anxiety but is particularly striking in patients suffering from tetany and hypocalcaemia.

The response of muscle to stretch (muscle tone) is also of diagnostic importance. Increased tone (spasticity or rigidity) implies disease in the central nervous system, whereas diminished tone (limpness or hypotonia) can be due to cerebellar dysfunction and other central lesions, but it can also be a consequence of many primary disorders of peripheral nerve and/or muscle.

Careful testing of the power of individual muscles, combined with an attempt at quantitative assessment, is one of the most important facets of the clinical examination. Different diseases show different patterns of muscular involvement and selective atrophy, and weakness of certain muscles with sparing of others may be one of the most important clues to the precise nature of the patient's illness. The tendon reflexes in muscle disease are usually diminished or lost when the muscles subserving the particular reflex being examined are involved in the disease process. In muscular dystrophy the tendon reflexes tend to disappear early but in myasthenia gravis and in polymyositis they often remain unexpectedly brisk even in the presence of substantial weakness.

Some important methods of differential diagnosis

The differential diagnosis of neuromuscular disease depends first upon the clinical history and examination as discussed above, secondly upon electromyographic and other neurophysiological evidence, thirdly upon the biochemical findings, and fourthly upon pathological changes in muscle as revealed by biopsy.

ELECTROMYOGRAPHY (EMG)

Electromyography is a technique of recording the electrical activity produced by muscle at rest and during contraction. Surface electrodes are of value only for physiological studies in determining which muscles or muscle groups contribute to a particular movement or for recording the frequency of involuntary movements (e.g. tremor). For diagnostic work the electrical activity is recorded from bipolar needle electrodes inserted into the muscle under test. The signal is amplified and then presented for interpretation both on a cathode-ray screen (Fig. 8.14) and in a loudspeaker. Sometimes the visual trace is more valuable, sometimes the auditory pattern, but the combination is more valuable than either alone. Normal voluntary muscle is electrically silent at rest, but on contraction motor-unit action potentials are seen and appear in increasing number and frequency as contraction increases to give a continuous trace across the cathode-ray screen and a low-pitched rumble in the loudspeaker. These potentials are smooth monophasic, diphasic or triphasic waves, each about 5–8 ms in duration and about 0.5–2 mV in amplitude. These potentials are most probably due to the contraction of only a few component fibres of the motor unit which happen to lie close to the recording electrode (a 'sub-unit').

When a muscle is denervated, spontaneous fibrillation or contraction of individual muscle fibres begins within 14–21 days and can be recorded from the relaxed and resting muscle. This takes the form of a series of repetitive small spikes on the cathode-ray screen with a ticking sound in the loudspeaker. If the muscle has lost only a part of its nerve supply, some motor unit potentials will still appear on attempted contraction, but the pattern of voluntary effort will be much reduced. During reinnervation following nerve regeneration, complex polyphasic potentials of long duration appear, called recovery potentials. The long duration of these units is due to the fact that regenerating nerve sprouts, which reinnervate previously denervated muscle fibres, conduct at different rates. In patients with disease of the motor neuron at any point from the anterior horn cell to the motor end-plate, the EMG will show spontaneous fibrillation and a reduced pattern of motor units on voluntary effort. When the lesion is in the anterior horn cells, some of the surviving motor unit action potentials may be unusually large (up to 5 mV in amplitude and 10 ms in duration, referred to as 'giant' units). This is because collateral axonal sprouts from surviving neurons may 'adopt' and reinnervate some denervated muscle fibres. In disorders of the anterior horn cell there are sometimes spontaneous fasciculation potentials which look like normal motor unit potentials but which are recorded from resting muscle.

In primary diseases of muscle, such as muscular dystrophy and other myopathies, the pattern of the EMG is different. There may be little or no spontaneous activity, but on volition the motor unit

NORMAL ELECTROMYOGRAM

Submaximal contraction individual motor units visible

1 mV
50 msec

Maximal contraction
Full recruitment pattern

1 mV
50 msec

A

ELECTROMYOGRAM IN MYOPATHY

Submaximal contraction
Full recruitment pattern
Low amplitude polyphasic units

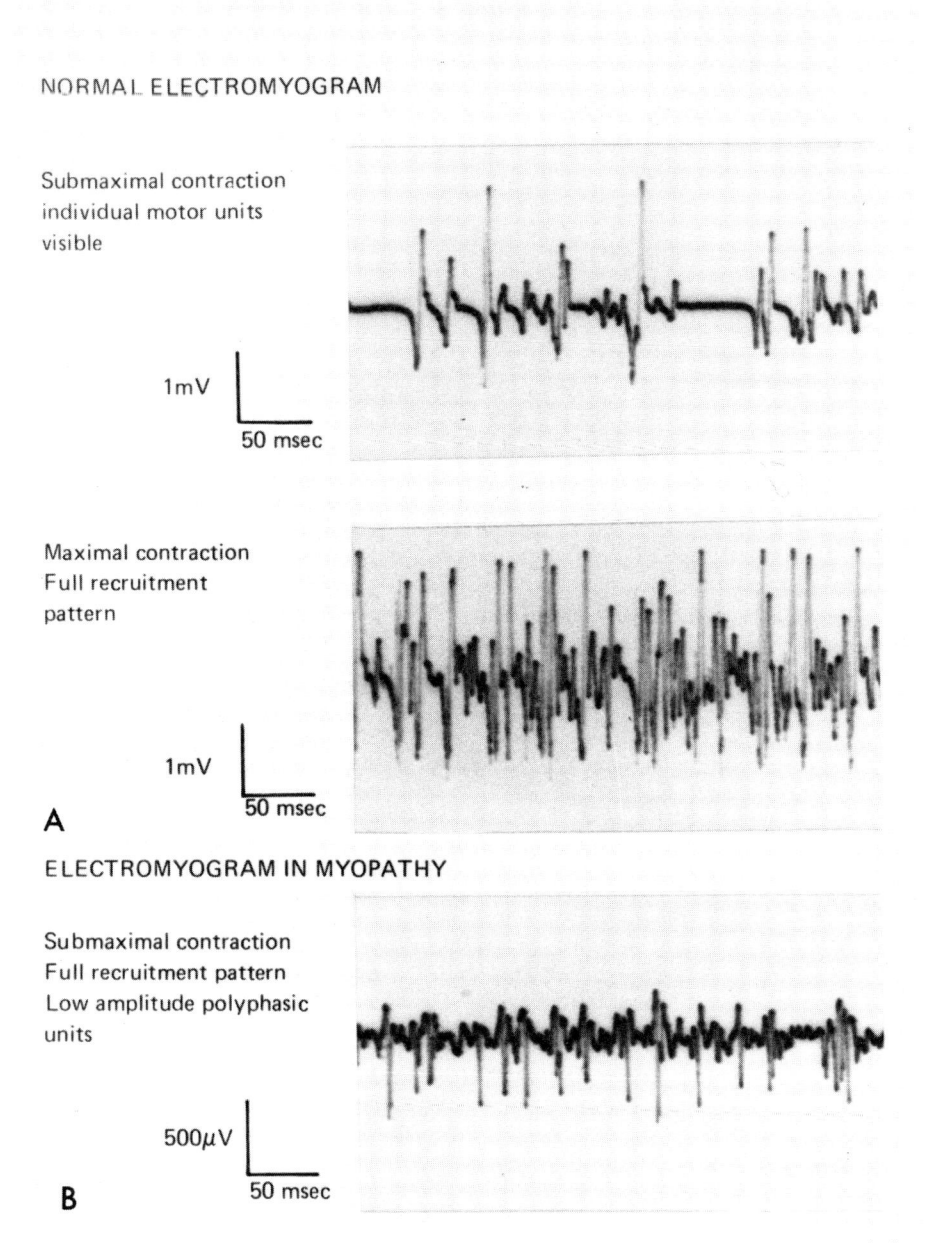

500 μV
50 msec

B

Figure 8.14 A, The normal electromyogram. Upper: Submaximal contraction. Note that the individual motor units here vary between 1.5 and 3 mV in amplitude and are of approximately 5–7 ms duration. Lower: During maximal contraction there is a full 'interference pattern'; the spikes of greater amplitude represent action potentials derived from motor units lying relatively close to the recording electrode, while those of lower amplitude are derived from motor units lying some distance away.

B, The electromyogram in myopathy. The constituent motor units are greatly reduced in amplitude and duration and many are polyphasic.

Illustration continued on the following page

potentials are seen to be broken up, polyphasic and of short duration. The pattern is complex and spiky, and the noise in the loudspeaker is a crackling sound, like hail on a tin roof. The phenomenon of myotonia also gives a characteristic EMG. Chains of oscillations of high frequency are seen which give a typical 'snarling' or 'dive-bomber' sound.

The EMG is of particular use in the investigation of peripheral nerve and root lesions and in the study of cases of muscular wasting and weakness. It is

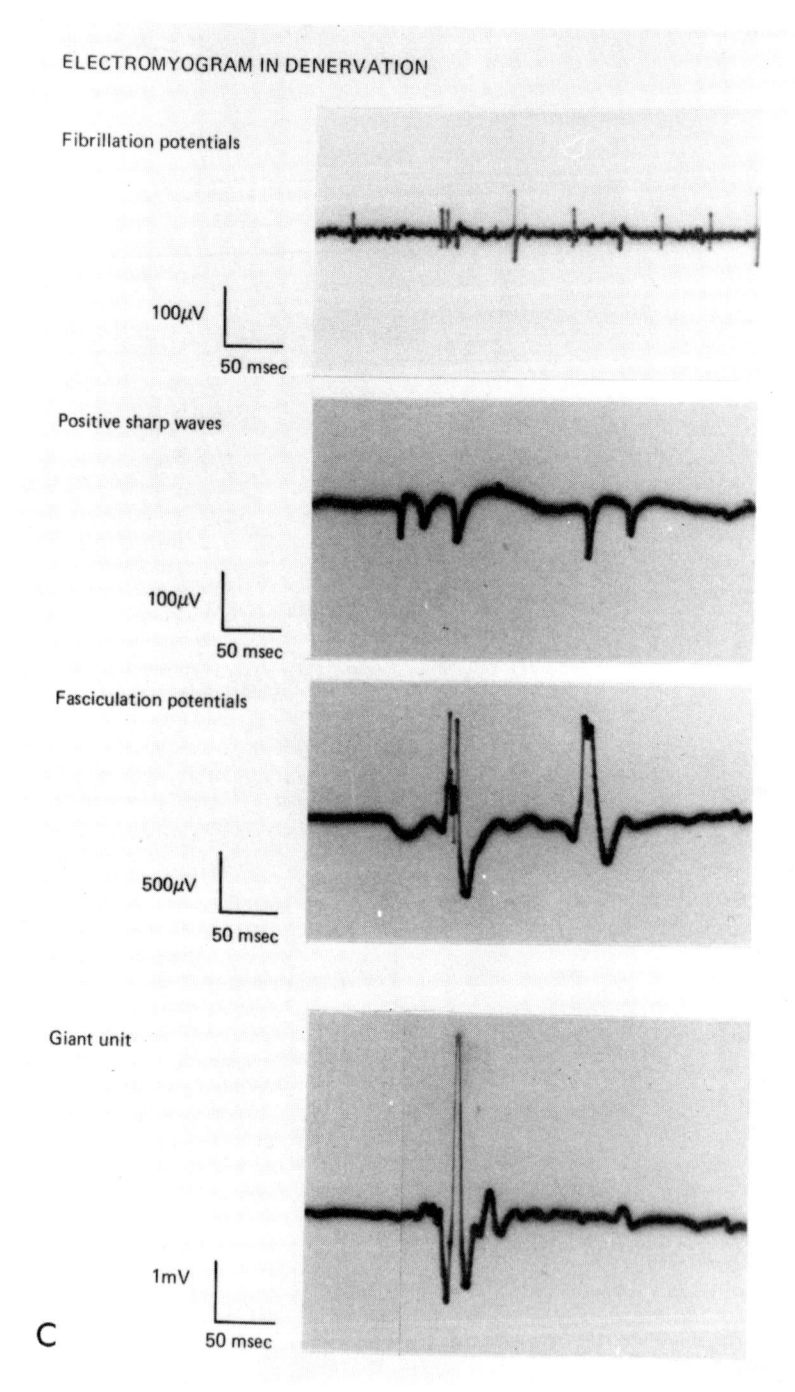

Figure 8.14 (*continued*) C, The electromyogram in denervation. From top to bottom: (1) Spontaneous fibrillation. This is recorded from relaxed resting muscle; the individual potentials measure no more than about 100 μV in amplitude and are of about 1 msec duration. (2) Positive sharp waves (saw tooth potentials); also recorded from relaxed resting muscle. This phenomenon is occasionally seen in denervated muscle. (3) Fasciculation potentials firing spontaneously; also recorded from relaxed resting muscle in a patient with motor neuron disease; these potentials are morphologically indistinguishable from motor unit action potentials. (4) A giant motor unit action potential of approximately 5 mV in amplitude occurring during volitional activity in a patient with motor neuron disease. [Reproduced from Walton (1985) *Brain's Diseases of the Nervous System*, 9th edn, by kind permission of the publisher, the originals having been kindly provided by Dr R. Weiser.]

especially helpful in distinguishing disease of the muscle from that of the motor nerve.

NERVE CONDUCTION VELOCITY

The rate of conduction of an impulse along a nerve can be calculated by stimulating a motor nerve at two separate points along its course and by recording the time intervals before the action potentials are evoked in an appropriate muscle (Fig. 8.15). For accurate recording the temperature of the limb must be carefully controlled. Nerve conduction has been found to be low in those forms of polyneuropathy which cause demyelination. The technique can also be utilized to localize focal lesions in the nerves, such as compression of the median nerve in the carpal tunnel, of the ulnar nerve at the elbow, or of the common peroneal (lateral popliteal) nerve at the neck of the fibula. For example, if one applies a supramaximal stimulus to the median nerve in the cubital fossa and records the compound muscle action potential so produced in the opponens pollicis, a similar action potential can be evoked by stimulating the nerve at the wrist. By measuring the stimulus–contraction latency in each case and the distance between the stimulating electrodes, the conduction velocity in the forearm segment of the nerve can be calculated. If the nerve is compressed in the carpal tunnel, then 'terminal latency' (normally 4.5 ms or less) is increased. Other more sophisticated techniques, including methods of measuring conduction over short segments of nerve in presumed entrapment neuropathies, are now available (Kimura, 1983).

The normal motor conduction velocity in the adult is 50–68 m/s in the median and ulnar nerves and 45–55 m/s in the lateral popliteal. Conduction in sensory nerves is significantly faster but the velocity in all nerves is somewhat lower in infants and children. In demyelinating peripheral neuropathies conduction is markedly slowed, while in those accompanied by axonal degeneration the surviving axons conduct at a normal rate but the amplitude of the evoked muscle action potential is reduced. Measurement of the conduction velocity in sensory fibres, stimulated by ring electrodes on a digit and picking up the sensory volley by an electrode over the nerve trunk, is also helpful in diagnosis.

OTHER METHODS

Many more sophisticated techniques of clinical neurophysiological examination have been introduced in recent years, including methods of recording tendon and other reflexes electrically, 'single fibre' electromyography, assessment of the response of the muscle to applied vibration, and recording of the so-called 'H' and 'F' reflexes, which can give useful information relating to muscle spindle activity and reflex dysfunction resulting from central and peripheral lesions (Kimura 1983). Some of these methods are also used in order to assess conduction velocity in proximal as distinct from distal segments of peripheral nerves. The H reflex is a contraction (which can be recorded electrically) in the calf muscles which can be elicited by stimulating the medial popliteal nerve. It follows the immediate contraction of these muscles resulting from such stimulation of their motor nerve, and the wave form associated with that contraction (the M response). The H response is a monosynaptic reflex evoked by stimulation of Group I afferent fibres in the nerve. The latency of this reflex can be used to estimate conduction in proximal segments of both the sensory and motor nerves involved in the reflex. The F wave, by contrast, which also follows the M response, and which is often recorded from the small hand muscles, is a late muscle potential resulting from an impulse spreading antidromically up the motor axons and inducing 'backfiring' in anterior horn cells.

It is also possible, by measuring spinal somatosensory-evoked potentials, to determine whether lesions of the brachial plexus lie proximal or distal to the dorsal root ganglia, while even in recording cerebral somatosensory-evoked potentials it has been shown that selective abnormalities of early peaks with relative preservation of late peaks can be seen in some patients with peripheral nerve lesions. These techniques are highly specialized and do not as yet form part of the routine investigation of neuromuscular dysfunction, except in the most specialized centres.

STUDIES OF SENSORY NERVE FUNCTION

If a nerve is rendered ischaemic, by inflating a sphygmomanometer cuff around a limb to above the systolic blood pressure, ischaemic paraesthesiae develop in the skin areas supplied by the nerve concerned within 5–10 minutes. On release of the cuff, postischaemic paraesthesiae are experienced. If the blood supply of the nerve concerned is already embarrassed by pressure, ischaemic paraesthesiae appear earlier, perhaps within 1 or 2 minutes, and postischaemic paraesthesiae are more severe. This technique is useful in diagnosing pressure lesions of peripheral nerves, of which median nerve compression in the carpal tunnel is a good example.

MOTOR END-PLATE DYSFUNCTION

Motor end-plate dysfunction may be studied by applying repetitive supramaximal shocks to the ulnar

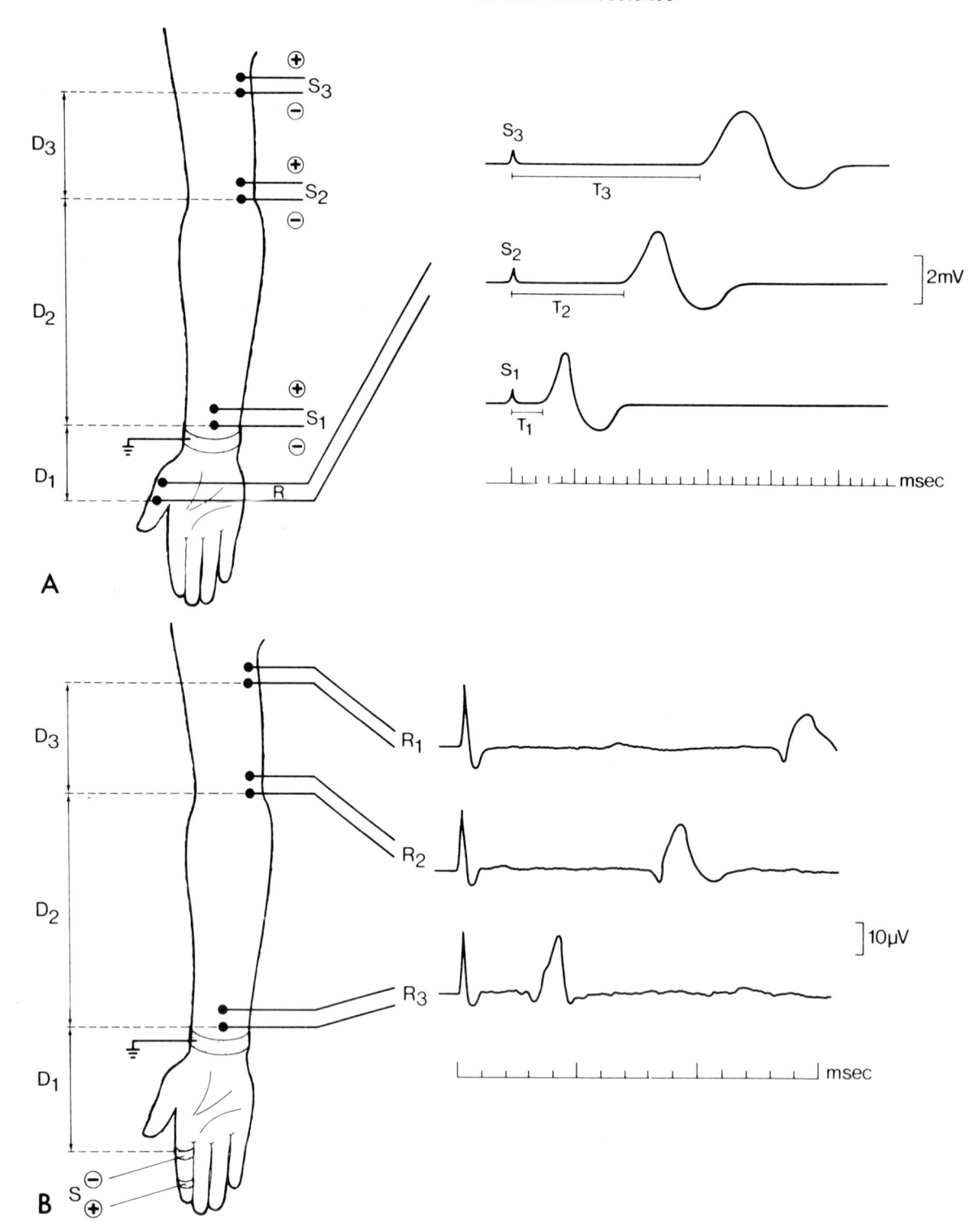

Figure 8.15 A, Diagrammatic representation of the technique of measuring maximum motor conduction velocity in the median nerve. B, Diagrammatic representation of the technique for measuring maximum sensory conduction velocity in the median nerve by orthodromic stimulation. [Reproduced from Walton (1985) *Brain's Diseases of the Nervous System*, 9th edn, and previously published in Bradley (1974) *Disorders of Peripheral Nerves* (Oxford: Blackwell) by kind permission of the author and publishers.]

nerve at the elbow at a rate of 3–5 shocks per second and recording the evoked motor action potential from the hypothenar muscles. In a patient with myasthenia gravis in whom these muscles are affected by the disease, there may be a progressive decrement in the amplitude of the evoked potential. This abnormality may be corrected temporarily by an intravenous injection of edrophonium hydrochloride (Tensilon). A similar decrement usually occurs at fast rates (50/s) of stimulation, which give a muscle tetanus. By contrast, in the myasthenic–myopathic syndrome that may occur in some cases of bronchial carcinoma, the evoked potential is initially of low amplitude, and a striking increment in amplitude is obtained at fast stimulation frequencies. Weakness in the latter disorder is little influenced by edrophonium but may be corrected by guanidine hydrochloride. Patients with myasthenia gravis also show certain abnormal responses to muscular relaxant drugs, and these were once used for diagnostic purposes. Patients with true myasthenia are abnormally sensitive to curare and resistant to decamethonium iodide, but the response is different in patients with the myasthenic–myopathic syndrome. Generally it is now agreed that such pharmacological tests are potentially dangerous and outmoded. Increased 'jitter' and 'blocking' observed in single-fibre electromyography give invaluable evidence of defective neuromuscular transmission; but in the diagnosis of myasthenia, estimation of circulating serum antibodies against the acetylcholine receptor is much more helpful than any electrophysiological test in diagnosis.

BIOCHEMICAL DIAGNOSIS

In the various endocrine and metabolic myopathies, many tests related to the diagnosis of individual endocrine and metabolic disorders may be required. In the periodic paralysis syndromes, serial estimations of serum potassium levels and measures designed to precipitate attacks for diagnostic purposes may be required. In addition there are cases in which the sodium and potassium output in the urine, and even sodium and potassium balance, may need to be measured. In patients with generalized muscle pain and weakness, myoglobin must be sought in the urine, while in individuals suffering muscle pain after effort, it may be necessary to exclude certain forms of glycogen storage disease by measuring the lactate and pyruvate in venous blood distal to a tourniquet following a period of ischaemic work. In such cases estimations of phosphorylase and of many other glycolytic enzymes in muscle biopsy samples may also be needed. Many complex biochemical studies on muscle biopsy samples may also be needed for diagnosis in other forms of glycogen storage disease which do not impair lactate production (such as Pompe's glycogenosis due to acid maltase deficiency) and in the large group of mitochondrial myopathies in which various defects of the electron transport chain may be identified. There are also various myopathies due to the abnormal storage of lipid within the muscle fibres in which carnitine and/or carnitine palmityl transferase must be estimated.

In cases of muscle disease in general, there may be an excessive urinary output of creatine and diminished creatinuria, but these findings are non-specific. The serum aldolase and the serum transaminases (aminotransferases) may be substantially raised in various forms of myopathy, including the more rapidly progressive varieties of muscular dystrophy and polymyositis. The most useful enzyme in the diagnosis of muscle disease is creatine kinase (normal, 60–75 IU/l in most laboratories, although much depends upon the technique employed). In early cases of muscular dystrophy of the Duchenne type, a 300-fold increase in the serum activity of this enzyme may be found, and changes of similar magnitude are observed in certain cases of acute and subacute polymyositis. Less striking rises in activity may be observed in patients suffering from other more indolent forms of myopathy and from the more benign varieties of muscular dystrophy. In some of the endocrine and metabolic myopathies and in the benign congenital myopathies, the activity of this enzyme is not infrequently normal, as is sometimes the case in patients suffering from muscular weakness secondary to disease of the anterior horn cell or motor nerve. However, in many chronic denervating diseases, such as long-standing spinal muscular atrophy, secondary myopathic change develops in the affected muscles with a consequential (and sometimes substantial) rise in serum creatine kinase activity.

MUSCLE BIOPSY

It is generally possible on the basis of the findings observed in sections of muscle obtained by biopsy to distinguish with reasonable confidence between muscular atrophy secondary to denervation on the one hand and that resulting from primary myopathic processes on the other. Differential diagnosis between the various forms of myopathy is sometimes much less exact. Modern techniques, including intravital staining of the motor end-plate, histochemistry, tissue culture and electron microscopy, have yielded information of considerable value from the point of view of research, and have also added considerable precision to the histological diagnosis of many disorders. As an example, 'fibre type grouping' (large groups of fibres of uniform histochemical type) is usually diagnostic of chronic denervation atrophy. The histological features observed in cases of muscular dystrophy are somewhat similar in all varieties of the disease, though varying considerably in severity. However, in early or preclinical Duchenne type dystrophy, in contradistinction to the other varieties, scattered hyaline or 'waxy' fibres, as seen in transverse sections stained with haemalum and eosin, are almost diagnostic together with other evidence of fibre necrosis and abortive regeneration. The most common changes in more advanced dystrophy of all types are marked variations in fibre size, fibre-splitting, the central migration of sarcolemmal nuclei, patchy atrophy of individual muscle fibres, the formation of nuclear chains, the presence of segmental areas of necrosis within muscle fibres with phagocytosis of necrotic sarcoplasm, and basophilia of sarcoplasm with an enlargement of sarcolemmal nuclei showing prominent nucleoli (changes construed as being regenerative in character). There is also a progressive infiltration by fat cells and connective tissue. In subacute or chronic polymyositis, the changes may be very similar, but in this condition signs of muscle fibre destruction and repair (necrosis, phagocytosis and regeneration) are usually more striking and widespread. In addition, in this disease there are usually interstitial or perivascular infiltrations of inflammatory cells such as lymphocytes or plasma cells. There are some cases in which such inflammatory cells are not found; distinction between muscular dystrophy on the one hand and polymyositis on the other then becomes impossible on histological grounds alone. In some cases of myasthenia gravis and in thyrotoxic and other endocrine myopathies, focal collections of lymphocytes (lymphorrhages) may be seen, either around blood vessels or between fibres. When these are seen, the possibility of polymyositis may be raised, but in endocrine myopathy and myasthenia, fibre necrosis is usually slight or absent.

Vacuolar change within muscle fibres, if striking and widespread, may imply the storage of abnormal metabolites within the cells, a pattern particularly seen in cases of glycogen storage disease and in some of the rare lipid storage myopathies. Widespread but less striking vacuolar change is often seen in muscle biopsies taken from patients with periodic paralysis during the attacks and (rarely) in patients with systemic lupus erythematosus or in others suffering from a myopathy resulting from long-continued chloroquine administration. In some of the rare benign congenital and non-progressive myopathies described in recent years, special stains of muscle biopsy sections may be required in order to demonstrate the specific morphological abnormalities of the muscle fibre which have been described in these various disorders.

CONCLUSIONS

Although the organization of voluntary movement is a complex mechanism which still holds many mysteries, a careful analysis, based upon anatomical and physiological knowledge of the ways in which it may be disorganized, can be of the greatest value in localizing the lesion responsible. Changes in muscle tone and in the reflexes may give invaluable aid. Once localized, reconsideration of the method of evolution of the lesion or pathological process will often indicate its nature.

References

de Jong, R. N. (1979) *The Neurologic Examination*, 4th edn. Hagerstown, Md.: Harper and Row.
Denny-Brown, D. (1962) *The Basal Ganglia and Their Relation to Disorders of Movement*. Oxford: Oxford University Press.
Dubowitz, V. and Brooke, M. H. (1974) *Muscle Biopsy*. Philadelphia: W. B. Saunders Company.
Edström, L. and Kugelberg, E. (1968) Histochemical composition, distribution of fibres and fatiguability of single motor units. *J. Neurol. Neurosurg. Psychiat.* **31**:424.
Fitzgerald, M. J. T. (1985) *Neuroanatomy, Basic and Applied*. London: Baillière Tindall.
Gardner, E. (1975) *Fundamentals of Neurology*, 6th edn. Philadelphia: W. B. Saunders Company.
Gilman, S., Bloedel, J. R. and Lechtenberg, R. (1981) *Disorders of the Cerebellum*. (Contemporary Neurology Series, vol. 21). Philadelphia: F. A. Davis.
Holmes, G. (1968) *An Introduction to Clinical Neurology*, 3rd edn, revised by W. B. Matthews. Edinburgh: Churchill Livingstone.
Kandel, E. R. and Schwartz, J. H. *Principles of Neural Science*, 2nd edn. London: Edward Arnold.
Kimura, J. (1983) *Electrodiagnosis in Diseases of Nerve and Muscle*. Philadelphia: F. A. Davis.
Lance, J. W. and McLeod, J. G. (1981) *A Physiological Approach to Clinical Neurology*, 3rd edn. London: Butterworths.
Marsden, C. D. (1985) The basal ganglia. In Swash, M. and Kennard, C. (eds) *Scientific Basis of Clinical Neurology*. Edinburgh: Churchill Livingstone.
Martin, J. P. (1967) *The Basal Ganglia and Posture*. London: Pitman Medical.
Mastaglia, F. L. and Walton, J. N. (eds) (1982) *Skeletal Muscle Pathology*. Edinburgh: Churchill Livingstone.
Medical Research Council (1976) *Aids to the Examination of the Peripheral Nervous System*. London: H.M.S.O.
Patten, J. (1977) *Neurological Differential Diagnosis*. London: Harold Starke.
Patton, H. D., Sundsten, J. W., Crill, W. E. and Swanson, P. D. (1976) *Introduction to Basic Neurology*. Philadelphia: W. B. Saunders Company.
Peachey, L. D. (1968) Muscle. *Ann. Rev. Physiol.* **30**:401.
Pearlman, A. L. and Collins, R. C. (1985) *Neurological Pathophysiology*, 3rd edn. Oxford: Oxford University Press.
Schaumburg, H. H., Spencer, P. S. and Thomas, P. K. (1983) *Disorders of Peripheral Nerves* (Contemporary Neurology Series, vol. 24). Philadelphia: F. A. Davis.
Sharrard, W. J. W. (1955) The distribution of the permanent paralysis in the lower limb in poliomyelitis. *J. Bone Jt Surg.* **37B**:540.
Sherrington, C. (1906) *The Integrative Action of the Nervous System*. New Haven: Yale University Press.
Snider, R. S. (1972) The cerebellum. In Critchley, M., O'Leary,

J. L. and Jennett, W. B. (eds) *Scientific Foundations of Neurology*. London: Heinemann.

Spillane, J. D. and Spillane, J. A. (1982) *An Atlas of Clinical Neurology*, 3rd edn. Oxford: Oxford University Press.

Tomlinson, B. E., Irving, D. and Rebeiz, J. J. (1973) Total numbers of limb motor neurones in the human lumbosacral cord and an analysis of the accuracy of various sampling procedures. *J. Neurol. Sci.* **20**:313.

Walshe, F. M. R. (1965) *Further Critical Studies in Neurology*. Edinburgh: Churchill Livingstone.

Walton, J. N. (ed.) (1980) *Disorders of Voluntary Muscle*, 4th edn. Edinburgh: Churchill Livingstone.

Walton, J. N. (1982) *Essentials of Neurology*, 5th edn. London: Pitman Medical.

Walton, J. N. (1985) *Brain's Diseases of the Nervous System*, 9th edn. Oxford: Oxford University Press.

Wartenberg, R. (1945) *The Examination of the Reflexes*. Chicago: Year Book Medical Publishers.

Wilkinson, J. L. (1986) *Neuroanatomy for Medical Students*. Bristol: John Wright.

9

THE SENSORY SYSTEM

INTRODUCTION

Somatic sensory input is of two principal types: first, there are impulses which lead to motor responses through the segmental reflex systems (discussed earlier) and secondly there are impulses which ascend to reach those centres in which sensory experiences are recorded and enter perception. The latter are known as sensory responses. These two processes are not totally independent as a single primary afferent nerve fibre may initiate reflex responses, while its long ascending collateral branches may also convey sensory information which reaches consciousness (sensory awareness). Generally the term 'sensory' relates only to those neurons and pathways that convey impulses to levels of the nervous system (thalamus and cortex) at which the sensation conveyed evokes conscious awareness, and not to the segmental reflex system. The distinction is not always useful in clinical practice, since proprioceptive sensory information, relating to the position and interrelationship of the parts of the body, does not as a rule enter consciousness, yet defects of this sense produce striking clinical manifestations. Not only will sensory mechanisms in the strict sense outlined above be considered but also some of the pathophysiological consequences of impaired reflex responses due to dysfunction of afferent pathways.

THE ANATOMICAL AND PHYSIOLOGICAL ORGANIZATION OF SOMATIC SENSATION

The sensory apparatus consists of (a) a series of sensory receptors in the skin and other organs, (b) the first sensory neuron, whose unipolar cells are located in the posterior root ganglia, and (c) secondary sensory neurons which are responsible for the conduction of impulses through the spinal cord and brain stem to the thalamus; further neurons then relay certain forms of sensation to the cerebral cortex. Cells in the substantia gelatinosa of the spinal cord and the network of internuncial neurons to which they relate probably play a major role in modulating sensory input. Visceral sensation, which is conveyed initially alongside fibres of the autonomic nervous system, enters the spinal cord along with somatic sensory impulses and is conveyed centrally in a similar manner.

Receptors

Sensory receptors can be divided into exteroceptors, which are largely situated in the skin and which are concerned with recording information about the external environment of the body, and proprioceptors and interoceptors, which are situated in muscles, tendons, joints and viscera and which inform us of the position and condition of these deeper structures. For many years controversy abounded over the question as to whether there were specific cutaneous sensory receptors responding to specific stimuli or whether different forms of sensation were related to patterns of stimulation of relatively undifferentiated networks of fine nerve endings terminating in the skin. This dispute has now been settled in favour of the specificity theory which accepts that individual cutaneous sensory receptors are most sensitive to a particular form of natural stimulation but that this specificity is not absolute and other types of stimuli may also excite the ending (Iggo, 1985a). Three broad classes of receptors can be distinguished in mammals, namely *mechanoreceptors*, which respond to mechanical displacement of the skin, *thermoreceptors*, which respond to temperature change, and *nociceptors*, which are insensitive to stimuli that excite the other two varieties but which are excited by higher intensity, potentially damaging stimuli.

Of the mechanoreceptors, some are rapidly-adapting. These include the large subcutaneous pacinian corpuscles which respond to vibration or tickle, the Meissner corpuscles and hair follicle receptors which respond to tapping, and the Krause end-bulbs whose function is still not entirely clear though they probably respond to similar stimuli. There are also slowly-adapting receptors, including Merkel cells and Ruffini endings that also respond to touch and pressure, which indent the skin but which continue to discharge during continuing indentation. The Merkel discs and cells are specifically pressure receptors, but no specific perceived sensation is associated with stimulation of Ruffini endings. Most mechanoreceptors are supplied by large myelinated axons, whereas the smaller myelinated (Aδ) and non-myelinated (C) axons innervate a variety of thermoreceptors, nociceptors and (a few) mechanoreceptors which are known as C-mechanoreceptors and which are excited by lightly moving hairs or light pressure on the skin.

Thermoreceptors are relatively or absolutely insensitive to mechanical stimuli but respond to changes in skin temperature. Cold receptors are excited by a fall in temperature, warm receptors by a rise in temperature, and these receptors can discharge continuously and more or less indefinitely at a constant temperature within their range of sensitivity, the rate of discharge depending upon the actual temperature. Most cold units have myelinated fibres, while warm units have non-myelinated fibres, and each have spot-like receptive fields corresponding to the warm and cold spots on the skin which can be identified clinically with fine thermal stimulators.

Nociceptors, which are innervated either by small myelinated (Aδ) or non-myelinated (C) afferent fibres, have small receptive fields. Some are mechanical and are excited by very firm pressure or by penetrating the skin with a sharp object; those responsible for pain sensation are often called fine C-terminals. Others are thermal or mechanothermal receptors, innervated by C-fibres; they can be excited by severe mechanical stimuli but are principally responsive to high skin temperatures (i.e. 42°C or above), well above the normal threshold (about 40°C) that stimulates warm thermoreceptors. Algogenic chemicals such as bradykinin, 5-HT and prostaglandins E_1 and E_2 produced in the skin during inflammation either excite or enhance the excitability of C-nociceptors.

Proprioceptive sensory input comes from the muscle spindles, the muscles themselves, the joint capsules, and the Golgi tendon organs. This information is conveyed by fibres of group Ia afferents (carrying impulses from muscle spindle primary afferents), group Ib afferents (from Golgi tendon organs) and group II afferents (from spindle secondary afferents). Some information also comes via somatosensory afferents from joint capsules and via slowly conducting afferents originating in muscle (the flexor reflex afferents). Comparatively few proprioceptive stimuli reach consciousness; most are concerned with reflex activity mediated through the spinal cord and cerebellum by means of which posture and movement are controlled.

Somatic sensation: its nature, coding and measurement

SENSORY PARAMETERS

Somatic sensation is not a uniform sensory experience. It is a fusion of several qualities which cannot be consciously dissociated but which may be differentially affected by disease or dysfunction. Each sensory experience has a quality or modality (touch, pain, heat and cold, etc.); the various sensory modalities will be considered below. Different receptors respond to different modalities. Similarly some secondary sensory neurons in the posterior horn of spinal cord grey matter, some fibres in the ascending sensory tracts, some thalamic neurons, and, to a lesser extent, neurons in the cortex are modality-specific. Thus, for example, in the dorsal horn of grey matter there are mechanoreceptive neurons, multi-receptive neurons (receiving stimuli from both mechanoreceptors and nociceptors) and nociceptive neurons (excited only by afferent input from nociceptors); but as yet neurons responding to thermoreceptors have not been identified. The substantia gelatinosa of the dorsal horn contains a very large number of small neurons, and most non-myelinated cutaneous axons end within it. The cells of this area clearly receive an excitatory input from a large number of synapses and there is an interplay of excitation and inhibition from mechanoreceptors and nociceptors. Several neuropeptides, notably substance P (which clearly has an important function in relation to pain sensation) have been identified in this region. Clearly, therefore, the dorsal horn provides a site of excitation and inhibition of activity in dorsal horn neurons, thus modulating sensory input before it enters ascending tracts leading to higher levels of the neuraxis (Iggo, 1985a).

Intensity is another parameter of importance, enabling us to distinguish between a light pinprick and a fierce jab. Intensity discrimination is pattern coded, i.e. it depends upon frequency of firing in sensory receptors and in neurons and afferent fibres at all levels of the nervous system. Phasic (on–off) receptors, such as those concerned with light touch, are more complex, intensity being little if at all related to frequency. The normal human subject is also skilled at the localization of sensory stimuli. This faculty is clearly related to the segmental organization of cutaneous sensory input. Localization of visceral sensation is less accurate, though even this may be aided by the interpretation, for instance, of referred pain. Specific groups of neurons can be excited by specific sensory stimuli applied to specific areas of the body surface. There is a clear, consistent and precise somatotopic localization in the posterior roots of the spinal cord and their ganglia, in the posterior horns of grey matter, in the ascending pathways in the spinal cord, in the principal sensory nuclei of the brain stem, in the thalamus, and in the sensory cortex. The density of sensory receptors differs in different areas of skin. This variability of distribution accounts for the striking differences observed in the ability to discriminate between two points applied at set distances apart (two-point discrimination). The receptive fields of somatosensory cortical neurons show an inverse relationship to sensory acuity in that these fields are small, for instance, in respect to sensory input from the tips of the fingers, and large for many areas of the trunk.

The nervous system is also capable of recognizing the duration and temporal pattern of sensory stimuli. The onset and the termination of a stimulus and its reaction time (the time taken for its conscious perception) can be recognized, as can recurring stimuli such as the perception of vibration. Different fibres in peripheral nerves conduct at different rates, depending upon their diameter and upon whether or not they are myelinated, and different modalities of sensation are therefore conducted at different rates. Reaction time is directly related to conduction velocity in both the peripheral and the central nervous systems. The mechanism of perception of vibration is more complex. Such recurrent stimuli specifically excite phasic (on–off) mechanoreceptors (especially pacinian corpuscles), each oscillation exciting a single spike, but different thalamic and cortical neurons may respond to different frequencies so that both place and pattern coding are involved.

Most somatic sensations evoke affective responses which determine whether the sensation perceived is pleasant (warmth), unpleasant (pain, excessive heat or cold) or neutral (touch, light pressure, change of position, etc.). The influence of cerebral and hypothalamic centres concerned with pleasure, reward and punishment upon somatic sensation has been considered earlier. Sedative drugs such as barbiturates and phenothiazines, for example, and surgical procedures such as prefrontal leucotomy or lesions which interrupt connections between the prefrontal cortex and subcortical centres may all diminish or even abolish affect, while leaving intact the ability to recognize sensory modalities. The patient continues to feel and to recognize pain but it no longer disturbs him.

The coding of sensory information allows the subject to recognize the nature of the somatic stimulus which he perceives, its intensity, where it is situated, how long it lasts and whether it is repetitive, and its character and emotional connotations.

EXAMINATION AND MEASUREMENT

Methods of examining the commoner sensory modalities will be mentioned below. Much depends upon the cooperation of the patient or subject, and upon his state of consciousness, intellectual capacity and emotional state. Areas of spurious cutaneous sensory impairment, especially to light touch and pin-prick, are often elicited by even the most skilled observer. Intelligent, obsessional or introspective patients often perceive relatively slight variations in intensity of stimulation which are almost impossible for the examiner to avoid and which prove in the end to be of no pathological significance. In addition, individuals vary considerably in their affective response to sensory stimuli, a sensation which appears acutely painful to one being well tolerated by another.

Considerable advances have been made in methods of measuring somatic sensory perception, both in animals and in man, but the techniques involved are generally too complex for use in clinical practice. Weber, assessing the ability of subjects to recognize differences in the weights of a series of test objects, introduced the concept of 'just noticeable difference' (j.n.d.), and Weber's law stated that $j.n.d./I = k$, where I was the weight of a reference object and k a constant found to be $1/30$. Thus with a 30 g reference weight, the difference between weights of 29 and 31 g could be perceived, but if the reference weight was 60 g, the subject could only discriminate between weights of 58 and 62 g. Subsequently Fechner concluded that the magnitude of the sensation perceived is directly proportional to the log of the physical stimulus. While the accuracy of this postulate has subsequently been called into question, Fechner's law remains a useful guide.

THE SIMPLER SENSORY MODALITIES

A number of clearly definable forms of somatic sensation can be recognized whose integrity is customarily assessed during the course of a neurological examination. Touch is commonly tested with a light application to the skin of a pledget of cotton wool. It may be assessed quantitatively by using von Frey hairs, so graduated that differing pressures are needed to bend them. The threshold for the appreciation of touch varies considerably on different parts of the surface of the body, depending upon such variables as the thickness of the epidermis and the number of hair follicles present. Pain sensation is generally assessed by means of a pin-prick, which can also be of graduated severity if an algesiometer is used. Care must be taken that the patient is asked to assess the painful quality of this stimulus and not the sensations of pressure or touch which may be simultaneously evoked. Squeezing of the tendo Achilles or of other deep tendons will determine whether the appreciation of deep pressure is intact, but this sensation can also be painful. Thermal sensation is generally tested by applying metal test tubes to the skin, one filled with ice, the other with water at 45° C. Again the patient must be told that it is the feeling of heat or cold he is being asked to note and not the sensation of touch or pressure. The assessment of position and joint sense is generally carried out by moving the terminal phalanx of the forefinger or the great toe in a vertical plane and by asking the patient, whose eyes are closed, to describe the direction of movement each time the digit is moved. After making an initial movement of considerable amplitude it must then be decided whether the patient can appreciate movements through a very small range (about 1 mm). Another test of position and joint sense is to ask the patient, with his eyes closed, to point towards a part of his body, when the position of the part in space has been altered by the examiner. Vibration sense, as tested with a tuning fork of 128-frequency applied to bony prominences, is not a physiological sensation, being compounded of both touch and pressure, but nevertheless absence of the ability to perceive this form of somatic sensibility is of considerable significance in clinical neurology. Tactile discrimination is assessed by recording the threshold distance at which the two blunt points of a compass, simultaneously applied, are independently perceived (Fig. 9.1). The normal threshold for two-point discrimination on the tip of the tongue is 1 mm, on the tips of the fingers 2–3 mm, on the palm of the hand or sole of the foot 1.5–3 cm, and in the centre of the back 6–7 cm. The appreciation of the texture, weight, size and shape of objects can also be assessed, somewhat crudely, by asking the patient, with his eyes closed, to identify objects placed in the hand, while tactile localization is tested by asking him to identify on a diagram or model, or on the examiner, the point or points on his body which had been stimulated. He may also be asked to identify figures or letters which are traced with a blunt point on his skin (graphaesthesia). There is considerable individual variation in the ability to perceive and interpret these more complex sensations, but retention of these functions on one side of the body and their absence on the other is always a finding of pathological significance.

The sensory pathways

The cells of the first sensory neuron are situated in the posterior root ganglia and have peripheral axons which convey afferent impulses from the sensory receptors, and central axons which enter the spinal cord in the posterior nerve roots. The sensory fibres in the peripheral nerves vary in diameter and in their rate of conduction. The large, heavily-myelinated rapidly-conducting A fibres are primarily concerned with the conduction of impulses subserving touch, pressure and proprioceptive sensation, but some (the Aδ fibres) undoubtedly transmit painful and thermal sensations. The most slowly-conducting unmyelinated C fibres are largely concerned with temperature and pain sensation, but some also convey touch. Thus, while there is some relationship between the size and myelination of sensory axons and their function, this is not absolute. Certain diseases of the peripheral nerves, and particularly various forms of peripheral neuropathy, may have a selective effect upon fibres of one particular size or degree of myelination. The result may be some cases in which the appreciation of painful stimulation is more severely affected than that of touch or vice versa. Whereas cutaneous and pressure sensations travel in pure sensory (cutaneous) nerves and later in mixed sensory and motor nerves, some proprioceptive stimuli, especially those concerned in reflex activity, travel centrally first of all in motor nerves.

As the central axons of the first sensory neuron enter the spinal cord, some degree of regrouping of these fibres occurs, according to their function. Initially most fibres enter the posterior column, lying just medially to the posterior horn of grey matter. At this point internuncial neurons arising from cells in the substantia gelatinosa exert a modifying or 'gating' influence (see below), especially upon painful sensations. The fibres concerned with proprioception, position and joint sense, vibration sense, and tactile discrimination, as well as some of those conveying touch, turn immediately upwards in the posterior columns and travel to the nuclei of Goll and Burdach in the medulla. Entering fibres continually

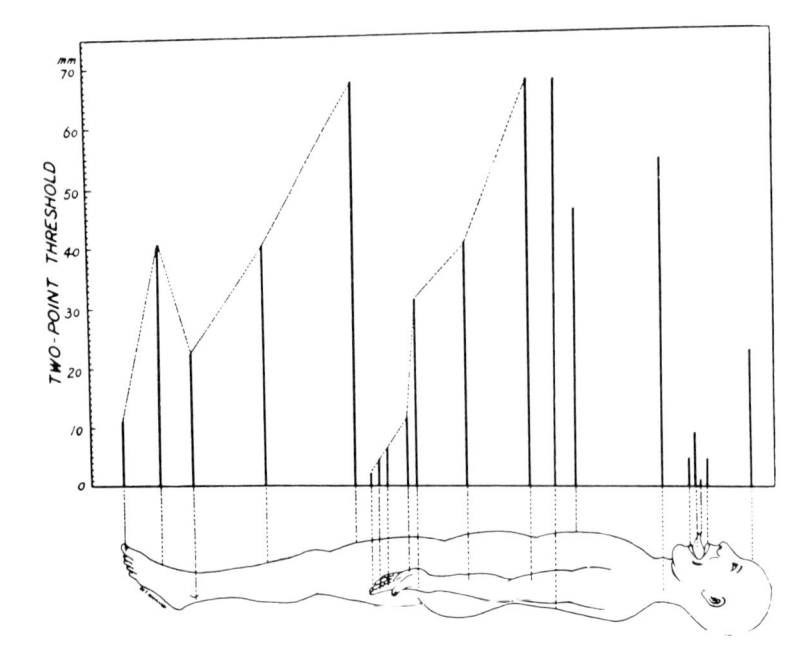

Figure 9.1 Regional variation in tactile two-point threshold in man. [Reproduced from Patton et al (1976) *Introduction to Basic Neurology*, and previously published in Ruch and Patton (eds) (1965) *Physiology and Biophysics* (Philadelphia: W. B. Saunders Co.) by kind of permission of the authors and publisher.]

displace medially those which have entered the cord at a lower level. The fibres from the lower limbs lie in the medial part of the posterior column (the fasciculus gracilis or column of Goll), while those from the upper limbs lie more laterally (the fasciculus cuneatus or column of Burdach) (Fig. 9.2).

The group of entering fibres concerned with the appreciation of touch also enters the most lateral part of the posterior column, where they ascend for several segments before entering the posterior horn of grey matter to synapse with cells in this area. The axons of these cells then cross the midline close to the central canal to end in the ventral spinothalamic tract. Fibres subserving pain and temperature sensation ascend in the posterior column for only a few segments before crossing the midline in the white commissure close to the central grey matter and canal to end in the more lateral portion of the spinothalamic tract in the opposite lateral column of the cord (Fig. 9.2). As in the posterior columns, there is some lamination of sensory fibres in the spinothalamic tracts, those from the lower limbs lying posterolaterally, and those from the upper limbs being situated anterolaterally. Fibres carrying thermal sensations lie most centrally, nearest to the anterior horn of grey matter. This may explain why a lesion giving rise to spinal cord compression often impairs pain sensation first in the lower limbs. The sensory 'level' then ascends steadily but finally becomes arrested on the trunk several segments below the location of the lesion. Presumably the fibres situated nearest to the surface of the cord are the first to be affected by pressure.

The spinothalamic fibres enter the medulla oblongata laterally and travel directly up through the pons and midbrain to reach the thalamus. The fibres of the posterior columns, however, terminate in synapses in the nuclei of Goll (nucleus gracilis) and Burdach (nucleus cuneatus). From the cells of these nuclei new axons arise which immediately cross the midline and then travel upwards as the medial fillet or lemniscus, again to enter the thalamus.

The pathway followed by sensory impulses from the face deserves special mention. The fibres of the trigeminal nerve, which carry touch and tactile discrimination, enter the main trigeminal nucleus; from that nucleus the quintothalamic tract, carrying these modalities, arises, crosses the midline and joins the medial fillet. Those subserving pain and thermal sensation enter the pons but then travel downwards in the descending root of the trigeminal nerve to end in a nuclear mass which extends downwards as far as the second cervical segment of the cord. Then they too cross the midline and travel upwards in the spinothalamic tract. 'Representation' of the parts of the face in the descending root of the trigeminal nerve is inverted. A lesion of the lower end of the root in the upper cervical cord will give loss of pain and temperature sensation only, but not of touch, over the area supplied by the ophthalmic division on the same side of the face. Proprioceptive stimuli from the face travel centrally in the facial nerve, so that sense of position in the facial muscles (a difficult faculty to test) is not abolished by a lesion of the trigeminus.

All sensory pathways ascending as far as the brain stem terminate in the thalamus. Throughout their

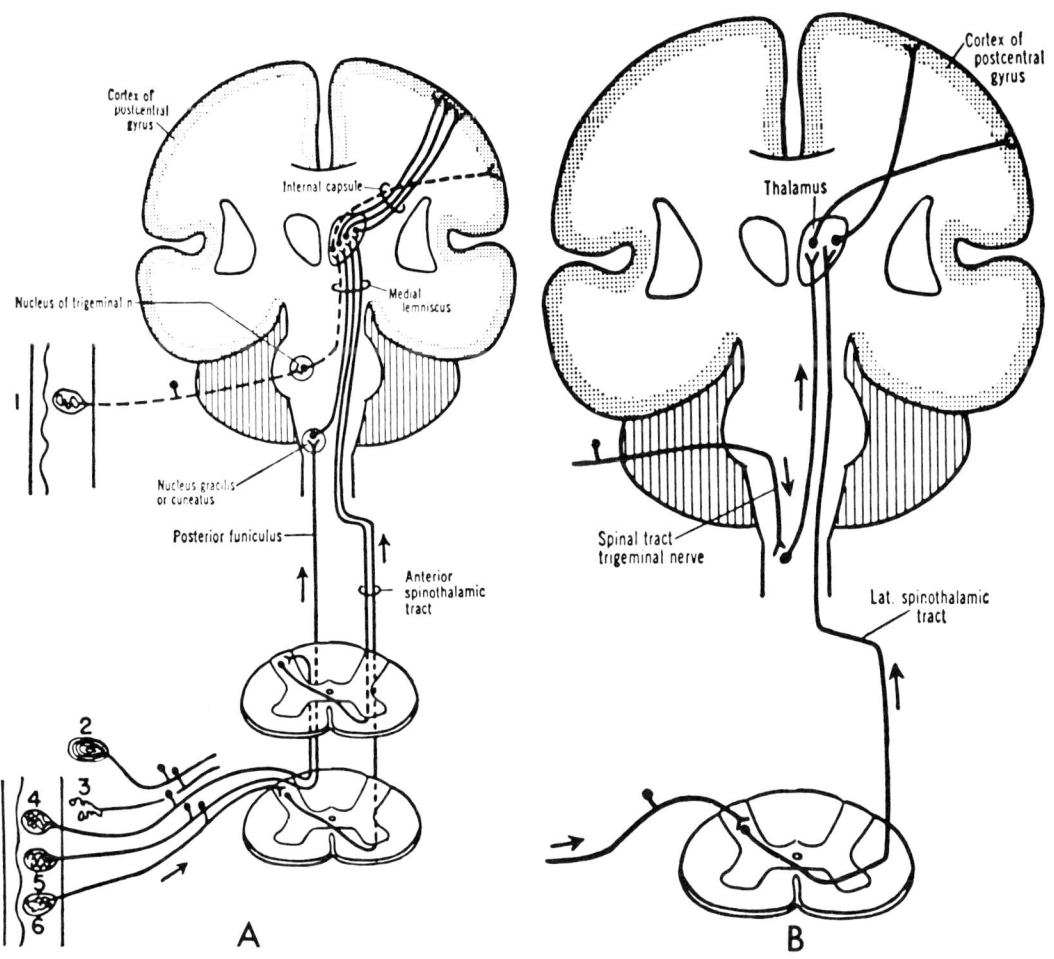

Figure 9.2 A diagram of the principal pathways of the sensory system. A, The pathways followed by impulses subserving touch, tactile discrimination, position and joint sense and related sensations. 1, 4, 5, and 6 represent Meissner's corpuscles; the pathways from 2 (Pacinian corpuscle) and 3 (joint receptor) are similar to those followed by impulses from 5. B, The pathways followed by impulses subserving pain and temperature sensation. [Reproduced from Walton (1985) *Essentials of Neurology*, 5th edn, and previously published in Gardner (1975) *Fundamentals of Neurology*, 6th edn, by kind permission of the authors and publishers.]

course in the spinal cord and brain stem these fibres give off collaterals or synapse with internuncial neurons. These connections complete the sensory side of the arcs concerned with those spinal and brain-stem reflexes which are necessary for the maintenance of posture and other functions. There are many sensory fibres which ascend the spinal cord in the dorsal and ventral spinocerebellar tracts and which are largely concerned with supplying the information through which the cerebellum exerts control over posture and movement.

The thalamus is the principal sensory relay station of the brain. The principal nuclei of the thalamus and their cortical projections in the cerebral hemisphere are illustrated diagrammatically in Fig. 9.3. The sensory relay nuclei that receive input from the ascending pathways conveying somatic and visceral sensation are the nuclei ventralis posterolateralis (VPL), which receive afferent stimuli from the trunk and limbs, and the ventralis posteromedialis (VPM), which is similarly concerned with input from the face. Both in turn send corticothalamic neuronal projections to the somatosensory and parietal association areas of the cortex and receive corticothalamic projections from the same areas. The lateral and medial geniculate bodies are concerned with vision and hearing respectively, the ventralis lateralis (VL) with cerebellar and extrapyramidal function, the ventralis anterior (VA) with activity of the basal ganglia, and the nucleus anterior (A) with hypothalamic function. The dorsomedial nucleus (DM), which projects to the prefrontal cortex, is not primarily concerned with the awareness of somatic sensation but appears to have a role relating to the affective response to

jections and even more so in the primary sensory cortex of the postcentral gyrus (Fig. 9.4). It also exists to a lesser extent in projections to the other (association) areas of the parietal lobe.

The cortex is concerned with the appreciation of most of those stimuli which enter consciousness. The integrity of the sensory cortex is particularly important in recognition of form, texture, size, weight and consistency of objects, or in changes in position of parts of the body. It is also essential for the accurate localization and recognition of the nature of stimuli applied to the body, for discrimination between two simultaneously applied stimuli, and even more for the ability to relate sensory experiences to others experienced previously, or to sense data perceived through the special senses. Clearly, numerous association pathways are concerned in the interpretation and recognition of these more complex sensory experiences, which may nevertheless be grossly deranged if there is a lesion of the primary sensory cortex, an important cell station in all sensory association mechanisms. Specific portions of the postcentral gyrus are concerned with the appreciation of sensations from particular areas of the opposite side of the body (Fig. 9.4). 'Representation' in the sensory cortex corresponds topographically with that in the motor area. A lesion of the lower end of the postcentral gyrus will impair sensory perception in the contralateral face and hand, while a lesion on the superior and medial aspect of the hemisphere will result in a failure to appreciate 'cortical' forms of sensation in the opposite leg.

Cortical or subcortical lesions, even if they divide all thalamocortical fibres, do not destroy completely the ability to perceive sensory experiences in the opposite half of the body. In the presence of such a lesion, sensitivity to pain and temperature is affected comparatively little. Crude touch will still be felt, though finer forms of sensory experience may be greatly impaired. The cruder varieties of sensation are in some way recorded in consciousness at a thalamic level.

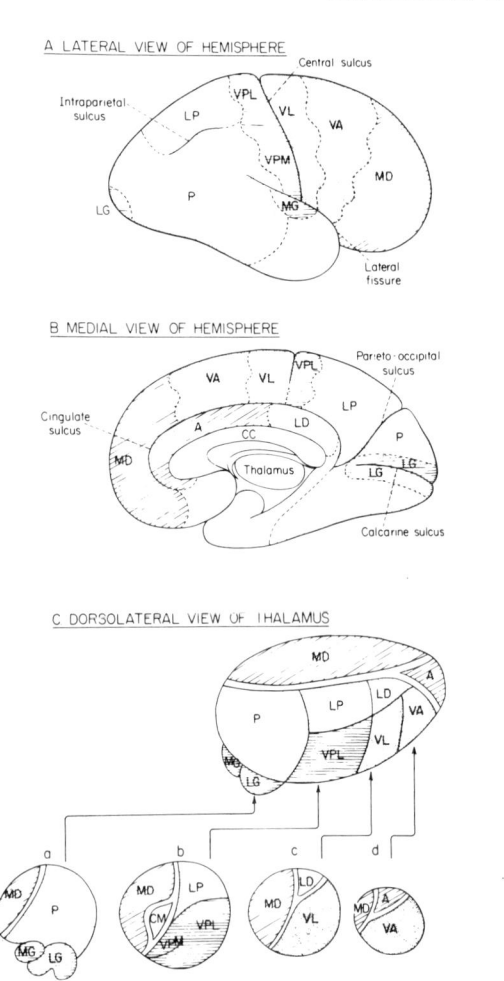

Figure 9.3 Thalamic nuclei and their cerebral cortical projection sites. A and B, The right cerebral hemisphere, the dotted lines represent approximate projection boundaries that cut across different cortical gyri. C, The right thalamus and representative frontal sections (a to d) through it. The thalamic nuclei and their projection areas are shaded according to categories as follows: somatosensory and special sensory, horizontal shading; cerebellar and striatal, dense stippling; hypothalamic, oblique shading; and 'association', light stippling.

Thalamic nuclei: A, anterior; CM, centromedian; LD, lateralis dorsalis; LG, lateralis geniculate; LP, lateralis posterior; MD, medialis dorsalis; MG, medial geniculate; P, pulvinar; VA, ventralis anterior; VL, ventralis lateralis; VPL, ventralis posterolateralis; VPM, ventralis posteromedialis.
[Reproduced from Patton et al (1976) *Introduction to Basic Neurology*, by kind permission of the authors and publisher.]

sensory input, especially of pain. There is a clear somatotopic representation of parts of the body in the sensory relay nuclei of the thalamus, with caudal areas projecting to the lateral part of the VPL, rostral segments more medially, and the face most medially in the VPM.

A similar and precise somatotopic representation continues in the thalamocortical neuronal pro-

Cutaneous sensory segmentation

Early in its development the human fetus demonstrates metameric segmentation, and each somatic segment, or metamere, is linked to the corresponding segment of the neuraxis by a pair of spinal nerves. In the course of evolution with specialization of the anterior end of the human organism to form the head and with the growth of the complicated motor and sensory functions of the limbs, this metameric segmentation of the nervous system has been disrupted, persisting only in the dorsal region. After the fusion of ventral and dorsal roots to form a spinal nerve,

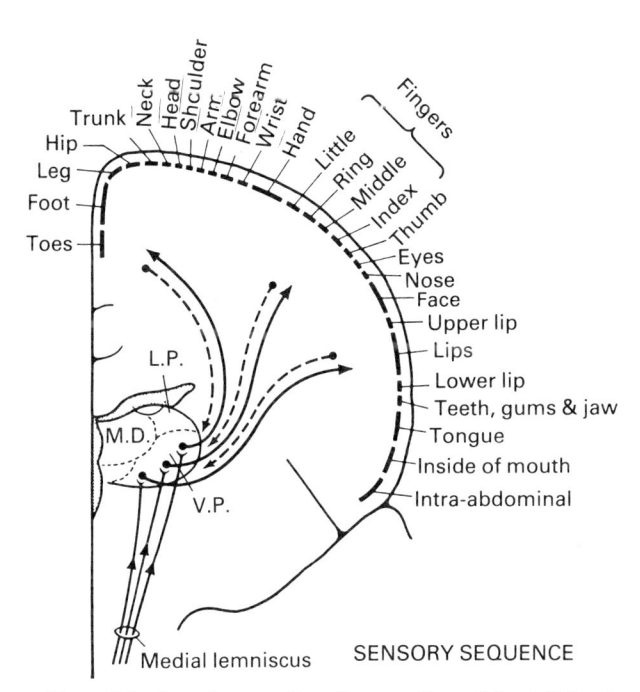

Figure 9.4 Somatic sensation. Cross-section of the left hemisphere along the plane of the postcentral gyrus. The afferent pathway for tactile and kinaesthetic sensation is indicated by the unbroken lines coming up, through the medial lemniscus and the posterolateral ventral nucleus of the thalamus, to the postcentral gyrus. [Reproduced from Walton (1985) *Brain's Diseases of the Nervous System*, 9th edn, by kind permission of the publisher.]

the dorsal primary division conveys motor fibres to the spinal muscles and sensory fibres to the overlying cutaneous area. In the mid-dorsal region the ventral primary division supplies motor fibres to the intercostal muscles and sensory fibres to a narrow zone extending more or less horizontally around the thorax on one side as far as the midline. In the cervical and lumbosacral regions the arrangement is complicated by the formation of the limb plexuses in which several ventral primary divisions unite and subsequently subdivide to form the peripheral nerves supplying the limbs. Through the intervention of the plexuses a single spinal nerve may send both motor and sensory contributions to several peripheral nerves, and, conversely, a single peripheral nerve may receive contributions from several spinal nerves. It follows that the sensory loss resulting from interruption of a peripheral nerve differs in its distribution from that produced by interruption of a posterior root or spinal nerve. A segmental or radicular cutaneous area—a dermatome—is an area of skin which receives its sensory supply from a single dorsal root and spinal nerve. In the trunk these segmental areas still exhibit a metameric arrangement. In the limbs this has been modified, but as a rule the segmental areas occupy elongated zones in the long axis of the limb (Fig. 9.5). Owing to the specialization of the ventral primary divisions of the lower cervical and first thoracic spinal nerves in the innervation of the upper limb, these have lost their cutaneous supply to the trunk anteriorly. At the level of the second rib the fourth cervical segmental cutaneous area is contiguous with the second thoracic. The lower six thoracic spinal nerves supply the abdominal wall as low as the inguinal ligament. The dorsal primary divisions of the spinal nerves take no part in the formation of the limb plexuses, so that all spinal segments appear to be represented in the cutaneous supply of the back.

There is considerable overlapping of contiguous segmental cutaneous areas. The division of a single dorsal root does not cause any sensory loss detectable by ordinary clinical methods. Each root supplies fibres for pain, heat and cold to a larger area than that to which it supplies fibres for light touch.

In the sensory innervation of the head the trigeminal nerve represents a fusion of the sensory supply of several segments, though the seventh, ninth and tenth cranial nerves still possess rudimentary sensory branches distributed to the neighbourhood of the auricle. The posterior and inferior boundaries of the trigeminal cutaneous area are contiguous with those of the first and second cervical segments respectively.

Some common abnormalities of sensation

In the description of disorders of sensation, the word numbness can have a variety of meanings. When a patient says that a part of the body is numb he may mean that sensation in the part is abnormal, but sometimes the term is used to denote weakness or clumsiness. Hence careful enquiry is needed in order to determine the significance of this symptom. In patients with neurological disease, one of the commonest symptoms is pain. Pain may result from inflammation or compression of any pain-sensitive structure. If it is due to irritation of a sensory nerve or root, the distribution of the pain will be in the cutaneous area supplied by the nerve or root concerned. Pain can also be felt in an organ or organs which are diseased, while if it is arising in a viscus or in a muscle, it can be referred to an area of skin which sometimes overlies the viscus but may be anatomically remote. The mechanism of referred pain is not fully understood, though it seems to be due to a spread of impulses to contiguous sensory neurons within the cord (see below). Spontaneous pain in the limbs or trunk can result from discrete thalamic lesions, usually due to infarction. It has a peculiarly unpleasant burning character, often with

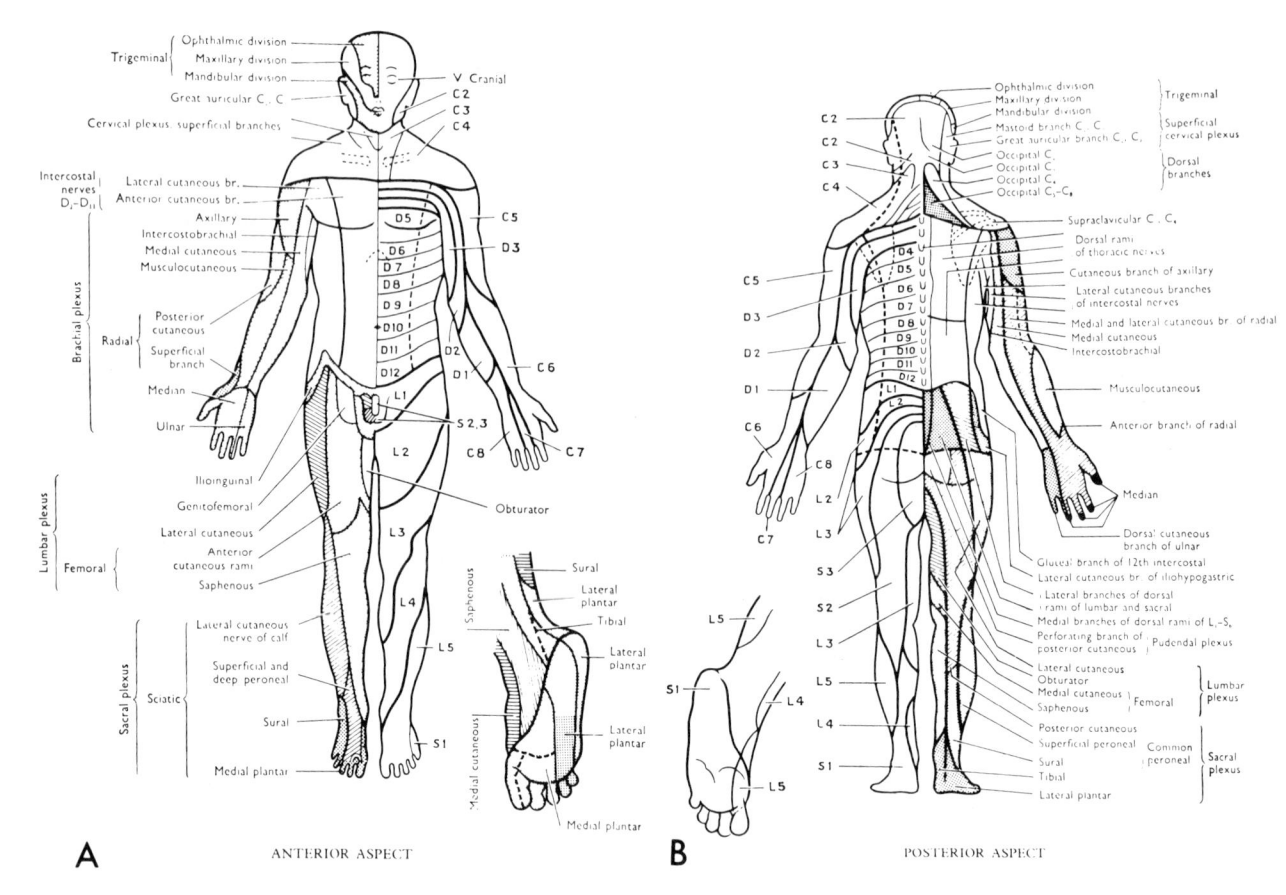

Figure 9.5 Cutaneous areas of distribution of spinal segments and of the sensory fibres of the peripheral nerves. A, Anterior aspect. B, Posterior aspect. [Reproduced from Walton (1985) *Brain's Diseases of the Nervous System*, 9th edn, by kind permission of the publisher.]

additional 'grinding' or 'tearing' qualities. This so-called thalamic pain is most often felt in the face, around one angle of the mouth, and in the hand and foot on the affected side. A closely related sensation of continuous burning or pricking, or warmth or even cold may result from a spinothalamic tract lesion, but tends to be more diffusely felt in the area of impaired cutaneous sensation. Disordered sensations of this type, occurring spontaneously, are often referred to as dysaesthesiae. In addition to these abnormal sensations, patients with lesions of the spinothalamic tract often observe that they are unable to feel pain or temperature in the affected part. They may injure or burn a limb without discomfort or they may be unable to assess the temperature of bath water.

Paraesthesiae include feelings of tingling, pins and needles, or swelling of a limb, sensations suggesting that tight strings or bands are tied around a part of the body, or as if water were trickling over the skin. Sensory experiences of this type result from disordered function in the pathways conducting the finer and discriminative aspects or sensibility. Tingling or pins and needles can result from ischaemia of peripheral nerves, from polyneuropathy, from transient ischaemia of the sensory cortex, or from sensory jacksonian epilepsy due to a cortical lesion. Similar symptoms are experienced by patients with lesions of the posterior columns of the cord, and it is usually in such individuals that the 'tight, constricting band' or the 'trickling' type of sensation is felt. Often the affected part feels swollen, or the patient may feel as if the limb is encased in a firm glove or plaster cast. If there is a lesion of the posterior columns in the cervical region, sudden flexion or extension of the neck may give an 'electric shock' sensation which travels rapidly to the hands and feet. This sign (*Lhermitte's sign*) is commonly observed in multiple sclerosis and in cervical spondylosis. Similarly, tapping or pressure over the trunk of an ischaemic nerve (as in patients with median nerve compression in the carpal tunnel) or over a sensory nerve which has been injured in some other way, will often give paraesthesiae which shoot along the cutaneous distribution of the nerve concerned. A comparable sign produced by tapping a nerve in which regeneration is occurring is known as *Tinel's sign*.

Patients with disordered function of the posterior columns of the cord or of the sensory cortex often observe that the affected part has become clumsy or even useless. If a hand is affected they may be unable to use it except under careful visual supervision and cannot recognize objects felt in a pocket or handbag, unless they can be taken out and examined visually. Fine movements such as fastening buttons or threading needles are grossly impaired. If both lower limbs are affected, then the patient is unsteady. He feels as if he were walking on cotton wool, and is worse in the dark.

The term anaesthesia is generally used to describe a cutaneous area in which the sensation of touch is totally lost, while hypaesthesia implies impaired touch appreciation. Similarly, analgesia refers to absence and hypalgesia to diminution of the appreciation of painful sensations. Hyperalgesia is allegedly an increased sensitivity to painful stimuli, while hyperaesthesia is a heightened perception of touch. In fact, however, careful examination will generally reveal that in the one case the pain threshold, and in the other the touch threshold, is actually raised above normal, owing to a disorder of the pain or touch pathways. The apparent over-reaction is due to some abnormal and often unpleasant additional quality added to the primary sensation which is in itself impaired. For this reason the term hyperpathia is generally preferred to hyperalgesia, which is semantically incorrect.

Romberg's sign is an important physical sign of impaired position and joint sense in the lower limbs. The preservation of the upright position depends upon labyrinthine, cerebellar and visual postural reflexes as well as upon those reflexes whose afferent pathway is from the proprioceptors of the lower limbs. So long as the eyes are open, and even if the conduction of proprioceptive stimuli from the lower limbs is grossly impaired, the patient is able to maintain his position, but once the eyes are closed he will sway or fall. Cerebellar or labyrinthine disease will also cause the patient to sway excessively, but severe instability and a tendency to fall when eliciting this sign results only from a serious impairment of position and joint sense in the lower limbs. The same patient will show sensory ataxia when he walks. Being unsure of the position of his feet in relation to the ground, he lifts them unusually high and then bangs them down heavily (the steppage gait). He is also unsteady, and owing to loss of visual control of posture, is much more so in the dark.

Ataxia of sensory type is also apparent in the upper limbs if they are affected by similar lesions. The hands are clumsy, and fine movements cannot be performed, particularly when the hands are out of sight (e.g. fastening a button behind the back). If the affected arm is held outstretched with the eyes closed, it tends to 'wander' in space, upwards or sideways or indeed in any direction, unlike the downward drift of the limb showing motor weakness from pyramidal tract disease. Often there are also purposeless movements of the fingers, of which the patient is unaware, and these may have a writhing character (pseudoathetosis).

Abnormalities of the finer and discriminative aspects of sensibility are more difficult to assess. In a patient with a lesion of the sensory cortex, the threshold for two-point discrimination is much greater on the abnormal than on the normal side, and there may be a total inability to recognize figures or letters drawn on the skin. Sensory stimuli are also incorrectly localized on the affected side. Lesions of the parietal lobe of less severity can be demonstrated by the phenomenon of so-called sensory inattention. The patient is well able to appreciate stimuli when applied independently to the two sides of the body, but when two similar stimuli are applied simultaneously to homologous points on the skin of the two sides, one may then be ignored, a finding which implies a disturbance in function of the sensory area of the contralateral cerebral cortex. Following amputation of a limb it takes time for the brain to realize that the limb is no longer there. There is generally a clear-cut 'phantom' sensation as if the amputated part were still present and were able to move. Sometimes the phantom is painful. A phantom limb can be abolished by a lesion of the contralateral sensory cortex.

Patients with lesions of the arm area of the opposite sensory cortex may be unable to appreciate the form and texture of objects placed in the hand (stereoanaesthesia). Strictly speaking, the term astereognosis, which is often used to identify this sign, should be reserved for a failure to recognize the nature of objects when the primary sensory modalities are intact. This is an agnosic defect, due to a disorder of sensory association and akin to the other more complex disorders of parietal lobe function which were described earlier.

THE PATHOPHYSIOLOGY AND CLINICAL SIGNIFICANCE OF SENSORY ABNORMALITIES

Abnormalities of sensation may result from lesions or pathological processes affecting the peripheral nerves, the sensory roots, the spinal cord, the brain stem, the thalamus, or the sensory cortex.

Accurate identification of the sensory abnormalities which result from peripheral nerve lesions or from lesions of the brachial and lumbosacral plexuses depends upon a knowledge of the cutaneous distribution of the various peripheral nerves and of the components of the plexuses (Fig. 9.5). Section of a nerve results in a central area of sensory loss to all forms of sensation and a surrounding zone in which tactile loss is more extensive than that for pain and temperature sensation. There is considerable overlap in the cutaneous supply of the individual peripheral nerves so that section of a small cutaneous nerve may produce no definable sensory abnormality. This is even more true of the dermatomes innervated by the individual sensory roots. Although these have a strictly segmental distribution (Fig. 9.5), section of a single root does not result in any area of sensory impairment. When more than one root is interrupted, however, there is usually some cutaneous sensory loss whose distribution will clearly indicate which roots are involved. With a knowledge of the dermatomes it is relatively easy to distinguish the sensory loss resulting from a root lesion from that due to abnormality of a peripheral nerve. Associated signs of a lower motor neuron lesion can be of great value in confirming the distinction.

The sensory loss resulting from an ulnar nerve lesion affects mainly the little finger and the ulnar half of the ring finger, while that due to a disorder of the median nerve involves chiefly the thumb, the first two fingers, and the radial half of the ring finger. An ulnar nerve lesion will also give wasting of most of the small hand muscles, while median nerve damage will affect only those in the lateral part of the thenar eminence. By contrast, compression of the medial or inner cord of the brachial plexus, which can also give wasting and weakness of the small hand muscles, produces sensory impairment in the medial aspect of the arm and forearm and only occasionally in the little finger.

When multiple peripheral nerves are symmetrically involved, as in polyneuropathy, the longest sensory fibres tend to be most severely affected. Hence sensory impairment, which generally affects all forms of sensation, is most severe in the periphery of the limbs. This type of sensory impairment is often described as of 'glove and stocking' distribution. The borderline between normal and abnormal areas of sensory perception is not usually abrupt; there is generally a gradual transition. When there is widespread disease of posterior spinal roots (as in the Guillain–Barré syndrome of postinfective polyneuropathy) there is occasionally an ascending level of sensory loss which eventually involves the entire trunk and all four limbs. The condition may mimic a transverse lesion of the spinal cord, as motor paralysis is often severe. A rare variety of hereditary sensory neuropathy exists (one of the so-called acrodystrophic neuropathies) in which pain fibres are affected almost exclusively. There is peripheral insensitivity to pain, often resulting in perforating ulcers of the feet and in extensive destruction of bones and joints (*Morvan's syndrome*).

Sensory abnormalities resulting from spinal cord disease depend upon which sensory pathways are principally affected. Total transection of the spinal cord will give rise to a total loss of all forms of sensation below the dermatome level on the trunk corresponding to the segment at which the cord transection took place. Often there is a zone of so-called 'hyperaesthesia' in the skin area supplied by the segment immediately above the lesion. In hemisection of the spinal cord (the *Brown-Séquard syndrome*) there is loss of tactile discrimination, impaired touch perception, and loss of position and joint sense on the same side of the body as that on which the cord has been divided, up to the dermatome of the cord segment at which the lesion is present. There are also signs of pyramidal tract dysfunction on the same side. On the opposite side of the body there is loss of pain and temperature sensation. The sensory level for these modalities is a few segments lower, in view of the fact that pain fibres ascend in the posterior horn for a few segments before crossing to the spinothalamic tract on the opposite side.

The principal lesion of tabes dorsalis lies in the root entry zone of the posterior nerve roots. There is ascending degeneration of the posterior columns, and to a lesser extent of the spinothalamic tracts. Patients with this disease show severe sensory ataxia and there is often pain loss and impairment of deep pressure sensation over the bridge of the nose, centre of sternum, perineum and Achilles tendons, while position and joint sense and vibration sense are greatly impaired in the lower limbs. The tendon reflexes are lost owing to a break on the sensory side of the reflex arc. Similar impairment of deep reflexes in the lower limbs with other evidence of sensory neuropathy may be seen in subacute combined degeneration of the cord (combined system disease or vitamin B_{12} deficiency neuropathy), in which disease sensory ataxia is also usual and vibration and position sense are commonly lost in the lower limbs. Signs of pyramidal tract disease are also present as a rule. The cavity of syringomyelia usually damages the central grey matter of the spinal cord in the cervical region. The decussating pain and temperature fibres are interrupted, resulting in dissociated anaesthesia, i.e. loss of pain and temperature sensation, but preservation of touch and of position and joint sense. Commonly this sensory loss is unilateral, affecting the whole of one upper limb and shoulder and ending on the trunk at the midline and with a sharp lower level like the edge of a cape. As the anterior horns of the cord and the pyramidal tracts may also be compressed or invaded by the cavity, there is often wasting of upper limb muscles with loss of reflexes in the affected arm or arms and a spastic paraparesis.

Lesions of the brain stem may give sensory abnormalities which can easily be interpreted on an anatomical basis. Dissociated sensory loss in the face can result from syringobulbia, owing to involvement of the descending root of the trigeminal nerve, while lesions of the pons and medulla can give facial sensory impairment on one side (due to a lesion of the trigeminal nucleus) with hemianaesthesia and/or hemianalgesia of the trunk and limbs on the opposite side due to involvement of the ascending sensory tracts. A lesion of the upper pons or midbrain, however, can give a complete contralateral hemianaesthesia. More often such unilateral sensory loss is dissociated, involving only pain and temperature sensation, owing to selective involvement of the spinothalamic tract.

A patchy contralateral hemianaesthesia and hemianalgesia can also result from a thalamic lesion. There will often be in addition spontaneous pain of a peculiarly unpleasant and disturbing nature on the partially anaesthetic side, most frequently in the face, arm and foot. Fortunately this thalamic syndrome, which usually results from cerebral infarction, is rare.

Lesions of the sensory cortex can cause sensory jacksonian epilepsy, often taking the form of spreading paraesthesiae whose 'march' corresponds closely to the cortical anatomical 'representation' of the parts of the body (Fig. 9.4). This symptom is easy to confuse with the paraesthesiae which often occur during the aura of migraine, or during transient cerebral ischaemic attacks. Destruction of a part of the postcentral gyrus does not impair pain sensibility and affects touch very little in the corresponding part of the opposite half of the body. The appreciation of position, of tactile discrimination and localization, and of form and texture, however, is profoundly impaired. Figures written upon the skin cannot be recognized, and the threshold for two-point discrimination is raised. In a less severe cortical lesion, there may simply be tactile inattention on the affected side. Defects of recognition and interpretation of sense data which may be noted in parietal lobe lesions have already been discussed.

Hysteria must often be considered as a possible cause of sensory abnormalities discovered on clinical examination. A total hemianaesthesia affecting all modalities of sensation and even vibration sense over one half of the skull is a common hysterical manifestation. Anaesthesia of the palate or of the limbs in 'glove and stocking' distribution may also occur. Commonly such sensory loss is found in one limb only, particularly after minor injury in a compensation setting. There is usually associated hysterical weakness, and the sensory impairment often ends at the level of a joint (e.g. the elbow, shoulder, knee or hip). Unlike the findings in polyneuropathy, there is an abrupt line of demarcation between the area of complete sensory loss and that where all sensation is normal. In a patient with hysterical sensory loss it may be possible to 'find' (with suggestion) a small area within the anaesthetic region (impossible to explain on an anatomical basis) where a pin-prick is felt acutely.

Sensory examination is a technique which can only be learned by experience and which even so is full of pitfalls. Nevertheless, consistent and clear-cut sensory abnormalities can be of great value in achieving accurate anatomical localization of a lesion within the nervous system, while the precise nature and evolution of the changes may give invaluable aid in determining the character of the lesion.

PAIN

General considerations

Pain is one of the most common and disturbing of human experiences. While it can have many causes, the appreciation of painful sensations depends upon the stimulation of pain-sensitive nerve endings in the skin, muscles, skeleton, blood vessels, viscera and membranes, and upon the conduction of nerve impulses into the central nervous system where the sensation finally enters consciousness. The central pathways along which impulses conveying painful sensations travel and the effect of disease of the central nervous system upon its appreciation have been considered above. In this section a number of common neurological syndromes of which pain is a prominent symptom will be mentioned, with particular reference to the pathophysiological mechanisms involved.

Patients vary widely in their response to painful experience, some remaining relatively impassive when experiencing sensations which would produce in others an intense reaction. Although the threshold intensity of stimulus required to give the appreciation of pain (the pain threshold) is relatively constant, the reaction to painful stimuli which exceed the threshold intensity may be specific to the individual and can even vary in the same patient, depending upon circumstances.

Painful sensations: their recording and modulation

As was mentioned above, painful stimuli applied to the skin stimulate specific nociceptors, which respond to stimuli of such intensity that they 'threaten to damage the skin' (Iggo, 1985b), just as thermoreceptors respond to warm and cold stimuli. Painful sensations are then conveyed by Aδ or C fibres to the posterior horn of grey matter to synapse with interneurons. In the so-called *gate theory* of Melzack and Wall it was proposed that interneurons in the substantia gelatinosa of the spinal cord exercise a modulating effect upon sensory input before this activates the first central transmission (T) cells in the dorsal horn of the cord which in turn stimulate central mechanisms responsible for response and perception. Tonic activity in small C fibres is thought to keep open the 'gate' and to allow the onward transmission of painful sensation. Activity in large A fibres, by contrast, is essentially inhibitory and tends to close the 'gate'. The final discharge from the T cells and the perception of pain is thus dependent upon the relative activity in large and small fibres. Counter-irritation, as by scratching or rubbing, increases large fibre discharge and so reduces pain. Not all of the recent physiological evidence supports the gate theory in its entirety, but it is a useful working hypothesis (Bonica, 1986).

Wall (1985) has indeed suggested that in future we shall need to modify the classical view that nerve impulses which signify the presence of injury are reliably transmitted by specified and automatic relay cells. He suggests that at least four different modifying mechanisms may generate chronic and intractable pains, as follows:
1. With a latency of milliseconds, combinations of afferent signals and of descending controls operate a rapid and powerful gate control.
2. With a latency of minutes, impulses in C fibres change the excitability of peripheral endings and of spinal cord circuits.
3. With a latency of days, chemical transport in C fibres from areas of damage further modifies cord connectivity with the disappearance of inhibitors and an expansion of receptive fields.
4. With a latency of weeks or months, anatomical degeneration produces secondary changes in deafferented cells with atrophy, but also sprouting and abnormal firing patterns.

On the basis of this theory, so-called hyperalgesia, better called hyperpathia, can be explained by an excessive continuing stimulation of C fibres, keeping the gate open, or by a selective loss of A fibres, reducing inhibition. Similarly, the phenomenon of referred pain (see below) can be explained by central summation effects, as there is a widespread, diffuse monosynaptic input to the T cells, often from relatively distant efferents.

The role of the cerebral cortex in the perception and localization of pain remains to be considered. Cortical lesions which impair the ability to localize touch sensation similarly disrupt the faculty of localizing painful stimuli. There are few cortical neurons which show any selective response to painful stimuli. Electrical stimulation of the sensory cortex fails to evoke painful sensations, though similar stimulation of cells in the posterior or thalamus and intralaminar reticular substance may do so. The receptive fields of the latter cells are immense and would appear to be incapable of recording spatial information, even though it seems that the perception of pain occurs at this level. It is probable that the localization of painful stimuli recorded by nociceptors with high stimulus thresholds depends upon the simultaneous activation of other contiguous receptors of lower threshold which, with their central pathways, have precise localizing capabilities. In other words the ability to localize painful sensations appears to depend, at least in part, upon the fact that nociceptive stimuli such as pain invariably stimulate other nearby receptors concerned with touch. It is now thought, in addition, that the simultaneous stimulation of mechanoreceptors by noxious stimuli plays a part in pain localization. These views receive support from clinical evidence which shows that patients with lesions of the lemniscal system do not localize pain well.

Some recent developments in the neuropharmacology of pain

Many neurons concerned with pain perception possess morphine (or other opiate) receptors with which morphine and its analogues combine to produce their analgesic effects. The cells of the periaqueductal grey matter of the brain stem seem to possess many such receptors, and it is believed that this area is a principal site of action of such analgesic drugs. It is thought that the action of morphine upon neurons in this region produces analgesia by activating a descending serotoninergic system which inhibits the transmission of pain sensation in the spinal cord, but the exact mechanism of this action is still poorly understood. The brain produces its own endogenous analgesic in the form of a pentapeptide called encephalin, which has an action similar to morphine. The naturally-occurring C-fragment of β-lipotropin (also called β-endorphin) contains the encephalin sequence and has been isolated from the pituitary. It has been shown to have a particularly powerful analgesic effect when administered intraventricularly in animals. The part played by encephalin and by the endogenous ligands which are formed when it is combined with various cerebral lipoproteins in disorders of the central nervous system that produce abnormalities of pain perception remains to be clarified. However, it is now known that one important action of encephalin is to inhibit the release of substance P, which is believed to be a neurotransmitter/neuromodulator of nociceptive primary afferent neurons. In the dorsal spinal cord encephalin-containing interneurons make axoaxonic synapses with the central projections (laminae I and outer II) of these primary afferent neurons. Encephalin released from these interneurons inhibits the release of substance P from the primary afferents by presynaptic inhibition.

Types of pain and their causation

Analysis of the pain which follows cutaneous stimulation has shown that it has two components, the first immediate and the second delayed. These two forms of the sensation are probably conveyed by nerve fibres which conduct at different rates. A sensation of deep pain is also experienced after stimulation of deeper structures such as tendons, blood vessels and the periosteum. Painful lesions of the muscles or viscera sometimes give pain in the overlying skin, or else this symptom can be experienced in a cutaneous area which is comparatively remote (referred pain). Such painful sensations are felt as if they were coming not from the viscus involved but from the body surface. This apparent error in localization is systematic and not random, as the reference is always to the dermatomes innervated by the same dorsal roots that supply the diseased viscus. Afferent pain fibres from the myocardium enter the T1–T5 dorsal root ganglia, and myocardial pain is therefore referred to the anterior chest wall and down the inner aspect of the left or of both arms. Similarly, pain fibres from the diaphragm travel in the phrenic nerve (C3–C4) so that diaphragmatic pain is often referred to the C3 and C4 dermatomes in the neck and shoulder.

Many different types of lesion or pathological process can give rise to pain, through stimulation of pain-sensitive nerve endings in the diseased organ or organs. Trauma and inflammation are two of the most important causes of cutaneous pain, while pain of skeletal origin is often similarly produced. Malignant disease, including metastases in bone, can also be very painful. Visceral pain, particularly that arising in the abdominal organs, most often results from excessive contraction of smooth muscle, giving rise to the passage of pain-carrying impulses along afferent fibres accompanying sympathetic nerves. Distension of hollow organs or inflammation of their enveloping membranes (such as the peritoneum) can also be painful. In the latter case the impulses are carried by somatic afferents. Pain arising in skeletal muscle is commonly due to prolonged overactivity, cramp or fatigue, though repeated activity of a muscle with an inadequate blood supply (ischaemic work) can also be responsible. This principle applies also to cardiac muscle (angina of effort).

The sensory nerve fibres and central structures concerned in the reception and appreciation of painful stimuli are themselves sensitive to inflammation or irritation. There are a number of other pain-sensitive structures within the cranium and spinal canal. Pain is a relatively common symptom of disease of the nervous system.

HEADACHE

Headache is produced by the stimulation of pain-sensitive structures within the cranium or in the extracranial tissues of the head and neck. Sensitive structures lying extracranially include the occipital, temporal and frontal muscle groups, the skin of the scalp, the arteries which traverse the subcutaneous tissue, and the periosteum. The cranial bones themselves are insensitive. Within the skull the sensitive areas are the meninges, particularly the basal dura mater and that which forms the walls of the venous sinuses, as well as the large arteries which lie at the base of the brain, forming the circle of Willis and its branches. The greater part of the cerebral substance itself is relatively insensitive to stimuli that are normally painful if applied to appropriate receptors.

Emotional tension is one of the commonest causes of headache of extracranial origin. So-called tension headaches are characteristically occipital but sometimes frontal in location, and result from continuous partial contraction of the muscles attached to the scalp. Typically, headaches of this nature come on towards evening when the patient is tired. The posterior neck muscles are often tender and this symptom may be relieved by rest if the patient can be taught to relax properly. The headaches of so-called eye strain are probably similar in aetiology. If an uncorrected visual refractive error is present, then the continuous effort required to compensate for this defect will also result in muscular tension, giving rise to headaches which can be relieved by appropriate spectacles. Headache of purely psychogenic origin, of the type which occurs in neurotic, hypochondriacal or hysterical individuals, is often vertical in situation and is typically described in overelaborate terms, perhaps in order to impress. Not uncommonly such patients also experience true tension headaches towards the end of the day. Headaches described as being like 'a sense of pressure' or like 'a tight constricting band' are usually of this type, and depressed patients may complain of headaches occurring in the mornings, when depression is often at its worst.

Disorders of the extracranial arteries can also give rise to headache. The symptoms of migraine, a common cause of headache, to be discussed later, may be attributed in part to alterations in calibre occurring in the branches of the external carotid artery. Other 'vascular' headaches, such as those of hypertension, can probably be attributed at least in part to dilatation of extracranial rather than intracranial arteries. The pain of temporal or giant cell arteritis is also extracranial in origin, being the result of inflammatory changes in the temporal arteries. Other causes of headache which must also be considered to be in a sense extracranial are paranasal sinusitis and middle-ear disease, in which the pain results either from the increasing tension of pus in a confined space or from the spread of inflammation to the bone and its coverings.

Headache of intracranial origin is due to inflammation, compression and distortion of or traction upon the pain-sensitive meninges and blood vessels within the skull. Such headaches are usually referred to the frontal or occipital regions or both, though a unilateral lesion will sometimes produce a unilateral headache. When this is the case it can be assumed with reasonable confidence that the lesion concerned probably lies upon the side of the head where the headache is experienced.

The headache of diffuse meningeal inflammation, as in meningitis, is generally severe, continuous, unvarying and associated with neck stiffness. Like the headache of increased intracranial pressure, it is characteristically made worse by sudden movements of the head, by stooping, or by coughing and straining. Each of these mechanisms will increase the distortion of pain-sensitive structures which is already present, either through movement or through a sudden brief increase in the intracranial pressure produced by delaying the outflow of venous blood from the cranium. Typically this type of headache is throbbing in nature, due to the transmission of arterial pulsation to tissues already under increased tension. It is present as a rule on waking but tends to improve as the day wears on.

In cases of reduced intracranial pressure a headache may occur which is similar in character to that described above and due to a comparable mechanism. There is again traction upon pain-sensitive arteries and meninges. This is the basis of the post-lumbar puncture headache which is presumed to be due to continued leakage of cerebrospinal fluid through the hole in the spinal dura left by the exploring needle. The headache of dehydration has a similar cause and some believe that a clinical syndrome of intracranial hypotension, characterized by this type of headache, can occur spontaneously. Dehydration caused by the diuretic effect of alcohol probably contributes to the 'hangover' headache. A severe headache, typically of the intracranial type, may accompany coughing (benign 'cough headache'). Some such patients have emphysema and may be presumed to have an unusually large increase in intracranial pressure during coughing owing to delayed venous return to the heart. Others have no evidence of severe chest disease and in them the aetiology of the syndrome remains obscure.

Migraine

Migraine is one of the commonest neurological disorders and may at the same time be one of the most disabling. More common in women, it generally begins in adolescence or early adult life and attacks are particularly liable to occur during or just before the menstrual periods. Rarely, migrainous headaches may begin first at about the time of the menopause, usually in hypertensive women. Often there is a strong family history of the condition. It has been thought by some to occur most often in the more intelligent and industrious, though intense and obsessional, members of the community, though this view has been disputed recently. Attacks of migraine tend to be more frequent during or after episodes of overwork or emotional stress.

Migraine has been defined as a paroxysmal unilateral headache, preceded by visual and sensory phenomena and accompanied or followed by nausea and vomiting. While this is a description of a 'typical' case, there are many patients with undoubted migraine in whom no visual or sensory aura is ever experienced and in whom the headache is never one-sided. Its paroxysmal occurrence is its most important feature. Some patients experience an aura alone, without subsequent headache but with vague malaise only, in certain attacks.

The mechanism of production of the migrainous headache is now quite well understood. The initial disturbance is one of vasospasm in the extra- and intracranial arteries and their branches, often on one side of the head. This is followed some 10–30 minutes later by a dilatation of the same vessels. The arterial constriction is responsible for the symptoms of the aura, the dilatation for the headache. The aetiology of these alterations in vascular tone, however, remains obscure. There is evidence of excessive fluid retention in the body before each attack, followed by a subsequent diuresis, a finding which raises the possibility of a metabolic or endocrine cause. There is no evidence that allergy or a disorder of the autonomic nervous system is responsible. Biochemical studies have demonstrated an increased urinary excretion of 5-hydroxyindolacetic acid (5-HIAA) during attacks, suggesting an intermittent release of 5-hydroxytryptamine (serotonin) into the circulation, and other evidence suggests a possible role of prostaglandins in the attacks. Paroxysmal headaches of migrainous type can be a prominent symptom in patients harbouring intracranial arteriovenous angiomas or even aneurysms, but in these individuals the headache is usually strictly unilateral, occurring on the same side of the head as the vascular anomaly. The reason for this association is not known.

Usually the migrainous attack begins soon after waking in the morning. A visual aura is the most common first symptom, resulting from spasm of the retinal arteries or of branches of the posterior cerebral artery supplying one or both occipital lobes. The patient will then experience a hemianopic field defect, a less well-defined scotoma, or, rarely, transient blindness, jagged lines, or bright dancing or shimmering lights in one half-field. Alternatively a sensory aura may occur with paraesthesiae in the corner of the mouth and in the arm, or less commonly in the leg on the same side, presumably due to spasm of those branches of the middle cerebral artery which supply the sensory cortex. In occasional patients the aura (vertigo, diplopia, bilateral paraesthesiae) suggests that the hindbrain rather than the forebrain circulation is involved (basilar artery migraine), and sometimes fainting occurs either during the aura or at the height of the headache. Very rarely there is actual transient weakness of one arm and leg (hemiplegic migraine) or a paresis of one oculomotor nerve (ophthalmoplegic migraine).

As the aura passes off, the headache usually begins and mounts in intensity. The headache can be unilateral and frontal (above one of the eyes), bifrontal, bioccipital or generalized. Sometimes it is comparatively mild, though accompanied by lassitude and depression, but more often it is prostrating, and there is photophobia, so that the patient must lie down in a darkened room. Typically the headache will last all day, passing off after a night's sleep, but sometimes it wanes in an hour or two. Less often, the headache can persist, though declining in severity, for several days. Characteristically the headache is accompanied by nausea and sometimes by vomiting. The condition tends to improve as the patient approaches middle age and to disappear at the menopause, but the form which first develops in postmenopausal women may be particularly intractable.

Periodic migrainous neuralgia
There are some patients who experience episodes of severe and continuous pain, often burning in character, in, around or behind one eye or in the cheek, forehead and temple. These attacks accur in bouts lasting a few weeks or months, and during a bout the patient suffers one or several attacks, lasting from 15 minutes to several hours, each day. Not uncommonly the attacks recur at the same time of day or night and may waken the patient from sleep. There is often suffusion of the conjunctiva and blocking of the nostril on the affected side during the attacks. The aetiology of this condition, which has been variously referred to as histamine headache, ciliary neuralgia or cluster headache, is unknown, but it has certain affinities with migraine and is probably best referred to as periodic migrainous neuralgia. Not only may typical attacks be reproduced in susceptible individuals by injections of histamine, but they are often precipitated by the ingestion of alcohol.

FACIAL PAIN

Pain in the face is a common symptom which may be difficult to understand and interpret. It sometimes results from obvious local causes such as sinusitis, neoplasia, dental disease, or parotitis. It can also be due to a variety of pathological lesions involving the trigeminal nerve and its branches and central connections. A plaque of demyelination or a syrinx (cavity) in the brain stem may give a continuous unilateral facial ache through irritation of the central connections of the trigeminus, as may a tumour or aneurysm which is compressing the gasserian ganglion or the sensory root of the fifth cranial nerve. Similarly, herpes zoster of the gasserian ganglion, which tends to affect particularly the ophthalmic division of the nerve, gives severe and continuous pain in the eye and forehead. Even more frequent, however, are the syndromes of intermittent facial pain, including trigeminal neuralgia and atypical facial neuralgia. Pain provoked by the taking of hot or cold foods or liquids is almost invariably of dental origin, while the pain of paranasal sinusitis is often accentuated by stooping and there may be local tenderness over the affected sinus.

Trigeminal neuralgia (tic douloureux)
Trigeminal neuralgia is an intermittent, brief, lancinating pain in the face, confined to the area of cutaneous distribution of one trigeminal nerve, and often evoked by movement of the face or by touching the skin. It is equally common in the two sexes and is most commonly seen after middle age, particularly in the elderly.

The aetiology of the 'idiopathic' form of the syndrome is becoming clearer. Its increasing incidence in the elderly once gave rise to the suggestion that ischaemia of the trigeminal nerve or ganglion, resulting from atherosclerosis, was the principal cause, but comparatively few cases were studied pathologically and no consistent histological changes were demonstrated. More recently, however, it has become apparent that in many syndromes of paroxysmal cranial nerve dysfunction, including hemifacial spasm and glossopharyngeal neuralgia (see below), as well as tic douloureux, the principal cause is one of compression of the trunk of the nerve, usually in the subarachnoid space, produced by an artery, sometimes aberrant, which may actually groove the nerve trunk.

The pain of tic douloureux is typically sudden, excruciating and brief, 'like the stab of a red-hot needle'. A continuous pain in the face, or one lasting for several minutes, is not tic douloureux, though some patients experience a background of dull aching between the paroxysms. The pain does not extend outside the territory supplied by the trigeminal nerve, nor does it cross the midline. It can occur in the distribution of any one or all of the divisions of the trigeminus. If the ophthalmic division alone is involved, this syndrome is often referred to as supraorbital neuralgia. The intensity of the pain can be judged from the apparently involuntary spasm of the facial muscles on the affected side and the agonized expression which often accompany each attack. The patient commonly holds one hand in front of the face to protect it and will not allow it to be touched, as he knows that movement, as in speaking, chewing, touching the face, or in shaving or washing, may provoke an attack. Neurological examination is rarely informative, though a few patients have very slight objective diminution of sensory perception on the affected side of the face.

Characteristically, tic douloureux is a periodic disorder. It tends to occur in bouts lasting for several weeks or months, during which the pain occurs with variable frequency and severity. Long remissions of weeks, months or even years may separate the bouts, but these remissions tend to become progressively shorter. The condition, though intensely distressing, is essentially benign, and does not shorten life, though some few patients were in the past driven to suicide to find relief from their agony. Fortunately, many patients respond to treatment with carbamazepine, but in unresponsive cases it was usual in the past to employ alcohol injection of the gasserian ganglion or neurosurgical division of the trigeminal sensory root at the expense of permanent facial anaesthesia. Now surgical decompression of the sensory root in the posterior fossa at the point where it is being compressed by a blood vessel is being used increasingly and usually affords a permanent and uncomplicated cure.

Atypical facial neuralgia
This condition, seen most often in young or middle-aged women, is characterized by continuous, dull, aching pain on one side of the face, usually in the region of the upper jaw. Typically the pain is unvarying throughout the day and often persists for months or years. Most affected individuals are chronically anxious, hypochondriacal or depressed and the condition often responds to treatment with a combination of antidepressive and tranquillizing remedies.

GLOSSOPHARYNGEAL NEURALGIA

This rare condition resembles trigeminal neuralgia in many respects, as the pain occurs in periodic bouts and is brief and lancinating in character. It occurs in the tonsillar fossa, the back of the throat, and the larynx, and may radiate to the ear on the affected side. Swallowing is the stimulus most likely to produce the pain. As mentioned above, it is most often due to vascular compression or irritation of the intracranial trunk of the nerve. Like trigeminal neuralgia it may respond to carbamazepine, but if intractable it can be cured by decompression or division of the affected glossopharyngeal nerve in the posterior fossa.

PAIN IN THE SPINAL COLUMN AND LIMBS

There are many skeletal and ligamentous lesions which can produce pain in the spinal column; some lesions involving nervous tissues also cause pain in this location. Diffuse inflammatory conditions such as ankylosing spondylitis, or metabolic disorders producing osteoporosis, may give dull, aching pain involving the greater part of the spine, while osteomyelitis of a vertebral body or a metastasis in one or more vertebrae gives severe and continuous pain which is localized to the affected site. As a secondary effect of these conditions, distortion and deformity of the bony architecture can occur, resulting in compression of the spinal cord (this is in general painless) or spinal roots (giving pain in the distribution of the root concerned). Similarly, lesions of the spinal cord and its roots, whether they be intramedullary, intrathecal or extradural, can irritate or compress sensory fibres or nerve roots, producing similar pain. A neoplasm such as a neurofibroma which begins by producing pain due simply to compression of its parent spinal root, may later grow sufficiently large to erode the bone of the vertebral body, giving a dull continuous 'skeletal' type of pain in the affected spinal area. Root irritation often produces a 'protective' spasm of the overlying spinal muscles which may itself be painful, while the muscles concerned become tender. Voluntary contraction of these muscles will then increase the pain, as will nervous tension.

NERVE AND NERVE-ROOT COMPRESSION

When nerve fibres or trunks concerned with the transmission of pain-carrying impulses are compressed or irritated, whether in the spinal cord, spinal roots or peripheral nerves, a characteristically intolerable, continuous, burning pain is produced. If fibres concerned with touch and proprioception run in the same nerve, then associated paraesthesiae (tingling, numbness, pins and needles) also occur. Some of these features may be due to direct nerve compression, others to ischaemia. Paradoxically, vasodilatation due to warmth can so increase the volume of the tissues which are compressing the nerve, or the nerve itself, that its effective blood supply is further reduced and the pain is made worse, while excessive cold, resulting in vasoconstriction, will also increase ischaemia and hence the symptoms. Pain due to peripheral nerve compression is referred to the cutaneous area from which the nerve concerned receives sensory fibres (projected pain). Root pain radiates throughout the dermatome of the root concerned, but it is less well recognized that deep muscular pain due to the same cause may be more widespread, corresponding broadly to the muscles supplied by the homologous motor root. Root pain has other special characteristics. It is affected by sudden movements of the spinal column which would be likely to cause movement of the root, or of the pathological lesion which is compressing or irritating it. A sudden increase in cerebrospinal fluid pressure, as in coughing or straining, will cause a sharp, shooting paroxysm of pain in the appropriate distribution. When symptoms of this type are of long standing, the trunks of peripheral nerves which contribute to the sensory root or roots involved often become tender on pressure.

CAUSALGIA

Causalgia is the name given to a particularly unpleasant burning type of continuous pain which may follow peripheral nerve injuries, or root lesions, particularly those in which severance of a nerve has been incomplete and in which some regeneration has occurred. This type of pain is most common in the hand and arm but does occur occasionally in the leg. It is most frequent after lesions of the median nerve. The skin area in which this spontaneous pain occurs in usually shiny and the seat of excessive perspiration. The patient will not allow the skin to be touched as this greatly accentuates the pain. Although the exact mechanism of this syndrome is not fully understood, it is clear that autonomic pathways play an important role as blocking or section of somatic sensory nerves from the skin area concerned does not relieve the pain, but sympathectomy is usually effective.

PHANTOM-LIMB PAIN

After amputation of a limb (or removal of an ear or some other member), sensations may be experienced for several months or years, suggesting that the part concerned is still in situ. Not infrequently, pain of a curiously unpleasant and intolerable nature, resembling causalgia in many respects, develops in the phantom member. Usually such patients are found to have plexiform neuromas in the amputation stump, resulting from regeneration of fibres from the severed ends of peripheral nerves, and digital compression of such a neuroma will often reproduce the patient's spontaneous pain. Repeated percussion or sometimes excision of the neuroma may relieve the pain.

POSTHERPETIC NEURALGIA

Pain in the distribution of the affected root, whether it be the ophthalmic division of the trigeminus, or one or more cervical, dorsal or lumbar posterior roots, is a striking feature of herpes zoster. In younger patients the pain generally resolves within a few weeks at the most, but in the elderly a severe continuous burning pain may persist for years afterwards. It seems that this pain must depend upon the reception of sensory stimuli from the skin area concerned, since in the early stages it can sometimes be relieved by subcutaneous infiltration with a local anaesthetic agent. Relief from these measures is only temporary, and it seems that a progressive facilitation of synapses occurs in the central nervous system with opening of the 'gate' due to selective damage to inhibitory A fibres. Eventually the pain continues to occur apparently spontaneously, despite division of the peripheral pathways. The pain may be so intolerable that some patients are driven to suicide.

THALAMIC PAIN

A lesion of the thalamus (usually an infarct) may be the cause of severe pain in the contralateral face, arm and leg. So-called thalamic pain is intense, burning and continuous in character and has other peculiarly unpleasant qualities, often described by the patient with such adjectives as 'tearing' or 'grinding'. Typically it is felt around the angle of the mouth and cheek and in the affected hand and foot. Pain of this type is fortunately rare as it is relatively unaffected by any but the most powerful analgesics.

References

Bickerstaff, E. R. (1981) *Neurological Examination in Clinical Practice*, 4th edn. Oxford: Blackwell Scientific Publications.

Bonica, J. J. (ed.) (1980) *Pain* (ARNMD Research Publications, vol. 58). New York: Raven Press.

Bonica, J. J. (1986) Pain. In Walton, J., Beeson, P. B. and Bodley Scott, R. (eds) *Oxford Companion to Medicine*. Oxford: Oxford University Press.

Dalessio, D. J. (1980) *Wolff's Headache and Other Head Pain*, 4th edn. Oxford: Oxford University Press.

Dostrovsky, J. O. and Deakin, J. F. W. (1977) Periaqueductal grey lesions reduce morphine analgesia in the rat. *Neuroscience Letters* **4**:99.

Feldberg, W. and Smyth, D. G. (1977) C-fragment of lipoprotein—an endogenous potent analgesic peptide. *Br. J. Pharmacol.* **60**:445.

Gardner, E. (1975) *Fundamentals of Neurology*, 6th edn. Philadelphia: W. B. Saunders Company.

Head, H. (1920) *Studies in Neurology*. Oxford: Oxford University Press.

Holmes, G. (1968) *Introduction to Clinical Neurology*, 3rd edn, revised by W. B. Matthews. Edinburgh: Churchill Livingstone.

Iggo, A. (1985a) Cutaneous sensations. In Swash, M. and Kennard, C. (eds) *Scientific Basis of Clinical Neurology*. Edinburgh: Churchill Livingstone.

Iggo, A. (1985b) Sensory receptors in the skin of mammals and their sensory functions. *Rev. Neurol.* (Paris) **10**:599.

Kuffler, S. W. and Nicholls, J. C. (1976) *From Neuron to Brain*. Sunderland, Mass: Sinauer Associates.

Lance, J. W. (1982) *The Mechanism and Management of Headache*, 4th edn. London: Butterworth.

Mayo Clinic, Section of Neurology (1981) *Clinical Examinations in Neurology*, 5th edn. Philadelphia: W. B. Saunders Company.

Melzack, R. (1973) *The Puzzle of Pain*. Harmondsworth, Middlesex: Penguin Education.

Melzack, R. and Wall, P. D. (1965) Pain mechanisms: a new theory. *Science* **150**:971.

Mountcastle, V. B. (1974) Neural mechanisms in somesthesia. In Mountcastle, V. B. (ed.) *Medical Physiology*. St. Louis: C. V. Mosby, 1974.

Noordenbos, W. (1968) Physiological correlates of pain syndromes. In Soulairac, A., Cahn, J. and Charpentier, J. (eds) *Pain*. London and New York: Academic Press.

Patton, H. D., Sundsten, J. W., Crill, W. E. and Swanson, P. D. (1976) *Introduction to Basic Neurology*. Philadelphia: W. B. Saunders Company.

Pearce, J. (1969) *Migraine: Clinical Features, Mechanisms and Management*. Springfield, Ill: Charles C. Thomas.

Ruch, T. C. (1979) Neural basis of somatic sensation. In Ruch, T. C. and Patton, H. D. (eds) *Physiology and Biophysics*, 20th edn. Philadelphia: W. B. Saunders Company.

Sunderland, S (1968) *Nerves and Nerve Injuries*. Edinburgh: Churchill Livingstone.

Wall, P. D. (1985) Future trends in pain research. In Iggo, A., Iversen, L. L. and Cervero, F. (eds.) Nociception and pain. *Phil. Trans. R. Soc.* **B308**:217.

Walton, J. N. (1985) *Brain's Diseases of the Nervous System*, 9th edn. Oxford: Oxford University Press.

10

CEREBRAL METABOLISM AND ITS DISORDERS

INTRODUCTION

Many specific diseases, symptom complexes and syndromes result from alterations in the chemical composition or metabolic activity of the brain or of other parts of the central or peripheral nervous system. Some of these, as in the many inborn errors of metabolism which primarily involve the nervous system, give rise to the storage of abnormal metabolites within neurons, glial cells, axons and/or myelin. Many such disorders are then accompanied by recognizable morphological abnormalities which can be identified histologically or ultrastructurally. Disorders of neuronal, glial or myelin structure and metabolism are sometimes classified as primary or endogenous metabolic encephalopathies. By contrast, abnormal function of the central and/or peripheral nervous system may result from an extracerebral disorder which affects the brain only indirectly. These disorders, which are called secondary or exogenous metabolic encephalopathies, include anoxia, ischaemia, hypoglycaemia, deficiencies of vitamin cofactors, liver disease, renal failure, endocrine dysfunction, diabetes, cancer, porphyria, toxic disorders due to infection, abnormalities of fluids, electrolytes, or the acid–base environment of the nervous system, and syndromes due to a wide variety of drugs and exogenous poisons. Many of the primary metabolic encephalopathies cause dementia. The secondary encephalopathies are more often characterized, at least initially, by disordered consciousness, leading to confusion, delirium, stupor or coma. In each group there may be many other additional manifestations of neurological disease, depending upon which components of the nervous system are predominantly affected. In this chapter a number of pathophysiological principles will first be outlined, and will be followed by a brief commentary upon the commoner and more important metabolic and deficiency states which produce major neurological manifestations.

SOME GENERAL PRINCIPLES

The pathophysiology of the cerebral circulation was described in chapter 1. In the resting state the brain receives about 15% of the cardiac output, i.e. about 55 ml of blood/100 g brain tissue/min. This provides the brain with about 3.5 ml of O_2/100 g brain tissue/min and about 5.5 mg (0.31 mM) glucose/100 g/min, the latter being carried across the blood–brain barrier by a process of active transport. When the haemoglobin content of the blood falls below about 8 g/dl, cerebral blood flow must increase to maintain an adequate oxygen supply to the brain. Even if the haemoglobin is normal, a fall in the cerebral blood flow to about half the normal value results in the oxygen supply being adequate to maintain normal cerebral metabolism, and consciousness is lost. When the P_{aO_2} value falls below 50 mmHg for whatever cause, delirium occurs, and at a figure of 25 mmHg coma ensues. If the blood glucose concentration falls below 30 mg/dl (1.66 mM/l), confusion develops, and at a level of 10–15 mg/dl (0.56–0.83 mM/l) the result is usually coma. Under aerobic conditions about 85% of the glucose which is the brain's principal energy supply is metabolized in the presence of oxygen to water, CO_2 and energy, and the remainder produces lactic acid. Lactic acid accumulates in excess in anaerobic conditions and, unlike glucose, is incapable of maintaining neuronal function.

In addition to glucose and oxygen, the brain requires amino acids to form peptides and proteins, lipids to form myelin, electrolytes to maintain impulse generation and transmission within neurons and their axons, and a variety of biogenic amines to form transmitter substances concerned with synaptic transmission (see p. 15). Energy derived from oxidative metabolism helps in maintaining the sodium pump, and a fine balance of extra- and intracellular electrolytes (especially Na and K) is needed for the generation and transmission of action potentials. Alterations in the extracellular sodium concentration, or partial replacement of this ion by another such as lithium, can cause confusion, delirium or even coma. Many disorders of behaviour and/or consciousness have been shown to result from overdosage with the many psychotropic drugs which mimic, potentiate or inhibit the activity of the various biogenic amines that fulfil a transmitter function in the nervous system. There is still some dispute as to whether cortical neurons or those of the reticular substance are the more sensitive to diminution in oxygen and/or glucose supply. Different groups of neurons demonstrate varying sensitivity and/or resistance to such influences, but other factors, including local cerebral blood flow and variations in energy requirements under different conditions, are also of importance. The situation is complex and in the present state of knowledge generalizations are invalid.

THE PATHOLOGICAL SUBSTRATE OF CEREBRAL METABOLIC DISORDERS

In patients dying in a state of severe delirium of relatively brief duration, few if any pathological changes may be demonstrable in the brain. More prolonged dysfunction lasting for hours or days may, however, result in recognizable physical changes. And total circulatory failure, as in cardiac arrest, can produce irreversible anoxic damage within a few minutes. Anoxia, ischaemia and hypoglycaemia first produce mitochondrial swelling in neuronal cytoplasm, a change which is probably reversible. This is followed by dissolution of the Nissl substance, nuclear shrinkage, and pallor of the affected cells (changes which are irreversible), leading on to necrosis and neuronophagia. These changes are maximal in the cortex, in the neurons of Ammon's horn of the hippocampus, in the globus pallidus, and in the Purkinje cells of the cerebellum. Later there may be demyelination in cerebral subcortical white matter. The brain stem and spinal cord are relatively resistant to these influences. The cerebellar Purkinje cells are peculiarly sensitive to the effects of hypoglycaemia, so that many survivors from severe hypoglycaemic insults are rendered ataxic.

In many of the secondary metabolic encephalopathies (such as those of uraemia, hyponatraemia or CO_2 narcosis), diffuse brain swelling is usual, and light-microscopic and ultrastructural studies of brain sections reveal marked interstitial oedema of both grey and white matter. In hepatic encephalopathy, the presence of enlarged and multilobular astrocytes in the cortex and basal ganglia is a characteristic finding, while in many of the toxic encephalopathies perivascular infiltrates of inflammatory cells are found.

The peripheral nerves as well as the central nervous system are susceptible to many metabolic insults. Axonal damage and primary or secondary demyelination may each be found, depending upon the cause. Many of the metabolic neuropathies (such as those due to deficiencies of vitamins B_1 or B_{12} or to uraemia or porphyria), are predominantly axonal in type, though secondary demyelination may appear later. In diabetic neuropathy demyelination is usually more prominent from the outset.

Of the many inborn errors of metabolism, there are a number of so-called storage diseases (including the many lipidoses and mucopolysaccharidoses) in which neuronal perikarya become ballooned with abnormal metabolites, producing characteristic histological and ultrastructural appearances. Special histochemical stains of these cells may be diagnostic. There are other genetic diseases (such as metachromatic leucodystrophy) in which there is either dysmyelination or destruction or degeneration of myelin in the cerebral white matter and often also in peripheral nerves, due again to the accumulation of abnormal substances.

THE BIOCHEMICAL SUBSTRATE OF CEREBRAL METABOLIC DISORDERS

I propose to consider successively disorders of carbohydrate, nucleic acid, amino acid, and protein and lipid metabolism, underlining the major biochemical mechanisms involved. The rare inherited syndromes will be tabulated briefly, highlighting those disorders of greater clinical importance. Finally, some of the commoner deficiency states and other toxic and metabolic disorders in which the nervous system is often involved will be considered.

Carbohydrate metabolism and its disorders

Glucose is the principal source of energy in the nervous system. The enzymes hexokinase and phosphofructokinase which are concerned in its breakdown are present in high concentration in neurons, the latter especially being influenced in its activity by concentrations of cyclic AMP, phosphate, ammonium ion and citrate, which assist in controlling the metabolic requirements of the cells. The glucose-6-phosphate formed after glucose enters the cell is mainly converted to fructose-6-phosphate, but about 5% of the glucose is metabolized through the pentose phosphate cycle. The glycogen content of brain (6.2 μmol/kg) is considerably lower than that of many other tissues such as skeletal muscle, and at present little is known of the function and method of breakdown of cerebral glycogen.

Among the commoner clinical disorders of cerebral carbohydrate metabolism are hypoglycaemia, whether due to the administration of insulin or to organic hyperinsulinism as in islet cell adenoma of the pancreas, and the hyperglycaemia of diabetes mellitus. Excess circulating glucose may be converted to sorbitol which, with its metabolite fructose, can exert an osmotic effect in brain tissue, causing cerebral oedema and coma. Spontaneous hypoglycaemia can give rise to abnormal behaviour, confusion, convulsions and coma, and if not rapidly reversed, irreversible brain damage. The effects of dietary deficiency of thiamine (vitamin B_1), an essential cofactor in carbohydrate metabolism, will be discussed later, along with the other deficiency disorders. Among the rare inherited abnormalities of carbohydrate metabolism are the glycogen storage diseases, most of which affect clinically the liver and/or skeletal and cardiac muscle, though some involve the brain, producing hypoglycaemia and seizures. In progressive myoclonic epilepsy (Lafora body disease), cerebral and especially cerebellar dentate neurons contain PAS-positive inclusions, representing the storage within the affected neurons of a product of carbohydrate metabolism which reacts histochemically as if it were a protein-bound mucopolysaccharide but which proves on chemical analysis to be a glucose polymer (polyglucosan) linked in the 1,4 and 1,6 positions, which is chemically, but not structurally, related to glycogen. There are also many other neuronal disorders, most of which are associated with mental retardation, in which a variety of mucopolysaccharides are stored in the affected cells, and heparan, dermatan, keratan or chondroitin sulphate are excreted in the urine. All but one (Hunter's disease, an X-linked recessive trait) are of autosomal recessive inheritance. The glycogen storage diseases and other rare inherited disorders of carbohydrate metabolism are tabulated in Table 10 and the mucopolysaccharidoses in Table 11. Some of the latter are closely associated with certain lipid storage diseases classified in Table 14.

SUBACUTE NECROTIZING ENCEPHALOMYELOPATHY (LEIGH'S DISEASE)

This autosomal recessive disorder is associated with raised blood pyruvate levels and a metabolic acidosis. It is due to a deficiency of pyruvate carboxylase, the enzyme which converts pyruvate to oxalacetate, but in some cases this enzyme is normal and it now appears that different enzymatic defects may be responsible in different cases. Biochemically pyruvate and lactic acidaemia are relatively constant. An inhibitor which blocks the synthesis of thiamine triphosphate has been identified in blood, urine and CSF. Pathologically the brains of affected individuals show widespread cellular necrosis with capillary proliferation in the optic nerves and chiasm, basal ganglia and brain stem, thus resembling the changes of Wernicke's disease (see below), although the corpora mamillaria are spared. Clinically the affected children show failure to thrive, poverty of movement, hypotonia and spasticity, loss of tendon reflexes, nystagmus and optic atrophy. Convulsions sometimes occur and the condition is usually fatal in 6–12 months. Occasionally less severe cases occur in adolescence and even in adult life.

Nucleic acid metabolism and its disorders

In neurons, messenger RNA is produced by transcription from a nuclear DNA template, and in the cytoplasm it is contained mainly in ribosomes which form the Nissl substance seen on light microscopy. The principal building blocks of nucleic acids are pyrimidines and purines, but the brain, unlike many other tissues, seems to be incapable of synthesizing pyrimidines from CO_2 and glutamine. Rather, it appears to convert uridine to uridine monophosphate (UMP) and then to uridine triphosphate (UTP) and cytidine triphosphate (CTP), all of which are important in nucleic acid, lipid and mucopolysaccharide metabolism. Similarly there is salvage synthesis of purine nucleotides, especially in the basal ganglia, where guanine and hypoxanthine are converted to their corresponding nucleotide derivatives.

In the rare clinical syndrome of hereditary orotic aciduria, due to combined deficiencies of orotidine-5'-phosphate decarboxylase and pyrophosphorylase, enzymes which are concerned in the synthesis of pyrimidines from CO_2 and glutamine, neurological abnormalities do not occur. The disorder gives rise to growth retardation and a megaloblastic bone

TABLE 11. Glycogen storage diseases and some other inherited disorders of carbohydrate metabolism*

Disease	Enzyme defect	Clinical manifestations
Glycogen storage diseases		
O Glycogen synthetase deficiency	Glycogen synthetase	Hypoglycaemia, convulsions
I von Gierke's disease	Glucose-6-phosphatase	Hypoglycaemia, convulsions
II Pompe's disease	Acid maltase (amylo-1-4-glucosidase)	Severe infantile myopathy and cardiomegaly or subacute adult myopathy
III Debranching enzyme deficiency (Cori)	Amylo-1-6-glucosidase Amylo-1,4-1,4-glucan transferase	Mild hypoglycaemia, convulsions Mild myopathy, cardiac failure
IV Branching enzyme deficiency (Anderson)	Amylo-1,4-1,6-transglycolase	Hypotonia, hepatic failure
V McArdle's disease	Muscle phosphorylase	Muscle pain on exertion, cramps, myoglobinuria, contracture, subacute myopathy in adults
VI Hers' disease	Hepatic phosphorylase	Mild hypoglycemia (as in von Gierke's disease)
VII Muscle phosphofructokinase deficiency	Muscle phosphofructokinase	Identical with McArdle's disease
VIII Phosphohexoisomerase inhibitor deficiency	Phosphohexoisomerase inhibitor	Identical with McArdle's disease
IX Hepatic phosphorylase kinase deficiency	Hepatic phosphorylase kinase (X-linked or autosomal recessive)	Mild hepatomegaly
X Muscle phosphorylase kinase deficiency	Muscle phosphorylase kinase	Similar to McArdle's disease of late onset
Other disorders of carbohydrate metabolism		
Fructose intolerance (fructosuria)	Fructose-1-phosphate aldolase	Hypoglycaemia, mental retardation
Idiopathic leucine-induced hypoglycaemia	? Pancreatic leucine sensitivity	Hypoglycaemia, mental retardation
Galactosaemia	Galactose-1-phosphate uridyl transferase	Cataract, mental retardation

* Modified from Appel, 1977.

TABLE 12. The mucopolysaccharidoses*

Disease	Enzyme defect	Clinical features
Hurler's (gargoylism)	α-L-iduronidase	Mental retardation, distinctive facial appearance, corneal opacities, skeletal deformities, hepatosplenomegaly
Hunter's	Iduronosulphate sulphatase	Moderate retardation, skeletal abnormalities, deafness, no corneal clouding, hepatosplenomegaly
Sanfilippo's	Type A Heparan N-sulphatase B α-N-acetylglucosaminidase C α-glucosaminidase	Severe retardation, mild skeletal abnormalities, mild hepatosplenomegaly
Morquio's	N-acetyl galactosamine-6-sulphatase	No retardation, severe skeletal changes with epiphyseal dysplasia
Scheie's	α-L-iduronidase	No retardation, mild skeletal changes, severe corneal opacities
Maroteaux-Lamy	H-acetyl galactosamine-4-sulphatase	No retardation, severe skeletal changes, corneal opacities, moderate hepatosplenomegaly
Mannosidosis	α-Mannosidase	Retardation, corneal opacity, hepatosplenomegaly
Fucosidosis	α-Fucosidase	Severe retardation, progressive dementia, paresis, rigidity of limbs
I-cell disease (sialidosis type 2, see Table 14)	? Increased lysosomal enzymes	Severe mental retardation; similar to Hurler's disease

* Modified from Appel, 1977.

marrow correctable by the administration of uridine. This fact gives some support to the view that the brain depends more upon the conversion of uridine to UMP.

The Lesch–Nyhan syndrome is a rare X-linked disorder. Affected boys show mild to moderate mental retardation and choreoathetosis, usually beginning in the second year of life, followed by the development of spastic tetraparesis. A typical unexplained feature is self-mutilation leading often to progressive destruction of the digits. The condition is due to a deficiency of hypoxanthine-guanine phosphoribosyl transferase. The serum uric acid is raised, and the urinary uric acid:creatinine ratio is usually greater than 2. The pathogenesis of the neurological disorder has not been established, although the administration of methyl xanthines may cause self-mutilation in rats. Allopurinol may reduce the hyperuricaemia but does not produce clinical improvement.

Amino acid and protein metabolism and their disorders

Some amino acids are synthesized within the neurons themselves; others enter from the blood. The brain possesses a number of preferential transport systems for neutral, acidic and basic amino acids. The role of the blood–brain barrier and the processes which control the influx and efflux of amino acids into and out of neurons are not well understood. It is known that glutamate, lysine, leucine and proline do not increase within neurons even when their blood levels rise; tyrosine, glutamine, methionine and phenylalanine do so. Glutamic acid, glutamine, aspartic acid and gamma-aminobutyric acid (GABA), which is formed by the decarboxylation of glutamate, are the principal free amino acids of the brain. The role of many of these substances which act as excitatory or inhibitory neurotransmitters at different levels of the nervous system was considered earlier (p. 19). GABA, for instance, is found only in the brain and spinal cord and not in other tissues. It appears to modulate intracellular activity and to act as a natural anticonvulsant in the central nervous system. The decarboxylated amine derivatives of 5-hydroxytryptophan and of dihydroxyphenylalanine, namely 5-hydroxytryptamine (serotonin) and dopamine respectively, are other important transmitter substances, as is glycine.

Brain tissue demonstrates a striking ability to synthesize proteins from amino acids, especially during infancy and childhood. This fact presumably explains at least in part the powerful adverse influence of protein-calorie malnutrition upon cerebral development and ultimate brain size in childhood. Even in adult life there is evidence that a substantial synthetic capacity persists. Although this is largely centred upon cytoplasmic polyribosomes, proteins are also formed in nuclei, mitochondria, axons and presynaptic terminals in both the central and peripheral nervous systems.

In both the brain and peripheral nerves, a number of specific proteins have been identified which may be altered as a result of disease. Neurotubules, corresponding to the microtubules found in the cells of other tissues, are found in the perikarya of neurons but more particularly in axonal processes in both the central and peripheral nervous systems. Neurofilaments are present in both axons and dendrites. The neurotubules in particular play an important role in the axoplasmic flow of proteins, and the protein 'neurotubulin' has two subunits, differing slightly in amino acid composition. Drugs such as colchicine and vincristine bind to neurotubular protein, interrupt axoplasmic flow, and may cause polyneuropathy. The protein composition of neurofilaments is now known to differ from that of the neurotubules, but the composition and function of these structures are still incompletely understood. However, recent work using monoclonal antibodies raised against neurofilaments has shown that these label a subpopulation of dorsal root ganglion neurons, and other neuronal somata so labelled have been found in the Gasserian (trigeminal) ganglion, vagal ganglia and the mesencephalic nucleus of the fifth nerve (all primary afferent neurons derived either completely or partially from the neural crest) (Lawson et al., 1984). This antibody has also been used to study the 'axon reaction' in motor and sensory neurons which follows peripheral nerve division (Moss and Lewkowicz, 1983). It is known that neurofilamentous proliferation produces the argyrophilic neurofibrillary tangles that occur in many cortical neurons with progressive ageing and are especially prominent and widespread in Alzheimer's disease. They can also be produced experimentally by the administration of aluminium.

Two other acidic proteins are also found in high concentration in brain tissue: the S-100 protein, which is presumed to be of glial origin and which is present in high concentration in experimentally induced astrocytomas, and the 14–3–2 protein, which is thought to be of neuronal origin, being found in excess in cultures of neuroblastoma cells. The functions of these two proteins are as yet unknown.

Myelin contains three different classes of protein. One class, a basic protein whose amino acid composition is now fully characterized, is the myelin fraction which can produce experimental allergic encephalomyelitis (encephalitogenic factor, or EF) and which constitutes about 30% of myelin protein.

The other two protein components are both conjugated with lipid, namely a proteolipid with a high content of neutral and aromatic amino acids (50–60% of myelin protein) and an acidic proteolipid (10–20%).

There are few, if any, specific disorders of cerebral metabolism demonstrably due to, or associated with, specific abnormalities of cerebral protein concentration. There are now many disorders, mainly of autosomal recessive inheritance, which have been recognized to be associated with the excretion of abnormal amounts of various amino acids in the urine. Most of these are associated with mental retardation and/or other profound abnormalities of cerebral development or function, presumably because the enzyme defects involved impair amino acid transport or activation, thus affecting peptide assembly, protein synthesis and neuronal function. Many of these disorders can now be recognized by means of specific biochemical tests, and several can be effectively controlled by the early institution of appropriate dietary restrictions. The principal aminoacidurias and their effects are summarized in Table 12, and in Table 13 the clinical effects of many of the aminoacidurias giving rise to symptoms in the neonatal period and early infancy are compared with those of some other inborn errors of metabolism which have already been mentioned (Adams and Lyon, 1982).

Lipid metabolism and its disorders

There is a high concentration of lipids in the nervous system, about half being present in myelin, the remainder being located mainly in plasma membranes and intracellular membranes. Many structural lipids are present in a static state, and lipid metabolism, especially of cholesterol, cerebrosides, ethanolamine, phospholipids and sphingomyelin is slow, although the turnover of phosphatidylcholine and of phosphatidylinositol is much more rapid.

PHOSPHOLIPIDS

The principal phospholipids of the nervous system are phosphatidylcholine, phosphatidylethanolamine, phosphatidylserine and phosphatidylinositol. They are mainly synthesized in brain from bases activated by cytidine triphosphate (CTP). These compounds form an important constituent of cell membranes. The rapid conversion of phosphatidic acid to phosphatidylinositol and vice versa is a process which is significantly enhanced by neuronal activity, and phosphatidylinositol metabolism is believed to be important in processes of membrane reconstitution or repair. The only known inborn metabolic error of phospholipid metabolism is Niemann–Pick disease (Table 14) in which there is a defect of sphingomyelin metabolism due to inability to cleave phosphorylcholine from acylsphingosine.

SPHINGOLIPIDS

Sphingosine is formed in the brain from palmitic acid and can be acylated to form ceramide. Cerebrosides, glycosphingolipids and gangliosides may then be formed by the addition of carbohydrate. In adult brain 90% of cerebrosides are found in myelin (sphingomyelin), while gangliosides are predominantly neuronal but are also present in glial cell membranes. Cerebrosides and sulphatide synthesis are most active during myelination of the developing nervous system. The total ganglioside concentration in brain doubles between birth and maturity, and during development the relative concentrations of specific gangliosides also change greatly. Within the last 20 years there have been major advances in the characterization of inborn errors of sphingolipid metabolism. The great majority are due to inherited deficiencies of lysosomal degradative enzymes so that abnormal concentrations of lipid accumulate within neurons. For this reason, Adams and Lyon (1982) have suggested that these conditions should be called the lysosomal storage diseases. However, some of the glycogen storage diseases and the mucopolysaccharidoses are also lysosomal, so the term lipid storage disease is retained, appreciating that some of the diseases classified in this group may yet prove not to be true lipidoses. The basic unit of the material stored in many cells is usually one of the four principal sphingolipids, namely sphingomyelin, neutral glycosphingolipid, sulphoglycosphingolipid or ganglioside. A classification of the commoner lipid storage and related diseases is given in Table 15 (Walton, 1985). While the gangliosidoses are generally characterized by progressive cerebral degeneration and often visual loss, in the metachromatic and globoid-cell leucodystrophies there is severe destruction of myelin in the central and peripheral nervous system with relatively little storage in restricted neuronal groups. The lesions of Fabry's disease are largely non-neuronal, while those of Farber's disease do involve neurons but also joints and connective tissue. And the sialidoses, types 1 and 2 (often called the mucolipidoses) are clearly closely related to the mucopolysaccharidoses discussed above. Most of these conditions are due to autosomal recessive genes, but Fabry's disease, Pelizaeus–Merzbacher disease and Addison–Schilder disease are all X-linked recessive traits.

TABLE 13. The principal hereditary aminoacidopathies (and related disorders) producing neurological symptoms in the neonatal period

Disorder	Clinical peculiarities	Significant biochemical abnormalities (usual laboratory tests)	Amino acid accumulation in serum and plasma	Abnormal enzyme
Disorders of branched-chain amino acids (BCAA)				
Classical				
Maple syrup urine disease	Specific urine odour	Ketoaciduria	Leucine, isoleucine valine (partition chromatography)	Branched-chain ketoacid decarboxylase
Disorders of BCAA oxidation without accumulation of free amino acids; accumulation of ninhydrin-negative 'organic acids'				
Isovaleric acidaemia	Cheesy odour of urine	Severe metabolic ketoacidosis 'anion gap'; ketonuria; short-chain fatty acids	Isovaleric acid (gas chromatography)	Isovaleryl-CoA dehydrogenase
Propionic acidaemia	Neutropenia; thrombopenia	Severe metabolic ketoacidosis 'anion gap'; hypoglycaemia; hyperammonaemia (butanonuria); short-chain fatty acids	Propionic acid, glycine (gas chromatography)	Propionyl-CoA carboxylase
Methylmalonic aciduria B_{12} responsive B_{12} unresponsive	Neutropenia; thrombopenia	Severe metabolic ketoacidosis 'anion gap'; hypoglycaemia; hyperammonaemia; ketonuria (butanonuria)	Methylmalonic acid, glycine (gas chromatography)	Methylmalonyl-CoA mutase Defective conversion of B_{12} to deoxyadenosyl B_{12} and methyl B_{12}
Disorders of urea cycle				
Hyperammonaemia, type I	Very rare in neonate	Hyperammonaemia	Glycine	Carbamyl-phosphate synthetase
Hyperammonaemia, type II	X-linked dominant hepatomegaly ±; no effective therapy available	Marked hyperammonaemia; respiratory alkalosis	Glutamine Orotic aciduria	Ornithine transcarbamylase
Citrullinaemia		Hyperammonaemia; respiratory alkalosis	Citrulline	Argininosuccinate synthetase
Argininosuccinic aciduria	Hepatomegaly ±	Hyperammonaemia	Argininosuccinic acid	Argininosuccinate lyase
Non-ketotic hyperglycinaemia	Severe seizures; no effective therapy available		Glycine	Glycine decarboxylase?
Congenital hyperlactic acidaemia	Tachypnoea; hepatomegaly ±	Severe lactic acidosis		Variable
3-Ketoacid CoA-transferase deficiency	Tachypnoea very rare	Severe ketoacidosis		3-Ketoacid CoA-transferase

* Modified from Adams and Lyon (1982).

TABLE 14. Aminoacidurias and other metabolic diseases giving an onset of clinical manifestations in the neonatal period or early infancy*

Disease	Vomiting and acidity	Failure to thrive (from poor feeding)	Mental retardation	Other neurological signs	Liver dysfunction	Renal tubular dysfunction	Odour
Maple syrup urine	+	+	+	+	−	−	Maple syrup
Ketotic hyperglycinaemia	+	+	+	±	−	−	−
Non-ketotic hyperglycinaemia	−	−	+	+	−	−	−
Argininosuccinic aciduria	±	+	+	+	+	−	−
Congenital hyperammonaemia	+	+	+	+	+	−	−
Citrullinaemia	+	+	+	+	−	−	−
Hyperornithinaemia, type II	−	+	+	−	+	+	−
Hereditary tyrosinaemia	−	+	+	−	+	+	±
Isovaleric aciduria	+	+	+	+	−	−	Sweaty feet
Methylmalonic aciduria	+	+	+	−	−	−	−
Pyruvic and lactic acidaemia	+	+	+	+	−	−	−
Galactosaemia	+	+	+	+	+	+	−
Fructose intolerance	−	+	+	+	+	+	−

* Modified from O'Brian, D. and Goodman, S. I. (1970).

TABLE 15. Classification of the commoner lipid storage and related diseases*

Disease	Lipid accumulated	Enzyme defect	Age of onset	Clinical features
Infantile amaurotic idiocy				
Tay–Sachs disease	GM_2 ganglioside	Hexosaminidase A	<1 year	Megalencephaly, convulsions, dementia, cherry-red spot in retina
Sandhoff's disease	GM_2 ganglioside plus globoside	Hexosaminidase A and B	6 months	As above, but more severe
Late infantile amaurotic idiocy (Batten–Bielschowsky group)				
Generalized GM_1 gangliosidosis	GM_1 ganglioside	β-Galactosidase	1–3 years	Retinal pigmentation, macular degeneration, convulsions, dementia
Juvenile GM_2 gangliosidosis	GM_2 ganglioside	Hexosaminidase A (partial)	2–10 years	Convulsions, psychomotor retardation
Late infantile form with curvilinear bodies	Ceroid and lipofuscin	Unknown	1–3 years	As late infantile above
Juvenile amaurotic idiocy (Spielmeyer–Vogt)	Often ceroid and lipofuscin (in occasional cases GM_2 ganglioside)	Usually unknown (in occasional cases hexosaminidase A—partial)	2–10 years	As juvenile above
Neuronal ceroid-lipofuscinosis	Ceroid and lipofuscin	Unknown	Variable	Variable, but principally dementia and convulsions
Late onset lipidosis (Kufs)	Lipofuscin	Unknown	20–30 years	Dementia, myoclonus, convulsions, ataxia
Niemann–Pick disease, type A	Sphingomyelin	Sphingomyelinase	<1 year	Severe retardation, hypotonia, hepatosplenomegaly
Gaucher's disease, infantile	Glucocerebroside	Glucocerebrosidase	<1 year	Hepatosplenomegaly, sometimes epilepsy, dementia
Gaucher's disease, juvenile	Lactosylceramide, GM_3 ganglioside and glucocerebroside	Lactosylceramide β-Galactosidase	3–20 years	

Disease	Lipid accumulated	Enzyme defect	Age of onset	Clinical features
Krabbe's disease	Galactocerebroside	β-Galactosidase	6 months	Mental retardation, megalencephaly, peripheral neuropathy
Metachromatic leucodystrophy (sulphatide lipidosis)	Sulphatide	Arylsulphatase A	Congenital—1–2 years	Retardation, convulsions
			Adult—20–40 years	Dementia, convulsions, polyneuropathy
Lipoprotein abnormalities				
A-β-lipoproteinaemia (Bassen–Kornzweig disease)	None	Not known	Variable often <2 years	Ataxia, retinal pigmentation, acanthocytosis, steatorrhoea
Hypo-α-lipoproteinaemia (Tangier disease)	Cholesterol esters	Not known	Variable	Peripheral neuropathy
Xanthomatoses				
Hand-Schüller-Christian disease	Cholesterol	Unknown	Infancy or early childhood	Exophthalmos, diabetes insipidus, psychomotor retardation
Farber's disease	Ceramide and gangliosides	Ceramidase	<6 months	Psychomotor retardation, hoarse cry, cutaneous nodules, arthropathy, hepatosplenomegaly
Wolman's disease	Triglyceride and esterified cholesterol	Unknown	1 year	Hepatosplenomegaly, mental retardation, calcified adrenals
Sialidosis, type 1	Sialylated oligosaccharides	α-Neuraminidase	Early or late childhood	Resembles Hurler's disease
Sialidosis, type 2	Sialylated oligosaccharides	α-Neuraminidase and β-galactosidase	Neonates	Psychomotor retardation, abnormal facies, hyperplastic gums, bone and joint changes
Fabry's disease	Trihexosyl ceramide	α-Galactosidase	>10 years	Skin changes, corneal opacity, renal failure, painful autonomic neuropathy
Refsum's disease	Phytanic acid	Phytanic acid α-hydroxylase	5–15 years	Retinal pigmentation, nerve deafness, ataxia, hypertrophic neuropathy
Pelizaeus–Merzbacher disease	Unknown	Unknown	<1 year	Spastic paresis, psychomotor retardation, impaired ocular movement
Adrenoleucodystrophy (Addison–Schilder's disease) (X-linked recessive)	Unknown	Unknown	5–12 years	Dementia, spastic paresis, visual loss, convulsions, features of Addison's disease
Alexander's disease	Unknown	Unknown	<18 months	Megalencephaly, mental retardation, spastic paresis
Canavan–van Bogaert–Bertrand disease	Unknown	Unknown	<6 months	Retardation, blindness, megalencephaly, spastic paresis

* Modified from White, H. H. Diseases due to inborn metabolic defects. In Merritt, H. H. (ed.) (1973) *A Textbook of Neurology*, and Menkes, J. H. (1980) *Textbook of Child Neurology*, 2nd edn.

FATTY ACIDS

Fatty acids of long hydrocarbon chain length turn over more slowly in the nervous system than do those with fewer carbon atoms. The fatty-acid composition of certain lipids varies depending upon their localization in the nervous system. The sphingomyelin of axonal terminals consists predominantly of fatty acids of short chain length and hence turns over rapidly, while that of myelin has many more long-chain acids and is more stable. Gangliosides also show rapid fatty-acid turnover whereas the cerebrosides of myelin are much more stable.

Refsum's disease (heredopathia atactica polyneuritiformis) is an autosomal recessive disorder due to phytanic acid α-hydroxylase deficiency, and is characterized clinically by the onset in childhood of retinal pigmentation, nerve deafness, cerebellar ataxia, and hypertrophic polyneuropathy. Phytanic acid (3, 7, 11, 15-tetramethylhexadecanoic acid) accumulates in the central nervous system and in peripheral nerves. If recognized early, the condition can be controlled, at least partially, by dietary restriction of foods containing phytol (a chlorophyll derivative), which is a precursor of phytanic acid.

ADRENOLEUCODYSTROPHY (ADDISON–SCHILDER DISEASE)

This appears to be due to a disorder of very long-chain fatty acid metabolism. It is an X-linked recessive disorder, manifest in males and transmitted by unaffected carrier females. It begins in childhood, giving rise to progressive visual impairment, dementia, spastic paresis of all four limbs, and often epileptic seizures. The affected individuals show adrenal atrophy and many develop the typical endocrinological and biochemical manifestations of Addison's disease. Sometimes (adrenomyeloneuropathy) the brunt of the disease falls upon the spinal cord and peripheral nerves, while in others the condition presents as X-linked Addison's disease without evidence of nervous system involvement.

An autosomal recessive disorder of carnitine synthesis results in a subacute proximal myopathy, in which there is accumulation of neutral lipid within skeletal muscle fibres. Carnitine is necessary for the transport of fatty acids into mitochondria.

Disorders of serum lipoproteins

A-β-lipoproteinaemia (the Bassen–Kornzweig syndrome), due to an autosomal recessive gene, usually presents between the ages of 2 and 16 years with atypical retinitis pigmentosa, progressive cerebellar ataxia, mental retardation and steatorrhoea. The red blood cells show a typical 'thorny' malformation (acanthocytosis) and the serum levels of cholesterol, carotenoids, vitamin A and phospholipids are invariably depressed, with absence of the β-lipoprotein moiety. There is now some evidence that early treatment with vitamin E may prevent or delay the development of neurological manifestations (Walton, 1985).

Hypo-α-lipoproteinaemia (Tangier disease), another rare autosomal recessive disorder, usually produces peripheral neuropathy and retinitis pigmentosa. There is almost total absence of high-density plasma lipoproteins. The liver, spleen, lymph nodes and tonsils are usually enlarged and demonstrate storage of cholesterol esters.

MYELIN

In the brain about 40% of the myelin that ensheaths the majority of long axons is made up of water. Lipid comprises 70–80% of its dry weight, and protein comprises 20–30% of its dry weight. Lipids are present in a proportion of 4:3:2 of cholesterol:phospholipid:galactolipid respectively. In the adult, all the cholesterol is unesterified, the predominant phospholipid is phosphatidylethanolamine, and the main galactolipid is cerebroside. Plasmalogens (glyceryl phospholipids) make up about one-third of myelin phospholipids. The myelin of peripheral nerves (see p. 49) is similar in constitution but contains a higher concentration of sphingomyelin and less phosphatidylcholine. In developing myelin the cholesterol precursor desmosterol is found in amounts which decrease with age. Gangliosides and phosphoinositides are present in much lower concentrations in myelin than in grey matter and may depend, at least in part, upon contamination of myelin preparations with axonal membranes. In many of the diseases listed in Table 14, other than the 'pure' neuronal storage disorders, there are enzymatic defects of genetic origin which impair the development of myelin (dysmyelination) or result in its destruction (demyelination). This group of diseases, which includes Krabbe's diffuse sclerosis (globoid body disease), the sudanophilic forms of diffuse sclerosis (including Pelizaeus–Merzbacher disease), metachromatic leucodystrophy and adrenoleucodystrophy (Addison–Schilder's disease) are generally grouped together under the title of 'the leucodystrophies'. Cholesterol esters are normally present while myelin is developing, but disappear during maturation. They reappear in inherited diseases which principally affect myelin, such as the sudanophilic leucodystrophies, or in acquired demyelinating disorders such as multiple sclerosis.

MEMBRANES

The plasma membranes of neuronal perikarya, axons and dendrites, and glial cells play a vital role in cell-to-cell interactions, in the transport of material from and into the extracellular environment, and in many other aspects of nervous function. Most mammalian plasma membranes consist of 60% protein, 40% lipid and 5–10% carbohydrate. Phospholipids are an important constituent of the membrane lipid fraction, but so too is cholesterol. Disorders of lipid metabolism are likely to derange membrane function while at the same time impairing the function of cells and/or myelin. Normal biochemical function may be disrupted and there may be morphological distortion of normal structure. Relatively little is known as yet about mechanisms of membrane dysfunction in diseases of the nervous system in man.

Some other inborn errors of CNS metabolism

DISORDERS OF COPPER METABOLISM

Hepatolenticular degeneration (Wilson's disease)
Hepatolenticular degeneration, first clearly defined by Kinnier Wilson in 1912, is described in standard neurology textbooks. Wilson's disease is due to an autosomal recessive gene, so that it can affect several members of a sibship, but there is generally no history of the disease in previous generations. It is characterized by the appearance of symptoms indicating progressive degeneration of the basal ganglia, by the development of liver cirrhosis, and by the presence of a ring of brown pigment around the margin of the cornea, the Kayser–Fleischer ring. The primary defect is one of copper metabolism, and copper is deposited in the brain and liver as well as in the periphery of the cornea. Characteristic biochemical features include aminoaciduria, an excessive output of copper in the urine (normal upper limit 30 μg/24 h) and a reduction of the serum copper level (normal range 86–112 μg/dl). The serum copper oxidase is also reduced. The primary defect, the presumed abnormal gene product, of Wilson's disease has not been established. Usually there is deficiency of caeruloplasmin, the copper-binding protein of the serum. The primary defect may lie in the ability of the liver to excrete copper rather than in caeruloplasmin deficiency. Kayser–Fleischer rings have been seen in a few patients with biliary cirrhosis, so they are not pathognomonic for Wilson's disease. The mechanism by which copper deposition is injurious to tissue has not been established.

Menkes' kinky hair disease (trichopoliodystrophy)
In 1962 Menkes et al described an X-linked recessive disorder characterized by early and severe retardation of growth, peculiar white and 'kinky' hair, frequent epileptic seizures, and focal cerebral and cerebellar degeneration particularly involving the white matter. The condition is usually fatal in early childhood. Low serum copper and caeruloplasmin have been found in these cases, together with a direct demonstration of impaired copper absorption by the gut. The concentrations of copper in the serum, liver and brain are all low, there is reduced cytochrome oxidase A1 and A3 activity in liver, brain and leucocytes, and dopamine β-hydroxylase activity is also reduced in blood and CSF. It now appears that neonatal copper deficiency causes the pathological changes in the brain. Antenatal diagnosis can be achieved by studying the incorporation of radioactive copper into amniotic cells, but copper injections, once thought to be of benefit, do not appear to produce clinical improvement, however early the condition is diagnosed and treated.

PORPHYRIA

The porphyrias are a group of disorders involving the metabolism of porphyrins and porphyrin precursors. They may be symptomless, may cause skin lesions, or can give rise to acute manifestations (acute porphyria) with mental, neurological and abdominal manifestations.

In acute intermittent porphyria, dysfunction of the nervous system predominates. Though seen in both sexes, it occurs more often in females between 16 and 50 years, and acute attacks are often precipitated by drugs, especially barbiturates, sulphonamides, phenytoin, diazepam and its analogues, and alcohol. There is a high urinary excretion of porphobilinogen and of δ-aminolaevulinic acid. The disorder is caused by reduced activity of uroporphyrinogen-I-synthetase, most readily measured in red blood cells. There is a greatly increased activity of δ-aminolaevulinic acid synthetase, the first specific enzyme of haem biosynthesis.

Pathologically, the predominant changes found in fatal cases are those of axonal degeneration with secondary demyelination in somatic and autonomic nerves. The cardinal clinical manifestations are episodes of acute abdominal pain, often misdiagnosed as being due to an acute abdominal emergency, episodes of mental confusion, and signs of a predominantly motor peripheral neuropathy which may be extensive and severe. The biochemical mechanism through which this disorder of porphyrin synthesis injures the nervous system has not been established.

Intravenous haematin may be helpful in terminating acute attacks (Walton, 1985).

OTHER IMPORTANT DISORDERS OF CEREBRAL METABOLISM

In the introductory section to this chapter, a distinction was made between endogenous and exogenous metabolic encephalopathies. In the preceding section we have considered disorders of carbohydrate, purine, protein and lipid metabolism successively, concentrating primarily upon endogenous disorders, especially those due to inborn errors of metabolism. It will now be appropriate to consider the following:
1. some metabolic encephalopathies and other disorders of the nervous system due to primary abnormalities in other systems of the body
2. deficiency disorders
3. disorders due to drugs or specific toxins or poisons

Metabolic encephalopathies and related disorders of the nervous system due to disease in other systems

PORTOSYSTEMIC ENCEPHALOPATHY

Neurological symptoms can appear as the result of hepatic failure from any cause. They may arise spontaneously or be precipitated in patients with chronic liver disease by gastrointestinal haemorrhage, acute alcoholic intoxication, the administration of morphine or barbiturates, paracentesis, diuretics or surgery. They may also follow the operation of portacaval anastomosis.

The causes of the neurological symptoms are complex. As an essential factor nitrogenous material intended for the liver enters the systemic circulation through abnormal anastomoses between the portal and systemic arterial systems, either arising naturally or produced by surgery. Similar symptoms have been observed after liver transplantation. Measurement of the blood ammonia sometimes gives a rough index of the severity of the condition. It has been shown that α-ketoglutaramate, a metabolite of glutamine not previously demonstrated in mammalian tissue, is increased four- to tenfold in patients with hepatic encephalopathy. This substance may exert a toxic effect on the nervous system by competing for glutamic acid receptors in the brain. It also seems that hyperammonaemia and increased circulating aromatic amino acids together induce cerebral depletion of dopamine and noradrenaline and also cause an accumulation of false neurotransmitters (octopamine and phenylethanolamine) (*Lancet*, 1982).

One of the most constant pathological features in the brain is the presence in the cortex and in the basal ganglia of Alzheimer type 2 astrocytes, which show no cytoplasm with ordinary staining methods. These cells are also present in Wilson's disease. The astrocytic abnormality may be due to a defect in function of the mitotic spindle. There is also evidence of microtubular dysfunction which may give a lead not only to the nature of the metabolic abnormality but also to new concepts of astrocytic function.

Neurological symptoms in chronic hepatic disease may be intermittent, and sometimes predominantly psychiatric, for long periods. In other cases, and especially in acute hepatic failure, they develop rapidly and progressively. Psychiatric symptoms consist of changes in personality, abnormalities of mood and behaviour, and drowsiness deepening into stupor and coma. Speech is likely to be slurred, and there may be dysphasia. A 'flapping' tremor (asterixis) is characteristic when the arms are outstretched, but may also occur in other toxic states. Neurological signs suggestive of focal cerebral damage or dysfunction are occasionally seen. Extrapyramidal rigidity and tremor may be present with or without signs of corticospinal lesions or cerebellar deficiency. A chronic choreo-athetotic syndrome has also been reported. Muscle twitching may occur, and myelopathy with spasticity and increased limb reflexes but with flexor plantar responses has been described; however, neuropathological studies suggest that this syndrome is more likely to be due to a restricted form of encephalopathy with descending degeneration of the corticospinal tracts rather than to a myelopathy.

In severe cases delta waves which may be triphasic will be present in the EEG. In milder cases there is a slowing of the dominant frequency. The EEG can be used as a sensitive indicator of the response to treatment as well as for diagnosis, but measurement of the blood ammonia or mercaptan is even more helpful. The cerebrospinal fluid is usually normal.

KERNICTERUS

Kernicterus is a disorder of infancy in which pathological examination of affected brains reveals canary-yellow staining of the meninges, choroid plexus, basal ganglia, dentate nuclei, vermis, hippocampus and medullary nuclei, associated with widespread degeneration of neurons and secondary astrocytosis. The condition is associated with an elevated blood level of indirect bilirubin to 200 mg/l or more in the neonatal period. Many reported cases have been due to Rh or other rare forms of blood-group incompatibility. An infant with an Rh-positive father is affected by the passage of antibodies across the placenta from a previously sensitized but Rh-negative mother, which results in haemolysis and overproduction of bilirubin. With increasingly effective prevention of this disease using anti-Rh gamma globulin, the incidence of kernicterus due to this cause has declined, but cases of kernicterus due to other factors (prematurity, haemolytic anaemia of other types, sepsis, acidosis) are still occasionally seen. A high circulating bilirubin alone will not damage the developing brain. Other factors which affect the vulnerability of the damaged cells are not clearly understood, but may include anoxia or exposure to drugs (via placental transfer) such as benzodiazepines, or possibly vitamin K or gentamicin (Menkes, 1980). The development of kernicterus in the deeply jaundiced neonate is usually heralded by coma, convulsions and a decerebrate posture with extensor spasms alternating with hypotonia. The survivors typically demonstrate nerve deafness, variable degrees of mental retardation, defects of vertical conjugate gaze, and bilateral choreoathetosis and/or dystonia.

URAEMIC ENCEPHALOPATHY

Uraemic encephalopathy may occur in acute or chronic renal failure. The metabolic changes so produced are complex, and clearly a raised blood urea or non-protein nitrogen, though a useful index of severity, is not the main cause of impaired consciousness. There is usually metabolic acidosis. Water intoxication, due to fluid retention, with a serum osmolality of less than 260 mosmol/l is a factor in some cases. The blood calcium may be subnormal and the administration of alkalis to correct the acidosis may precipitate tetany. The serum pyruvate is usually raised and the cerebral consumption of oxygen is reduced. None of these chemical derangements, however, represents a satisfactory explanation for most cases of uraemic encephalopathy. Headache, vomiting, dyspnoea, confusion and drowsiness or restlessness and insomnia are early symptoms, and later, muscular twitchings or generalized convulsions may precede coma. Coma due to uraemia must be distinguished from that due to hypertensive encephalopathy, as arterial hypertension is common in patients with chronic renal disease. Recently a fatal progressive spongiform encephalopathy giving rise to dysarthria, dementia, seizures, myoclonus, asterixis, apraxia and variable focal neurological signs has been described in patients with chronic renal disease undergoing regular haemodialysis in certain centres. This syndrome has been shown to be due to aluminium deposition in the brain related to a high concentration of this trace element in the tap water used for dialysis. This progressive disorder must be distinguished from the dialysis dysequilibrium syndrome, which is commoner in children, and usually occurs when rapid changes in blood solutes are taking place. It is a temporary condition, correctable by careful control of serum electrolytes and osmolality during dialysis (Plum and Posner, 1980).

DIABETIC ENCEPHALOPATHY

Diabetic coma is usually associated with ketoacidosis, a blood sugar greater than 250 mg/dl, and massive ketonuria. Lactic acidosis is an occasional cause of metabolic acidosis in diabetic subjects (especially during treatment with hypoglycaemic agents) and must be distinguished from the lactic acidosis that may result from severe anoxia or from poisoning with methyl alcohol or paraldehyde. Hyperosmolality due to hyperglycaemia (hyperglycaemic non-ketotic diabetic coma) has also been described and a similar syndrome has been reported in non-diabetic subjects with severe burns. The patient is usually wasted, pale and dehydrated, the rate and amplitude of respiration are increased, ocular tension is low, the pulse is rapid and feeble, and the blood pressure is often low. There are often signs of associated diabetic polyneuropathy. Encephalopathy in the uncontrolled diabetic tends to parallel the degree of hyperosmolality.

HYPOGLYCAEMIA

Coma due to hypoglycaemia is not difficult to recognize in the diabetic subject if due to an overdose of insulin, but it is less easily diagnosed when due to factitious self-administration of insulin in the doctor or nurse. Spontaneous hypoglycaemia due to an adenoma of the islets of Langerhans may give intermittent convulsions, confusion or abnormal behaviour for months or years before producing coma, but occasionally in such cases deep coma develops without warning in a previously healthy individual. Spontaneous hypoglycaemia is particularly common in the premature infant, and in the adult it may also be a consequence of liver disease, alcoholism, hypopituitarism or hypoadrenalism. Episodic hypoglycaemia in infancy and early childhood is also a common feature of several of the urea-cycle disorders and aminoacidurias and can also occur in systemic carnitine deficiency. The affected patient is usually pale and perspiring profusely, the pupils are dilated, and the plantar responses are extensor. In occasional cases focal neurological manifestations (a 'stroke-like' presentation) are seen. A predominantly motor polyneuropathy is a rare complication of organic hyperinsulinism.

DISORDERS OF WATER AND ELECTROLYTE METABOLISM

Hyponatraemia or water intoxication has been increasingly recognized as a cause of delirium, often leading to coma. It is most often due to inappropriate ADH secretion (as may occur in cases of bronchial carcinoma) or to organic lesions (e.g. neoplasia) in the region of the hypothalamus and/or pituitary, but it sometimes occurs without evident cause. Sometimes water intoxication results from compulsive drinking in psychotic or alcoholic individuals, or else it may complicate renal failure.

Hypernatraemia may also cause delirium and, less often, coma. It is seen in children with severe diarrhoea or the rare condition of nephrogenic diabetes insipidus, but rarely in adults with true diabetes insipidus, and can also be iatrogenic, resulting from the administration of excessive quantities of intravenous saline. These causes of delirium, drowsiness or coma are recognized by measurement of the serum osmolality.

ENCEPHALOPATHY AND OTHER NEUROLOGICAL MANIFESTATIONS OF ENDOCRINE DISEASE

Hypopituitarism

Confusion leading to coma in hypopituitarism is usually due to several interrelated factors including hypoglycaemia, hypotension, diminished adrenal cortical function, and occasionally hypothermia. The onset of coma is often precipitated by infection, less often by exposure to narcotic drugs, in many such cases. The blood pressure and blood sugar are usually low, the body temperature is often subnormal (as in myxoedema), and the serum cortisol is very low in such cases. The syndrome of pituitary apoplexy with headache, neck stiffness and rapid loss of consciousness in some cases, due to infarction and rapid swelling of a chromophobe adenoma of the pituitary gland, must be remembered as an alternative cause of coma in patients showing clinical manifestations of pituitary failure.

Cushing's disease

The adrenocortical overactivity of Cushing's disease not uncommonly results in depression, paranoid ideas and confusional episodes. In occasional cases there is diffuse cerebral oedema with headache and papilloedema. A subacute proximal myopathy, sometimes painful and usually involving thigh muscles predominantly, is common and resembles iatrogenic steroid myopathy.

Thyroid disease

Hypothermia is a common complication of hypothyroidism (myxoedema) and must be borne in mind in elderly subjects living in poorly heated accommodation in the winter months. It is described further on p. 228. In hyperthyroidism (Graves' disease), a severe confusional state occasionally occurs in acute cases but this is uncommon. The more usual neurological complications of this condition are ophthalmic Graves' disease (exophthalmic ophthalmoplegia or infiltrative autoimmune ophthalmopathy) and subacute proximal myopathy, a frequent complication which resolves after treatment of the thyroid disease. When external ocular or bulbar muscles are weak in such cases, the possibility of associated myasthenia gravis must be borne in mind. Attacks of hypokalaemic periodic paralysis, also resolving after effective treatment of the thyroid disorder (thyrotoxic periodic paralysis), occur especially in patients of Chinese or Japanese ancestry.

Adrenocortical failure

Mild delirium is not uncommon in untreated Addison's disease, but stupor and coma as a rule develop only in addisonian crises, sometimes precipitated by stress or by infection. In such cases, papilloedema, presumably due to cerebral oedema, is rarely seen. Acute adrenal failure due to meningococcal septicaemia is now a very rare cause of sudden collapse and coma in infants and young children.

Abnormalities of blood calcium

Hypercalcaemia as a cause of confusion or coma may be missed if the blood calcium is not examined routinely. It may be due to excessive ingestion of vitamin D, hyperparathyroidism, carcinoma (with or without bone metastases), myelomatosis or sarcoidosis. Hypocalcaemia, as in hypoparathyroidism, can also give rise to coma, but much less often, though papilloedema and cerebral oedema have been described in such cases. Tetany and/or convulsions are more common. In idiopathic hypoparathyroidism, mental retardation, recurring major convulsions, and calcification of the basal ganglia are frequent features. A subacute proximal myopathy, typically with brisk tendon reflexes, is a common manifestation of hyperparathyroidism, and, paradoxically, also of some forms of metabolic bone disease associated with hypocalcaemia, including osteomalacia.

ANOXIA AND HYPOXIA

The commonest varieties of anoxia met with in clinical practice are those in which there is deficient oxygenation of the arterial blood due either to a failure of adequate quantities of oxygen to reach the lungs (high altitudes, suffocation, drowning) or to diminished oxygenation resulting from pulmonary disease (emphysema). These causes are grouped together as anoxic anoxia. In anaemic anoxia there is a deficiency in circulating haemoglobin or a chemical alteration in the haemoglobin (as in carbon monoxide poisoning) which prevents it from carrying oxygen. Cardiac arrest occurring as a result of heart disease or during anaesthesia may also be followed by irreversible anoxic brain damage, which is also sometimes seen as a complication of open-heart surgery. In the latter situation air or gas embolism is an additional hazard. Local anoxia of the tissues can also be due to arterial disease producing ischaemia (ischaemic anoxia). Local infarction of the brain, spinal cord or peripheral nerves may result from focal vascular occlusion due to atheroma, thrombosis or embolism, and then gives rise to focal neurological signs depending upon the site of the lesion. Diffuse ischaemic anoxia can also be due to fat embolism (in severe limb fractures) or to widespread disease of small arteries and arterioles. Oxygen lack has a profound effect upon the brain. The spinal cord and peripheral nerves on the other hand seem capable of resisting degrees of anoxia that produce irreversible cerebral damage. When the oxygen supply to the brain is moderately reduced over a long period, the most frequent symptoms are fatigue, drowsiness, apathy and failure of attention, followed later by impairment of judgement, memory, ataxia, and incoordination. Sudden profound anoxia produces almost instantaneous loss of the senses, and normally the brain cannot withstand more than 3 minutes of total anoxia after cardiac arrest. If the period of anoxia is much more prolonged, respiration ceases and death rapidly ensues. After a period of from 5 to 15 minutes of cardiac arrest, even if the circulation is re-established, the patient may survive for a time in a semicomatose decerebrate state, but full intellectual function is never restored. After less prolonged periods of anoxia the patient may regain full control of his limbs, and consciousness is restored after several hours or days, but there is commonly some degree of permanent intellectual deficit. Epileptic seizures of the temporal-lobe type are a frequent sequel, resulting from the pathological changes which anoxia produces in Ammon's horn and in contiguous areas of the hippocampus. In some cases of carbon monoxide poisoning the patient is initially unconscious but then may regain his senses at least to some extent after 24 or 48 hours. A relatively lucid interval may then be followed by progressively deepening coma and death (postanoxic encephalopathy). Many cases showing partial recovery from an anoxic insult, however caused, show permanent dementia and severe behaviour disorders. Cortical blindness and/or various apraxic or agnosic syndromes are common. They may also exhibit cerebellar ataxia (due to Purkinje cell damage), variable extrapyramidal features superficially resembling those of parkinsonism, and spastic weakness of the limbs with extensor plantar responses. In occasional cases there may be a surprising degree of recovery even after prolonged unconsciousness, so that the prognosis is difficult to predict in any single case.

CARBON DIOXIDE INTOXICATION

In some patients with chronic bronchitis and emphysema the respiratory centre appears to become increasingly insensitive to retained carbon dioxide. The syndrome can also result from chronic respiratory insufficiency of neuromuscular origin or from depression of respiration by morphine or other sedative drugs. In chronic cases headache, drowsiness and confusion may persist over many months. Sometimes an acute syndrome develops, characterized by intense headache, vomiting, convulsions and papilloedema, not infrequently precipitated by the administration of oxygen. As in chronic CO_2 retention, the respiratory centre fails to react to the raised level of CO_2, and respiration is then maintained by the receptors which respond to oxygen lack. Administering oxygen then removes the stimulus to respiration, raises the blood CO_2 still further, and hence causes coma. The chemical basis of suppression of brain function caused by carbon dioxide has not been established.

ELECTRICAL INJURIES

Electrocution, occurring either as a result of accidental contact with an electrical supply or from being struck by lightning, can be immediately fatal due to cardiac arrest. In such cases there are extensive pathological changes in the brain, muscles and peripheral nerves as well as in other tissues. Less severe and more localized injuries commonly produce extensive burning or electrical necrosis of the tissues. It is not uncommon in such cases for a temporary flaccid paralysis of the lower limbs to occur, with sensory loss. This usually passes off in 24 hours and is believed to be due to profound vasoconstriction in the arteries of the spinal cord. A variety of other syndromes resulting from focal injury to the brain, spinal cord or peripheral nerves may occur in other cases.

DECOMPRESSION SICKNESS (CAISSON DISEASE)

This condition, which is commonest in divers and in tunnel workers who work in an atmosphere of compressed air, is due to the release of bubbles of nitrogen into the bloodstream during decompression. Nitrogen is soluble in many lipids under conditions of pressure, but is released during decompression, especially in the nervous system. Many neurological symptoms, including hemiplegia, paraplegia, visual scotomas, vertigo and diplopia can occur in such cases, presumably as a result of gas embolism of the arteries of the brain or spinal cord. Symptoms of this type developing in those working in a compressed-air environment demand immediate recompression in a compressed-air chamber, a measure which will almost invariably relieve the symptoms. Subsequently, decompression must be repeated much more slowly. Non-neurological symptoms include chest pain, dyspnoea, cough, aching in the limbs, and infarction of bones, with subsequent arthropathy, particularly of the hip joints.

HEAT STROKE

In an individual exposed to a consistently high environmental temperature, the typical manifestations of heat stroke are a rapidly mounting temperature and a hot, dry skin with total absence of sweating. The patient is at first apathetic, and later stuporous or comatose, and convulsions are common. Circulatory collapse soon follows if rapid cooling is not instituted. Variable degrees of cerebral damage may persist even in those patients who recover. Variable confusion, slurring dysarthria, and ataxia are common in the recovery phase. The Purkinje cells of the cerebellum are particularly sensitive to heat injury, and a severe cerebellar ataxia, often with mild dementia and polyneuropathy, may be permanent sequelae.

HYPOTHERMIA

Accidental hypothermia is usually due to prolonged exposure to cold or immersion in cold water. Hypothermic coma is, however, an occasional complication of myxoedema as noted above. Diagnosis depends upon careful measurement of the rectal temperature, which may be less than 34°C (90°F). Indeed, hypothermia was commonly used in the past as an adjunct to anaesthesia and occasionally produced untoward complications and sequelae. Unduly prolonged hypothermia can lead to convulsions, irreversible coma, cardiac arrest and death, while less severe and prolonged episodes can give sequelae similar to those of cerebral anoxia. Confusion and alternating rigidity of the limbs with coarse myoclonic jerking are sometimes seen during recovery. Immersion foot is a syndrome of local hypothermia involving the lower limbs, seen in shipwreck survivors and common in the trenches in the first world war. It gave manifestations of severe peripheral neuropathy with necrosis of muscles and sometimes gangrene. By contrast, in frostbite the principal pathological changes are in the blood vessels, and evidence of injury to peripheral nerves and skeletal muscle is relatively unobtrusive.

RADIATION INJURY

The nervous system is relatively resistant to the effects of ionizing radiation. After a dose of radiation exceeding 40 Gy (4000 rad) and more often between 60 and 80 Gy, late radiation encephalopathy has been described, but it is rare as doses of radiation of this magnitude are rarely delivered to the brain. Radiation myelopathy following irradiation of the neck or mediastinum for malignant disease is not uncommon, usually giving rise to a slowly progressive paraparesis, developing 1–4 years after the course of treatment. Pathologically there is vacuolation and degeneration of neurons, myelin breakdown, and thickening of the walls of spinal arterioles and capillaries with narrowing of their lumina.

Deficiency disorders

DEFICIENCIES OF SPECIFIC VITAMINS

Although many specific syndromes occurring in man have been ascribed to an insufficient dietary intake of certain vitamins, these syndromes are not solely dependent upon vitamin deficiency. Total starvation does not as a rule cause scurvy, pellagra or beri-beri, while symptoms and signs of thiamine deficiency are greatly enhanced if the diet contains large amounts of carbohydrate. Some food must be taken before characteristic clinical evidence of vitamin deficiency can develop. Even so, the resultant clinical syndrome varies greatly in the individual cases. It is not clear as yet, for instance, why thiamine (vitamin B_1) deficiency will produce Wernicke's encephalopathy in some cases, beri-beri in others, and optic neuritis or perhaps even 'burning feet' in yet others. Conditions such as pregnancy, or infective illnesses, which enhance the body's demands for vitamins, may accentuate symptoms attributable to deficiency which were previously minimal. The vitamins of the B group, particularly thiamine, nicotinic acid, pyridoxine and vitamin B_{12}, are of greatest importance to the nervous system. Clinical syndromes resulting from vitamin C deficiency (scurvy) and from lack of the fat-soluble vitamins (A, D and K) are not usually attended by symptoms of nervous disease. However, vitamin A deficiency causing night blindness and xerophthalmia can also be associated with protein-calorie malnutrition in young children in tropical countries, with impaired cerebral development and/or myopathy and polyneuropathy. And osteomalacia resulting from vitamin D deficiency can cause a reversible proximal myopathy. Hypervitaminosis A due to excessive consumption of polar bear or seal liver (in Arctic explorers) or of cod liver oil, may produce headache, drowsiness and vomiting, while excess vitamin D can cause hypercalcaemia with neurological symptoms.

Thiamine deficiency
Thiamine (vitamin B_1) consists of two moieties—a pyrimidine and a thiazole ring. Most vegetable foods contain free thiamine, while in meats it is present as thiamine diphosphate. Further phosphorylation of ingested thiamine, carried out mainly in the liver, is needed to form thiamine pyrophosphate (TPP or cocarboxylase), which is the active cofactor. It has a wide range of activity in intermediary carbohydrate metabolism, acting mainly in the decarboxylation of α-keto acids (e.g. pyruvate to acetaldehyde) and in oxidative decarboxylation (e.g. pyruvate to active acetate). It is also involved in the pentose phosphate pathway or hexose monophosphate shunt, an important pathway in the synthesis of pentose nucleic acid. In this pathway transketolase, an enzyme which requires thiamine pyrophosphate as a cofactor, acts as a catalyst. Transketolase activity is markedly depressed in the erythrocytes of thiamine-deficient rats and in human subjects with Wernicke's disease (see below), but increases within hours after the administration of thiamine. The estimation of transketolase before and after TPP activation is a sensitive test for thiamine deficiency.

Primary dietary deficiency of thiamine is now relatively uncommon in developed societies except as a complication of chronic alcoholism. While chronic alcoholism acts mainly by reducing the dietary intake of thiamine, there is also evidence that alcohol may impair the absorption of this vitamin.

WERNICKE'S ENCEPHALOPATHY

Wernicke's encephalopathy is characterized by mental disturbance, disorders of eye movement and ataxia. It is most often observed in chronic alcoholic patients in whom alcoholic beverages have gradually replaced other forms of food and in whom gastrointestinal irritation has contributed by producing anorexia. However, it can develop as a result of thiamine deficiency arising from any cause and has been described as a consequence of repeated vomiting in pregnancy or of gastrectomy. There is usually an associated polyneuropathy. The principal pathological features are focal areas of haemorrhage and neuronal degeneration in the corpora mammillaria and upper midbrain. Although in severe cases consciousness may be impaired, the characteristic mental symptoms are (a) transient delirium and hallucinatory experiences, occurring particularly in alcoholic patients and resulting from alcoholic withdrawal, (b) apathy, listlessness, and variable confusion, and (c) most characteristic of all, the *Korsakov syndrome*. The principal abnormality in this syndrome is a severe memory defect giving inability to record new impressions, from which springs disorientation in time and place, together with confabulation. The principal neurological abnormalities which accompany these mental changes are coarse nystagmus, present in all directions of gaze, and ophthalmoplegia, which may consist merely of paralysis of both lateral recti or more often of disorders of conjugate ocular movement, leading in some cases to total immobility of the eyes. A severe truncal ataxia is also present as a rule, even though signs of cerebellar incoordination in the limbs are often inconspicuous. The neurological abnormalities generally remit promptly when the patient is treated with thiamine, although the mental disturbances, particularly those of the Korsakov syndrome, may take weeks or months to resolve.

BERI-BERI

Although thiamine deficiency is clearly important in the aetiology of beri-beri, some additional factor is probably necessary in view of the rarity of the fully developed syndrome in European or American chronic alcoholics. It rarely occurs in its entirety except in populations fed upon milled rice. Polyneuropathy due to vitamin B deficiency is not uncommon in Western countries, not only in alcoholics but also in patients with prolonged anorexia due to mental disease and in elderly people living alone.

The principal clinical features of beri-beri are those of polyneuropathy. Distal muscular atrophy and sensory loss occur but are common to all varieties of peripheral neuropathy. A characteristic feature of beri-beri is that the patients often complain of intense burning and tingling in the extremities and especially in the feet. Touching the skin is often particularly unpleasant, so that walking becomes impossible, not as a result of muscular weakness, but because of sensory disturbance. In some individuals, these are the only manifestations ('dry' or 'neuritic' beri-beri), but generally peripheral oedema, breathlessness, tachycardia and cardiac enlargement also occur, indicating myocardial involvement. The administration of thiamine in large doses usually gives gradual improvement and eventually complete recovery.

Other nutritional neuropathies

NUTRITIONAL AMBLYOPIA

In some individuals existing on diets low in vitamin B content, progressive blurring of vision develops and the visual fields show central or paracentral scotomas, at first for coloured objects and later for white. The optic disc is now swollen, but if the condition is untreated, optic atrophy follows. This disorder clearly resembles clinically and perhaps aetiologically the forms of amblyopia which have been attributed to alcohol and tobacco. Nutritional amblyopia was once thought to be due to a deficiency of riboflavin and it certainly responds to treatment with vitamins of the B group in high dosage. Recent work suggests that vitamin B_{12} deficiency is the principal factor. The condition resembles the optic atrophy which may complicate subacute combined degeneration.

TROPICAL ATAXIC NEUROPATHY

Optic atrophy, presumed in the past to be due to nutritional deficiency, is also a feature of the syndrome of tropical ataxic neuropathy which has been described in many parts of Africa, particularly in Nigeria. In this condition there is also progressive unsteadiness in walking, with impairment of vibration and position and joint sense in the legs. It is now known to be due to the excessive ingestion of dietary cyanide, which is present in cassava, the tuber of manioc.

WEST INDIAN AND SOUTH INDIAN SPASTIC PARAPLEGIA

A form of progressive spastic paraplegia of unknown origin has been observed both in the West Indies and in Southern India. Often there is associated evidence of posterior column dysfunction, and optic atrophy as well as nerve deafness is occasionally seen. There is no evidence that this condition is due to cyanide intoxication. Inflammatory changes of granulomatous type have been found in the spinal cords of some patients. Toxic dietary factors (e.g. bush tea) and nutritional deficiencies have been postulated, but the cause remains unknown. A similar clinical picture occurs in lathyrism due to the consumption of lathyrus peas containing β-aminoproprionitrile.

TOBACCO/ALCOHOL AMBLYOPIA

This condition has been reported particularly in heavy pipe-smokers who customarily smoke thick dark tobacco. Slow visual deterioration occurs and paracentral or centrocaecal scotomas are usually found. There is some evidence that an abnormality of B_{12} metabolism may be involved, but the visual symptoms have been thought to disappear completely if the individual gives up smoking or changes to a more innocuous tobacco. It has been postulated that cyanide in the tobacco or some form of sensitivity may cause an impairment of the utilization of vitamin B_{12}. Sometimes improvement has followed the administration of hydroxocobalamin even if the patient continued to smoke. In the United States it has long been believed that alcohol is also a factor of importance, but recent evidence strongly suggests that nutritional factors are of primary importance as some subjects recovered who continued to smoke and drink but who were given a full and nutritious diet.

PYRIDOXINE DEFICIENCY

The group of related compounds with vitamin B_6 activity, including pyridoxol (pyridoxine), pyridoxal and pyridoxamine, are found in almost all foods, especially meats, fish and vegetables. In the body they are converted into pyridoxal phosphate, which is coenzyme to a large number of apoenzymes, including the aminotransferases, amino acid decarboxylases, tryptophan synthase, and many more. Pyridoxal phosphate is necessary for the formation, through amino acid decarboxylation, of serotonin, GABA and the catecholamines. Pyridoxine (vitamin B_6) deficiency in early infancy may result in repeated convulsions thought to be due to GABA deficiency. Recurrent epileptiform seizures developed in a large number of infants in the United States who were fed upon artificial milk which, through an accident of manufacture, was deficient in this vitamin. Nutritional pyridoxine lack can also cause polyneuropathy, less often optic atrophy or microcytic anaemia, and polyneuropathy due to isoniazid, hydrallazine or penicillamine is due to metabolic antagonism of pyridoxine and may be corrected by giving high doses of this vitamin. Some inborn errors of metabolism, especially cystathioninuria, can be corrected by massive doses of vitamin B_6.

PELLAGRA

Nicotinic acid occurs mainly as its amide (nicotinamide), which is involved in the formation of physiologically active nucleotides (NAD and NADP), which serve as coenzymes in fundamental oxidation–reduction reactions. Pellagra is generally attributed to dietary deficiency of nicotinic acid, but a secondary factor is often defective protein intake, as the amino acid tryptophan is a chemical precursor of nicotinic acid. Pellagra occurs in individuals who are existing on a predominantly vegetable or cereal diet deficient in animal protein. It is not uncommon in alcoholics and in vegetarians who refuse all food derived from animal sources. The skin lesions of pellagra consist initially of erythema on the face, hands and other exposed surfaces, and later give rise to vesiculation, pigmentation and thickening of the skin. The lesions are precipitated by exposure to sunlight. The symptoms of nervous system involvement, which almost invariably develop in such cases, are predominantly mental. Sometimes the clinical picture is that of severe confusion, while in other cases there is memory impairment, apathy, fatigue, depression and insomnia. Evidence of polyneuropathy is often found, but is probably due to an associated deficiency of other B vitamins. In some cases of apparently uncomplicated pellagra there are symptoms and signs of spinal cord involvement, with spastic paresis of the lower limbs and with variable evidence of disease in the posterior columns.

VITAMIN B_{12} DEFICIENCY

Vitamin B_{12} is converted into a coenzyme that is involved with tetrahydrofolate in synthesizing labile methyl groups. One specific metabolic site lies in the conversion of homocysteine to methionine. It is also a coenzyme for the mutase which converts methylmalonyl-CoA into succinyl-CoA, so that methylmalonate is excreted in the urine in deficiency states.

Although a primary dietary deficiency of vitamin B_{12} has been observed in vegetarians and its absorption may be impaired in various gastrointestinal disorders (especially intestinal 'blind-loop' syndromes, or previous gastrectomy), the clinical effects of vitamin B_{12} deficiency upon the nervous system are most often seen in patients with pernicious anaemia. In this condition the dietary intake of the vitamin is adequate but its absorption is prevented by the absence of intrinsic factor in the gastric juice. Histamine-fast achlorhydria is invariable and usually there are changes in the blood or in the bone marrow to indicate a diagnosis of pernicious anaemia. Rarely, however, neurological symptoms and signs antedate any recognizable change in the blood and even in the bone marrow. Although the principal neurological symptoms and signs indicate disease of the spinal cord, there are occasional cases in which cerebral symptoms are predominant, at least initially. These symptoms include defects of intellect, memory and concentration or episodes of confusion or paranoia. It may at times be difficult to distinguish these cerebral manifestations of vitamin B_{12} deficiency from the clinical features of early presenile dementia or from those resulting from any organic confusional state. Occasionally there is progressive bilateral visual loss with central scotomas, and optic atrophy is found.

SUBACUTE COMBINED DEGENERATION OF THE SPINAL CORD (COMBINED SYSTEM DISEASE)

Symptoms and signs of involvement of the nervous system occur in about 80% of cases of pernicious anaemia. The principal sites of pathological change, in which initial loss of myelin with subsequent axonal degeneration occurs, are the posterior columns and the pyramidal tracts. The disease process often involves the posterior roots and peripheral nerves, giving clinical and pathological features of a predominantly sensory demyelinating polyneuropathy.

The clinical features of the illness depend upon which tracts of the spinal cord are principally affected. Since the lesions in the posterior columns usually predominate, the principal initial symptoms are generally paraesthesiae, tingling, numbness and pins and needles in the extremities. Commonly, patients describe sensations of having a tight band of constriction around one toe, around a limb, or about the waist, or they say that the hands and feet feel swollen or as if encased in tight bandages. Feelings suggesting that cold water is trickling down the legs may also occur. Physical signs may be minimal, but usually vibration sense is impaired early. Romberg's sign is positive, the appreciation of position in the toes and fingers is defective, and the threshold for two-point discrimination is raised. As evidence of posterior column involvement becomes more severe, the patient develops sensory ataxia. Locomotion and maintenance of the upright posture are particularly difficult in the dark or when the eyes are closed. Impairment of appreciation of light touch in the periphery of the limbs is sometimes seen, together with tenderness of the calves. These features, along with depression or absence of tendon reflexes (usually the ankle jerks), as well as evidence of impaired sensory nerve conduction, have shown that peripheral nerves or posterior nerve roots are often involved. Rarely, pain and temperature sensation are impaired, owing to changes in pain-conducting fibres of the peripheral nerves or in the spinothalamic tracts, and there may even be a sensory 'level' on the trunk.

Disturbances of motor function result from damage to the pyramidal tracts. This gives the characteristic stiffness and slowness of the gait which develops in any case of spastic paraparesis, however caused. The abdominal reflexes are lost, and the lower limb reflexes may be exaggerated, with clonus, unless the lesions in the sensory pathways have interrupted the reflex arc. The plantar responses are usually extensor.

The condition is very variable in presentation. Usually sensory symptoms are predominant and the earliest signs may simply be those of a sensory neuropathy. Spasticity of the lower limbs may be striking, whereas signs of posterior column involvement, though present, may be relatively slight. Hence this diagnosis should be seriously considered in any case of sensory neuropathy or spastic paraparesis which develops subacutely in adult life. Even if examination of the blood and bone marrow reveals no abnormality, it is essential to estimate the level of vitamin B_{12} in the serum. A result of less than 100 $\mu\mu g/ml$ of serum is virtually diagnostic of B_{12} deficiency. A Schilling test, examination of the gastric juice for histamine-fast achlorhydria, and estimation of gastric parietal-cell antibodies will then be necessary to confirm that B_{12} absorption is impaired and that the diagnosis is one of pernicious anaemia. When gastric acidity is normal and intestinal malabsorption or a small bowel 'blind-loop' syndrome is suspected, appropriate radiological and other studies will be needed. It is of the greatest importance to recognize B_{12} deficiency because early treatment can lead to complete resolution of the neurological manifestations. Sensory symptoms and signs are usually the first to improve and may be relieved completely. If there is a spastic paraparesis of moderate severity before treatment is begun, there is usually some persistent residual disability.

FOLATE DEFICIENCY

The term folic acid is applied to a group of substances of which the parent compound is pteroylglutamic acid. It is probably absorbed across the intestinal mucosa as a monoglutamate and is then converted to tetrahydrofolate, which is involved in the synthesis and degradation of many compounds, including the conversion of serine to glycine, purine, pyrimidine, methionine and choline synthesis, and the degradation of histidine. A deficiency of folate caused by malabsorption or the use of anticonvulsant drugs has long been known to cause megaloblastic anaemia. It has also been found that some patients with polyneuropathy and/or myelopathy, and even some with dementia, have serum folate levels of less than 2 $\mu g/ml$. However, the role of folate deficiency in the aetiology of these syndromes is yet to be defined.

VITAMIN E DEFICIENCY

Until comparatively recently there was relatively little evidence to implicate vitamin E in the pathogenesis of human disease. However, as mentioned above, the administration of this vitamin can be strikingly beneficial in preventing or partially reversing the neurological manifestations of abetalipoproteinaemia (the Bassen–Kornzweig syndrome) and it also appears to improve some of the neurological manifestations of some of those conditions which cause severe malabsorption of fat. In such cases severe vitamin E deficiency has been reported to cause spinocerebellar degeneration with dysarthria, ataxia, severe proprioceptive loss and diminished tendon reflexes (Harding et al, 1982).

Disorders due to drugs, toxins and other chemical agents

Many drugs will, if taken to excess, produce manifestations of disordered nervous activity. Among those commonly encountered in practice as a cause of intoxication or poisoning are alcohol (usually ethyl or rarely methyl), hypnotic or sedative drugs, opiates, amphetamine and its derivatives, and heavy metals. Intoxication may result from excessive and prolonged indulgence or it may be acute, as in a suicide attempt. In the case of heavy metals, it is usually due to accidental ingestion, often in the course of the patient's occupation. Not only are the specific symptoms induced by some of these drugs of considerable importance, but a characteristic clinical syndrome may follow their sudden withdrawal. Since addiction, clinical pharmacology and toxicology could only be dealt with fully in a larger volume, only a number of points of importance in neurological pathophysiology will be mentioned here.

ALCOHOLISM

Chronic alcoholism due to excessive ethyl alcohol consumption is one form of drug addiction, and as a rule has potent psychological causes. It can develop insidiously in an individual who is at first merely a social drinker. Gradually the intake of alcohol increases so that any excuse or opportunity, however trivial, is regarded as a reason for having a drink, or several drinks. When the patient begins to drink alone, when alcoholic beverages take the place of meals, and when there is a compulsive and irresistible urge to drink, regardless of the time of day, he becomes an alcoholic. The individual who indulges in occasional episodes of excessive drinking with intervals of abstinence is not strictly an alcoholic, though he may become so if the intervals between the episodes shorten progressively, or if his debauches last for days rather than hours (a 'lost weekend'). Only occasionally does alcoholism develop quickly as a result of acute emotional stress; when it does, this usually implies a basically insecure personality. Even small quantities of alcohol can significantly impair the performance of skilled motor activity as well as mental functions. Although the individual who has taken one or two drinks may be elated and may feel himself to be in a state of heightened perception, his reaction time is increased and his senses are dulled. Alcohol also increases water and electrolyte excretion by the kidneys and thus has a diuretic effect. Dehydration and gastrointestinal irritation are largely responsible for 'hangover' symptoms, including headache.

The nervous symptoms of alcoholism can be divided into those resulting from acute intoxication and those which follow alcohol withdrawal. The symptoms and signs of acute intoxication are well known. The speech is slurred, the gait unsteady, and the patient is either jocular and inattentive, noisy and aggressive, or dulled, confused and retarded. More severe degrees of intoxication result in stupor or coma. The diagnosis must be made not only upon the flushed face and alcohol-laden breath, but upon the absence of signs of nervous disease. It must be remembered that subarachnoid haemorrhage, for instance, or head injury, can occur during an alcoholic debauch. Pure alcoholic coma, however, is rarely deep or prolonged, and there are no focal neurological signs. Although an estimation of blood alcohol level may indicate the amount of alcohol that the individual has consumed, it may not be closely related to the degree of clinical intoxication, as individual tolerance varies widely and depends to some extent upon habituation.

Many symptoms and physical signs may follow the withdrawal of alcohol after prolonged intoxication or after several days of heavy drinking. The commonest feature is a state of nervousness or intense tremulousness ('the shakes'), which is relieved by a further drink, but which returns more severely when once again the patient abstains. The patient is alert, jumpy and easily startled, and has a marked tremor of the limbs. Sometimes these symptoms settle within a few days, but occasionally there is a superadded hallucinosis in the form of vivid visual experiences, or less commonly auditory hallucinations, involving voices, motor cars, radios, etc. Occasionally, too, a series of convulsions ('rum fits') occur either at the height of a drinking bout or on withdrawal. The most severe of all the syndromes of alcoholic withdrawal is *delirium tremens*. It commonly develops 2–4 days after the last drink and especially in individuals who have been excessive drinkers for several years. Often it is seen when the patient develops an intercurrent illness such as pneumonia or is admitted to a hospital for an operation, or following an accident. The patient is typically restless, voluble and sleepless, living in a state of intense physical and mental activity both day and night. There are tremors of the limbs, intermittent muscular twitching, confusion, and, as a rule, hallucinations. A fatal outcome, resulting from circulatory failure or even, in some cases, from exhaustion despite sedation, is not uncommon. Usually the illness lasts for 3–4 days, and the patient at last falls into a calm sleep and awakens lucid but amnesic, having no recollection of the illness.

Alcoholic cerebellar degeneration is a progressive, symmetrical cerebellar ataxia of subacute type which is now presumed to be due to thiamine deficiency. Degeneration of the corpus callosum (Marchiafava–Bignami disease) is a syndrome of progressive dementia with fits and eventual spastic paralysis, which develops almost exclusively in Italian males who are heavy wine drinkers and of which the cause is unknown. Even less common is central pontine myelinolysis, which gives pseudobulbar palsy and quadriparesis. Acute and chronic varieties of alcoholic myopathy have also been described. Acute myopathy usually develops at the height of a debauch and produces phosphorylase deficiency, muscle necrosis and often myoglobinuria, while the subacute variety is more often progressive and resembles other metabolic varieties of muscle disease. Alcoholic polyneuropathy is virtually identical with the predominantly sensory neuropathy of dry beri-beri described above. Wernicke's encephalopathy and the Korsakov syndrome, each described above, are other common complications of chronic alcoholism, and it has also become clear that a subacute progressive dementing process is another important complication of prolonged and severe alcohol addiction (Walton, 1985).

The syndrome produced by the ingestion of methyl alcohol is characterized by an acute acidosis and by nausea, vomiting, visual loss, muscle pains and impairment of consciousness. If large quantities have been taken, permanent visual loss due to optic nerve damage is common. Some patients remain blind, while others show bilateral central scotomas.

HYPNOTIC AND SEDATIVE DRUGS

Drugs of the barbiturate group were once in such common use that they were frequently used in suicide attempts by the depressed patient. While acute or chronic intoxication with barbiturates still occurs, habituation to remedies of the benzodiazepine group is now much commoner and produces similar effects. Accidental excessive dosage is also seen, when a patient awakens during the night, and being bemused as a result of a tablet taken on retiring, proceeds to take several more. Alcohol can greatly potentiate the action of these drugs. There are also some individuals to whom they have been given as sedatives who have gradually increased their habitual dose and thus developed a syndrome of chronic intoxication.

Symptoms of acute poisoning depend upon the dose taken. Mild intoxication results from taking about two or three times the maximum recommended dose. The patient is drowsy, but easily awakened, and often shows nystagmus, dysarthria and ataxia. When the dose of barbiturates taken was 5–10 times the normal, the patient is semicomatose and can be awakened only by vigorous stimulation, when he may mutter a few words and will then lapse again into unconsciousness. The patient who has taken from 15 to 20 times the usual dose or more is comatose with shallow respiration, absent reflexes and extensor plantar responses. Treatment is urgent, as this condition can be fatal. The safety margin with the benzodiazepine hypnotics is very much greater than it was with older remedies such as the barbiturates, and fatal poisoning with the newer drugs is uncommon.

The clinical features of chronic benzodiazepine and barbiturate intoxication and those of withdrawal are similar to those of alcoholism. Increasing tolerance can be considerable, so that the patient who is habituated can take many times the recommended dose with comparatively little effect. Characteristically the addict is slow in his mental reactions, his perception is dulled, and he is slovenly in dress and habits. The physical signs are nystagmus, dysarthria and cerebellar ataxia. Withdrawal of the drug is followed by a few hours of temporary improvement, but later by tremulousness, nervousness, weakness and confusion. There may be a phase of delirium with hallucinations and delusions, and convulsions are common after barbiturate withdrawal, less so after stopping benzodiazepines.

AMPHETAMINE INTOXICATION

Amphetamines and related compounds were once commonly used not only for their stimulant and antidepressive effects but also in order to reduce appetite in patients who were attempting to lose weight. Such individuals often steadily increased the dose up to a point where symptoms of intoxication or chronic addiction appeared. The principal symptoms of overdosage are restlessness and overactivity, dryness of the mouth, tremor, palpitations and tachycardia, hallucinations, irritability and profound insomnia. Very heavy dosage can give fits, hypertension and fatal ventricular arrhythmia. Withdrawal is followed by an acute delirious state with severe hallucinations, and sometimes by a delusional psychosis which may last for days or weeks.

MARIJUANA (CANNABIS)

This drug, used for many years in the Orient, was introduced more recently into Western countries, often being smoked in cigarettes. It produces a temporary sense of well-being and is a drug of habituation rather than of addiction. Its principal danger is that it may introduce the user to more harmful narcotic drugs. Recent work suggests that long-continued use in high dosage may produce dementia and cerebral atrophy, but this has not been firmly established.

HALLUCINOGENIC AGENTS

The hallucinations induced by mescaline and LSD are often terrifying and rarely pleasurable. Rarely, continued use may lead to irreversible psychosis. Addiction to these and related agents is increasing.

OPIATES

Among the drugs of the opiate group that have been known to cause symptoms of intoxication or addiction are opium itself and its tincture (laudanum), morphine, heroin (diacetylmorphine), dilaudid (dihydromorphine) and codeine (methylmorphine). Synthetic analgesics such as pethidine (demerol), methadone and dromoran are similar pharmacologically and can also be addictive. They may conveniently be considered together with the opiates.

Acute poisoning with these drugs is relatively uncommon except as a result of accidental ingestion, mistakes in dispensing, or illicit use, as their issue is carefully controlled by law. The usual clinical features are stupor or coma, pinpoint pupils, shallow respiration and bradycardia.

Chronic opiate intoxication or addiction is characterized by an initial phase of tolerance in which increasing doses of the drug are required to produce the desired effect, whether it be the pleasurable feeling of detachment which first encourages the eventual addict to use them, or the relief of symptoms for which they were initially prescribed. Prolonged therapeutic use of these drugs in illness is a potent cause of addiction, which is also a serious and widespread problem among doctors and nurses owing to their easy access to the drugs. The phase of tolerance is followed by one of dependence in which attempted withdrawal gives a series of characteristic symptoms. Some 12 hours or so after the last dose the patient begins to yawn repeatedly, and there is lacrimation and running of the nose. This is followed by restlessness, insomnia, muscular twitching, generalized aching and shivering, and then by nausea, vomiting and diarrhoea. Commonly, these acute symptoms last for 2 or 3 days, but insomnia and weakness can persist for days or even weeks. Even when the stage of withdrawal and physical dependence has passed, emotional dependence or habituation remains and is an important cause of relapse. Physical, mental and moral dilapidation is invariable in the established addict, and most addicts will resort to any measure, including lying, feigning illness, stealing and many other subterfuges, in order to obtain supplies.

COCAINE

Cocaine as a drug of addiction may be injected, drunk as coca wine, smoked or taken as snuff. Addicts suffer from progressive mental deterioration, sometimes confusional psychosis, hallucinations and fits. Unlike the opiates, withdrawal does not produce severe symptoms, but nevertheless addiction is difficult to treat.

HEAVY METALS

Although poisoning with any one of a number of heavy metals is accompanied by symptoms of involvement of the nervous system, the most important in clinical practice are arsenic, lead, manganese and mercury.

Arsenic poisoning
Though not strictly a heavy metal, arsenic combines with sulphydryl (SH) groups of coenzymes, notably thiamine, thus interfering with cellular oxidative processes. The principal symptoms of acute arsenical poisoning are gastrointestinal, namely vomiting, diarrhoea and acute abdominal pain, though convulsions may occur. In chronic arsenical poisoning, however, whether resulting from criminal intent, from the excessive use of therapeutic arsenical preparations, or from contamination of food with arsenical insecticides, the main symptoms are neurological. The nervous symptoms include headache, drowsiness, confusion and a symmetrical polyneuropathy that gives burning paraesthesiae in the extremities followed by muscular weakness and atrophy, distal sensory loss and absence of the tendon reflexes. Hyperkeratosis, pigmentation and desquamation of the skin are also common.

Lead poisoning
Industrial lead poisoning was at one time common, but has now been greatly reduced by legislative restrictions, though it may still be seen in painters and battery-makers. Water which had passed through lead pipes was an important source of poisoning in the past, and beer and cider were sometimes similarly contaminated. Sucking or chewing articles covered in lead paint and pica are still the commonest causes of lead poisoning in children. In all of these conditions absorption occurs mainly through the gastrointestinal tract. Lead tetraethyl, contained in certain brands of petrol, may be absorbed through the lungs and skin and has been known to cause encephalopathy. Because of its potential environmental effect, many countries have introduced legislation to reduce the lead content of motor fuel.

At least 90% of ingested lead is not absorbed, but that which *is* absorbed from the intestine enters the erythrocytes and is then stored in liver, kidney and bone. That stored in liver and kidney is later transferred to bone, and in chronic lead poisoning its storage in bone as an insoluble phosphate is facilitated by a calcium-rich diet. In states of acidosis or as a result of increased secretion of parathormone, the stored lead may be released into the bloodstream. Lead combines with essential SH-groups of certain enzymes involved in porphyrin synthesis and carbohydrate metabolism. In particular it depresses δ-aminolaevulinic acid dehydratase and enzymes concerned with haem synthesis, causing anaemia and impaired renal tubular function. In the central nervous system it causes cerebral oedema, and in experimental lead encephalopathy in primates epilepsy is common. In peripheral nerves combined axonal degeneration and demyelination occur. In children, the principal symptom of lead poisoning is encephalopathy, giving somnolence, convulsions and sometimes coma, and a correlation between infantile ingestion of lead and mental retardation has been postulated. In adults, particularly in painters using lead-containing paint, agonizing colicky abdominal pain and anaemia are the commonest presenting symptoms. A peripheral neuropathy is also common, but is rarely symmetrical and more often affects one limb. A worker who is making batteries may develop a unilateral wrist-drop in the arm most often used, and the presence of a blue line on the gums and of punctate basophilia in the red blood cells will suggest that this is due to lead. Confirmation depends upon measurement of lead in the serum and in the urine. Sometimes lead in the bones gives a characteristic increased density in radiographs.

Manganese poisoning
This industrial disease, seen almost exclusively in manganese miners, results from inhalation of dust and is observed particularly in Chile and in some parts of central Europe. It gives a clinical syndrome almost indistinguishable from parkinsonism, but there is often associated lethargy, irritability and somnolence. Marked improvement follows the use of levodopa.

Mercury poisoning
Acute mercury poisoning gives severe vomiting and diarrhoea followed by anuria and uraemia due to renal tubular necrosis. In infants, however, chronic mercurial poisoning due to excessive use of calomel teething powders probably caused most cases of pink disease (acrodynia). A syndrome of chronic mercurial poisoning in adults has been described, due to the inhalation of mercury vapour, to the ingestion of fish that have fed on the effluent from a mercury factory (Minimata disease), or, in police officers, to working with outdated fingerprint powders containing mercury. In some instances this produces cerebellar ataxia, but more often a syndrome characterized by excessive salivation, tremulousness, vertigo, irritability and depression or erethism (childish over-emotionalism) occurs.

SOME OTHER POISONS AFFECTING THE NERVOUS SYSTEM

Other metals
Apart from the heavy metals mentioned above, other elements have been reported to cause neurological manifestations when absorbed to excess. Many of these, including antimony, bismuth, copper, phosphorus and thallium, have been reported to cause polyneuropathy on occasion. Thallium poisoning produces symptoms varying from mild alopecia to irreversible coma and death. Skeletal fluorosis due to the excessive dietary ingestion of fluoride has been known to give spastic paraparesis due to spinal cord compression. Chronic cyanide intoxication is now known to cause one form of tropical ataxic neuropathy, as noted above.

Other drugs, organic chemicals and toxic substances
Atropine and related anticholinergic drugs taken in excess produce nervous excitation and confusion, which may progress to mania as a result of uncontrolled activity in cholinergic neurons. Bromism, now rarely encountered, is characterized by drowsiness, lethargy, dysarthria and occasionally psychosis. Chloral hydrate has an effect similar to that of alcohol, and antihistamines can give lethargy and coma and sometimes convulsions in childhood. Toxic symptoms due to overdosage with anticonvulsant drugs such as phenytoin include drowsiness, dysarthria, nystagmus, and sometimes diplopia with cerebellar ataxia which is occasionally irreversible, in addition to the well-known megaloblastic anaemia due to folate antagonism. Long-continued use of phenothiazines can give drug-induced parkinsonism and/or irreversible facial and limb dyskinesias.

The number of chemical substances known to cause polyneuropathy are now legion. Among them are acrylamide, aniline, 'bush tea', carbon monoxide, carbon bisulphide, carbon tetrachloride, chloral, chloretone, chloroquine, clioquinol, cyanogenetic glycosides, cytotoxic agents (including vincristine sulphate), DDT, dinitrobenzol, dimonosulfiram, emetine, ethionamide, glutethimide, immune sera, isoniazid, n-hexane, nitrofurantoin, pentachlorphenol, phenytoin, stilbamidine, streptomycin, sulphanilamide and its derivatives, sulphonal, tetrachlorethane, thalidomide, trichlorethylene and tri-orthocresylphosphate. For details of the effects of these and of many other drugs and toxic agents the reader is referred to Spencer and Schaumburg (1980) and Walton (1985).

TOXIC DISORDERS

There are many bacterial infections in which exotoxins produced by the infective agents have profound effects upon the functioning of the nervous system. Tetanus produces, among other manifestations, spasms of intense muscular rigidity due to the effect of its exotoxin upon inhibitory interneurons in the spinal cord. Botulism causes widespread muscular weakness and/or paralysis of ocular, bulbar and limb muscles, owing to the fact that the toxin acts presynaptically at the neuromuscular junction, impairing the release of acetylcholine. Diphtheria exotoxin spreads from the site of infection in a retrograde manner along nerve trunks, producing a demyelinating polyneuropathy in which muscles close to the site of infection are predominantly involved. There are many other bacterial, viral and auto-immune or hypersensitivity disorders in which encephalopathy, encephalomyelopathy, polyneuropathy or less often myopathy have been described as complications. Toxic encephalopathy is especially common as a complication of infection in childhood, but specific toxins have not yet been isolated. These conditions are dealt with in depth in standard textbooks of infectious diseases.

Saxitoxin is a powerful neurotoxin, acting particularly at the neuromuscular junction. It may produce symptoms in human subjects eating mussels or other shellfish contaminated by dinoflagellates of the genus *Gonyaulax* which occur in the sea only at certain times of the year and in certain weather conditions. Epidemics have been reported from the Pacific Coast of the United States and from many places in Europe. Symptoms usually develop within 30 minutes to 12 hours after eating mussels and include paraesthesiae in the limbs and circumoral distribution, muscular weakness, ataxia, headache, vomiting and choking sensations. Recovery is usually complete in 24–72 hours, but rare fatal cases have been described. Many snake venoms are also powerful neurotoxins, acting upon synapses both in the central nervous system and at the neuromuscular junction. Snakebite is often followed by widespread muscular weakness and especially by respiratory paralysis, though the bite of various sea snakes can cause widespread necrosis of skeletal muscle and hepatic and renal damage.

References

Adams, R. D. and Foley, J. M. (1953) The neurological disorder associated with liver disease. In *Metabolic Disorders of the Nervous System*. Baltimore: Association for Research in Nervous and Mental Disease.

Adams, R. D. and Lyon, G. (1982) *Neurology of Hereditary Metabolic Diseases of Children*. Washington, DC: Hemisphere Publishing.

Appel, S. H. (1977) Introduction to metabolic diseases of the nervous system, In Goldensohn, E. S. and Appel, S. H. (eds) *Scientific Approaches to Clinical Neurology*, chap. 1, p. 2. Philadelphia: Lea & Febiger.

Barbeau, A., Growdon, J. H. and Wurtman, R. J. (eds) (1979). *Choline and Lecithin in Brain Disorders* (Nutrition and the Brain, vol. 5). New York: Raven Press.

Cavanagh, J. B. (1974). Liver bypass and the glia. In Plum, F. (ed.) *Brain Dysfunction in Metabolic Disorders*, vol. 53. New York: Association for Research in Nervous and Mental Disease.

Davies, D. M. (1981). *Textbook of Adverse Drug Reactions*, 2nd edn. Oxford: Oxford Medical Publications.

Essig, C. F. (1972) Chronic abuse of sedative-hypnotic drugs. In Zarafonetis, C. J. D. (ed.) *Drug Abuse*. Philadelphia: Lea & Febiger.

Fahn, S., Davis, J. N. and Rowland, L. P. (1979) *Cerebral Hypoxia and its Consequences* (Advances in Neurology, vol. 26). New York: Raven Press.

Garland, H. and Pearce, J. (1967) Neurological complications of carbon monoxide poisoning. *Quart. J. Med.* **36:** 445.

Goldensohn, E. S. and Appel, S. H. (eds) (1977) *Scientific Approaches to Clinical Neurology*. Philadelphia: Lea & Febiger.

Goulding, R. (1986) Poisoning. In Walton, J., Beeson, P. B. and Bodley Scott, R. (eds) *Oxford Companion to Medicine*. Oxford: Oxford University Press.

Harding, A. E., Muller., D. P. R., Thomas, P. K. and Willison, H. J. (1982) Spinocerebellar degeneration secondary to chronic intestinal malabsorption: a vitamin E deficiency syndrome. *Ann. Neurol.* **12:** 419.

Hunter, D. (1975) *The Diseases of Occupations*, 5th edn. London: Little, Brown & Company.

Lancet: False neurotransmitters and hepatic failure. *Lancet* **i:** 86.

Lawson, S. N., Harper, A. A., Harper, E. I., Garson, J. A. and Anderton, B. H. (1984) A monoclonal antibody against neurofilament protein specifically labels a subpopulation of rat sensory neurones. *J. Comp. Neurol.* **228:** 263.

Menkes, J. H. (1985) *Textbook of Child Neurology*, 3rd edn. Philadelphia: Lea & Febiger.

Merritt, H. H. (ed.) (1973) *A Textbook of Neurology*, p. 652. Philadelphia: Lea and Febiger.

Millar, J. A., Battistini, V., Cumming, R. L. C., Carswell, F. and Goldberg, A. (1970) Lead and delta-aminolaevulinic acid dehydratase levels in mentally retarded children and in lead-poisoned suckling rats. *Lancet* **ii:** 695.

Moss, T. H. and Lewkowicz, S. J. (1983) The axon reaction in motor and sensory neurons of mice studied by a monoclonal antibody marker of neurofilament protein. *J. Neurol. Sci.* **60:** 267.

Nakae, K., Yamamoto, S., Shigematsu, I. and Kono, R. (1973) Relation between subacute myelo-optic neuropathy (S.M.O.N.) and clioquinol: nationwide survey. *Lancet* **i:** 171.

Namba, T., Nolte, C. T., Jackrel, J. and Grob. D. (1971) Poisoning due to organophosphate insecticides. *Amer. J. Med.* **50:** 475.

O'Brian, D. and Goodman, S. I. (1970) The critically ill child (acute metabolic diseases in infancy and early childhood). *Pediatrics* **46:** 620.

Pallis, C. and Lewis, P. D. (1974) *The Neurology of Gastrointestinal Disease*. Philadelphia: W. B. Saunders Company.

Pant, S. S., Rebeiz, J. J. and Richardson, E. P. (1968) Spastic paraparesis following portacaval shunts. *Neurology* **18:** 134.

Plum, F. and Posner, J. (1980) *Stupor and Coma*, 3rd edn. Philadelphia: F. A. Davis.

Rosenberg, R. N. (ed.) (1983) *Neurology* (The Clinical Neurosciences, vol. 1). New York: Churchill Livingstone.

Rustam, H. and Hamdi, T. (1974) Methyl mercury poisoning in Iraq—a neurological study. *Brain* **97:** 499.

Seixas, F. A., Williams, K. and Eggleston, S. (1975) Medical consequences of alcoholism. *Ann. NY Acad. Sci*, 252.

Seneviratne, K. N. and Peiris, O. A. (1970) Peripheral nerve function in chronic liver disease. *J. Neurol. Neurosurg. Psychiat.* **33:** 609.

Spencer, P. S. and Schaumburg, H. (1980) *Experimental and Clinical Neurotoxicology*. Baltimore: Williams and Wilkins.

Spillane, J. D. (1973) *Tropical Neurology*. Oxford: Oxford University Press.

Victor, M. (1974) Neurologic changes in liver disease. In Plum, F. (ed.) *Brain Dysfunction in Metabolic Disorders*, vol. 53. New York: Association for Research in Nervous and Mental Disease.

Victor, M. and Silby, H. (1977) Thiamine deficiency. In Goldensohn, E. S. and Appel, S. H. (eds) *Scientific Approaches to Clinical Neurology*. p. 204. Philadelphia: Lea & Febiger.

Walton, J. N. (1985) *Brain's Diseases of the Nervous System*, 9th edn. Oxford: Oxford University Press.

11

THE CEREBROSPINAL FLUID, RAISED INTRACRANIAL PRESSURE, BRAIN OEDEMA, CRANIOCEREBRAL AND SPINAL TRAUMA, SPINAL CORD COMPRESSION AND RELEVANT INVESTIGATIONS—SOME PATHOPHYSIOLOGICAL PRINCIPLES

INTRODUCTION

The final chapter in this book on the pathophysiology of the nervous system brings together information about several disparate but in some respects interrelated disorders of nervous function. In order to appreciate the pathophysiological principles of importance in understanding the effects of raised intracranial pressure, it is essential to appreciate the principles which govern the formation, circulation and absorption of the cerebrospinal fluid. Such information is also of importance in appreciating the effects of physical injury to, or compression of, the brain and spinal cord. Finally it will be necessary to comment briefly upon the role of special neurological investigations, and especially of neuroradiology, in the elucidation of these mechanisms.

THE CEREBROSPINAL FLUID (CSF)

Formation, circulation and absorption

The choroid plexuses of the cerebral ventricles play an important part in the formation of the cerebrospinal fluid. Blockage of the aqueduct of Sylvius gives dilatation of the lateral and third ventricles, consequent upon the continued production of CSF for which there is no longer an outlet. Hydrocephalus can also follow blockage of the superior longitudinal sinus which impairs reabsorption of the fluid. The CSF is formed in the choroid plexuses, not by simple diffusion or dialysis but by a process of active secretion and transport. It is secreted in the lateral ventricles, from which it passes through the foramina of Monro, the third ventricle, the aqueduct and the fourth ventricle, to enter the basal cisterns of the subarachnoid space through the foramina of Magendie and Luschka. The CSF then flows upwards over the surface of the cerebral hemispheres, while some flows down into the spinal subarachnoid space. Reabsorption into the bloodstream occurs through the arachnoidal villi which protrude into the superior longitudinal and other venous sinuses. Work on the passage of radioactive substances into the CSF has confirmed this mechanism of secretion and reabsorption. The mean rate of formation and therefore of absorption is about 0.35 ml/min. A constant process of dialysis occurs across the arachnoid membrane at all levels, with exchange of chemical constituents between the CSF and blood. Large molecules fail to enter the CSF from the blood because of the interposition of the vascular endothelium that constitutes the blood–brain barrier, but there is a rapid exchange of small molecular weight substances between the CSF and the extracellular fluid of the brain and cord. The CSF acts in certain respects as a 'sink', preventing the extracellular fluid of the brain from achieving a true equilibrium with the blood plasma. The composition of the ventricular fluid is different from that in the lumbar subarachnoid space, and some constituents in the lumbar fluid are added to it by diffusion across the spinal arachnoid membrane.

Function

The CSF acts as a buffer or cushion protecting the brain and spinal cord against the effects of external pressure waves. It seems to have no nutritional role but does remove metabolites such as carbon dioxide, lactate and hydrogen ions from nervous tissue. CSF

TABLE 16 Composition of normal lumbar cerebrospinal fluid and serum*

	Cerebrospinal fluid		Serum			Cerebrospinal fluid		Serum	
Osmolarity	295	mosmol/l	295	mosmol/l	beta-trace protein	2.0	mg/dl	0.5	mg/dl
Water content	99%		93%		fibronectin	3.0	µg/ml	300	µg/ml
Sodium	138.0	mEq/l	138.0	mEq/l					
Potassium	2.8	mEq/l	4.5	mEq/l	Total free amino acids	80.9	µmol/dl	228.0	µmol/dl
Calcium	2.1	mEq/l	4.8	mEq/l					
Magnesium	2.3	mEq/l	1.7	mEq/l	Ammonia	24.0	µg/dl	37.0	µg/dl
Chloride	119.0	mEq/l	102.0	mEq/l	Urea	4.7	mmol/l	5.4	mmol/l
Bicarbonate	22.0	mEq/l	24.0	mEq/l	Creatinine	1.2	mg/dl	1.8	mg/dl
CO_2 tension	47.0	mmHg	41.0	mmHg	Uric acid	0.25	mg/dl	5.50	mg/dl
pH	7.33		7.41		Putrescine	184.0	pmol/ml		
Oxygen	43.0	mmHg	104.0	mmHg	Spermidine	150.0	pmol/ml		
Glucose	60.0	mg/dl	90.0	mg/dl					
Lactate	1.6	mEq/l	1.0	mEq/l	Total lipids	1.5	mg/dl	750.0	mg/dl
Pyruvate	0.08	mEq/l	0.11	mEq/l	free cholesterol	0.4	mg/dl	180.0	mg/dl
Lactate/pyruvate ratio	26.0		17.6		cholesterol esters	0.3	mg/dl	126.0	mg/dl
Fructose	4.0	mg/dl	2.0	mg/dl					
Polyols	340	µmol/l	148.0	µmol/l	cAMP	20.0	nmol/l		
Myoinositol	2.6	mg/dl	1.0	mg/dl	cGMP	0.68	nmol/l		
Total protein	35.0	mg/dl	7.0	g/dl	HVA	60.0	µg/ml		
prealbumin	4%		trace		5-H1AA	0.04	µg/ml		
albumin	65%		60%		Norepinephrine	200.0	pg/ml	350.0	pg/ml
alpha$_1$ globulin	4%		5%		MHGP	15.0	mg/ml		
alpha$_2$ globulin	8%		9%		Acetylcholine	1.8	mg/dl		
beta globulin (beta$_1$ + tau)	12%		12%		Choline	2.5	mmol/ml		
gamma globulin	7%		14%		Prostaglandin PGF$_2$ alpha	92.0	pg/ml		
IgG	1.2	mg/dl	987	mg/dl	Insulin	3.7	mu/ml	36.0	mu/ml
IgA	0.2	mg/dl	175	mg/dl	Gastrin	3.4	pmol/l		
IgM	0.06	mg/dl	70	mg/dl	Cholecystokinin	14.0	pmol/l		
kappa/lambda ratio	1.0		1.0		Beta endorphin	145.0	pmol/l	10.0	pmol/l
					Phosphorus	1.6	mg/dl	4.0	mg/dl
					Iron	1.5	µg/dl	15.0	mg/dl

* Average or representative values are given. Reproduced from Fishman (1980) by kind permission of the author and publisher; also reproduced in Walton (1985), p. 65.

pH, which is in equilibrium with the pH of the extracellular fluid of the nervous system, influences ventilation, cerebral blood flow and various other aspects of cerebral metabolism. The fluid also appears to distribute, by intracerebral transport, some biologically active substances such as hormones within the central nervous system.

Composition

The total volume of CSF in the normal adult is between 100 and 130 ml. The fluid is clear and colourless. It contains fewer than five white blood cells per cubic millimetre and all of these are lymphocytes. The protein content of the lumbar fluid is 15–45 mg/dl, the respective values for ventricular and cisternal fluid being 5–15 mg and 15–25 mg/dl. Most of the protein present is albumin. Normally, too, the fluid contains 50–80 mg glucose/dl and 120–130 mEq chloride/l. The concentrations of these and of other substances in the CSF as well as comparative concentrations in CSF and plasma are listed in Table 16. The protein and sugar content of the fluid is low when compared with that of the blood plasma, while the chloride content is higher. Sodium, potassium, urea and some drugs such as sulphonamides pass freely into the fluid and are found there in concentrations equal to those in the serum. Other substances such as antibodies, salicylates, penicillin and streptomycin pass into CSF in relatively minute quantities even if the serum concentration is high. Bromide, too, is found in the lumbar CSF in only about one-third the concentration in which it is present in the plasma. The entry of many chemicals into the CSF is selective and does not depend upon a simple process of diffusion across a semipermeable membrane. Disease, and particularly inflammation of the arachnoid, may influence this process. In some cases of meningitis, for example, penicillin and bromide enter the fluid more easily.

Lumbar puncture

Cytological and chemical examination of the CSF is of considerable value in neurological diagnosis, and specimens of fluid are most easily obtained by lumbar puncture. The exploring needle is inserted into the lumbar subarachnoid space below the termination of the spinal cord, and since the roots of the cauda equina are pushed aside by the needle, the risks of damage to nervous tissue are negligible. The investigation is, however, dangerous if the intracranial pressure is high (see p. 244), and particularly if a space-occupying lesion such as an intracranial tumour is present. In this circumstance reduction in the pressure of fluid in the lumbar subarachnoid space can result in impaction of the cerebellar tonsils in the foramen magnum or the medial aspects of one or both temporal lobes between the brain stem and the edge of the tentorium cerebelli, with fatal results. Papilloedema is almost always a contraindication, and the examination should also be avoided if the patient's symptoms suggest that the intracranial pressure is raised. Even in subarachnoid haemorrhage, a condition in which it was long thought that lumbar puncture was an essential diagnostic step, if only to distinguish the condition from meningitis, there is now evidence that the procedure may be dangerous, especially when there is extension of bleeding into the brain substance or cerebral infarction and brain swelling due to arterial spasm. Hence, when CT scanning is freely available and shows blood in the subarachnoid space, it may be possible in many cases to avoid the examination, with its attendant risks. Should manometry reveal that the pressure is unexpectedly high, it may be wise to remove the needle at once. Even this precaution, however, will not always avoid cerebellar or tentorial herniation as persistent leakage of fluid may occur through the hole in the spinal dura mater left by the exploring needle. The latter mechanism, with consequent reduction of the intracranial pressure below normal, probably causes the common post-lumbar-puncture headache.

It has long been common practice to measure the pressure of the fluid by attaching a manometer to the needle. The normal pressure in the recumbent adult is 60–180 mm of CSF fluid. When the patient is sitting upright the pressure in the lumbar subarachnoid space is about 200–250 mm. The patient must be comfortably relaxed during this procedure. Coughing or straining causes increased pressure in abdominal veins and consequently in vertebral veins. This displaces CSF from the spinal canal and its pressure therefore rises. If there is free communication between the cerebral and lumbar subarachnoid spaces, a temporary increase in the intracranial pressure is reflected in the manometer. Such an increase may be produced by compressing one or both internal jugular veins in the neck, thus reducing venous outflow from the cranium. In carrying out this procedure (Queckenstedt's test), there is usually a sharp rise in pressure to 300 mm or more, with an equally rapid fall to normal when the pressure is released. If there is a block to the free passage of fluid in the subarachnoid space, then no rise in pressure occurs during the manoeuvre, while if the block is partial the rise and fall are both abnormally slow.

Queckenstedt's test was often used in the past to identify the presence of lesions causing complete or partial obstruction to CSF circulation and flow. It was also used in the diagnosis of thrombosis of one lateral sinus, when pressure upon the affected (but not on the unaffected) jugular vein failed to produce a rise in CSF pressure. The increasing sophistication of radiological techniques such as angiography, and, above all, the CT scan, as well as the relative imprecision of Queckenstedt's test, which gives too many false-negative results to be reliable, have sharply restricted its utilization. It may still be of limited value when neuroradiological facilities are not immediately available, but even then, if a spinal tumour is suspected and transfer to a neurological or neurosurgical unit is possible, lumbar puncture is better avoided as withdrawal of CSF distal to a spinal block may render subsequent myelography difficult or impossible. And, in addition, the performance of Queckenstedt's test may increase the hazards of lumbar puncture as described above, when an intracranial space-occupying lesion is present.

Samples of fluid are usually collected, depending upon the clinical situation, for microbiological, cytological and chemical studies. Failure to obtain fluid (a dry tap) usually means that the puncture has been incorrectly performed. A genuine dry tap, when the needle is in the subarachnoid space but no fluid can be withdrawn, means either that the space is blocked at a higher level or that the lumbar sac itself is filled by a neoplasm or developmental lesion such as a lipoma.

Cisternal puncture

Cisternal puncture is a more difficult and dangerous procedure than lumbar puncture. If the needle is inserted too far into the cisterna magna, the lower part of the medulla oblongata is pierced. This approach is used only if lumbar puncture is impossible owing to spinal deformity, if an opaque substance must be injected to define the upper level of a spinal lesion causing a block, if it is necessary to compare the chemical constitution of the lumbar and cisternal fluids, or if intrathecal injections of therapeutic agents are to be given and there is a block in the spinal subarachnoid space.

Ventricular puncture

Direct needle puncture of the lateral cerebral ventricles is occasionally necessary in order to relieve symptoms of increased intracranial pressure prior to an operation for intracranial tumour, and was often used in the past in order to inject air for ventriculography. When there was severe inflammatory exudate in the subarachnoid space and lumbar or cisternal puncture failed to produce a free flow of CSF, this route was also occasionally used for the administration of antibiotics. In infants the ventricles can be entered directly by a needle which is inserted in the lateral angle of the fontanelle and which is then passed through the cerebral substance. In older children and in adults, cranial burr-holes must first be made. In view of the hazards which may result from passing a needle through brain tissue, this technique is one for the specialist, but in any event, the advent of effective means of reducing the intracranial pressure with drugs and with CT scanning and newer antibiotics mean that it is rarely used.

Examination of the CSF and some common abnormalities

PRESSURE

An increase in the pressure of the CSF above 200 mm in a relaxed, recumbent patient usually implies raised pressure inside the cranium. This is usually due to brain swelling or oedema or to a space-occupying lesion such as a tumour, abscess, infarct or haematoma. A moderate rise occurs in severe arterial hypertension. An unusually low pressure is much less significant if there is no other evidence of spinal block and is generally of no diagnostic value.

NAKED EYE APPEARANCE

Turbidity of the fluid usually indicates a neutrophil pleocytosis. Excess lymphocytes, even in large numbers, rarely give visible changes. Some specimens which contain excess protein may clot on standing. A fine cobweb-like fibrin deposit appearing after a few hours also implies an increased protein content. Frank blood in the CSF may be present owing to puncture of a vertebral vein, in which case the contamination of the fluid becomes less as it flows. If two test tubes are filled, the second is less stained than the first, and if the specimen is centrifuged the supernatant fluid is clear. Uniform blood-staining occurs in subarachnoid haemorrhage or following extension of a primary cerebral haemorrhage to the subarachnoid space. In such cases, the supernatant generally shows a yellow colouration or xanthochromia. A faint colour, generally orange, appears within 4 hours of a subarachnoid bleed and is then due to oxyhaemoglobin. Within 48 hours the deep yellow colour of bilirubin appears. This colour may persist for 6 weeks after a haemorrhage but usually disappears in from 2 to 3 weeks. Xanthochromia is also seen in CSF with a very high protein content (as in spinal tumour), in some patients with subdural bleeding, and in others who are deeply jaundiced. Spectrophotometric analysis of samples of fluid has shown that methaemalbumin is another pigment occasionally found in the CSF, but it only appears as a rule in the presence of extensive brain damage (as in severe head injury or cerebral haemorrhage).

CYTOLOGY

Many techniques of counting the white cells in the CSF are in common use. That most commonly used is to draw up 0.1 ml of methyl green diluting fluid in a white-cell-counting pipette and to fill the pipette with CSF. After mixing, the number of cells seen in the entire lined area of a Neubauer counting chamber is counted; this gives the number of cells per cubic millimetre of fluid. Staining is usually good enough for red cells, lymphocytes and neutrophil leucocytes to be identified. Tumour cells, yeasts and other abnormal cells are occasionally found but require specialized cytological techniques and skilled scrutiny for their recognition and interpretation.

A small number of red cells may be present owing to the trauma of the puncture, but if they persist in several specimens they usually indicate bleeding directly or by extension into the subarachnoid space. After a subarachnoid haemorrhage cells may disappear within 7 days or persist in small numbers up to 6 weeks, depending upon the severity of the bleed. An increase in white cells generally implies inflammatory changes in the meninges. These can be primary, as in meningitis, or secondary to diffuse cerebral disease, as in encephalitis. In general, neutrophil leucocytes are predominant in pyogenic infections such as coccal or influenzal meningitis, and many thousands of cells may be present per cubic millimetre of fluid. As the condition resolves, the neutrophils are gradually replaced by lymphocytes in decreasing numbers. In a case of cerebral abscess, but without obvious meningitis, it is usual to find between 20 and 200 cells/mm^3 of which most are neutrophils. In tuberculous meningitis there is a neutrophil reaction at the onset of the illness, but within a few days the pleocytosis is generally entirely mononuclear (lymphocytes and histiocytes) and usually of the order of from 200 to 1000 cells/mm^3. Meningovascular syphilis generally gives a mononuclear pleocytosis of up to 200 cells/mm^3, but some neutrophils are present in the more acute cases. Patients with tabes dorsalis rarely show an excess of cells in the fluid, but in patients with general paresis, counts of from 5 to 50 lymphocytes/mm^3 are usual. Plasma cells are inconstantly present in many inflammatory disorders, especially in those running a subacute or indolent course, but have little diagnostic significance.

In virus infections such as encephalitis, lymphocytic meningitis and poliomyelitis, a moderate lymphocytic reaction (up to 1000 cells/mm^3) is general, but in poliomyelitis a number of neutrophils and even a predominance may be observed in the first few days of the illness.

A slight pleocytosis, nearly always of lymphocytes, may also be found in many miscellaneous disorders, including cerebral tumour (primary or secondary), cerebral infarction, venous sinus thrombosis and multiple sclerosis. Only rarely in these conditions does the count exceed from 40 to 50 cells/mm^3. In subarachnoid haemorrhage, too, the aseptic meningitis produced by blood in the CSF excites a moderate lymphocytic pleocytosis, and the number of white cells is proportionately greater than would be expected from the number of red cells present. In occasional cases of intracranial tumour, particularly medulloblastomas in childhood, neoplastic cells, which look very like lymphocytes, are present in the fluid in comparative profusion. Specialized cytological techniques may be helpful in identifying other types of tumour cell and are particularly useful in diagnosing carcinomatosis of the meninges, leukaemias and lymphomas. Even with the most precise modern cytological techniques, malignant cells are found in the fluid in only 10% of cases of glioma and in 20% of patients with intracranial metastases. Immunofluorescent techniques of examining fresh or cultured cells obtained from CSF are being increasingly used in the rapid diagnosis of viral encephalitis, meningitis and cryptococcosis and in differentiating T and B lymphocytes. In addition, monoclonal antibodies have been used to identify malignant cells in CSF (Coakham et al, 1984).

CHEMICAL ABNORMALITIES

Protein

An increase in total protein in the CSF is one of the commonest of abnormalities and also one of the most difficult to interpret. A rise to several hundred milligrams per decilitre is usual in inflammatory disorders of the meninges, such as meningitis, and persists for some time after the pleocytosis has disappeared. In subacute or granulomatous meningitis, as in sarcoidosis, the rise in protein may persist for months or years. In poliomyelitis a rise in protein without an increase in cells is sometimes noted only 4 or 5 days after the onset. A moderate increase, usually to about 100 mg/dl or less, may be found in a variety of cerebral disorders—encephalitis, cerebral abscess, cerebral infarction, neurosyphilis, intracranial venous sinus thrombosis and multiple sclerosis. Particularly high values, often of several hundred milligrams and sometimes as much as 1 g/dl are found in patients with postinfective polyneuropathy (the Guillain–Barré syndrome). In these cases there is typically no pleocytosis. Almost the only other circumstance in which similarly high readings are found in the lumbar CSF is in cases of spinal block, usually due to a neoplasm in the spinal canal, but occasionally due to other causes. Minor degrees of spinal cord compression without a complete block, as in cervical spondylosis, show less striking rises in the CSF protein, rarely to above 100 mg/dl. A lesser rise is also found sometimes in patients suffering from a recent prolapse of an intervertebral disc, either lumbar or cervical.

Albumin-globulin content

In the normal CSF the albumin-globulin ratio is approximately 8:1, but in many of the inflammatory conditions referred to above there is a selective rise in globulin. Various techniques of electrophoresis, immunoprecipitation and electroimmunophoresis are useful not only to estimate gamma globulin as a fraction of the total CSF protein but also to fractionate IgG, IgA, IgM and IgD. These methods have shown that the gamma globulin content of the fluid is usually raised in diseases such as multiple sclerosis, neurosyphilis and subacute sclerosing panencephalitis. Normally less than 14% of CSF protein is gamma globulin. Comparison of serum and CSF levels has shown that most of the excess IgG present in the CSF in multiple sclerosis and neurosyphilis is produced in the central nervous system. Variations in the kappa/lambda ratios of the IgG light chains may also prove to be of diagnostic value, and the terminal component of complement (C9) is also often raised in the fluid in multiple sclerosis. These techniques and those of isoelectric focusing of CSF proteins are being supplied increasingly for diagnostic purposes.

Hydrogen ion concentration
The hydrogen ion concentration of CSF is normally maintained within narrow limits at a pH of about 7.31. This is largely controlled by the level of $P\text{CO}_2$ in the fluid. The variation in CSF pH is much less than in the blood. Change in the CO_2 tension ($P_a\text{CO}_2$) of the arterial blood is the most important factor in controlling pulmonary ventilation through its effect upon chemoreceptors in the medulla. However, in experimental animals perfusion of the cerebral ventricular system with solutions of different pH and different $P\text{CO}_2$ concentration has been shown to produce changes in ventilation also. Clearly the pH of the CSF has some influence on respiration through its effect upon the pH of the cerebral extracellular fluid with which it is in equilibrium. In metabolic acidosis induced by administering ammonium chloride, the pH of the blood falls, that of the CSF rises, and a slight increase in ventilation occurs, presumably due to the CSF alkalosis. In chronic hypercapnia the brain produces increased amounts of ammonia, which is reflected in the CSF not by an increase of ammonia but of glutamine. The CSF pH and hence that of the cerebral extracellular fluid also influence cerebral vascular resistance. As is well known, hypercapnia is followed by vasodilatation, hypocapnia by vasoconstriction.

Glucose
Glucose may disappear almost completely from the CSF in patients with pyogenic meningitis. In tuberculous meningitis, in carcinomatosis of the meninges and sometimes in cerebral sarcoidosis, unlike lymphocytic meningitis, a moderate fall in glucose level to about 20–45 mg/dl is often found and is a valuable aid in diagnosis.

Amines
The CSF contains 5-hydroxyindoleacetic acid (5-HIAA), a metabolite of serotonin, and also homovanillic acid (HVA), a metabolite of dopamine. Both amines may be reduced in the fluid in cases of parkinsonism and may then rise after treatment with levodopa. Changes in certain mental diseases such as schizophrenia are now being reported, but many transmitters do not cross the blood–brain barrier and no place has yet been established for these estimations in relation to clinical diagnosis and management.

Other substances
Many other substances, including phospholipids, enzymes, sterols, amino acids, GABA, glutamine and a large number of other metabolites, have been estimated in CSF (Fishman, 1980) but such studies have not as yet yielded information of significant diagnostic value.

MICROBIOLOGICAL EXAMINATION

If turbid CSF is removed, a smear should be stained with Gram's stain and examined for microorganisms and another specimen cultured. In pneumococcal, staphylococcal, and *H. influenzae* meningitis the causal organisms are usually profuse in a direct smear, but meningococci may be difficult to find and culture. Fluorescent antibody techniques are now extensively used to assist in diagnosis. Tubercle bacilli should be sought in preparations stained by the Ziehl–Neelsen or auramine techniques and are usually found in cases of tuberculous meningitis after an assiduous search, particularly if a fibrin 'web' can be examined. If no bacilli are found, confirmation of the diagnosis depends upon finding the organisms on culture on Lowenstein–Jensen slopes or on guinea-pig inoculation, but these measures take about 6 weeks. In some cases of chronic meningitis, special culture media (e.g. Sabouraud's medium for cryptococcosis and Korthof's for leptospirosis) are required for the identification of less common infections. Virological studies carried out on CSF have often tended to give results only when the illness is over, but are useful even at this stage in establishing the nature of the virus responsible for a number of obscure infections of the nervous system. Techniques of immunofluorescent staining for viral antibodies have also added precision to early diagnosis. Serological tests for syphilis, such as the Wasserman, Kahn, VDRL and treponema immobilization, and the even more specific fluorescent treponemal antibody absorption (FTA-ABS) reactions, are sometimes positive in the CSF but negative in the serum in cases of neurosyphilis.

RAISED INTRACRANIAL PRESSURE—PATHOPHYSIOLOGY

Many pathological processes may cause an increase in intracranial pressure (ICP), but the commonest are diffuse swelling of the brain (cerebral oedema, p. 248), hydrocephalus and intracranial space-occupying lesions of which the most common are tumours. The brain is unique among the viscera in being confined within a rigid box, the cranium. The total volume of the intracranial contents, namely the brain and its coverings, the blood vessels and the blood, and the CSF, is normally constant, so that an increase in any one of these can occur at the expense of the others. The intracranial contents do not respond passively to changes in their volume or pressure but react in a number of complicated ways.

As an intracranial mass lesion increases in size there is initially a compensatory reduction in the intracranial CSF and blood volume, and only when this compensatory process is exhausted does the ICP increase. In this first, or compensated state, there is little change in the clinical condition of the patient. In the second stage, as the compensatory process becomes increasingly ineffective, headache and drowsiness develop. The third stage of increasing intracranial pressure is characterized by increasing depression of consciousness, increased systemic arterial blood pressure, bradycardia and irregular respiration. In the fourth or terminal stage there is deep coma and a progressive fall in systemic arterial pressure, and the pupils are fixed and dilated.

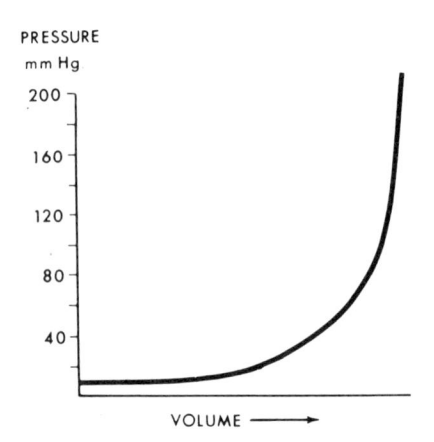

Figure 11.1 Relationship between intracranial pressure and volume of space-occupying lesion. [Reproduced from Miller and Adams (1972) in Critchley et al (eds) (1972) *Scientific Foundations of Neurology*, by kind permission of the authors, editors and publisher.]

The effects of mass lesions on intracranial pressure

GENERAL EFFECTS

The direct local effects of the increased mass of the brain produced by a tumour play a comparatively small part initially in raising intracranial pressure. Owing to the partial division of the cranial cavity into compartments by the falx and tentorium, the local rise of pressure is partly confined to the cranial compartment. This is in contrast to the increased pressure throughout the craniospinal axis which is usually produced by diffuse cerebral oedema, or to that which can be produced in experimental animals by infusing saline into the lumbar subarachnoid space. As the mass of the lesion increases and compensation fails, a volume/pressure curve can be derived, confirming the initial slight rise in ICP followed by an exponential increase as it grows larger (Fig. 11.1). Recent work upon methods of continuous monitoring of the ICP has shown that there are at least three periodic wave forms superimposed upon baseline pressure, one due to the arterial pulse, one to respiration, and the other comprising slow waves of increased pressure ('X' waves) whose cause is still unknown. The higher the ICP, the greater the amplitude of the arterial pressure waves and the greater the increase in ICP produced by small increments in volume. By contrast, the respiratory and 'X' waves remain relatively constant in amplitude whether the ICP is normal or increased. As the mass of a focal lesion increases, the communication of the resultant increase in pressure throughout the subarachnoid space is reduced by the progressive herniation of brain tissue from the compartment in which the mass lesion lies. The principal sites of such herniation (Fig. 11.2) are the cingulate gyrus beneath the falx cerebri (subfalcial herniation), the medial temporal lobe through the tentorial hiatus (tentorial herniation), and the cerebellar tonsils into the foramen magnum (the cerebellar pressure cone). In these circumstances pressure gradients develop between the various intracranial compartments, depending upon that in which the mass lesion lies. The effects of these lesions will be considered later.

An early effect of a mass lesion is to displace CSF from the cranial cavity, increasing pressure through the lumbar subarachnoid space. Depending upon their location, mass lesions can also obstruct the outflow of CSF from one lateral ventricle (due to pressure occlusion of one foramen of Monro), from the third ventricle (due to occlusion of the aqueduct), or less often from the fourth ventricle, giving rise to hydrocephalus with dilatation of one or more of the ventricles, thus causing an even greater increase in ICP.

The effect of ICP upon the cerebral circulation must also be borne in mind. Compression of venous sinuses and cortical veins increases venous pressure, thus contributing to the rise in intracranial pressure and to the induction of cerebral oedema, often most severe in the neighbourhood of the tumour. Pressure upon arteries may reduce blood flow focally or generally (if the rise in ICP is severe), and rarely infarction may result. An increase of ICP to over 30 mmHg has been shown to cause a reduction in cerebral blood flow. In such circumstances arterial hypertension

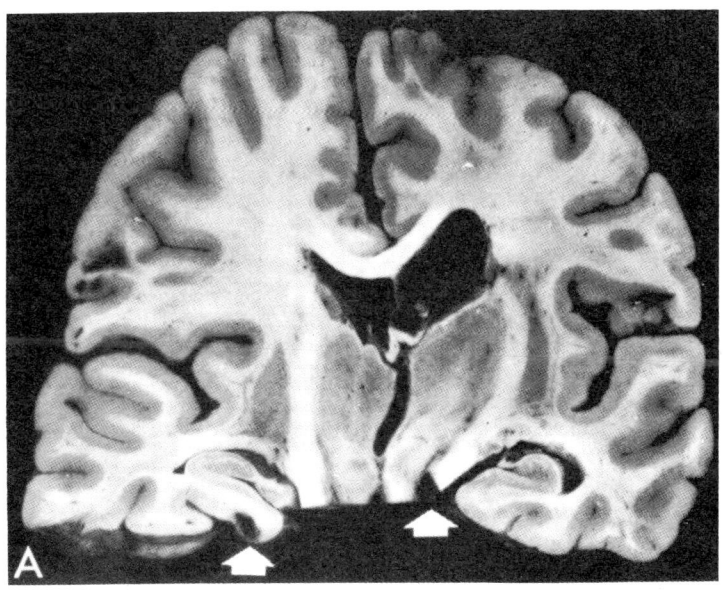

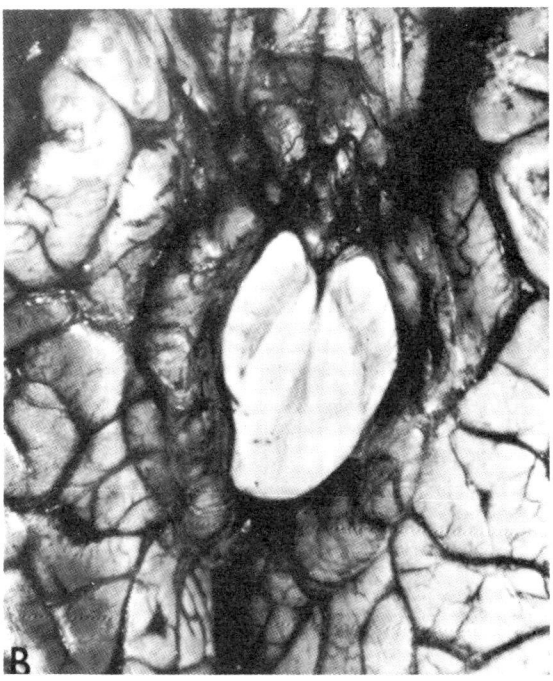

Figure 11.2 A, Internal herniae produced by a left subdural haematoma. In addition to lateral displacement, the cingulate gyrus has herniated under the falx to produce a supracallosal hernia. This has produced downward displacement of the roof of the left lateral ventricle and a selectively severe shift of the pericallosal arteries. There is also a haemorrhage in the left hippocampal gyrus (arrow) in the groove produced by a tentorial hernia, and a haemorrhagic infarct in the contralateral cerebral peduncle (arrow) where it has been compressed against the tentorium. B, There is a large tentorial hernia on the left of the illustration and a smaller one on the right. The midbrain is narrowed. [Reproduced from Miller and Adams (1972) in Critchley et al (eds) (1972) *Scientific Foundations of Neurology*, by kind permission of the authors, editors and publisher.]

usually develops, partially in an attempt to compensate for the increased cerebral arterial resistance and partially to increase perfusion pressure. This rise in systemic arterial pressure is thought to result at least in part from medullary ischaemia due to stretching of perforating branches of the basilar artery induced in turn by downward brain-stem displacement. These changes may also be accompanied by electrocardiographic abnormalities such as prominent U waves, ST-T segment changes, notched T waves and prolonged (or sometimes shortened) QT intervals. ICP may also be influenced by cerebral vasodilatation induced by hypercapnia, or by hypoxia which may in turn be a consequence of the respiratory irregularities induced by increased ICP. Conversely, hyperventilation and consequent hypocapnia reduce ICP, as do hypothermia, hyperbaric oxygen and some neuroleptic and analgesic drugs, especially the phenothiazines.

The adult skull is rigid and unyielding. As the ICP rises, downward pressure, often from a dilated third ventricle, upon the sella turcica may cause initially decalcification and later erosion of the posterior clinoid processes. Sometimes the sella turcica enlarges, and rarely clinical manifestations of hypopituitarism ensue. In infants, non-union of the cranial sutures provides a partial safety valve so that increased ICP leads to separation of the cranial sutures, and the skull may yield a 'crack-pot sound' on percussion. By contrast, premature union of the sutures (craniostenosis) causes a marked increase in ICP because skull growth is arrested while the brain is still increasing in size.

The headache associated with an increase in ICP, and especially that resulting from mass lesions, is mainly due to compression or distortion of the dura mater and of the pain-sensitive intracranial blood vessels. It is often paroxysmal, at first worse on waking, throbbing in character (due to the arterial pressure wave), and is accentuated by exertion, coughing, sneezing, vomiting, straining or sudden changes in posture. The headache is often frontal or occipital or both, and its distribution is usually of little localizing value. Lesions in the posterior fossa often give suboccipital headache, and if there is associated neck stiffness or if pain is increased by attempted neck flexion this may give warning of the presence of a cerebellar pressure cone.

The pathogenesis of papilloedema was considered in chapter 2. It develops more rapidly in patients with mass lesions in the posterior fossa because of their special tendency to cause obstructive hydrocephalus. Papilloedema is sometimes worse on one side, but is rarely unilateral.

The vomiting which often accompanies increased ICP often occurs in the mornings when the headache is at its height. It is generally attributed to compression or ischaemia of the vomiting centre in the medulla oblongata. Similarly bradycardia, which is also common, is a consequence of dysfunction in the cardiac centre. Effects upon the respiratory centre commonly produce disorders of respiration. A sudden rise in ICP giving disordered consciousness is often accompanied by slow and deep respiratory movements. Later, breathing may become irregular (e.g. Cheyne–Stokes respiration) and periods of apnoea then alternate with periods during which breathing waxes and wanes in amplitude. Central neurogenic hyperventilation or so-called apneustic or ataxic breathing are less common effects of brainstem compression or distortion, but in terminal coma the breathing is often rapid or shallow. These abnormalities of respiratory rate and rhythm result sometimes from compression or distortion of the brain stem but more often from median raphe haemorrhages or infarcts in the midbrain which may extend into the pons, resulting from tentorial herniation (see below).

So-called 'false localizing signs' may also arise as a consequence of a sustained rise in ICP. Unilateral or bilateral sixth nerve palsies may result from compression of the trunks of one or both nerves as they cross the apex of the petrous temporal bone. Bilateral extensor plantar responses or grasp reflexes may result from ventricular dilatation in hydrocephalus. A third nerve palsy or, more rarely, facial pain or sensory loss may occur due to compression of the gasserian ganglion in tentorial herniation. An ipsilateral extensor plantar response may represent compression of the opposite cerebral peduncle against the free tentorial edge in tentorial herniation (Fig. 11.2) (Kernohan's sign). Rarely, signs of cerebellar dysfunction may result from a massive frontal lesion owing to downward displacement of the brain stem. Bilateral fixed dilated pupils or defects of upward conjugate gaze may be due to a central cerebellar lesion displacing the midbrain upwards.

SUBFALCIAL HERNIATION

Herniation of the cingulate gyrus beneath the free edge of the falx cerebri can be identified radiologically, especially on angiography or in the CT scan. It is often associated with a reduced size of the ipsilateral lateral ventricle, but usually produces no specific clinical features. Focal necrosis of the cingulate gyrus may develop, or alternatively, extensive infarction may occur consequent upon compression of the pericallosal arteries.

TENTORIAL HERNIATION

Tentorial herniation most often develops as a consequence of lesions in the temporal lobe but may complicate any supratentorial mass lesion. As the herniated part of the medial temporal lobe descends in the tentorial hiatus, the midbrain is pushed to the opposite side and downwards, the opposite cerebral peduncle is compressed against the free edge of the contralateral tentorium, the aqueduct is also compressed, and the ipsilateral third nerve is compressed against the tentorial edge. The latter gives first a dilated fixed pupil on the same side and later other signs of a third nerve palsy. There may be grooving of the uncus and hippocampal gyrus with focal necrosis or infarction.

If herniation increases there is further downward displacement of brain-stem structures. The principal complications of this process are (a) paresis or paralysis of upward conjugate gaze due to compression of the tectal plate, (b) pressure upon one or both posterior cerebral arteries, giving unilateral or bilateral occipital lobe infarction with consequent hemianopia or cortical blindness, and (c) most important of all, median raphe haemorrhages or infarction in the brain stem due sometimes to venous obstruction but more often to shearing effects upon perforating branches of the basilar artery, giving rise to irreversible coma due to necrosis of the reticular substance.

TONSILLAR HERNIATION (CEREBELLAR PRESSURE CONE)

The principal effects of tonsillar herniation through the foramen magnum, which may complicate supratentorial, but more particularly infratentorial lesions, are haemorrhagic infarction of the cerebellar tonsils themselves and compression of medullary structures with respiratory and/or cardiac arrest and death. The latter results when there is associated downward displacement of the brain stem.

INFRATENTORIAL LESIONS

Infratentorial lesions, because of their effects upon the brain stem, aqueduct and fourth ventricle, tend to cause obstructive hydrocephalus early in their course, as well as tonsillar herniation. Medullary or cerebellar infarction may occur as a result of compression of the medulla in the foramen magnum or distortion of the posterior inferior cerebellar arteries. Sometimes reversed tentorial herniation occurs with displacement of the brain stem and the posterior fossa contents upward, with infarction of the superior aspects of the cerebellar hemispheres due to distortion of the superior cerebellar arteries. Distortion of the hippocampal gyri due to upward pressure is rarely seen.

HYDROCEPHALUS

Strictly, hydrocephalus means 'water on the brain'. This term has sometimes been used in the past to embrace cases in which the amount of CSF within the cranial cavity is increased in order to compensate for cerebral atrophy, whatever its cause. This dilatation of the cerebral ventricles with an increased volume of CSF overlying the cortex and within the sulci is generally seen in patients with various forms of dementia solely as a consequence of loss of brain substance. This finding is no longer regarded as a variety of hydrocephalus.

Hydrocephalus as now conventionally defined embraces those conditions in which there is at some stage an increased volume (and usually pressure) of CSF within the cranial cavity due to (a) increased production of CSF, (b) obstruction to the flow of fluid at some point between the choroid plexuses of the lateral ventricles from which it is secreted and the arachnoidal villi in the sagittal sinus through which it is reabsorbed, and (c) impaired absorption of the fluid due to inflammation of the arachnoid as in meningitis or as a result of thrombosis of the sagittal sinus.

Increased production of CSF may occur as one result of a rare tumour—a papilloma of the choroid plexus—which can also give rise to recurrent subarachnoid haemorrhage.

The commonest cause of hydrocephalus in infancy, childhood and adult life is obstruction to the flow of CSF. Conventionally this has been divided into that due to obstruction to the circulation at some point between the lateral ventricles and the exit foramina (of Magendie and Luschka) of the fourth ventricle ('obstructive') and that due to processes which impede flow throughout the subarachnoid space ('communicating'). Distortion of the cerebral aqueduct in particular, but also compression elsewhere, may cause secondary hydrocephalus in patients with intracranial mass lesions. Obstruction to the outflow of CSF from the fourth ventricle can cause hydrocephalus and/or syringomyelia because the fluid which cannot obtain egress into the subarachnoid space is forced, perhaps by intermittent pulse waves, into the central canal of the spinal cord which therefore dilates and may later lose its ependymal lining.

Communicating hydrocephalus with obstruction to the flow of CSF in the subarachnoid space overlying the cerebral hemispheres is usually a consequence of adhesions resulting from previous meningitis or subarachnoid haemorrhage, but it sometimes develops without evident cause. In adults, this condition may give rise to confusion or even dementia and often severe ataxia, a syndrome of so-called 'low- or normal-pressure hydrocephalus' as lumbar puncture in such cases frequently demonstrates a normal CSF pressure in the lumbar theca. In all forms of obstructive and communicating hydrocephalus, computerized transaxial tomography and/or pneumoencephalography or ventriculography (see p. 258) demonstrate cerebral ventricular dilatation, depending upon the site of the obstruction. In low- or normal-pressure hydrocephalus there is increasing evidence that at some stage the ICP was raised but that ultimately once ventricular dilatation reaches a certain stage a phase of adaptation develops in which, despite continuing symptoms, the pressure in the ventricles and especially in the lumbar theca is normal or low. In such cases pneumoencephalography has often shown that no air is able to enter the subarachnoid space. This procedure often causes dramatic clinical deterioration. Isotope encephalography has also proved helpful in diagnosis. Even though the pressure is low or normal, 'shunting' procedures through which CSF is drained from the lateral ventricles into the venous circulation sometimes produce dramatic improvement, as in obstructive hydrocephalus.

The terms 'brain oedema' and 'brain swelling' are synonymous, implying an increase in brain volume due to an increase in its water and sodium content. Oedema must be distinguished from enlargement due to an increase in the brain's blood volume caused by venous obstruction or vasodilatation, though the latter, if prolonged, can lead to the former. Fishman (1980) classified oedema into vasogenic, cellular or cytotoxic, and interstitial or hydrocephalic types. The vasogenic variety, associated with increased capillary permeability, is the commonest form observed in clinical practice in conditions such as tumour, abscess, haemorrhage, infarction, contusion, lead encephalopathy, purulent meningitis and benign intracranial hypertension (see below). The oedema is often localized around the primary lesion, producing focal symptoms and signs which are often due more to the oedema than to the primary lesion. Cellular or cytotoxic oedema, resembling that due to water intoxication in experimental animals, as in that induced experimentally by triethyl tin, is characterized by swelling of all the cellular elements of the brain (neurons, glia and endothelial cells) with an associated reduction in extracellular fluid. This occurs in diffuse hypoxia, acute hypo-osmolality (in dilutional hyponatraemia, sodium depletion or inappropriate ADH secretion) or in osmotic dysequilibrium syndromes (as in haemodialysis or diabetic ketoacidosis). The clinical manifestations are normally less localized than in vasogenic oedema, including drowsiness leading to stupor or coma and sometimes convulsions. Ischaemic states usually produce vasogenic oedema first, followed by cellular oedema. Interstitial or hydrocephalic oedema simply identifies the increased water content of the brain (largely extracellular) which occurs in hydrocephalus.

Cerebral oedema

A syndrome of benign intracranial hypertension (often erroneously called toxic hydrocephalus, or pseudotumour cerebri) results from diffuse cerebral oedema of unknown cause. It has been found in association with obesity in women and also with pregnancy or miscarriage. It also occurs in men, occasionally after infection or trivial head injury. Typically the cerebral ventricles are small. The condition is benign and self-limiting, but in the acute state, compression of the central retinal arteries due to papilloedema may be sufficiently severe to threaten sight. Headache is often relatively mild and there are few if any systemic symptoms or other neurological signs. A similar clinical picture can result from intracranial venous sinus thrombosis, especially of the sagittal sinuses but also of the lateral sinuses ('otitic hydrocephalus') in which the principal problem is probably one of CSF reabsorption. There also appears to be a component of cerebral oedema as well, as the cerebral ventricles are rarely enlarged. These conditions usually respond dramatically to treatment with large doses of glucocorticoids (e.g. dexamethasone 5 mg every 4 hours), which quickly shrinks the brain. Hyperosmolar solutions such as mannitol, sucrose, and urea, which have often been used in the past in conditions associated with brain swelling, are now largely outmoded, since although they may produce rapid shrinkage of the brain they quickly pass into the cerebral extracellular fluid and produce 'rebound' swelling. However, steroids are much more effective in the vasogenic variety of cerebral oedema than in the cellular form, in which hypertonic solutions given intravenously or, preferably, powerful diuretics such as frusemide, are more effective. Barbiturates had a temporary vogue, and calcium antagonists are being tested.

CRANIOCEREBRAL TRAUMA—PATHOPHYSIOLOGY

General considerations

In recent years head injuries have occurred with increasing frequency, most being due to direct trauma resulting from road traffic or industrial accidents. Penetrating wounds of the brain (e.g. gunshot wounds) are relatively rare except in wartime. There is no direct parallelism between the severity of an injury to the skull and the extent to which the brain is damaged. Though severe fractures of the skull are often associated with severe cerebral injury, the brain can be extensively damaged without skull fracture. Conversely, fracture may occur without severe damage to the brain. Compound fractures of the skull, especially those involving the base and extending into the nasopharynx, nasal air sinuses, middle ear and mastoid, carry the additional risk of infection of the intracranial contents, i.e. meningitis or intracranial abscess.

The factors operating upon the brain in head injury are multiple and complex, and their results often equally so. 'Compression, acceleration and deceleration may occur during the traumatic episode. Tissues are injured by compression, tension and shear. All of these modes of injury may occur simultaneously or in succession in the same accident' (Gurdjian et al, 1966). These factors, of which shearing forces may well be the most important, give widespread microscopic lesions throughout the brain and brain stem, microglial clusters and ischaemic or haemorrhagic lesions of the anterior hypothalamus. Rotational and accelerative forces may produce a graded centripetal progression of diffuse cortical-subcortical disconnection phenomena maximal at the periphery and enhanced at junctions between grey and white matter. After severe closed head injury there is widespread vascular spasm and slowing of the cerebral circulation, but these changes do not invariably correlate with the pathological finding of widespread ischaemic lesions which may occur in more than half of all cases of fatal head injury. Unexplained haemorrhages in spinal posterior root ganglia may also be found.

Concussion

Concussion was defined by Trotter as 'a condition of widespread paralysis of the functions of the brain which comes on as an immediate consequence of a blow on the head, has a strong tendency to spontaneous recovery, and is not necessarily associated with any gross organic change in the brain substance'. In practical terms concussion is a reversible impairment of consciousness of comparatively brief duration. Concussion cannot occur without some damage to nerve cells and fibres. It is now uncertain as to whether any physiological or anatomical distinction can be drawn between concussion as just defined and more prolonged states of unconsciousness resulting from head injury. Consciousness is dependent upon the integrity of the ascending reticular alerting formation (see p. 82), and there is evidence that this system can be reversibly blocked by acceleration concussion. The brain stem, attached above to the massive cerebral hemispheres and passing through an opening in the tentorium, is especially vulnerable to brief displacements of the cranial contents. Head injuries producing a decerebrate state or prolonged unconsciousness (the 'persistent vegetative state') probably result from primary injury to the brain stem, but brain-stem injury does not exist in isolation and is only one aspect of diffuse brain damage. A persistent vegetative state after head injury may be due to diffuse damage to the cortex, to subcortical structures or to the brain stem, but often to all three areas.

Cerebral contusion

The term cerebral contusion has traditionally been used to identify bruising of the brain, or a diffuse state more severe than concussion and characterized by diffuse nerve-cell and axonal damage, multiple punctate haemorrhages and oedema. It is doubtful

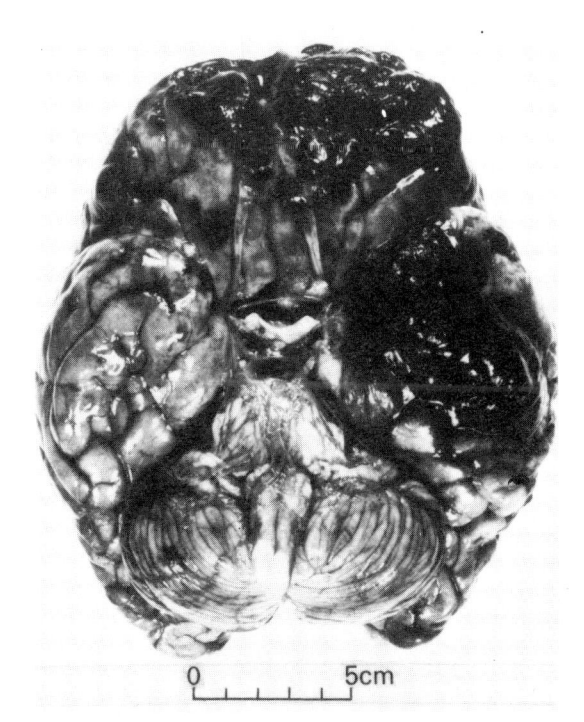

Figure 11.3 The brain in a case of fatal closed head injury. Extensive areas of superficial haemorrhage are seen over both temporal poles and in the left temporal region. [Reproduced from Walton (1985) *Brain's Diseases of the Nervous System*, 9th edn, by kind permission of the publisher.]

whether it is useful to distinguish this condition from concussion, as the pathological changes in the two conditions differ only in degree, depending upon the severity of the injury. Larger areas of laceration or intracerebral haemorrhage are sometimes found, either in the cortex beneath the site of the blow or in the contralateral hemisphere where the cortex has been driven forcibly against the interior of the skull vault (contre-coup injury). Superficial haemorrhages often occur in one or both frontal, temporal or occipital poles (Fig. 11.3), sometimes even after relatively minor injury, especially in the elderly. Diffuse degeneration of the cerebral white matter is an important sequel of severe injury.

Communicating hydrocephalus

The cerebral oedema which usually accompanies severe head injury generally causes a substantial rise in ICP with an accompanying increase in the pressure of the CSF in the ventricles and lumbar theca. Arachnoidal adhesions may subsequently form, resulting in disturbances of CSF formation and flow and even in communicating hydrocephalus; rarely, rupture of the arachnoid may allow CSF to enter the subdural space, producing a subdural hygroma.

Intracranial haemorrhage

Traumatic intracranial haemorrhage may be either intracerebral, subarachnoid, subdural or extradural. An intracerebral haematoma may develop immediately after the injury but is rarely delayed, giving symptoms after an asymptomatic interval of hours or days, especially in older patients. Bleeding into the subarachnoid space is generally associated with contusion of the cerebral cortex. Acute subdural haemorrhage is usually the result of a severe laceration, which may either involve the surface of the hemisphere or cause a large cavity filled with blood within its substance. Less often, acute subdural haemorrhage is due to rupture of venous tributaries of the superior sagittal sinus or to laceration of one of the venous sinuses. Chronic subdural haematoma usually develops after a latent interval following minor trauma, but sometimes arises spontaneously. Extradural haemorrhage is almost invariably the result of tearing of the middle meningeal artery or one of its branches due to a fracture of the skull vault crossing the groove in which it lies.

Clinical features of craniocerebral trauma

CONCUSSION AND CONTUSION

After a slight injury the patient may be dazed or unconscious for a few seconds only, but his higher mental functions can subsequently be impaired for a period lasting up to several hours, during which he may carry out complicated activities in an automatic fashion, after which he remembers nothing of these events. This is the period of post-traumatic amnesia, which is best measured from the time of the injury to the time of the beginning of continuous awareness. This loss of memory may also extend to incidents which occurred before the acccident, and is then known as retrograde amnesia. For example, a patient who sustains a head injury in an aeroplane crash may remember nothing that happened after he left the ground. Retrograde amnesia does not occur without post-traumatic amnesia.

In cases of more severe injury unconsciousness is more prolonged, and in addition the patient often exhibits signs of brain-stem dysfunction. The pupils may be dilated and may fail to react to light, and the cutaneous and tendon reflexes may be lost, the musculature being flaccid. In severe cases a decerebrate or decorticate state is present. The blood pressure is low and the pulse slow, or, in some cases, rapid and feeble or even imperceptible. Respiration may stop or it may be shallow and sighing. Death may occur in severe cases from medullary paralysis.

Recovery is manifest first in an improvement of visceral function. The volume of the pulse increases, respiration becomes deeper, and the pupils again react to light. Vomiting is common at this stage. On recovering consciousness the patient may be delirious, restless and irritable, and almost always complains of headache. In cases of mild concussion these symptoms, with the possible exception of headache, usually disappear within a few days. Even after mild injury the post-concussional syndrome (see below) may develop, especially in a compensation setting.

In recent years the Glasgow coma scale (Jennett and Teasdale, 1977), based upon the hierarchical scoring of responses to appropriate stimuli (eye-opening, limb movement and verbal response) has been widely used to assess the depth and severity of coma after head injury, and a similar Glasgow outcome scale has been devised to help in assessing the prognosis (Jennett and Bond, 1975). Among the factors which have an adverse influence on prognosis are age (children often recover remarkably, even from severe injury), decerebrate rigidity or extensor spasms, prolonged coma, hypertension, a low arterial $P\text{CO}_2$ and a body temperature persistently above 39°C (Walton, 1985).

TRAUMATIC ENCEPHALOPATHY

Focal brain damage can occur in the absence of clinical manifestations of concussion or contusion, especially when a localized blow causes a depressed fracture of the skull. The severity of the underlying damage to the brain may be dependent upon whether or not the dura is penetrated. In such cases, infection, haemorrhage and focal neurological symptoms and signs are the most important complications. In moderate or severe closed head injury, with or without linear skull fracture, consciousness is usually lost immediately. In the most severe cases the depth of coma steadily increases and the patient dies from medullary paralysis within a few hours. In less severe cases the patient, after recovering from concussion, passes into a state of stupor or confusion. He is usually drowsy and presents the picture long known as 'cerebral irritation', but better described as traumatic delirium. The patient lies in a flexed attitude, resenting interference, confused and disorientated when roused, and at times noisy and violent. This condition may last for days or even weeks with a corresponding duration of post-traumatic amnesia, and in favourable cases gradually passes away. The patient may remain in a state of stupor for many months. Symptoms of a focal lesion of the brain are usually absent, but focal convulsions, hemiparesis or aphasia may follow a contusion involving the cortex. Injury to the basal ganglia can cause mutism and extrapyramidal syndromes, and damage to the midbrain may result in quadriplegia, tonic convulsions and, in less severe cases, ocular palsies, diplopia and nystagmus. Other cranial nerve palsies may be present, and diabetes insipidus and disorders of hypothalamic function are rare complications. The 'persistent vegetative state' is one in which patients show periods of apparent wakefulness, random eye movements and primitive postural and reflex motor activity. They remain in this condition for weeks, months or even years. Those few who regain limited speech and volitional motor activity have severe residual intellectual and neurological deficits.

Though a patient may recover rapidly and completely from a cerebral contusion, persistent disabling symptoms are common. The three cardinal late symptoms are headache, giddiness and mental disturbances, and they usually develop out of the symptoms of the acute stage. Headache tends to be severe and to occur in paroxysms which may last for several hours, often against a background of continuous pain. It is brought on or exacerbated by activities such as stooping, sneezing, physical exertion, noise and excitement. The giddiness is not always a sense of rotation but a feeling of instability. Transitory vertigo and staggering on sudden head movement are frequent. Post-traumatic vertigo induced by change of posture is probably due to damage to the utricle and saccule of the internal ear and is accompanied by nystagmus which can be recorded in the electronystagmogram.

The commonest mental symptoms are inability to concentrate, fatigability and impairment of memory, together with nervousness and anxiety, and intolerance of alcohol. There are often symptoms of mild dementia of traumatic origin, and all grades are encountered between the common milder cases and the less frequent more severe examples. In the latter the patient passes from the initial stupor into a stage of profound disorientation and confusion with defects of perception and disorganization of speech. Sometimes a stage resembling Korsakov's psychosis develops with gross defects of memory for recent events and sometimes confabulation (see p. 107). The final picture depends on many factors, especially the psychological constitution of the patient. Residual intellectual impairment is not uncommon. Severe dementia is uncommon but not as rare as has been suggested. Moods of excitement or depression are not infrequent in cyclothymic individuals, while after severe head injury with prolonged unconsciousness, paranoid and other psychotic manifestations have been reported.

There has been considerable dispute as to whether the so-called post-concussional or post-traumatic syndrome as described above, when occurring in a setting which may involve financial compensation (e.g. in industrial accidents or road accidents), is largely an organic disorder or an 'accident neurosis'. Unquestionably headache, giddiness, impaired concentration and the other symptoms described, when occurring after moderate or severe head injury, are the result of organic brain damage and may take between 1 and 3 years to recover, if indeed they ever do so. These symptoms tend to be directly proportional in severity and duration to the duration of the post-traumatic amnesia, but may sometimes occur after relatively minor head injury. Nevertheless, neurotic and hysterical manifestations may certainly cloud the clinical picture, especially when prolonged disability follows minor or even trivial injury. Even frank malingering may be difficult to recognize, and considerable experience is necessary in the assessment of such cases. Detailed psychometric testing may be needed, but reliable objective measures are few and it may only be possible to talk of 'the balance of probabilities'.

'Punch-drunkenness' is a chronic traumatic encephalopathy which may occur in professional boxers. It leads to deterioration of the personality, impairment of memory, dysarthria, tremor, parkinsonian features and ataxia. Radiological studies in such cases often show not only cortical atrophy but also absence or cavitation of the septum pellucidum.

ACUTE TRAUMATIC CEREBRAL COMPRESSION

Cerebral compression leads to progressive deepening unconsciousness, indicated by the failure of the patient to respond to stimuli which have previously been capable of rousing him, and by loss of corneal reflexes. Deepening coma is of special importance when it follows a lucid interval after concussion. If tentorial herniation occurs, the pupil on the side of the haemorrhage often becomes dilated and fails to react to light. Papilloedema is relatively uncommon, though the optic discs and fundi may exhibit venous congestion. These manifestations must always raise the possibility of an extradural haematoma, which is a neurosurgical emergency. Similar symptoms may result from an acute subdural haematoma, an intracerebral haemorrhage, or even severe unilateral cerebral oedema associated with contusion or laceration, a fact which underlines the importance of skilled neurosurgical assessment and management of such cases. Symptoms and signs of a progressive lesion of the affected hemisphere, focal convulsions or a flaccid hemiparesis are more likely to be due to an intracerebral lesion, but rarely occur in extradural haemorrhage.

CRANIAL NERVE PALSIES

Cranial nerve palsies may be due to injury of the brain stem or the nerves, either in their intracranial or their extracranial course. Bilateral anosmia is a common complication resulting from tearing of the olfactory nerve filaments as they pass through the cribriform plate of the ethmoid. Ageusia is much less common. Contusion of the midbrain may cause permanent paresis of ocular movement, usually in the vertical plane, either unilaterally or bilaterally, resulting in diplopia and often associated with nystagmus. Intracranial injuries of the nerves are usually the result of fracture of the base of the skull. After the olfactory, the seventh is the nerve most frequently affected and then the eighth, sixth, second, third and fourth in that order. The facial nerve, or its branches, and branches of the trigeminal may be divided or contused as a result of wounds and blows upon the face. Traumatic cranial nerve palsies are usually permanent, but recovery occasionally occurs when intracranial or extracranial nerve trunks have been contused rather than divided.

THE SPINAL CORD—THE PATHOPHYSIOLOGY OF INJURY AND COMPRESSION

Spinal cord injury

AETIOLOGY

The spinal cord may be injured directly by penetrating wounds (e.g. stabs or gunshot wounds), but it is more often injured as a consequence of injuries to the vertebral column (especially fracture, dislocation or, more commonly, fracture-dislocation). Acute prolapse of an intervertebral disc, especially in the cervical region, may have a similar effect. The commonest sites of injury are the lower cervical region and the thoracolumbar junction, resulting sometimes from a blow leading to fracture at the site of impact, but more often from transmitted force such as that which may occur as a consequence of a fall from a height. Acute flexion of the spine and less often hyperextension, especially in the cervical region, are usually responsible. If there is pre-existing cervical spondylosis, which narrows the cervical canal, the effects of relatively minor injury of this type upon the cervical cord (cervical cord contusion) may be especially severe, even in the absence of fracture or dislocation. Spontaneous fracture-dislocation can occur as a consequence of vertebral disease (e.g. tuberculous osteomyelitis or metastatic neoplasm).

PATHOLOGY

The anatomy and blood supply of the spinal cord were described earlier (p. 32). The spinal cord, like the brain, may be 'concussed' as a consequence of transmitted violence (as in blast injury after an explosion) without vertebral fracture or displacement, but this probably cannot be distinguished from contusion, which can be defined as bruising of the cord without disruption of the pia mater. The contused cord is oedematous and may show small haemorrhages. Histologically there is swelling of axons and disintegration of myelin or even total necrosis at the site of injury, with secondary degeneration of ascending and descending tracts. Occasionally, transmitted force, resulting especially from falls on the feet from a height, causes a central area of haemorrhage extending upwards and downwards in the region of the central canal over several segments (haematomyelia). The 'central cervical cord syndrome', resulting most often from acute flexion or hyperextension of the neck and often thought in the past to be due to haematomyelia, is more often a consequence of softening in the central part of the cord due to contusion rather than haemorrhage. Injury to the spinal cord may also occur as a consequence of decompression sickness (Caisson disease). Ascending cavitation of the cord may develop in some patients with transverse cord lesions due to trauma, even several years after the injury (traumatic ascending syringomyelia).

CLINICAL FEATURES

The effects of spinal cord transection or less complete injury upon the motor, sensory and autonomic systems were described earlier in the chapters on 'The autonomic nervous system and hypothalamus', 'The motor system' and 'The sensory system'. Severe injury to the upper cervical cord is usually rapidly fatal because of diaphragmatic and intercostal muscle paralysis, but some patients may survive with mechanically assisted respiration. Complete transection of the cord leads immediately to flaccid paralysis with loss of all sensation and reflex activity below the level of the lesion, and paralysis of the bladder and rectum. As spinal shock passes off over a few weeks, paralysis of voluntary movement and sensory loss remain complete but reflex activity gradually returns to give the clinical picture of spastic paraplegia with automatic bladder and bowel activity.

Less severe lesions such as contusion may give equally severe paralysis and sensory loss at the outset, or else these features may even increase for a few days, owing to traumatic oedema. Subsequently there is gradual improvement and eventually partial or complete recovery, depending upon the severity of the pathological change. In haematomyelia and the commoner central cervical cord contusion, a common sequel is dissociated sensory loss for pain and temperature sensation with retention of tactile and proprioceptive sensibility in the upper limbs comparable to that which is seen in central cord tumours or cavitation (syringomyelia). This results from division of fibres of the spinothalamic tracts as they decussate in the neighbourhood of the central canal of the cord. Injury to one half of the spinal cord may give rise to the Brown-Séquard syndrome.

Fracture-dislocation of the spine below the first lumbar vertebra (i.e. below the termination of the spinal cord) damages only the cauda equina and not the cord itself. Paralysis of the bladder, rectum and sexual functions is usually complete and there is residual 'lower motor neuron' paralysis and sensory loss in the lower limbs depending upon the extent and distribution of the injury to the lumbar and sacral roots. Reflex activity is permanently lost because of division of the various reflex arcs so that the bladder and rectum remain atonic.

Spinal cord compression

The clinical manifestations of compression of the spinal cord depend upon (a) the location of the lesion which is responsible (whether it is extradural, extramedullary but intraspinal, or intramedullary, and whether it lies in the cervical or dorsal regions), (b) its nature and whether it involves spinal nerves or roots as well as the cord, and (c) the rate of its development. Acute compression gives clinical features directly comparable to those of injury as described above. Lesions which cause cord compression developing gradually over weeks, months or even years produce symptoms and signs which are usually much more insidious. The principles which govern the clinical nosology of cord compression and which aid in localization of the lesion have been described in the chapters on 'The motor system' and 'The sensory system', so that only brief further comment upon pathophysiology is necessary here.

Spinal compression, however produced, affects the cord in several ways. Direct pressure interferes with conduction in the spinal roots and in the cord itself. Pressure upon the ascending longitudinal spinal veins leads to oedema of the cord below the site of compression. It has been suggested that interference with venous drainage may explain symptoms and signs of low cervical cord dysfunction arising in patients with high cervical cord compression. Compression of the longitudinal and radicular spinal arteries also leads to ischaemia of the segments of the cord which they supply. These vascular disturbances cause local oedema of the cord with degeneration of the ganglion cells and the white matter. Areas of softening may develop—so-called compression myelitis. In general, slow spinal compression affects the pyramidal (corticospinal) tracts first, the posterior columns next, and the spinothalamic tracts last, but there are many exceptions to this rule. This sequence may be due to the fact that the pyramidal tracts are supplied by terminal branches of the anterior spinal artery which are thus most susceptible to compression ischaemia. Alternatively it has been suggested that the pyramidal tract lies closest to the attachments of the ligamentum denticulatum, which is subjected to traction when the cord is compressed. Finally, obstruction of the subarachnoid space causes loculation of the CSF below the point of compression and leads to characteristic changes in its composition as described above.

INVESTIGATIONS IN NEUROLOGY—SOME GENERAL PRINCIPLES

Introduction

In many patients with neurological disease, investigations are unnecessary either for diagnosis or to give guidance in management. Migraine, for instance, is a condition in which the diagnosis can usually be made on the clinical history alone and in which ancillary tests are rarely needed. In other cases investigations should be designed to establish or exclude the various diagnoses which are brought to mind by the patient's symptoms and signs.

Symptoms of neurological dysfunction may result from disease in another part of the body. The patient must therefore be viewed as a whole if he is not to be subjected to a series of prolonged and unpleasant tests designed to demonstrate a primarily nervous disease, when the lesion lies elsewhere. Investigations should always be planned to give the maximum required information about the patient's illness with the least possible discomfort and risk. It is reasonable to begin by carrying out the simpler tests which the doctor is capable of doing himself before proceeding, if necessary, to the more difficult methods which need specialized apparatus and skilled technical help.

In view of the fact that many diseases of other systems may present with neurological manifestations, numerous studies regularly used in the practice of internal medicine may be required in patients with symptoms and signs of nervous disease. Biopsy of skin, lymph nodes, liver, kidney and other organs has been used increasingly in diagnosis in internal medicine. By analogy there are various biopsy techniques which are of immediate relevance to neurology. Open or needle biopsy of muscle is used increasingly in the differential diagnosis of neuromuscular disease (see p. 188), and sural nerve biopsy has a much more limited role in distinguishing between various forms of polyneuropathy. Brain biopsy is widely used in the diagnosis of brain tumour and to a much lesser extent in the differential diagnosis of degenerative or inherited metabolic disorders of the brain in infancy and childhood and much less often in encephalitic and/or dementing processes in adult life. In some rare inherited disorders of the nervous system, such as the lipidoses, specific enzymatic abnormalities can be detected in skin fibroblasts or leucocytes in cultures. Similar techniques applied to amniotic cells obtained by amniocentesis can be used for antenatal diagnosis with a view to therapeutic abortion on eugenic grounds. Measurement of α-fetoprotein in amniotic fluid may similarly allow the antenatal diagnosis of serious neural tube malformations such as anencephaly and spina bifida.

Electroencephalography (EEG)

Electroencephalography is a method of recording the electrical activity of the brain through the intact skull. Electrodes are applied to the scalp and the potential changes so recorded are amplified and presented for interpretation as an inked tracing on moving paper. Machines in common use have eight, sixteen or more channels, so that the activity from many different areas of the head can be recorded simultaneously. The technique is simple and harmless and may give valuable diagnostic information.

In the normal adult with the eyes closed the dominant electrical activity in the EEG from the postcentral area is usually a sinusoidal wave form with a frequency of 8–13 Hz (the term cycles per second has now been replaced by the hertz, abbreviation Hz). This is the alpha rhythm. It usually disappears on attention, as when the eyes open. Normally there is often some faster so-called beta activity (14–22 Hz) in the frontal region. This is accentuated by the administration of sedative drugs such as barbiturates and sometimes by anxiety. In young infants the EEG is dominated by generalized slow activity of so-called delta frequency (up to 3.5 Hz). Gradually during maturation this is replaced by theta activity (4–7 Hz) and subsequently by the alpha rhythm. Theta activity disappears last from the posterior temporal regions, particularly on the right side, and the record is usually completely mature, showing no theta activity, by the time an individual is 12–14 years of age. During drowsiness and sleep in the normal individual, theta activity and later delta activity reappear. Some common appearances in the EEG are illustrated in Fig. 11.4.

The EEG is of particular value in the diagnosis of epilepsy. In cases of petit mal it often shows regular, rhythmical, generalized outbursts of repetitive complexes, each consisting of a spike and a delta wave ('spike-and-wave'), and recurring at a frequency of about 3 Hz. In idiopathic or 'centrencephalic' major epilepsy, the interseizure record may show brief generalized outbursts of spikes or sharp waves, or of mixed spikes and slow activity. In patients with focal epilepsy, including temporal lobe or 'complex partial' seizures, there are often spikes, sharp waves or rhythmic outbursts of slow (delta or theta) activity arising in the epileptogenic area of cortex. Unfortunately, a single record taken in an epileptic patient between attacks is often normal. Positive findings are more common in children and less common the older the patient. Many other patients show non-specific abnormalities such as excessive temporal theta activity, a finding often attributed to immaturity in the broadest sense. It may be necessary to take repeated recordings or else to use various activation techniques in order to uncover epileptic discharges. Overbreathing for a period of from 2 to 3 minutes is particularly effective in evoking the discharges of petit mal, while photic stimulation (repetitive light flashes of variable frequency) can also bring out epileptic discharges. Since temporal spikes or sharp waves often appear in early sleep it has become conventional to carry out recordings after oral or intravenous sedation in cases of suspected temporal lobe epilepsy. In some such cases, and particularly when the patient's symptoms are sufficiently severe for surgical treatment to be considered, recordings can be made from underneath the medial surface of the temporal lobe by inserting a needle electrode to lie in contact with the basisphenoid.

A single routine EEG is of limited value but should generally be performed, using simple activation techniques if necessary, in most patients who are suspected to be suffering from epilepsy. The demonstration of epileptic discharges will support the diagnosis, and the nature of the discharge may help in deciding upon appropriate treatment. Negative findings, however, cannot be taken to exclude the diagnosis of epilepsy.

The EEG is also of limited value in the diagnosis of focal cerebral lesions. A relatively acute lesion of one cerebral hemisphere usually gives a focus of delta activity in or around the area of the lesion. It is not the lesion itself which produces this abnormal discharge, but the changes which it has produced in the surrounding brain. A cerebral abscess usually produces a slow-wave focus of high amplitude, and similar though less striking abnormalities result from

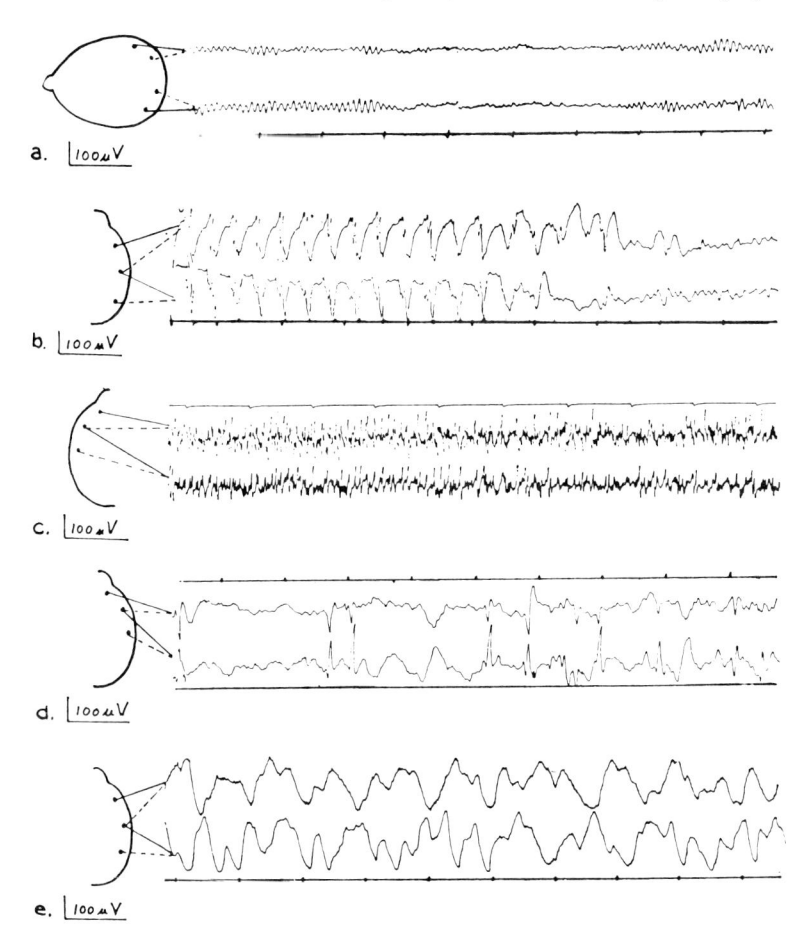

Figure 11.4 Some common appearances in electroencephalographic (EEG) recordings.
a. A normal alpha rhythm recorded from both occipital regions and disappearing (in the centre of the recording) when the eyes are open.
b. A 3 Hz spike-and-wave discharge of petit mal epilepsy, recorded in this illustration from the right temporal region.
c. High-frequency discharges (mainly muscle artefact) recorded from the left frontotemporal region during a major epileptic seizure.
d. A right anterotemporal focus of spike discharge in a patient suffering from temporal lobe epilepsy.
e. A focus of high-amplitude delta activity seen in the right mid-temporal region in a patient suffering from a cerebral abscess in this situation.
[Reproduced from Walton (1982) *Essentials of Neurology*, 5th edn, by kind permission of the publisher.]

tumour, haemorrhage, local injury or infarction. The EEG may help in localization but gives little guide to pathological diagnosis, which must depend upon other information. An abnormality due to a tumour will usually become worse, while that due to an infarct will tend to improve. In lesions which are more chronic or more deeply located in the cerebral hemisphere, focal theta activity of low amplitude, or even an absence of the alpha rhythm or of beta activity which is present on the other side, may be the only abnormality. Some localized abnormality of the EEG is generally found in about two-thirds of all patients with cerebral neoplasms, but a negative record is of no real value in excluding tumour.

There are some inflammatory, metabolic and degenerative diseases of the brain, however, in which the EEG is especially helpful in a diagnostic sense. The periodic complexes of subacute sclerosing panencephalitis, the less typical but also periodic focal triphasic waves of herpes simplex encephalitis, the diffuse irregular spike-and-wave activity of Creutzfeldt–Jakob disease, the somewhat similar spike-and-wave discharge (hypsarrhythmia) seen in children with infantile spasms and also in some of the lipidoses and phakomatoses, and the diffuse slow activity with triphasic waves seen in hepatic encephalopathy are just a few examples.

The EEG is of comparatively little value in psychiatric diagnosis although anxious and obsessional patients often show excessive frontal fast activity. Patients with personality disorder and children with behaviour disorders have typically immature records with excessive temporal slow activity. Patients with organic dementia often show a dominant rhythm of theta rather than alpha frequency. This is in a sense a reversion to the childhood pattern and may even occur naturally as a result of ageing.

In summary the EEG is of considerable value in the diagnosis of epilepsy and certain uncommon brain diseases in which relatively specific abnormalities are found. It is of limited value in the investigation of patients with cerebrovascular disease or intracranial space-occupying lesions. A single negative recording is of very little value.

Ultrasonic imaging

For many years echo-encephalography or sono-encephalography had a considerable vogue in the investigation of patients with suspected intracranial space-occupying lesions. Many simple and inexpensive machines have been commercially available and some are still used, though the technique is now used relatively infrequently.

An ultrasonic beam is passed horizontally through the intact skull and an 'echo' can be recorded from the midline structures (the A-scan). A 'shift' of the midline can readily be demonstrated, and this method, which carries no risk, has proved useful in confirming the presence of a space-occupying lesion in or overlying one cerebral hemisphere. The method was often used for the rapid screening of patients in whom a subdural or extradural haematoma or a tumour in one cerebral hemisphere was suspected. More complicated and refined techniques have been introduced in order to define the 'echoes' arising from intracranial structures other than those in the midline (the B-scan), but these have been largely supplanted by the more accurate technique of computed tomography (the CT scan).

As the use of echo-encephalography has declined, so the use of ultrasonic Doppler scanning (echotomography) has come to be used increasingly as a means of detecting arterial stenoses, especially in the carotid artery tree, and it can also be used, for example, to assess ophthalmic artery flow after total carotid occlusion.

Gamma-encephalography

Scanning of the radioactivity recorded over the skull surface following the intravenous injection of a suitable isotope (^{99}technetium has been most widely used) has also been a useful aid in the diagnosis of intracranial lesions. The blood vessels, and in all probability the cells of certain tumours, show a selective affinity for the isotope so that the tumour may be shown as an area of increased radioactivity. With lateral and anteroposterior 'scans', localization may be very accurate. Uptake may also be increased in vascular malformations, abscesses and infarcts. This technique has also proved particularly valuable in demonstrating multiple intracranial lesions (e.g. metastases). Although still used in some centres, this method, too, has been largely supplanted by CT and NMR scanning.

Isotope ventriculography

In a normal individual radio-iodinated serum albumin (RISA) injected by lumbar puncture is demonstrable a few hours later as radioactivity in the subarachnoid space over the surface of the brain and not, as a rule, in the cerebral ventricles. If the lateral ventricles soon show radioactivity, and if little or no isotope is seen to flow over the brain surface towards the superior longitudinal sinus, then some degree of communicating hydrocephalus is likely to be present. (However, obliteration of the subarachnoid space may also be demonstrated by the CT scan.) The technique is also useful in detecting fistulous communications between the subarachnoid space and the middle ear or paranasal sinuses. Measurement of the rate of clearance of the isotope into the systemic circulation has also been used as a method of detecting the rate of CSF absorption in a case of suspected hydrocephalus.

Radiology

Radiological methods are among the most helpful and widely used of all the ancillary techniques in neurological diagnosis. Final diagnosis has often depended upon specialized methods involving the use of air or other contrast media, but these techniques are time-consuming, expensive and often disturbing to the patient. The advent of CT and NMR scanning has increased immeasurably the accuracy of diagnosis and has greatly reduced the risk and discomfort to which patients in the past were often subjected. However, as will be shown below, the older contrast methods still have a part to play in certain circumstances, and even pneumoencephalography and ventriculography which are very rarely performed now in specialized neurological and neurosurgical units in developed countries may still sometimes be required in centres where CT and NMR scanning are not yet freely available. Valuable and even conclusive information can sometimes be obtained from plain radiographs of the skull and/or spine and even of other parts of the body. In patients with a clinical picture suggestive of intracranial tumour, for example, X-ray of the chest is vital, perhaps revealing either a bronchogenic carcinoma or evidence of pulmonary tuberculosis. In other cases skeletal changes will throw light upon the significance of neurological symptoms and signs as, for instance, in cases of prostatic carcinoma or multiple myelomatosis.

STRAIGHT RADIOGRAPHY OF THE SKULL

It is usual to take routine anteroposterior and lateral views of the skull, and in most specialized centres an anteroposterior view is also taken with the brow depressed some 35° so that the petrous temporal bones become visible (Towne's view), and still another is taken of the skull base. Usually the skull

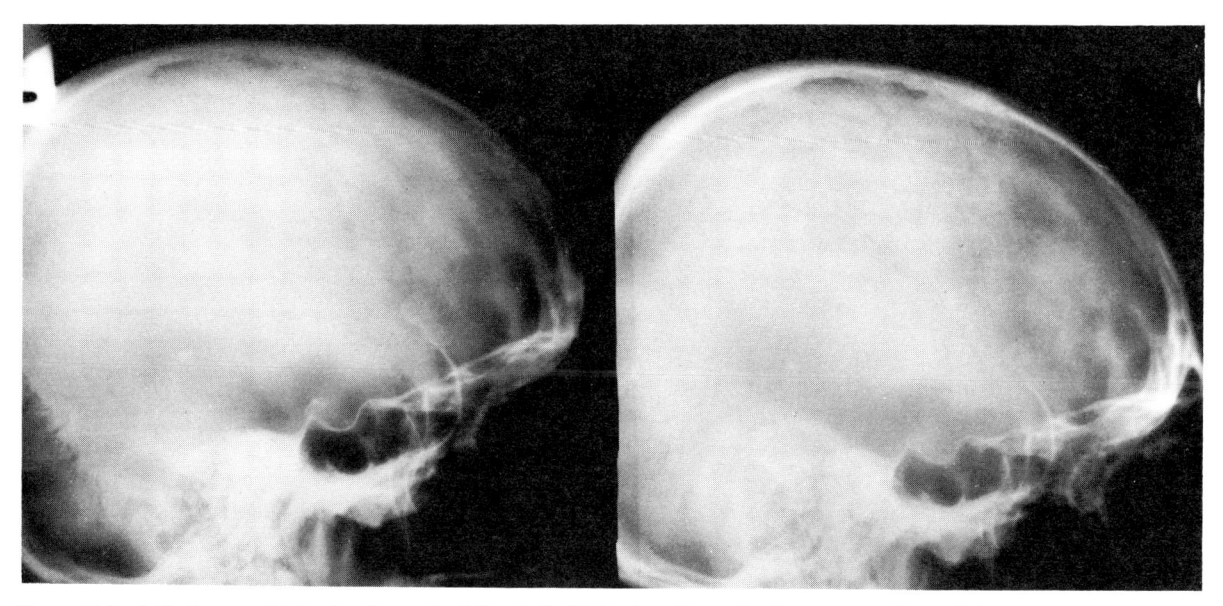

Figure 11.5 Left, A normal lateral radiograph of the skull. Right, A radiograph taken one year later of the same patient showing loss of the lamina dura of the dorsum sellae due to increased intracranial pressure. [Reproduced from Walton (1985) *Brain's Diseases of the Nervous System*, 9th edn, by kind permission of the publisher.]

vault is first examined to see if there is reasonable uniformity of bony thickness or whether there is any erosion or bony overgrowth (as may result from a meningioma) or abnormal vascular markings due to dilatation of the middle meningeal artery which is supplying a meningeal tumour or vascular malformation. Sometimes, as in myelomatosis or carcinomatosis, there are multiple areas of bony rarefaction in the skull vault or there is a general thickening or 'woolliness' of the bone as in Paget's disease. Frontal hyperostosis is not uncommon but is of no pathological significance. In young children, hydrocephalus due to any cause gives separation of the cranial sutures and a characteristic 'beaten copper' mottling of the bone. However, the latter appearance is so often seen in normal individuals, even in adult life, that in itself it is not diagnostic. It is also wise to examine the frontal, maxillary and sphenoidal paranasal sinuses for opacities which might suggest infection or neoplasia.

At the base of the skull the relationship of the upper cervical spine to the foramen magnum is observed, and the examiner should note whether there is any protrusion of the odontoid process of the axis above the line joining the posterior margin of the hard palate to the posterior lip of the foramen magnum (Chamberlain's line). If the odontoid protrudes above this line, or if there is an abnormal tilt of the body of the atlas implying invagination of the basiocciput, then basilar impression, which can give important neurological manifestations, is present. The most important structure in the skull base visible on the lateral projection is the sella turcica. The size and shape of the sella and the integrity and density of the anterior and posterior clinoid processes which form its lips are noted. In patients with pituitary neoplasms the sella is expanded or ballooned and partially decalcified. In those patients with suprasellar lesions the sella is also expanded, but is shallower and flattened and there is often erosion of the clinoid processes (Fig. 11.5). Moderate flattening and expansion of the sella with decalcification of the posterior clinoid processes can occur in any patient with increased intracranial pressure whether or not there is a lesion near the sella.

Also to be noted on the lateral projection is the presence or absence of intracranial calcification. If present, such calcification can then be more accurately localized by anteroposterior views, or by stereoscopic lateral projections. In about 50% of adults, and even in some normal children, the pineal gland is calcified and may measure up to 0.5 cm in diameter. If the gland is calcified it is important to measure its distance from the inner table of the skull on either side on anteroposterior radiographs, as displacement of the gland to either side may indicate the presence of a space-occupying lesion in one cerebral hemisphere. Other intracranial structures which occasionally calcify in the normal individual are the choroid plexuses, the falx cerebri and the petroclinoid ligaments. Pathological intracranial calcification, if mottled in type and suprasellar in location, may indicate a craniopharyngioma (Fig. 11.6), but many other intracranial tumours some-

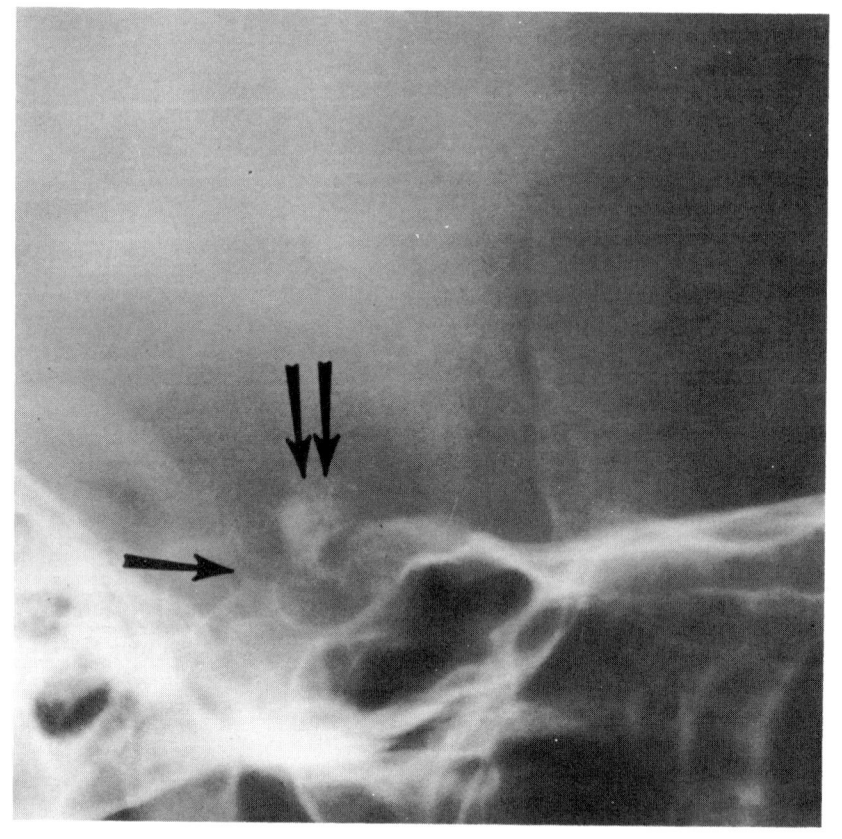

Figure 11.6 Lateral radiograph of skull in a child with a suprasellar craniopharyngioma showing calcification (double arrows) and erosion of the tip of the dorsum sellae (single arrow). [Reproduced from Walton (1985) *Brain's Diseases of the Nervous System*, 9th edn, by kind permission of the publisher.]

times show a fine spidery pattern of calcification. Rarely, fine curvilinear lines of calcification are seen in the wall of a large aneurysm, while calcific stippling or even dense calcification can occur in a haematoma or an arteriovenous angioma. Rare causes of intracranial calcification include cysticercosis (calcified cysts), toxoplasmosis (mottling in the basal ganglia) and hypoparathyroidism (also in the basal ganglia). A form of calcification outlining clearly the gyri of one occipital and/or parietal lobe occurs in diffuse cortical angiomatosis associated with a port-wine naevus of the face (the Sturge–Weber syndrome).

In anteroposterior, Towne's and the basal views it is important to look for enlargement or erosion of cranial exit foramina. Sclerosis and overgrowth of bone may also occur, particularly in the wings of the sphenoid, in patients with a meningioma in this region. It is usual to examine particularly the optic foramina, superior orbital fissures and internal auditory meati. A funnel-shaped erosion of one internal auditory meatus, revealed by Towne's views, is characteristic of acoustic neuroma.

COMPUTED TOMOGRAPHY SCANNING

This exciting technique of radiological diagnosis has transformed the practice of neuroradiology and has supplanted progressively some of the more traditional contrast methods. The equipment required is costly and requires considerable technical skill for its operation and maintenance but it has been gradually brought into general use throughout the world. It depends upon the transmission of photon beams across the head or body and recording with crystals instead of X-ray film. While the first generation scanners were head scanners only, this was quickly followed by the development of 'whole-body' machines which not only give images, for example, of intrathoracic or intra-abdominal structures and of the voluntary muscles, but also give precise and invaluable information about many intraspinal lesions. The sensitivity of the technique is such that small variations in X-ray absorption coefficients between the normal intracranial, intraorbital or intraspinal contents can be displayed, so that cortex white matter

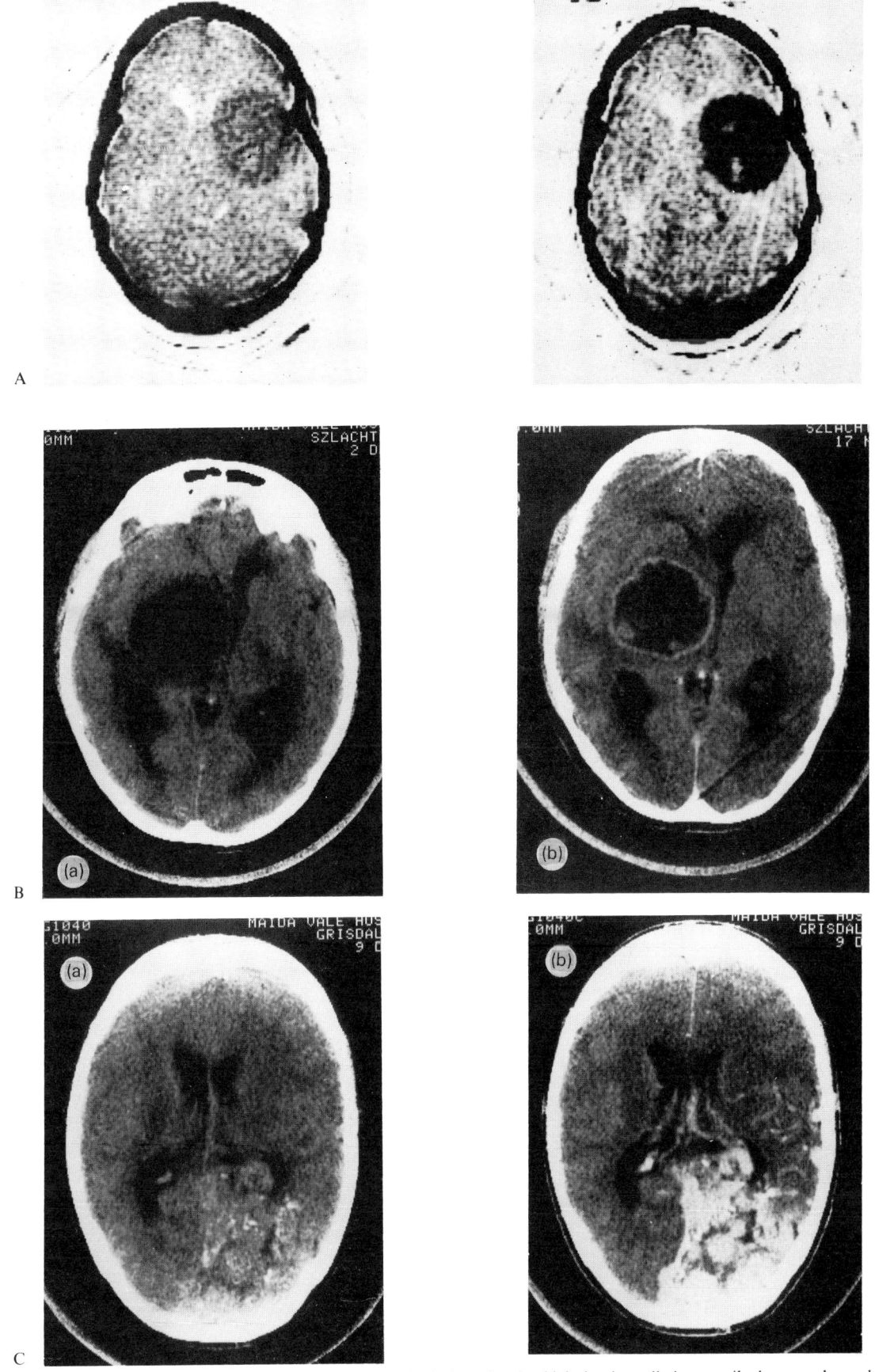

Figure 11.7 A, Meningioma, arising from the right sphenoidal wing, showing high-density well-circumscribed mass, enhanced (right). B, CT scan, cystic glioma, left hemisphere, with distorted and enlarged ventricles (a) unenhanced and (b) contrast-enhanced. C, CT scan, angioma with calcification, right parieto-occipital region (a) unenhanced and (b) contrast-enhanced.

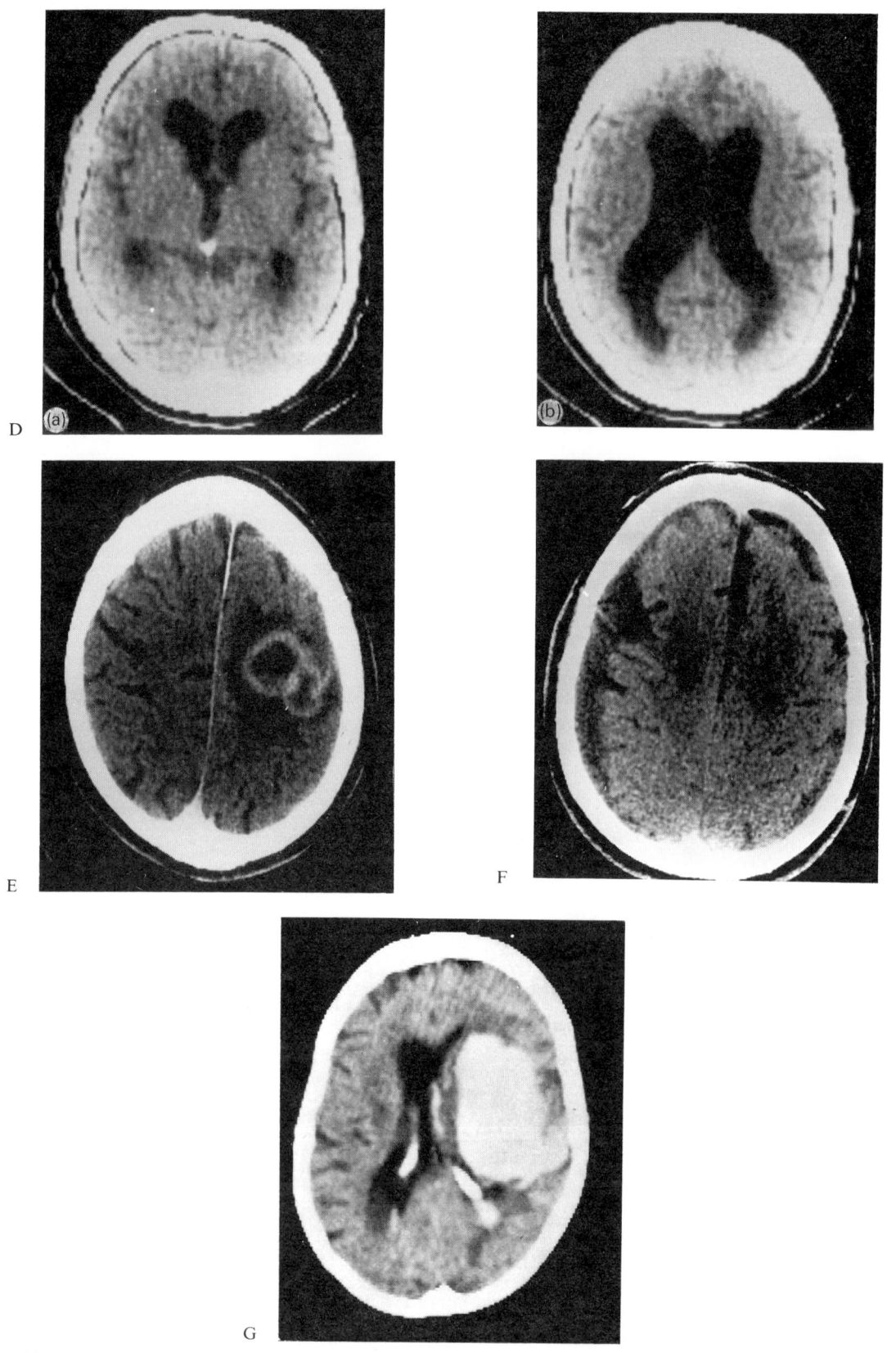

Figure 11.7 (*continued*) D, CT scans showing dilated lateral and third ventricles, widened sylvian fissures and cortical sulci. These scans demonstrate cerebral atrophy in a patient with Alzheimer's disease. E, CT scan, cerebral abscess, right hemisphere, biloculated, contrast-enhanced. F, CT scan, subdural haematoma. G, CT scan showing intraventricular haemorrhage with blood in the ventricles and shift of midline to the left. Reproduced from *Brain's Clinical Neurology*, 6th edition, by Sir Roger Bannister, Oxford University Press, 1985, with kind permission of the author and publisher.

(including internal capsule and corpus callosum) can be identified as well as the ventricles, cortical subarachnoid spaces and basal cisterns. Tumours, haematomas, infarcts, oedema and calcification have different absorption coefficients so that it is possible to determine the site and pathological characteristics of many intracranial and spinal lesions. The accuracy of the CT scan is greatly enhanced by the use of 60 ml of sodium iothalamate (Conray) given intravenously, which often increases image density in some lesions. The technique allows one to carry out rapid serial tomographic 'cuts' in multiple planes through the intact skull with no discomfort to the patient and no risk, as the radiation exposure is minimal. Some representative CT scans demonstrating various intracranial lesions are reproduced in Fig. 11.7. The use of this technique has greatly reduced the numbers of pneumoencephalograms, ventriculograms, and to a somewhat lesser extent angiograms carried out in neurological and neurosurgical centres where it is available.

NUCLEAR MAGNETIC RESONANCE (NMR)

Yet a further important dimension has been added to techniques of neuroimaging by NMR scanning which makes use of the magnetic properties of the hydrogen nucleus excited by radiofrequency radiation transmitted by a coil surrounding the head. The signals so produced are detected as induced electric currents in a receiver coil which lies within the transmitter coil. Fat and bone marrow appear white, while tissue or fluids with longer 'relaxation' times, like cortical bone which contains a low concentration of hydrogen, appear black. The NMR scan, which carries no hazard to the patient, gives better differentiation of grey from white matter than does the CT scan, can identify individual nuclei of the basal ganglia, distinguishes blood from CSF and can readily pick out, for example, plaques of demyelination. It is clearly complementary to, and often superior to, CT scanning, especially in diagnosing degenerative, toxic, metabolic and infective encephalopathies and multiple sclerosis. Some representative NMR scans are given in Fig. 11.8.

RADIOLOGY OF THE SPINAL COLUMN

Spinal radiographs give information concerning the vertebrae themselves, the intervertebral discs and the intervertebral foramina. Anteroposterior and lateral views are sufficient for study of the vertebrae and discs, but for examination of the intervertebral foramina, oblique views are needed. Bony erosion and enlargement of the relevant intervertebral foramen is typically seen in cases of spinal neurofibroma, often with the extraspinal soft tissue shadow of a dumb-bell tumour. Less striking but diagnostically important is a variation in interpedicular distance. The distance between the vertebral pedicles is large in the cervical region, diminishes gradually to a minimum in the mid-dorsal region, and then expands again in the lumbar region, corresponding to the cervical and lumbar enlargements of the cord. If one or more interpedicular distances fall outside the normal arithmetical progression, this indicates the presence of an expanding lesion in the cord or spinal canal. Dorsal meningiomas may produce no more radiological change than this, whereas neurofibromas often give bony erosion as well. Measurement of the anteroposterior diameter of the spinal canal is also of value. An unduly wide cervical canal is seen, for instance, in some cases of syringomyelia. An unusually narrow canal may contribute to the early development of symptoms of myelopathy in patients with cervical spondylosis or to the development of 'intermittent claudication of the cauda equina' in cases of lumbar canal stenosis.

Radiographs of the spine are often normal after an acute prolapse of an intervertebral disc, or simply reveal a narrowing of the disc space concerned. The prolapsed disc is not itself radiopaque. If one or more disc protrusions have developed gradually over months or years, the margins of the prolapsed tissue gradually become calcified, giving posterior (and often anterior) osteophyte formation at the upper and lower borders of the contiguous vertebrae (Fig. 11.9). As the prolapsed tissue often projects laterally as well, osteophytes may also encroach upon the intervertebral foramina and are then seen on oblique views. A combination of changes of this type, most often seen in the cervical and lumbar regions, is called spondylosis.

CONTRAST METHODS

The contrast methods most often used in the past in neurological diagnosis were pneumoencephalography, ventriculography with air or contrast medium, and carotid, vertebral and aortic arch angiography and myelography. Each method involves possible hazards to the patient and all produce some degree of pain or discomfort. They are not to be regarded as routine methods of investigation but should be utilized only when an accurate diagnosis can be reached in no other way. Sometimes it is necessary to carry out a number of these studies successively, but they should always be kept to the minimum necessary to give adequate information concerning the patient's disease. In general, pneumoencephalography was indicated, before CT or NMR scanning were available, in patients in whom

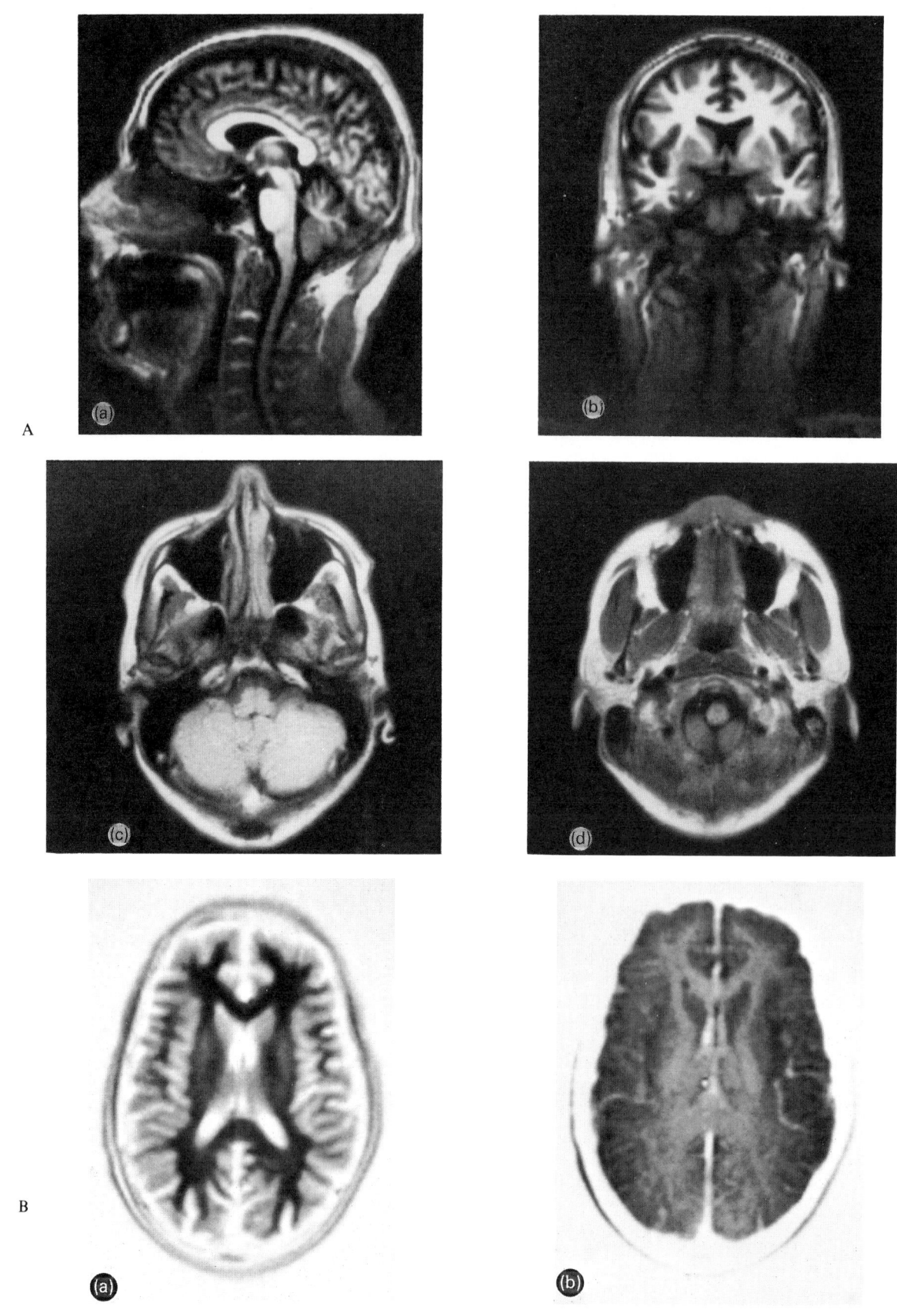

Figure 11.8 A, Nuclear magnetic resonance scans of normal brain to show brain anatomy of (a) sagittal, (b) coronal, (c) high medulla, and (d) low medulla (showing cerebellar tonsils). B, NMR scans: (a) inversion–recovery and (b) spin-echo. The spin-echo scan shows much less grey-white matter contrast but shows oedema in pathological brain.

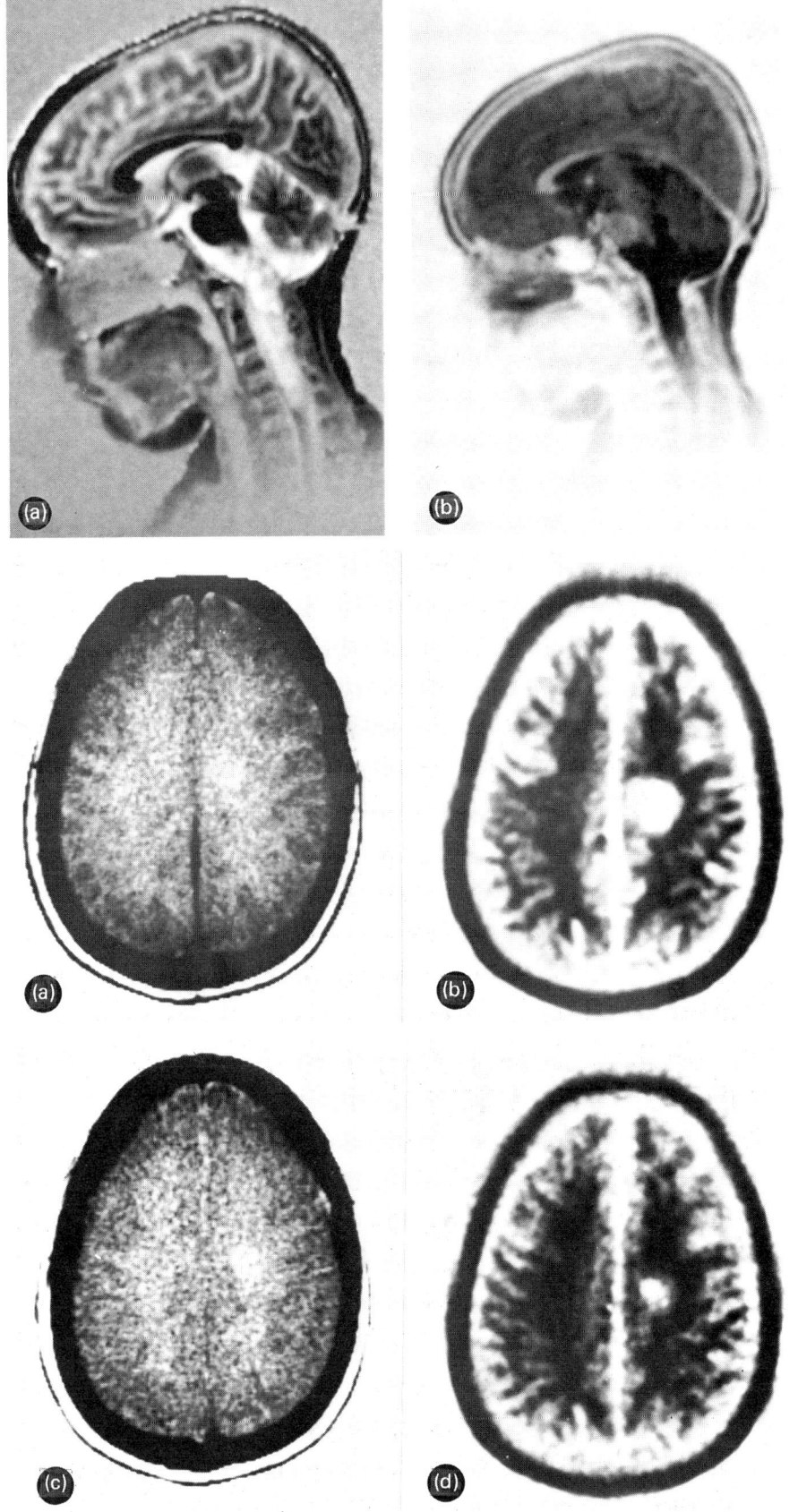

Figure 11.8 (*continued*) C, Astrocytoma of the medulla and spinal cord in an 8-year-old boy. (a) NMR (inversion–recovery) and (b) NMR (spin-echo) scans, showing the extent of the tumour. D, Acute multiple sclerosis: (a) initial contrast-enhanced CT scan. Low attenuation area on CT scan corresponds in position to lesion seen on (b) NMR (inversion–recovery) scan; (c) follow-up CT scan; (d) NMR (inversion–recovery) scans—lesion has diminished.

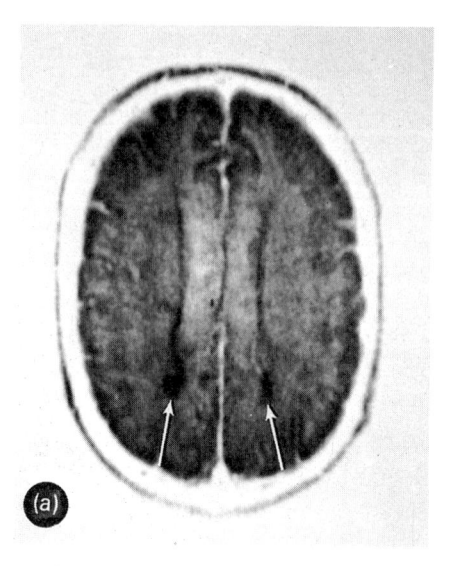

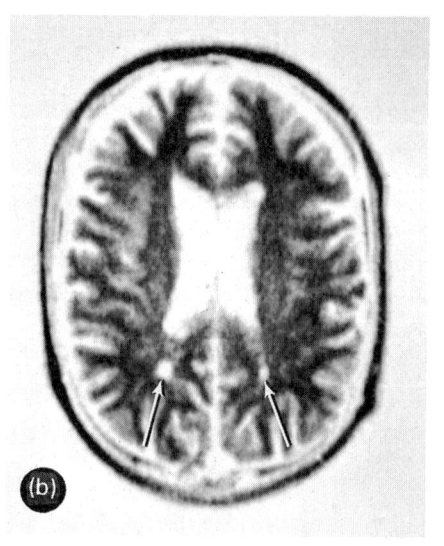

Figure 11.8 (*continued*) E, Multiple sclerosis. (a) NMR (inversion–recovery) and (b) NMR (spin-echo) scans. Two lesions are demonstrated. Reproduced from *Brain's Clinical Neurology*, 6th edition, by Sir Roger Bannister, Oxford University Press, 1985, with kind permission of the author and publisher.

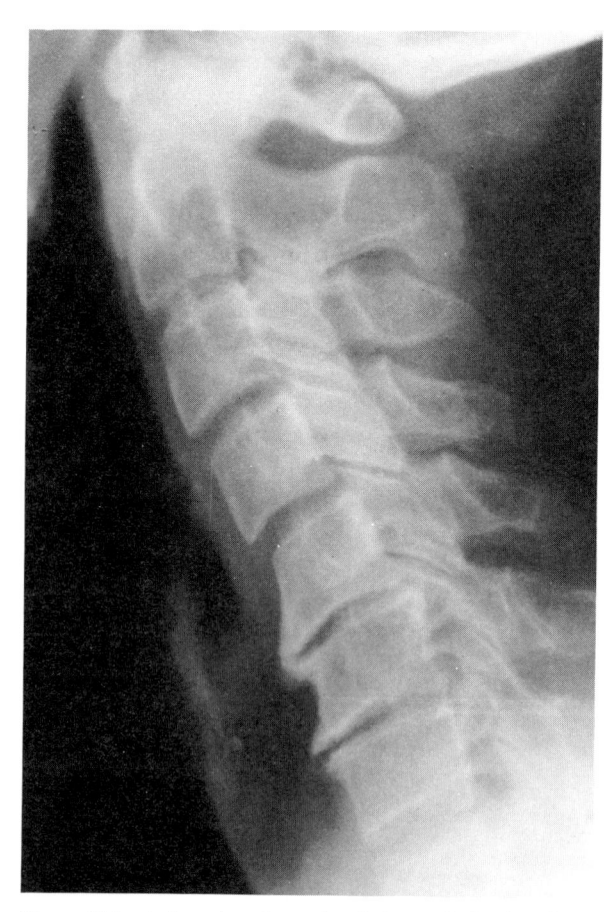

Figure 11.9 A lateral radiograph of the cervical spine demonstrating anterior osteophytes and narrowing of disc spaces at C5–C6 and C6–C7. [Reproduced from Walton (1985) *Brain's Diseases of the Nervous System*, 9th edn, by kind permission of the publisher.]

cortical atrophy, either focal or generalized, or communicating hydrocephalus was suspected. Usually this investigation was contraindicated in the tumour suspect, even when there were no focal neurological signs and no features suggesting raised intracranial pressure. Subarachnoid, subdural or intracerebral haemorrhage are now easily diagnosed as a rule by CT scanning as blood can readily be demonstrated in the brain substance, subdural or subarachnoid space. Sometimes, too, an aneurysm or angioma is also shown by this technique, but nevertheless for accurate identification and localization of the source of haemorrhage, especially in subarachnoid haemorrhage, carotid arteriography is usually necessary and may have to be followed by vertebral angiography if carotid injection gives negative results. Carotid angiography is also of considerable value in the diagnosis of other forms of cerebral vascular disease, especially when arterial occlusion, narrowing or venous thrombosis is suspected. In patients considered to have an intracranial space-occupying lesion it was often useful before CT scanning was possible. A 'wide sweep' of the anterior cerebral arteries might give evidence of hydrocephalus, or vascular displacement or a pathological circulation often confirmed the presence of a tumour. Aortic arch angiography is still very useful in the diagnosis of extracranial arterial occlusion or stenosis in the carotid or vertebral vessels. In patients with papilloedema or other evidence of raised intracranial pressure, especially when a tumour in the brain stem or posterior fossa was suspected, air ventriculography was generally indicated in the past if gamma-encephalography or carotid angiography failed to

The cerebrospinal fluid, etc.—some pathophysiological principles 265

localize or identify the lesion. Ventriculography with contrast medium was sometimes required, especially if the third and fourth ventricles were not adequately outlined by air. These were highly specialized investigations which required immaculate radiographic technique and skilled neuroradiological interpretation. They were carried out only in units where neurosurgical help was readily available, in case of unforeseen complications. Often ventriculography had to be followed by immediate craniotomy. Although, as mentioned above, these painful and hazardous techniques have been almost totally supplanted by CT and NMR scanning, they will be described briefly below, first for historical and anatomical interest, and secondly because there may still be very rare situations or circumstances in which one or other of these methods may still be required.

In the investigation of suspected spinal cord com-

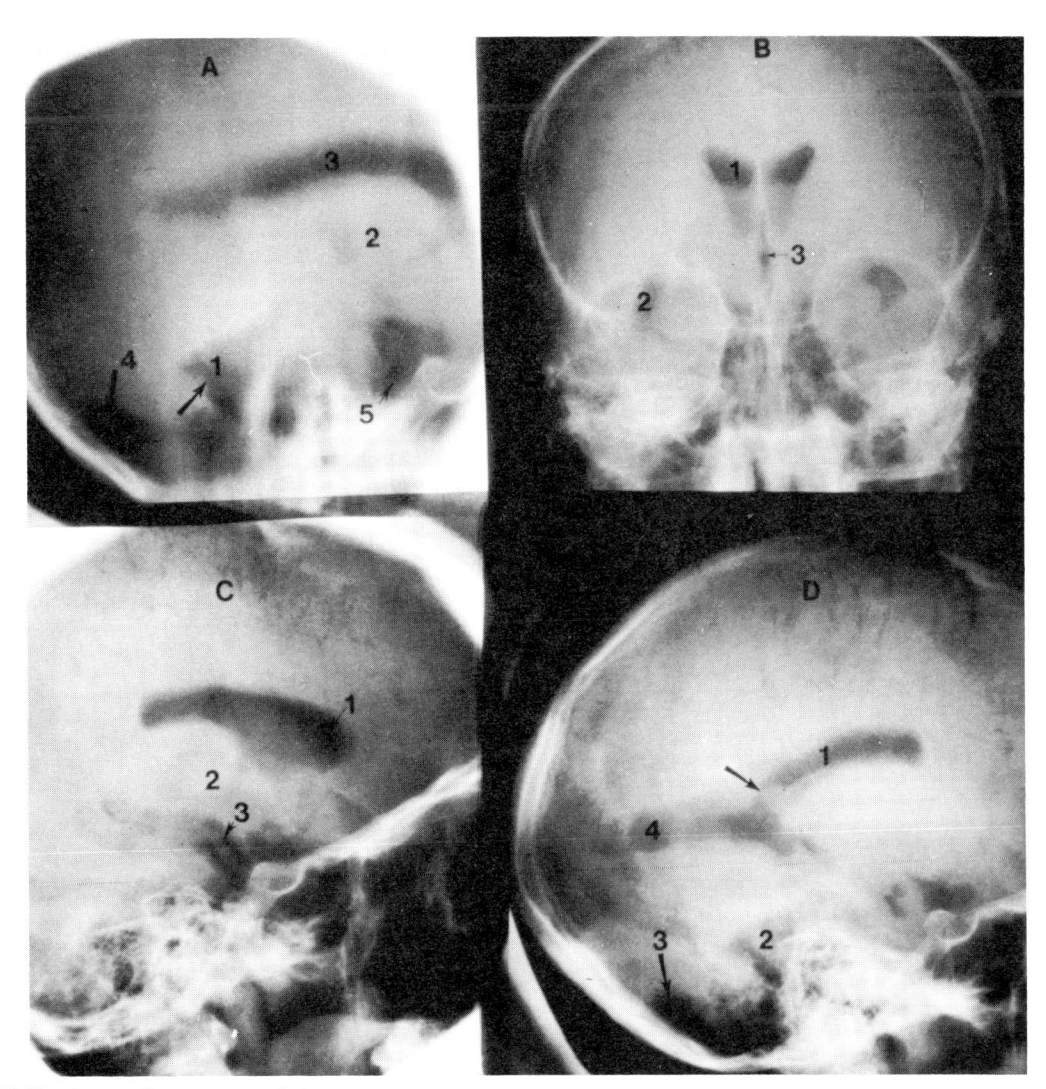

Figure 11.10 A normal pneumoencephalogram.
A, Erect midline tomogram.
   1. 4th ventricle (the choroid plexus is arrowed).
   2. 3rd ventricle.
   3. Lateral ventricle.
   4. Cisterna magna.
   5. Pre-pontine cistern.
B, Anteroposterior brow-up view.
   1. Body of lateral ventricle.
   2. Temporal horn.
   3. 3rd ventricle.
C, Lateral brow-up view.
   1. Frontal horn of lateral ventricle.
   2. 3rd ventricle.
   3. Temporal horn.
D, Lateral brow-down view.
   1. Lateral ventricle (choroid plexus arrowed).
   2. 4th ventricle.
   3. Cisterna magna.
   4. Occipital horn.

[Reproduced from Walton (1985) *Brain's Diseases of the Nervous System*, 9th edn, by kind permission of the publisher.]

pression, while whole-body CT scanning is now being used increasingly to localize and identify intraspinal lesions, myelography is still the technique of choice in many, if not most, cases and is usually performed by the lumbar route. Rarely, cisternal injection is required in order to define the upper limit of a spinal lesion prior to surgical exploration.

Pneumoencephalography

Pneumoencephalography, like lumbar puncture, is generally contraindicated in patients with papilloedema or other evidence of increased intracranial pressure, in view of the risk of cerebellar or tentorial herniation. It should be performed only if neurosurgical aid is immediately at hand in patients suspected of having an intracranial neoplasm, even if the CSF pressure in the lumbar region is normal.

To perform a pneumoencephalogram, a lumbar puncture is performed with the patient sitting upright. After a few drops of CSF have been allowed to flow, sufficient only to determine that the needle is in position, 5 ml of air is injected slowly and radiographs are taken as the bubble of air passes through the basal cisterns and fourth ventricle. Then 5 ml of CSF is removed, 10 ml of air is injected, and subsequently 10 ml of fluid is withdrawn. The procedure is continued until a total of 25–30 ml of air has been injected and adequate filling of the ventricular system has been obtained. Usually this amount of air is adequate and can be manipulated in order to give a complete demonstration of the entire ventricular system (Fig. 11.10) and of the basal cisterns. The procedure usually produces severe headache and sometimes even prostration and vomiting. The severity of these symptoms is usually in direct proportion to the amount of air injected.

Pneumoencephalography may define the upper limits of a pituitary neoplasm by distortion of the basal cisterns or a posterior fossa neoplasm by displacement of or encroachment upon the fourth ventricle. Neoplasms of the cerebral hemispheres are localized by evidence of distortion and displacement of the lateral and third ventricles. A localized dilatation of some part of the ventricular system may indicate localized cerebral atrophy, while enlargement of the cerebral ventricles and/or pooling of air in widened cortical sulci results from diffuse cerebral atrophy, as in presenile dementia. If air enters the ventricles but none appears over the cortex, this may indicate communicating hydrocephalus which was often then confirmed in the past by isotope ventriculography. Clinical deterioration following the procedure was often thought to be characteristic of cases of 'low-pressure' communicating hydrocephalus. While a failure to fill the cerebral ventricles may be indicative of obstruction to the exit foramina of the fourth ventricle, it is much more often due to technical failure.

Ventriculography

To perform ventriculography, air is injected into one lateral ventricle through a needle inserted through a burr-hole in the skull and then passed through brain tissue. The procedure is not without risk as the needle may pierce a vessel during its passage through brain tissue, while a sudden release of pressure in one lateral ventricle can result in herniation of the contralateral cerebral hemisphere across the midline beneath the falx cerebri. Immediate puncture of the other lateral ventricle or even operative decompression will then be required. The investigation should be carried out only when the appropriate neurosurgical operation can be performed without delay.

The information obtainable by this method is comparable to that derived from pneumoencephalography. It was usually performed in patients with suspected cerebral tumour in whom the intracranial pressure was high. A stenosis of the aqueduct of Sylvius, giving internal hydrocephalus, could also be demonstrated, as the air failed to pass through the aqueduct into the fourth ventricle. When it was impossible to demonstrate the fourth ventricle adequately, it was sometimes necessary to inject 1–2 ml of oily contrast medium into the lateral ventricle and to observe its flow downwards through the third and fourth ventricles. This technique was used only in carefully selected cases, as the medium sometimes acted as a cerebral irritant unless it was able to flow down into the spinal theca when the examination had been completed.

Cerebral angiography

In carotid arteriography the common carotid artery is injected with an iodine-containing contrast medium percutaneously under either local or general anaesthesia. The internal carotid artery and its branches (middle and anterior cerebral and their radicals) are demonstrated. Vertebral arteriography can also be performed by percutaneous injection of the vertebral artery in the neck, and the vertebral, basilar and posterior cerebral arteries are then filled. This method is used much less often than carotid injection. In skilled hands, complications are few, but undue trauma may cause arterial spasm. In the elderly, hypertensive or atherosclerotic individual this can lead to cerebral or brain-stem ischaemia or infarction with transient or even occasionally permanent sequelae. Most radiologists now prefer to inject contrast medium into the vertebral arteries through a catheter inserted into a limb artery such as the femoral or radial. A similar technique is utilized when it is

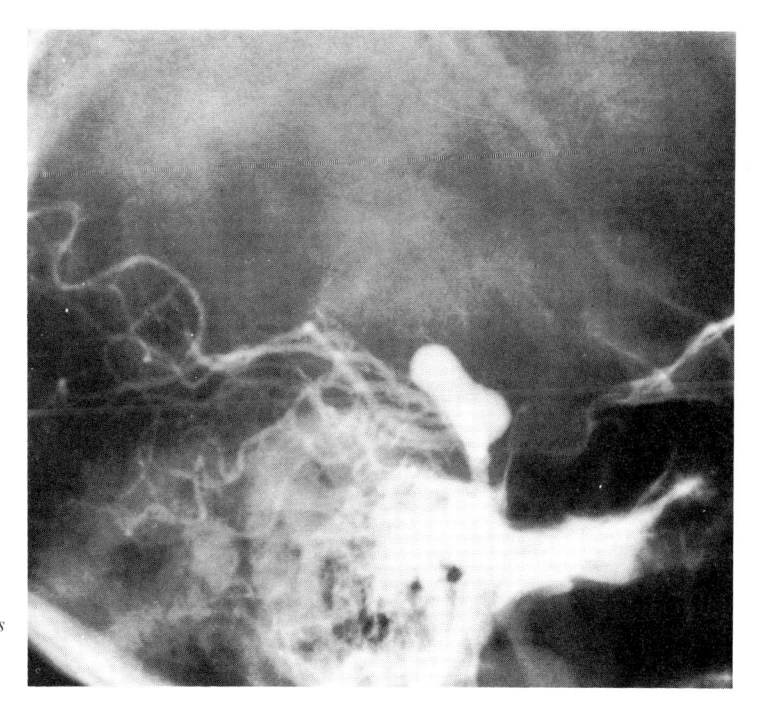

Figure 11.11 A large aneurysm at the bifurcation of the basilar artery demonstrated by vertebral angiography. [Reproduced from Walton (1985) *Brain's Diseases of the Nervous System*, 9th edn, by kind permission of the publisher.]

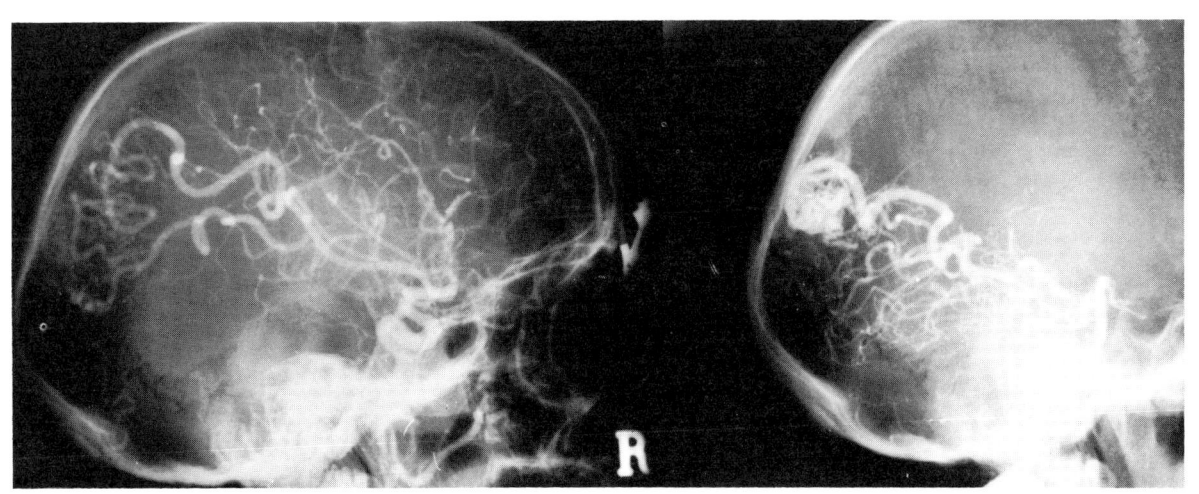

Figure 11.12 An occipital arteriovenous angioma supplied by both the carotid (left) and vertebral (right) systems. [Reproduced from Walton (1985) *Brain's Diseases of the Nervous System*, 9th edn, by kind permission of the publisher.]

necessary to demonstrate the aortic arch and its main branches in cases of presumed extracranial vascular disease.

Usually at least three lateral, anteroposterior and oblique views are taken at 1- or 2-second intervals to give early and late arterial and venous filling, but it is possible to obtain much more frequent pictures, giving a more comprehensive demonstration of the vascular tree (rapid serial angiography).

Angiography is particularly valuable in the diagnosis of vascular lesions. Thus intracranial aneurysms and arteriovenous angiomas (Figs. 11.11 and 11.12) are demonstrated and localized with considerable success. The technique must be used with caution in cases of presumed cerebral ischaemia or infarction because of the danger of complications, but in some such cases occlusion or stenosis of the internal carotid artery (Fig. 11.13) or of other major vessels in the neck or cranium are clearly demonstrated. Subdural haematoma can be confidently diagnosed by finding an avascular area beneath the skull in the anteroposterior view.

Carotid arteriography may also assist in the diagnosis and localization of space-occupying lesions of the cerebral hemispheres, though it is much less often used for this purpose than in the past, since the advent of CT scanning. Distortion and displacement of vessels will localize the lesion whether it be tumour, abscess or haemorrhage, while many tumours show a characteristic pattern of vascularization. Astrocytomas are relatively avascular, while glioblastomas commonly show a tangle of small abnormal blood vessels (Fig. 11.14). Meningiomas often give a characteristic 'blush' in the venous phase of the angiogram (Fig. 11.15), owing to retention of contrast medium in the vessels of the tumour. Vertebral arteriography may help in the diagnosis of tumours in the posterior fossa, and is especially useful in patients suspected of having vascular anomalies of the hindbrain circulation.

Conclusions

In patients in whom the symptoms and physical signs indicate a space-occupying lesion of one cerebral hemisphere, CT and/or NMR scanning is the investigation of choice, or else carotid arteriography if no CT scan is available. Where cortical atrophy or communicating hydrocephalus are suspected but there are no localizing signs and no evidence of increased pressure, and again, only in the absence of CT or NMR scanning, pneumoencephalography may be indicated. When, however, in such a case, the intracranial pressure is clearly raised and the angiogram or gamma scan have been uninformative, ventriculography may still very rarely be required. However, increasing use and availability of the CT scan has undoubtedly supplanted most of these traditional neuroradiological methods.

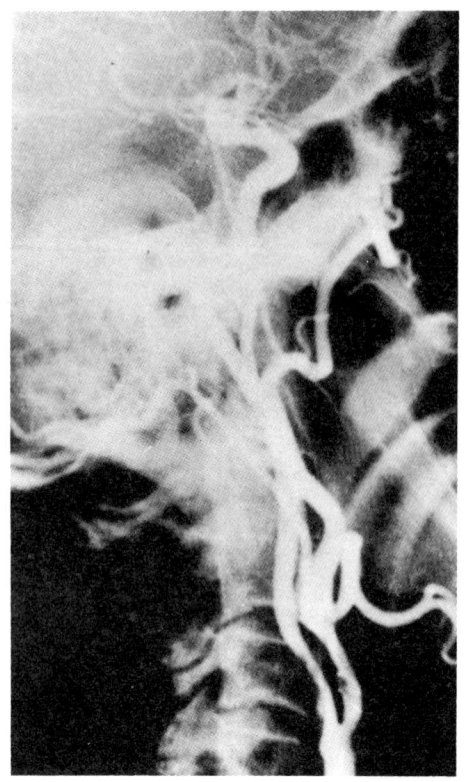

Figure 11.13 Left carotid arteriogram demonstrating stenosis at the origin of the internal carotid artery. [Reproduced from Walton (1982) *Essentials of Neurology*, 5th edn, by kind permission of the publisher.]

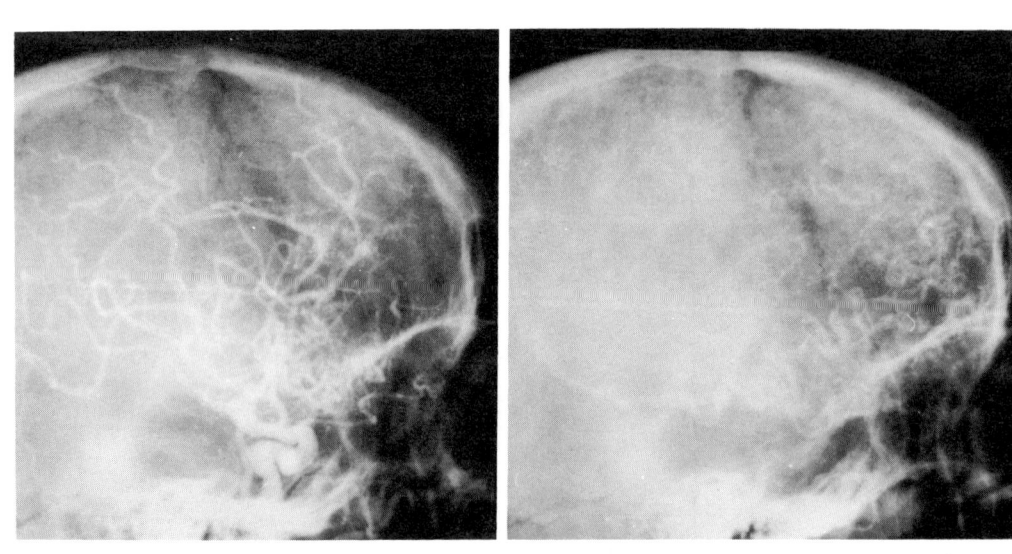

Figure 11.14 A pathological circulation in a large frontal lobe glioma. [Reproduced from Walton (1985) *Brain's Diseases of the Nervous System*, 9th edn, by kind permission of the publisher.]

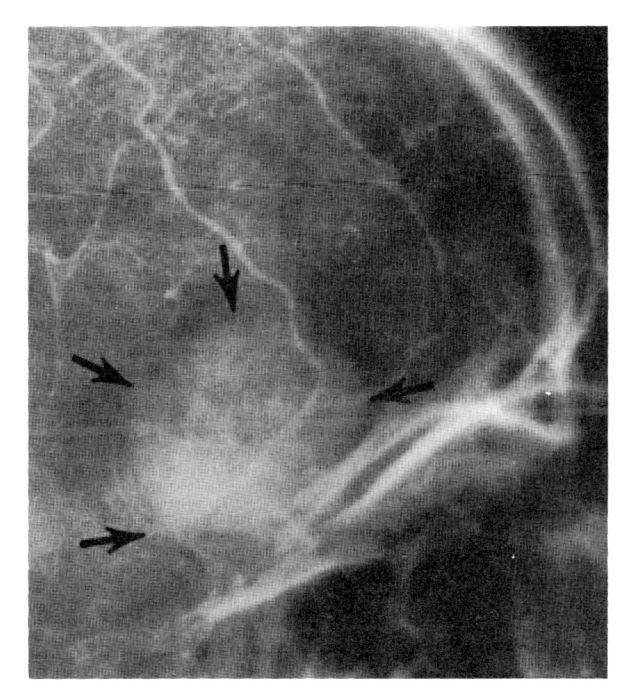

The cerebrospinal fluid, etc.—some pathophysiological principles 269

Figure 11.15 A subfrontal meningioma showing a typical 'blush' (arrows) in the late arterial phase. [Reproduced from Walton (1985) *Brain's Diseases of the Nervous System*, 9th edn, by kind permission of the publisher.]

Myelography

Myelography is an invaluable method of localizing lesions which are compressing the spinal cord. It is usual to inject 5–6 ml of appropriate contrast medium into the lumbar subarachnoid space and then to observe under the screen (fluoroscope) the flow of medium up and down the spinal canal on tilting the patient. Anteroposterior and lateral radiographs are also taken at intervals. It is necessary only to inject the medium cisternally when there is a block beyond which that injected in the lumbar region will not pass and information is required concerning the upper limit of the lesion, or when there is some other contra-indication to lumbar injection such as the probability of a space-occupying lesion in the lower lumbar canal. The investigation has few complications, though some pain and paraesthesiae in the lower back and legs, along with mild fever, may persist for a few days afterwards. Very rarely a transient 'cauda equina syndrome' occurs, or else lumbar or sacral root pain, presumably due to irritation or mild arachnoiditis, persists for some weeks or months. In Great Britain no attempt was made to remove oily media, when used, after the examination, but this was generally done in the United States and in some other countries, largely for medicolegal reasons. The

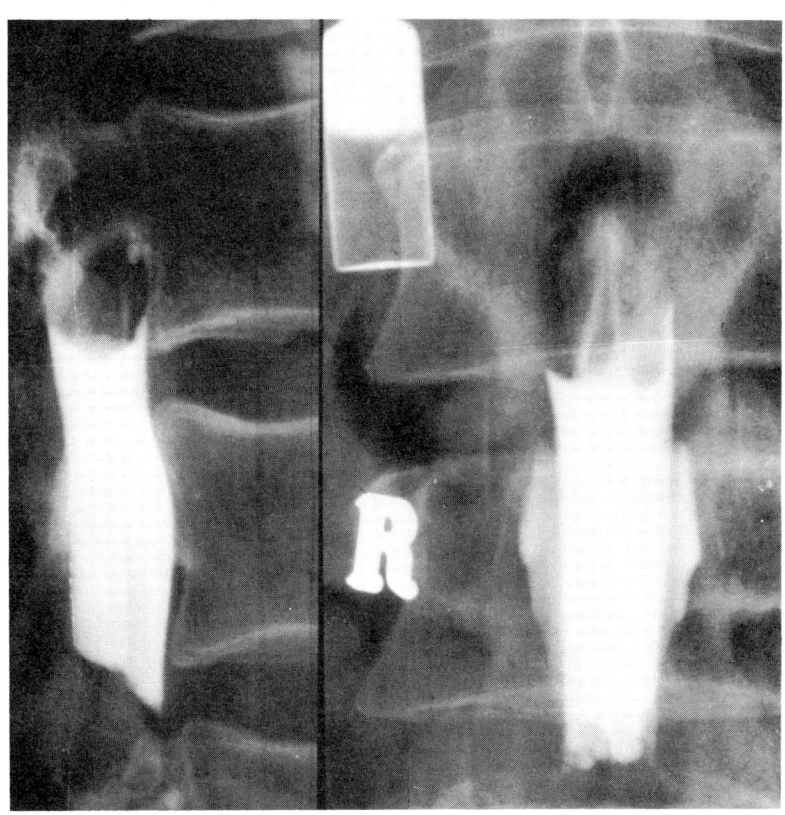

Figure 11.16 Lateral and anteroposterior views of a myelogram demonstrating a rounded filling defect due to a neurofibroma of the cauda equina. [Reproduced from Walton (1985) *Brain's Diseases of the Nervous System*, 9th edn, by kind permission of the publisher.]

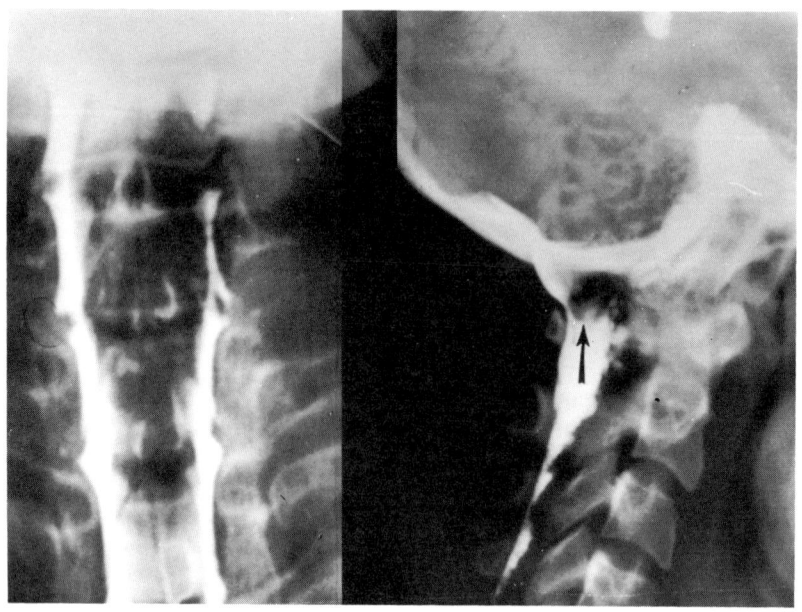

Figure 11.17 The myelographic appearances of communicating syringomyelia in association with a Chiari type I anomaly. The anteroposterior view (on the left) shows marked widening of the upper cervical cord, while the lateral supine view demonstrates the ectopic cerebellar tonsils (arrow). [Reproduced from Walton (1985) *Brain's Diseases of the Nervous System*, 9th edn, by kind permission of the publisher.]

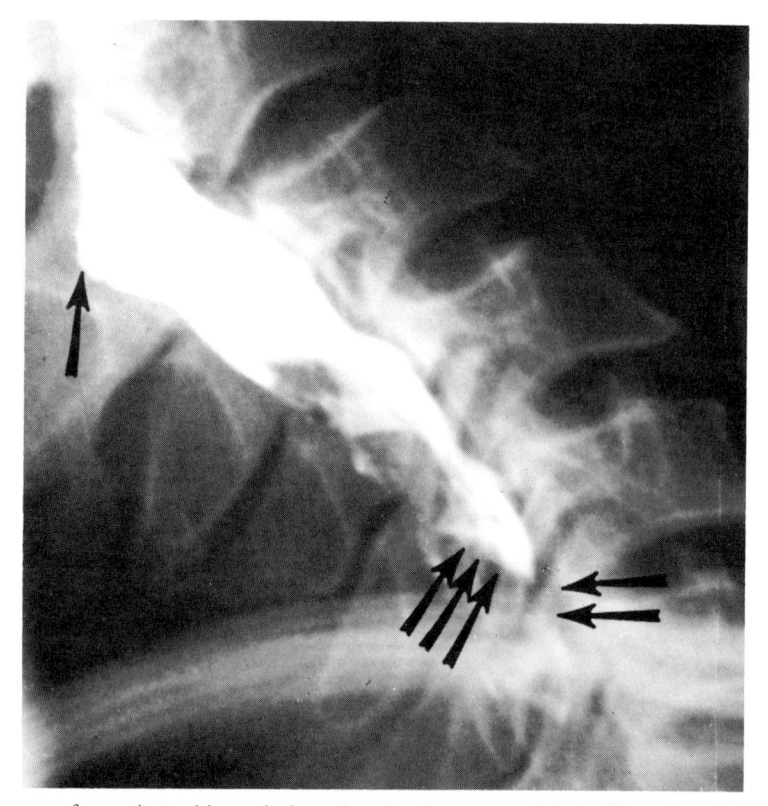

Figure 11.18 A myelogram of a patient with cervical myelopathy due to spondylosis. There is a fluid level (the single arrow demonstrates hold-up due to a narrow canal), posterior osteophytes with a disc protrusion (double arrows), and corrugation of the ligamentum subflavum (triple arrows). [Reproduced from Walton (1985) *Brain's Diseases of the Nervous System*, 9th edn, by kind permission of the publisher.]

increasing use of water-soluble media such as metrizamide has greatly reduced complications, although when this substance reaches the cranial cavity, it occasionally precipitates attacks of epilepsy.

An extramedullary neoplasm will almost always be localized accurately on myelography, either by the presence of a block or by a characteristic filling defect in the column of contrast medium (Fig. 11.16). Expansion of the spinal cord, indicative of an intramedullary neoplasm or syringomyelia (Fig. 11.17) can also be demonstrated, while an outline of abnormal vessels in patients with spinal vascular malformation may also be seen. Prolapsed intervertebral discs and spondylotic changes are demonstrated best in lateral views, when indentations in the column of contrast medium are seen opposite the disc space or spaces concerned (Fig. 11.18). Lateral protrusions may result in failure of certain root sleeves to fill with contrast medium, seen best in the anteroposterior view. Myelography is an essential preliminary (when the results of CT or NMR scanning of the spinal canal are equivocal or inconclusive) to any operation performed for the relief of spinal cord compression, as clinical signs in themselves are never sufficiently accurate for exact localization of the lesion.

Other methods
Spinal cord angiography, involving the injection of contrast medium by catheter into the aorta so as to visualize the spinal cord circulation, is of particular value in demonstrating vascular malformations. Extradural venography and lumbar discography (a technique involving the direct injection of contrast medium into the intervertebral disc itself) may also be used to demonstrate herniated intervertebral discs. Myeloscintigraphy, using radioactive isotopes, is on the whole less useful than gamma-encephalography but whole body CT and NMR scanners are being used increasingly in order to demonstrate spinal lesions.

References

Bannister, R. (1985) *Brain's Clinical Neurology*, 6th edn. Oxford: Oxford University Press.
Barnett, H. J. M., Foster, J. B. and Hudgson, P. (1973) *Syringomyelia* (Major Problems in Neurology Series, ed. J. N. Walton. Philadelphia: W. B. Saunders Company.
Cartlidge, N. E. F. and Shaw, D. A. (1981) *Head Injury*. Philadelphia: W. B. Saunders Company.
Coakham, H. B., Brownell, B., Harper, E. I. et al (1984) Use of monoclonal antibody panel to identify malignant cells in cerebrospinal fluid. *Lancet* i:1095.
Critchley, M., O'Leary, J. L. and Jennett, B. (eds) (1972) *Scientific Foundations of Neurology*. London: Heinemann.
di Chiro, G., Doppman, J. and Ommaya, A. K. (1967) Selective arteriography of arteriovenous aneurysms of spinal cord. *Radiology* 88:1065.
du Boulay, G. (1975) Myelography. In Vinken, P. J. and Bruyn, G. W. (eds) *Handbook of Clinical Neurology*, vol. 19, p. 179. Amsterdam, North-Holland.
Fishman, R. A. (1980) *Cerebrospinal Fluid in Diseases of the Nervous System*. Philadelphia: W. B. Saunders Company.
Gilland, O. (ed.) (1965) *Technical Progress in Neurological Diagnostics*. Amsterdam: Elsevier Publishing Company.
Graham, D. I. and Adams, J. H. (1971) Ischaemic brain damage in fatal head injuries. *Lancet* i:265.
Gurdjian, E. S., Lissner, H. R., Hogdson, V. R. and Patrick, L. M. (1966) Mechanism of head injury. In *Clinical Neurosurgery*, p. 112. Baltimore: Williams & Wilkins.
Guthkelch, A. N. (1972) High pressure hydrocephalus. In Critchley, M., O'Leary, J. L. and Jennett, B. (eds) *Scientific Foundations of Neurology*, p. 296. London: Heinemann.
Hopkins, A. and Rudge, P. (1973) Hyperpathia in the central cervical cord syndrome. *J. Neurol. Neurosurg. Psychiat.* 36:637.
Jennett, B. and Bond, M. (1975) Assessment of outcome after severe brain damage: a practical scale. *Lancet* i:480.
Jennett, W. B. and Plum, F. (1972) Persistent vegetative state after brain damage: a syndrome in search of a name. *Lancet* i:734.
Jennett, B. and Teasdale, G. (1977) Aspects of coma after severe head injury. *Lancet* i:878.
Kiloh, L. G., McComas, A. J. and Osselton, J. W. (1975) *Clinical Electroencephalography*, 3rd edn. London: Butterworth.
Krayenbuhl, H. A. and Yasargil, M. G. (1972) *Cerebral Angiography*, 3rd edn. London: Butterworth.
Mayo Clinic (1982) *Clinical Examinations in Neurology*, 5th edn. Philadelphia: W. B. Saunders Company.
Miller, D. and Adams, H. (1972) Physiopathology and management of increased intracranial pressure. In Critchley, M., O'Leary, J. L. and Jennett, B. (eds) *Scientific Foundations of Neurology*, p. 308 London: Heinemann.
Miller, H. (1961) Accident neurosis. *Br. Med. J.* 1:919, 992.
Miller, H. and Cartlidge, N. (1972) Simulation and malingering after injuries to the brain and spinal cord. *Lancet* i:580.
Newton, T. H. and Potts, D. G. (1974) *Radiology of the Skull and Brain*. St Louis: C. V. Mosby Company.
Ojemann, R. G. (1972) Normal pressure hydrocephalus. In Critchley, M., O'Leary, J. L. and Jennett, B. (eds) *Scientific Foundations of Neurology*, p. 302. London: Heinemann.
Ommaya, A. K. and Gennarelli, T. A. (1974) Cerebral concussion and traumatic unconsciousness. *Brain* 97:633.
Penning, L., Front, D., Bechar, M., Go, K. G. and Rodermond, J. M. (1973) Factors governing the uptake of pertechnetate by human brain tumours—a scintigraphic study. *Brain* 96:225.
Popp, J. A., Bourke, R. S., Nelson, L. R. and Kimelberg, H. K. (eds) (1979) *Neural Trauma* (Seminars in Neurological Surgery). New York: Raven Press.
Ramsey, R. G. (1977) *Computed Tomography of the Brain* (Advanced Exercises in Diagnostic Radiology, vol. 9). Philadelphia: W. B. Saunders Company.
Robertson, E. G. (1967) *Pneumoencephalography*, 2nd edn. Springfield, Ill.: Charles C. Thomas.
Rosenberg, R. N., Grossman, R. G., Schochet, S. S., Heinz, E. R. and Willis, W. D. (1984) *Neuroradiology* (The Clinical Neurosciences, vol. 4) Edinburgh: Churchill Livingstone.
Schäfer, E. R. (1975) The spinal compression syndrome. In Vinken, P. J. and Bruyn, G. W. (eds) *Handbook of Clinical Neurology*, vol. 19, p. 347. Amsterdam, North-Holland.
Shapiro, R. (1975) *Myelography*, 3rd edn. Chicago: Year Book Medical Publishers.
Stern, W. E. (1972) The cerebral edemas. In Critchley, M., O'Leary, J. L. and Jennett, B. (eds) *Scientific Foundations of Neurology*, p. 289. London: Heinemann.
Strich, S. J. (1956) Diffuse degeneration of the cerebral white matter in severe dementia following head injury. *J. Neurol. Psychiat.* 19:163.

Sweet, W. H. (1957) Formation, absorption and flow of cerebrospinal fluid. In Williams, D. (ed.) *Modern Trends in Neurology*, 2nd series. London: Butterworth.

Taylor, A. R. and Byrnes, D. P. (1974) Foramen magnum and high cervical cord compression. *Brain* **97**:473.

Thompson, R. A. and Green, J. R. (eds) (1980) *Critical Care of Neurologic and Neurosurgical Emergencies*. New York: Raven Press.

Tomlinson, B. E. (1964) Pathology. In Rowbotham. G. F. (ed.) *Acute Injuries of the Head*, 4th edn. Edinburgh: Churchill Livingstone.

Toole, J. F. (ed.) (1969) *Special Techniques for Neurologic Diagnosis*. Contemporary Neurology series, vol. 3. Philadelphia: F. A. Davis Company.

Walton, J. N. (1982) *Essentials of Neurology*, 5th edn., London: Pitman Medical.

Walton, J. N. (1985) *Brain's Diseases of the Nervous System*, 9th edn. Oxford: Oxford University Press.

INDEX

A fibres, 49
Abdominal reflexes, 70, 180
Abducens nerve (cranial nerve VI), 125
  nuclei, 138, 139
  palsy, 141, 246
Abetalipoproteinaemia, 221, 222, 232
Acalculia, 75
'Accident' neurosis, 251
Acetylcholine, 11, 13, 15
  drugs affecting action, 13–14, 15, 166–7
  epileptic seizures induced by, 91
  neuromuscular transmission, 164–6
  synthesis and breakdown, 15, 16
  see also Cholinergic neurons
Acetylcholine receptors, 12, 113–14, 166
  muscarinic, 12, 15, 114
  in myasthenia gravis, 167, 185
  nicotinic, 12, 15, 114
Acetylcholinesterase, 15
Achondroplasia, shape of skull in, 20
Acoustic neuroma, 151, 153, 258
Acrodynia (pink disease), 236
Action potentials
  compound nerve, 49–50
  motor unit, 186, 187
  muscle fibre, 166
  single nerve fibre, 8, 9, 10, 11
Adaptation
  of nervous tissue to lesions, 55
  of sensory receptors, 12
Addison–Schilder disease, 218, 221, 222
Addison's disease, coma in, 89, 226
Adenosine, 11, 18
Adenosine triphosphate (ATP), 8, 166
ADH, see Antidiuretic hormone
Adie's (Holmes–Adie) syndrome, 121, 137
Adiposogenital dystrophy, idiopathic, 123
Adrenaline, 13, 113
  behaviour and, 100
  drugs influencing activity, 13–14, 16–17, 114
  synthesis and breakdown, 15–16, 17
Adrenergic neurons, autonomic, 112, 113
Adrenergic receptors, 16, 114
Adrenocortical failure, 226
Adrenoleucodystrophy (Addison–Schilder disease), 218, 221, 222
Affective disorders, 107
Affective responses to sensory input, 196, 199–200
  see also Emotions
After-potential, 9, 10
Ageing of nervous tissue, 37, 55
Ageusia, 126–7, 252
Aggressive behaviour, 108
Agnosia, 63, 64–5, 79
  auditory, 79
  developmental, 80
  tactile (asterognosis), 79, 203
  topographical, 79
  visual, 79
Agraphia, 74, 75
Akinesia, 162
Akinetic mutism, 77, 86
Akinetic seizures, 94
Alanine, 11
Alar lamina, 23–4, 25
Albumin–globulin ratio in cerebrospinal fluid, 242–3

Alcohol
  acute intoxication, 89, 233
  amblyopia associated with, 134, 230
  interactions with hypnotics and sedatives, 234
  withdrawal symptoms, 233
Alcoholic myopathy, 233
Alcoholic polyneuropathy, 233
Alcoholism, 232–3
  delirium tremens, 90–1, 183, 233
  Korsakov syndrome in, 108, 229, 233
  vitamin B$_1$ (thiamine) deficiency in, 229
  Wernicke's encephalopathy in, 229, 233
Alexander's disease, 221
Alexia, 75
Algodystrophy, 123
Alpha-adrenergic receptors, 16, 114
Alpha motor neurons, 49, 50, 160, 163, 164, 172
  balance with gamma motor neuron activity, 163, 168–9, 175, 177
  type I and II, 166
Aluminium
  accumulation in dialysed patients, 225
  neurofibrillary tangles and, 217
Alzheimer type 2 astrocytes, 224
Alzheimer's disease (presenile dementia), 55, 217, 260
Amacrine cells, 128, 129, 132
Amaurotic idiocy, infantile and juvenile types, 220
Amaurosis fugax, 136
Amblyopia
  nutritional, 230
  tobacco, 134
  tobacco–alcohol, 134, 230
Amines, biogenic, 15–17
  in cerebrospinal fluid, 243
  see also Adrenaline; Dopamine; 5-Hydroxytryptamine; Noradrenaline
Amino acids
  brain metabolism, 217
  neurotransmitters, 11, 17–18, 217
Amino acidurias, 218, 219, 220
Amitriptyline, 13, 17, 105–6
Ammonia, blood levels in hepatic encephalopathy, 224
Amnesia, 106, 107–8
  hysterical, 108
  post-traumatic, 250, 251
  retrograde, 250
  transient global, 103, 107
'Amnestic syndrome', see Korsakov syndrome
Amphetamines, 13, 17
  intoxication, 234
  withdrawal states, 91, 234
Amputation of limbs, phantom sensations after, 203, 211
Amusia, 64, 74, 75
Amygdala, functions of, 101, 114
Amyotrophic lateral sclerosis, 184
Anaemia
  megaloblastic, 232
  pernicious, 231, 232
Anaemic anoxia, 227
Anaesthesia, 203
  hysterical, 205
Anal reflex, superficial, 70, 180
Anal sphincter reflex, 70
Analgesia, 203
Anarthria, 63, 65, 76
Anencephaly, 23, 254

Aneurysms, intracranial
  headache in, 209
  imaging techniques, 264, 266, 267
Angiography, 31, 261, 264
  cerebral, 266
  spinal cord, 271
Angiomas
  arteriovenous
    diagnostic investigations, 258, 267
    headache in, 209
  calcification of, 258, 259
  retinal, 136
Angiomatosis, diffuse cortical, in Sturge–Weber syndrome, 258
Anhidrosis (loss of sweating), 120, 121, 137
Ankle clonus, 180
Ankle jerk reflex, 70, 179
Anomia, 75
Anorexia, hypothalamic lesions causing, 123
Anosmia, 126, 252
  hysterical or factitious, 66, 126
Anosognosia, 79
Anoxia, 89, 227
  see also Cerebral anoxia
Anoxic anoxia, 227
Antenatal diagnosis, 61, 254
Anterior horn of spinal cord, 47, 49
Anticholinergic drugs, intoxication with, 236
Anticholinesterases, 14, 167, 185
Anticonvulsant drugs, overdose with, 89, 236
Antidepressant drugs, 16–17, 105–6
Antidiuretic hormone (ADH, arginine vasopressin), 84, 101, 114
  inappropriate secretion of, coma in, 89, 226
Antihistamines, 14, 236
Anton's syndrome, 79
Anxiety, 54, 106, 109
Aortic arch angiography, 261, 264, 267
Apathy, 108–9
Aphakia, 131
Aphasia, 63, 73–6
  auditory (word deafness), 74
  classification, 74
  conduction, 75
  developmental receptive, 78
  global, 74–5
  jargon, 74
  motor, expressive or Broca's, 65, 74
  nominal or amnestic, 75
  posterior or association, 75
  scheme of investigation, 75–6
  sensory, receptive or Wernicke's, 64, 65, 74
  visual, 75
Aphonia, 63, 65, 77
Apneustic breathing, 88, 246
Apnoea
  primary obstructive, 86
  sleep, 85–6
Apomorphine, 14
Appetite, excessive, 123
Apraxia, 63, 64, 78–9, 158
  constructional, 79
  developmental, 80, 107
  dressing, 79
  of gait, 79
  oculomotor, 79, 143
Arachnoid, 22
Arachnoiditis, 135
Archicerebellum, 163

Arcuate (U) fibres, 37
Arecoline, 15
Arginine vasopressin, see Antidiuretic hormone
Argininosuccinic aciduria, 219, 220
Argyll Robertson pupil, 137
Arousal, 82
Arsenic poisoning, 235
Arteries,
  cerebral, 26–31
  extracranial, 31
  headaches caused by disorders of, 208
  spinal cord, 32, 33
Arteriovenous angiomas, see Angiomas, arteriovenous
Arteritides, 58–9
  blindness in, 136
  headache of, 208
Aspartic acid, 11, 17
Association fibres, 37, 38
  verbal communication and, 73
Astereognosis, 79, 203
Asterixis, 89, 183, 224
Astigmatism, 128
Astrocytes, 5, 6, 7
  Alzheimer type 2, 224
Astrocytomas, investigation of, 263, 268
Ataxia, 63, 69, 158, 178–9
  Freidreich's, 61
  sensory, 68, 178, 203
  truncal or central, 163, 178
  see also Cerebellar ataxia
Ataxic breathing, 88, 246
Ataxic neuropathy, tropical, 230
'Ataxic nystagmus', 143
Atenolol, 14
Atherosclerosis
  cerebral, cerebral blood flow (CBF) in, 29
  of internal auditory artery, 151, 156
  ischaemia of inner ear, 152
  retinal arterial changes in, 136
Athetosis, 183, 184
Atriopeptin, 19
Atropine, 14, 15, 114, 137, 236
Audiometry, 151
Auditory agnosia, 79
Auditory (acoustic) cortex, 35, 150
Auditory evoked potentials, 151
Auditory nerve (cranial nerve VIII), 125, 148–9, 152
  assessment of function, 67, 150–1
  lesions (nerve deafness), 150, 151
  tinnitus and, 151–2
  see also Vestibular nerve
Autoimmune diseases, systemic, 58–9
Autonomic failure, progressive (idiopathic orthostatic hypotension), 97, 122
Autonomic nervous system, 47, 112–24
  anatomy, 115, 116–19
  bladder and bowel innervation, 119
  cerebral control, 114
  chemical transmission, 113–14
  disorders of, 121–3
  functions, 112–13, 118
  hypothalamic control, 100, 114–16
  reflexes, 120–1
  sexual activity controlled by, 119–20
  see also Parasympathetic nervous system; Sympathetic nervous system
Autonomic neuropathy, acute, 122

273

Index

Autonomous respiration, 88
Autoregulation of cerebral blood flow, 29
Autotopagnosia, 79
Axillary nerve, 173, 176
Axolemma, 3
Axon, 1, 3
  hillock, 3, 8–9
  regeneration, 57
Axonal degeneration, 55–7, 184
  in metabolic neuropathies, 214
  nerve conduction velocity in, 189
Axoplasm, 3
Axoplasmic flow, 3, 217

B fibres, 49, 50
Babinski response, 70, 177, 180
Baclofen, 14
Bacteria in cerebrospinal fluid, 243
Bacterial toxins, 236
Baillarger, lines of, 37
Barbiturates, 14
  electroencephalographic (EEG) changes, 83
  intoxication, 89, 234
  withdrawal states, 91, 234
Basal ganglia, 158, 162–3
  function, 100, 162–3, 177
  lesions in head injured patients, 250
  structure, 162
Basal lamina, 4
  of spinal cord, 23, 24, 25
Basilar artery, 26
Basilar artery migraine, 209
Basket cells, cerebellar, 40
Bassen–Kornzweig disease, 221, 222, 232
Behaviour, control of, 99–101
Bell's palsy, 145, 170
Benzodiazepines, 14, 16, 18, 234
Beri-beri, 229–30
Beta-adrenergic receptors, 16, 114
Betz cells, 37, 159, 161
Biceps jerk reflex, 69, 179
Bicuculline, 14, 17–18
Biopsy techniques, 253–4
Bipolar cells, retinal, 128, 129, 132
Bipolar neurons, 2, 3
'Blackouts', 91
Bladder
  control of micturition, 114, 119
  function in spinal cord and cauda equina lesions, 121–2, 252, 253
Blepharospasm–oromandibular dystonia, 184
Blindness
  causes of, 134, 135, 136
  denial of, 79
  methyl alcohol ingestion and, 233
  see also Amblyopia; Colour blindness; Vision; Visual acuity, Word blindness
Blood–brain barrier, 31, 238
Blood–nerve barrier, 50
Blood pressure, reflex responses of, 120–1
Body image, awareness of, 65, 79–80
Botulinum toxin, 13, 167, 236
Bowels
  control of evacuation, 114, 119
  function in spinal cord and cauda equina lesions, 121–2, 252, 253
Boxers, chronic traumatic encephalopathy in ('punch-drunkenness'), 251
Brachial plexus, 164, 172, 173
  lesions, 204
  muscles innervated by, 176
Bradykinesia, 162
Bradykinin, 195
Brain
  amino acid and protein metabolism, 217–18
  biopsy, 254
  blood supply, 26–32
    collateral channels, 26–7
  carbohydrate metabolism, 215
  development and growth, 22, 24–5, 26
  external appearance, 27
  lipid metabolism, 218, 222
  metabolic disorders, see Metabolic disorders
  metabolism, 213–14
  nucleic acid metabolism, 215
  space-occupying lesions, see Intracranial space-occupying lesions
  swelling, see Cerebral oedema
  ventricular system, 25–6, 28
  see also Cerebral abscess; Cerebral atrophy; Cerebral haemorrhages; Cerebral tumours etc.
Brain death, diagnosis of, 89–90
Brain stem
  anatomy and functions, 41–6
  auditory evoked potentials (BAEP), 151
Brain stem lesions, 87, 137, 151
  in head injury, 249
  localization in comatose patients, 88
  nystagmus in, 144, 153, 155
  ocular movement defects in, 88, 143
  sensory impairment in, 205
  vertigo in, 155
Breathing, see Respiration
Bretylium, 13
Broca's area, 73, 74, 75
Bromide in cerebrospinal fluid (CSF), 239–40
Bromism, 236
Bromocriptine, 14
Bronchitis, chronic, hypercapnia in, 227
Brown–Séquard syndrome, 204, 253
Brudzinski's sign, 65
Brueghel's syndrome, 184
Bulbar palsy, progressive, 172, 184
Bulbocavernosus reflex, 70
α-Bungarotoxin, 12
Burdach, nucleus of (cuneate nucleus), 41, 197, 198
Buspirone, 14
Butyrophenones, 14, 16

C fibres, 49, 50
Caisson disease, 228, 252
Calcification, intracranial, 257–8
Calcium, (Ca^{2+})
  abnormalities of blood levels, 226–7
  role in cell activation, 10, 15, 16
  role in photoreception, 131
Caloric tests of vestibular function, 144, 153, 154
Calvarium, 20
Canavan–van Bogaert–Bertrand disease, 221
Cannabis, 234
Carbachol, 13
Carbohydrate metabolism, 215
Carbohydrate metabolism, disorders of, 215, 216
Carbon dioxide (CO_2)
  intoxication, 227
  tension, cerebral blood flow (CBF) and, 29
  see also Hypercapnia; Hypocapnia
Carbon monoxide poisoning, 89, 227
Cardiac arrest, anoxic brain damage in, 227
Cardiac centre, 41
Cardiac muscle, nervous control of, 5

Carnitine synthesis, disorder of, 222
Carotid arteries, internal, 26–7
  occlusion or stenosis, 267, 268
Carotid arteriography, 261, 264, 266, 267, 268
Carotid sinus, pressure applied to, 121
Carotid sinus syncope, 97
Cataplexy, 85
Catatonic stupor, 89
Catechol-O-methyltransferase (COMT), 16
Catecholamines, see Adrenaline; Dopamine; and Noradrenalin
Cattell test, 107
Cauda equina
  intermittent claudication, 261
  lesions, 120, 121, 180, 253
Caudate nucleus, 35, 36, 162, 183
Causalgia, 123, 211
Cavernous sinus
  aneurysm in, 141
  thrombosis, 32
Central nervous system (CNS), morphology and organization, 19–49
Cerebellar ataxia, 178–9
  after heat stroke, 228
  alcoholic, 233
  gait in, 68, 178
Cerebellar dysfunction
  dysarthria in, 76–7
  hypotonia in, 178
  nystagmus in, 144, 178
  ocular movements in, 142
  testing for, 69, 178–9
  tremor in, 183
  vertigo in, 155
Cerebellar tonsillar herniation (cerebellar pressure cone), 87, 244, 246, 247
Cerebellum
  cellular structure and organization, 39–41
  development and growth, 25, 26
  general morphology, 38–9
  motor functions, 158, 161, 162, 163–4
  vestibular input to, 152–3, 163
Cerebral abscess, 89, 260
  cerebrospinal fluid (CSF) in, 242
  electroencephalography in, 254–5
Cerebral anoxia, 227
  coma in, 89, 213, 227
  pathological effects, 61, 214
  postanoxic encephalopathy, 227
Cerebral atrophy, diagnostic investigations in, 266, 268
Cerebral blood flow (CBF), 27–31, 213
  autoregulation, 29
  measurement, 29
  raised intracranial pressure and, 244–5
Cerebral compression, acute traumatic, 251
Cerebral contusion, 249, 250, 251
Cerebral cortex, 99
  autonomic activity controlled by, 114
  'bladder centres', 122
  electrical activity, 37
  functions, 34–6
  ocular movement control, 142
  pain perception and localization by, 206
  plasticity of function, 55
  structure, 36–7
  see also Auditory cortex; Motor cortex; Sensory cortex; Striate cortex
Cerebral haemorrhage
  coma in, 88
  diagnostic investigations, 255, 264

traumatic, 249, 250
Cerebral hemispheres
  disconnection syndromes, 73, 80
  dominance of, 36
Cerebral infarction, 29, 60–1, 155, 227, 242
'Cerebral irritation', 250
Cerebral ischaemia, 227
  cerebral blood flow (CBF) in, 29
  pathological changes, 61, 214
Cerebral oedema, 87, 214, 248, 249
Cerebral palsy, 174
Cerebral tumours, 59–60
  cerebrospinal fluid (CSF) in, 242
  coma in, 89
  electroencephalography in, 255
  imaging techniques, 257–8, 266–7
  see also Gliomas; Intracranial space-occupying lesions; Meningiomas; Pituitary tumours
Cerebrosides, 218
Cerebrospinal fluid (CSF), 25–6, 238–43, 247
  albumin–globulin content, 242–3
  amine in, 243
  circulation, 28, 238
  cisternal puncture, 240–1
  composition, 239–40
  cytology, 241–2
  formation and absorption, 238
  function, 238–9
  glucose in, 239, 243
  hydrogen ion concentration, 243
  lumbar puncture, 240
  microbiological examination, 243
  naked eye appearance, 241
  pressure, 240, 241
  protein content, 239, 242
  ventricular puncture, 241
  see also Hydrocephalus; Intracranial pressure
Cerebrovascular disease, 26, 58
  diagnosis, 263
  see also Cerebral infarction; Vascular lesions
Cerebrovascular resistance, 29, 243
Cerebrum, 33–7
  development and growth, 24–5, 26
  general morphology, 33–6
Cervical cord syndrome, central, 252, 253
Cervical spine, radiography of, 264
Cervical spondylosis, 261
Cervical sympathetic ganglia, 116, 118, 121
Charcot–Marie–Tooth disease, 137
Charcot's arthropathy, 123
Chemicals causing polyneuropathy, 236
Chemoreceptors, 12
Chiari malformation, 144
Children
  'clumsy', 80
  deafness in, 77, 151
  electroencephalography in, 254
  speech disorders, 77–8
Chloral hydrate, 236
Chloride ions, membrane permeability to, 8
p-Chlorophenylalanine, 84, 106
Chloroquine, long-term administration of, 192
Chlorpromazine, 14
Cholinergic neurons, 15, 164–6
  autonomic, 112, 113
  in striatum, 163
Cholinergic paralysis, 15
Cholinergic receptors, see Acetylcholine receptors
Chorda tympani, 42, 125, 126, 170
Chorea, 183
Choreoathetosis, 183

Index

Choroid plexuses, 238
  papilloma of, 247
Ciliary ganglion, 117, 118, 121
Ciliary nerves, 117, 136
Ciliospinal reflex, 137
Cimetidine, 14
Cingulate gyrus, 36
  functions of, 101–2, 114
  subfalcial herniation, 87, 244, 245, 246
Cisternal injection for myelography, 269
Cisternal puncture, 240–1
Cisterns, subarachnoid, 22
Citrullinaemia, 219, 220
Climbing fibres, 40–1
Clonidine, 14
Clonus, 69, 177, 179–80
Cocaine, 13, 137
  addiction, 235
Cochlea
  function of, 148
  structure of, 145, 146, 147
Cochlear nerve, 148–9
Cochlear nuclei, 149–50
Coeliac plexus, 116
Colchicine, 217
Collateral channels, 26–7
Colliculus
  inferior, 41, 150
  superior, 41, 142
Colour blindness, 61, 66, 133
Colour vision, 66, 132–3
Coma, 86–90
  in cerebral anoxia, 89, 213, 227
  common causes, 87
  diagnosis, 88–9
  diagnosis of brain death, 89–90
  in head injury, 88, 249, 250, 251
  mechanisms of, 86–7
  psychogenic, 89
Coma vigil, see Akinetic mutism
Combined system disease, see Subacute combined degeneration of the cord.
Commissural fibres, 36, 37, 39
Commissurotomy
  memory defects after, 103
  speech and, 73, 80
Compression myelitis, 253
Computerized tomography (CT scans), 263, 264, 268, 271
Concussion, 249, 250
  post-concussional syndrome, 250, 251
Cones, retinal, 128, 129, 130
Confabulations, 108, 251
Confusion, 91
  post-traumatic, 251
  postepileptic, 95
Consciousness, 82
  clouding of, 90
  disorders of, 82, 86–91, 213
  pathophysiology of, 82–3
  transient disorders of, 91–8
  see also Coma; Confusion; Stupor, Delirium, Sleep
Contractures, 68, 185–6
Contre-coup injury, 249
Conus medullaris, 46
Convulsions
  in alcoholism, 233
  epileptic, 92–5, 182
  see also Epilepsy
  hysterical, 97–8
  tonic, 94
'Convulsive threshold', 92
Coordination, testing, 69
Copper metabolism, disorders of, 223
Corneal reflexes, 70, 179
Corpus callosum, 24, 35, 36
  degeneration of (Marchiafava–Bignami disease), 233
  division of, 73, 80, 103
Corpus striatum, 36, 162, 163
  lesions, 183–4
Corti, organ of, 144–8

degeneration of, 152
Corticobulbar motor system, 158–61
Corticofugal fibres, 37
Corticospinal tract (pyramidal tract), 37, 158–61, 162
  function, 160–1
  lesions
    bladder control in, 122
    clinical features in, 170, 177, 179, 180, 181
    dysarthria in, 76, 172
    slow spinal cord compression and, 253
  structure, 159–60
Corticothalamic tract, 199
Cough headache, benign, 208
Cough syncope, 97
Cranial bruits, 65
Cranial nerves, 41–2
  autonomic effects of lesions, 121
  motor, 68, 169–72
  motor nuclei, 42, 160, 169
  raised intracranial pressure affecting, 246
  sensory nuclei, 42
  traumatic lesions, 251, 252
  see also Specific nerves
Craniocerebral trauma, see Head injury
Craniopharyngioma, 257, 258
Craniosacral outflow, see Parasympathetic nervous system
Craniostenosis, 20, 246
Creatine kinase, 191
Cremasteric reflex, 70, 180
Creutzfeldt–Jakob disease, electroencephalography in, 255
Crocodile tears, syndrome of, 121
CT scanning (computerized tomography), 263, 264, 268, 271
Cuneate nucleus (nucleus of Burdach), 41, 198, 199
Cuneocerebellar tracts, 163
Curare, 167, 191
Cushing's disease, 226
Cutaneous reflexes, 70, 120, 180
Cyanide, excessive ingestion of, 230, 236
Cyclic 3'5'-adenosine monophosphate (cAMP), 10, 18
Cyclic 3'5'-guanosine monophosphate (cGMP), 10, 131
Cyclothymic individuals, 107, 109, 251
Cyproheptadine, 14
Cystathioninuria, 231
Cysticercosis, 258
Cytoarchitectonics, 37

Dark adaptation of eyes, 131, 132
Deafness
  assessment of, 67, 150–1
  in childhood, 77, 151
  conductive, 150, 151
  lesions causing, 151–2, 156
  nerve, 150, 151
  sensorineural, 150, 151
  see also Hearing
Decamethonium, 167, 191
Decerebrate state, 249
  reflexes in, 69, 180
  rigidity, 177
Decompression sickness, 228, 252
Degenerative disorders, 61
Dehydration, headache of, 208
Deiters' (phalangeal) cells, 145
Deiters' nucleus, 161
Déjà vu, 105
Delirium, 86, 90–1
  in cerebral anoxia, 213
  traumatic, 250
Delirium tremens, 90–1, 183, 233

Delta sleep-inducing peptide (DSIP), 84
Delusions, 90, 105, 110
Dementia, 106, 110, 213
  presenile (Alzheimer's disease), 55, 217, 260
  senile, 55
  subacute progressive, in alcoholics, 233
  traumatic, 251
Demyelinating disorders, 57, 58, 184
  metabolic, 214, 222
  nerve conduction velocity in, 57, 189
Dendrites, 1, 3, 4
Dendritic spines, 3, 4
Denervation
  electromyography, 186, 188
  hypersensitivity to acetylcholine, 166
  investigations, 191, 192
Dental facial pain, 209
Dentate nuclei, 38, 39
Depersonalization, feelings of, 105
Depression, 106, 109
Dermatomes, 47, 201, 204
Desipramine, 13, 17
Developmental disorders, 58
Diabetes insipidus, 123
Diabetes mellitus, 215
  neuropathy, 214
  ophthalmoplegia in, 141
  pseudotabes, 137
  retinopathy, 136
Diabetic coma, 89, 225
Dialysis dysequilibrium syndrome, 225
Diaphragmatic pain, referral of, 207
Diencephalon, 24, 25
  function of, 99–101
Dihydromorphine, 234
Diisopropylphosphofluoridate, 15
Diphtheria exotoxin, 236
Diplegia, 63, 174
Diplopia, 67, 140–1
Disconnection syndromes, 73, 80
Disorientation
  post-traumatic, 251
  right–left, 65
  in time and space, 90
Dissolution, Hughlings Jackson law of, 55
Doll's head manoeuvre, see Oculocephalic reflexes
Dopamine, 11, 13, 217
  behaviour and, 100, 106
  -containing neurons, 16
  drugs influencing activity, 13–14, 16–17
  in parkinsonism, 163
  synthesis, 15–16, 17
Doppler ultrasonography, 31, 256
Down's syndrome, 110
Drop attacks, 97
Drugs
  acting on neuromuscular junction, 166–7
  addition, 234–5
  in cerebrospinal fluid (CSF), 239–40
  influencing activity of neurotransmitters, 13–14, 15–18, 166–7
  intoxication, 89, 183, 234–5, 236
  nystagmus caused by, 144
  porphyria and, 223
  producing unconsciousness, 82
  pupillary effects, 137
  vertigo caused by, 155
  withdrawal states, 83, 91, 234, 235
  see also Specific agents
Duane's syndrome, 141
Dura mater, 21, 22
Dynorphin, 19

Dysaesthesiae, 202
Dysarthria, 63, 65, 76–7, 173
  developmental, 77–8
Dysautonomia, familial (Riley–Day syndrome), 122
Dysdiadochokinesis, 179
Dyskinesias, drug-induced, 184, 236
Dyslalia, 78
Dyslexia, developmental, 78, 107
Dysmetria, 178
Dysmyelination, 222
Dysphasia, 63, 73–4
Dysphonia, 171
Dyspraxia, 63
Dystonia, 177
Dystonia musculorum deformans, 183–4
Dystrophia myotonica, 62, 185

Ear
  function, 148–50
  structure, 145–8
  see also Hearing; Vestibular system
Eaton–Lambert syndrome (myasthenic–myopathic syndrome), 185, 191
Echo-encephalography, 256
Echolalia, 77
Echotomography, 256
Edinger–Westphal nucleus, 117, 118, 138, 139
Edrophonium hydrochloride, 191
Eighth nerve, see Auditory nerve; Vestibular nerve
Ejaculation, premature, 120
Electrical injuries, 227–8
Electrocardiographic (ECG) changes in raised intracranial pressure, 245
Electrocorticogram (ECoG), 37
Electroencephalogram (EEG), 37, 254–5
  in epilepsy, 94, 95, 96, 97, 254, 255
  in hepatic encephalopathy, 224, 255
  in sleep, 83, 84
Electromyography (EMG), 186–9
  single fibre, 189, 191
Electronystagmography, 153
Electroretinogram (ERG), 131
Eleventh cranial nerve, see Spinal accessory nerve
Embolism, cerebral, 88
Embryonic development of nervous system, 22–6
Emotions
  control of, 100, 101–2
  instability or lability of, 108
Emphysema, carbon dioxide retention in, 227
Encephalins, 19, 101, 206–7
Encephalitis, 58, 88–9, 91
  cerebrospinal fluid (CSF) in, 241, 242
  herpes simplex, 58, 89, 103, 255
  lethargica, 86
Encephalitogenic factor (EF), 217–18
Encephaloceles, 20
Encephalomyelitis, 58
End-plate potential, 166
Endocrine diseases
  myopathies, 191, 192, 226, 227
  neurological manifestations, 226–7
Endocrine system, hypothalamic control of, 114
Endoneurium, 4
β-Endorphin, 84, 206
Endorphins, 101, 106
Enophthalmos, 67, 121, 137
Ependymal cells, 6
Ependymomas in fourth ventricle, 155
Ephedrine, 13, 14, 114

Index

Epidural space, 22
Epilepsy, 91–5
  aetiology of attacks, 92–3
  aggressive behaviour in, 108
  akinetic attacks, 94
  causes, 93, 98, 227, 271
  clinical classification of seizures, 93, 94
  coma after, 89
  complex partial, see Temporal lobe epilepsy
  constitutional influences, 62, 93
  electroencephalography in, 94, 95, 96, 97, 254, 255
  focal, 94, 96
  grand mal (major), 93–4, 95, 255
  idiopathic, 92
  jacksonian attacks, 94, 205
  myoclonic, 94–5, 97
  ocular movements in, 143
  pathophysiology, 91–2
  petit mal 'absence', 93, 95, 254, 255
  postepileptic paralysis, 95
  postepileptic stupor or confusion, 87, 95
  progressive myoclonic (Lafora body disease), 215
  symptomatic, 92
  temporal lobe, see Temporal lobe epilepsy
Equilibrium potential, 8
Eserine, 137
Euphoria, 109
Eustachian tube, 145, 146
Evoked potentials
  auditory, 151
  motor action, 189–91
  sensory, 37, 189
Excitatory postsynaptic potentials (EPSP), 10–11, 37
Excitement, 109
Exophthalmos, 67, 138
Exteroceptors, 5, 194
Extradural haematoma/haemorrhage, traumatic, 250, 251
Extrapyramidal disorders, 77, 177, 183
Extrapyramidal system, 160, 161, 162
Eye strain headaches, 207
Eyeballs, pressure applied to, 121
Eyelids, 137–8
  drooping, see Ptosis
  lagging/retraction of, 67, 138
Eyes, 126, 127
  abnormal position of globe, 67, 138
  dark and light adaptation, 131
  see also Ocular movements; Optic nerve; Retina; Vision

F reflex, 189
Fabry's disease, 218, 221
Facial nerve (cranial nerve VII), 42, 169–70
  parasympathetic outflow, 117, 118, 119
  sensory function, 125, 126, 198
  testing motor function, 68
Facial neuralgia, atypical, 210
Facial pain, 209–10, 246
Facial paralysis/palsy, 170, 252
  aberrant reinnervation after, 121, 170
  idiopathic (Bell's palsy), 145, 170
Facial spasm, clonic, 170, 182
Facial weakness, 170, 181
Facilitation, 11
Fainting, see Syncope
Falx cerebelli, 21
Falx cerebri, 21, 34
Farber's disease, 218, 221
Fascicles, nerve fibre, 50, 51
Fasciculation, 182
  potentials, 186, 188
Fastigial nucleus, 38, 163

Fatty acid metabolism, disorders of, 222
Femoral nerve, 175, 176
Fibrillation of muscle fibres, 182, 186, 188
Fifth cranial nerve, see Trigeminal nerve
Finger jerk reflex, 69, 179
Flaccidity, see Hypotonia
'Flare' reaction, 120
Fluorosis, spinal cord compression in, 236
Fluoxetine, 13
Flupenthixol, 14
Folate deficiency, 232
Fontanelles, 20
Foot-drop, 68
Foramen magnum, 20
Forebrain, development and growth, 24–5, 26, 28
Fourth cranial nerve, see Trochlear nerve
Freidreich's ataxia, 61
Fröhlich's syndrome, 123
Frontal gyrus, control of ocular movements, 142
Frontal lobes, 34, 104
'Frontal lobe syndrome', 104
Frostbite, 228
Fructose intolerance (fructosuria), 216, 220
Fucosidosis, 216
Functional disorders, 54
Fusiform cells, 37
Fusimotor system, 167–9

GABA, see Gamma-aminobutyric acid
Gait
  abnormalities of, 67–8, 178, 179
  apraxia of, 79
  steppage, 203
Galactosaemia, 216, 220
Gallamine, 167
Gamma-aminobutyric acid (GABA), 11, 13, 17–18, 217
  anticonvulsant activity, 91–2
  pyridoxine deficiency and, 230
Gamma-encephalography, 256
Gamma motor neurons, 49, 50, 160, 164, 168, 169, 172
  balance with activity of alpha motor neurons, 163, 168–9, 175, 177
Ganglion cells, retinal, 128–9, 132
Gangliosides, 218, 222
Gangliosidoses, 218, 220
Gap junctions, 5
Gasserian ganglion
  compression of, 246
  herpes zoster of, 209
Gate theory of pain, 206
Gating currents, 9
Gaucher's disease, 220
Gene-specific markers of disease, 61–2
General paresis, 58, 137, 242
Generator potential, 12
Geniculate bodies
  lateral, 133, 199
  medial, 150, 199
Geniculate ganglion, 170
  herpes zoster of (Ramsay Hunt syndrome), 170
  lesions, 126
Gennari, line of, 37
Gerstmann's syndrome, 79
Gilles de la Tourette's syndrome, 77, 184
Gitter cells (compound granular corpuscles), 7, 61
Glabellar tap sign, 69
Glasgow coma scale, 250
Glasgow outcome scale, 250
Glaucoma, 135
Glioblastomas, 268
Gliomas, 59–60, 123, 242, 259
Gliosis, 6, 57

Globoid-cell leucodystrophy (Krabbe's disease), 218, 221, 222
Globus pallidus (pallidum), 35, 36, 162, 163
Glossopharyngeal nerve (cranial nerve IX), 42, 121
  motor function, 170
  parasympathetic outflow, 117, 118, 119
  sensory function, 125, 126, 127
Glossopharyngeal neuralgia, 210
Glucose
  in cerebrospinal fluid (CSF), 239, 243
  metabolism, 213–14, 215
Glutamic acid, 11, 13, 17
Gluteal nerve
  inferior, 175, 176
  superior, 175, 176
Glycine, 11, 13, 17–18
Glycogen, cerebral, 215
Glycogen storage diseases, 191, 192, 215, 216
Gnosis, 36, 64–5, 72
Golgi cells, cerebellar, 40
Golgi neurons
  type I, 3, 4
  type II, 3, 4
Golgi tendon organs, 167–9, 195
Gracile nucleus, (nucleus of Goll), 41, 197, 198
Gradenigo's syndrome, 141
Granular corpuscles compound (gitter cells), 7, 61
Granule cells, 2
  cerebellar, 39–40, 41
Graphaesthesia, 197
Grasp reflex, 69, 180
Graves' disease, see Thyrotoxicosis
Guanethidine, 13, 114
Guanidine hydrochloride, 167, 185, 191
Guillain–Barré syndrome, 141, 204, 242
Gyri, 34

H reflex, 189
Habit spasm, 182
Haematomyelia, 252, 253
Haemorrhage
  in head injury, 249, 250
  intraventricular, 260
  in nervous parenchyma, 60
  subhyaloid, 136
  see also Cerebral haemorrhage; Extradural haemorrhage; Subarachnoid haemorrhage; Subdural haemorrhage
Hair cells
  auditory, 145–8, 149
  vestibular, 152
Hair follicle receptors, 195
Hallucinations, 90, 105
  in alcoholics, 233
  auditory, 105
  hypnagogic, 85
  olfactory, 126
  of taste, 127
  visual, 105, 123
Hallucinogenic drugs, 17, 105, 234
Haloperidol, 14
Hand–Schüller–Christian disease, 221
Harris's sign, 143
Head injury, 88, 248–52
  cerebral contusion, 249, 250
  clinical features, 250–2
  concussion, 249, 250
  hydrocephalus in, 249
  intracranial haemorrhage, 250
  loss of taste sensation in, 127, 252
  vertigo after, 156, 251
Headache, 207–9
  benign cough, 208
  eye strain, 207
  post-lumbar puncture, 208, 240

post-traumatic, 250, 251
psychogenic, 207–8
in raised intracranial pressure, 208, 246, 248
tension, 207
'vascular', 208, 209
Hearing, 125, 144–52
  assessment tests, 67, 150–1
  central auditory pathways, 149–50
  see also Auditory nerve; Deafness; Ear
Heart rate
  in raised intracranial pressure, 246
  reflex responses, 121
Heat stroke, 89, 228
Heavy metal poisoning, 232, 235–6
Hemiballismus, 184
Hemicholinium, 13
Hemifacial spasm, 170, 182
Hemiplegia, 63, 68, 174, 180–1
Hemiplegic migraine, 209
Hepatic disease
  chronic, 183, 224
  pathological changes in, 61, 214, 224
Hepatic encephalopathy, 89, 224
  electroencephalography in, 224, 255
Hepatolenticular degeneration (Wilson's disease), 61, 183, 223
Hereditary disorders, 61–2
Heredopathia atactica polyneuritiformis (Refsum's disease), 221, 222
Heroin, 234
Herpes simplex encephalitis, 58, 89, 103, 255
Herpes zoster, 58
  of gasserian ganglion, 209
  of geniculate ganglion (Ramsay Hunt syndrome), 170
  postherpetic pain, 211
Heterophoria, 139–40
Hindbrain, development and growth, 24–5, 26
Hippocampus, functions of, 101, 103, 114
Hippus, 137
Histamine, 11, 13, 18
Histocompatibility antigens (HLA), 62, 85
Hodgkin cycle, 11–12
Hoffmann's sign, 69
Holmes–Adie (Adie) syndrome, 121, 137
Homatropine, 137
Homovanillic acid (HVA), 243
Horizontal cells, retinal, 128, 129
Horner's syndrome, 121, 137
Hughlings Jackson, law of dissolution, 55
Hunter's disease, 215, 216
Huntington's chorea, 61–2, 183
Hurler's syndrome, 216
Hydralazine, polyneuropathy due to, 230
Hydrocephalus, 238, 247–8
  communicating, 247, 249
  diagnostic investigations, 256, 266, 268
  low- or normal-pressure, 247
  mass lesions causing, 244, 247
  obstructive, 247
  otitic, 247
  skull changes in, 20, 257
  toxic, 248
Hydrogen ion concentration in cerebrospinal fluid, 243
Hydromyelia, 26
5-Hydroxyindoleacetic acid (5-HIAA), 243
5-Hydroxytryptamine (serotonin), 11, 13, 217, 243,
  behaviour and, 100, 105–6

Index

drugs influencing activity, 13–14, 16–17, 105–6
migraine and, 209
nociception and, 195
sleep and, 84
synthesis, 15, 16
Hypaesthesia, 70, 203
Hypalgesia, 70, 203
Hyperacusis, 145
Hyperaesthesia, 203
Hyperalgesia, 203, 206
Hyperammonaemia, types I and II, 219, 220
Hypercalcaemia, 226–7
Hypercapnia, 227
chronic, 227, 243
intracranial pressure and, 245
Hyperglycaemia, 215, 225
in brain disease, 123
Hyperglycinaemia
ketotic, 220
non-ketotic, 219, 220
Hyperhidrosis (excessive sweating), 122, 123
Hypermetropia, 127–8
Hypernatraemia, 89, 226
Hyperopia, 127–8
Hyperornithinaemia, type II, 220
Hyperparathyroidism, 227
Hyperpathia, 63, 70, 203, 206
Hyperpolarization, 11
Hypersomnia, 85, 123
Hypersomnolence, idiopathic, 85
Hypertension, arterial
cerebral blood flow (CBF) and, 29, 244–5
headaches of, 208
retinal changes in, 135, 136
Hypertensive encephalopathy, 89, 225
Hyperthyroidism, see Thyrotoxicosis
Hypertonia, 69, 176
extrapyramidal, 177
see also Rigidity; Spasticity
Hyperventilation
in brain stem lesions, 88
cerebral blood flow (CBF) and, 29
hysterical, 98
intracranial pressure and, 245
Hypnagogic hallucinations, 85
Hypnotic drugs, 234
Hypo-α-lipoproteinaemia (Tangier disease), 221, 222
Hypoaesthesia, 63
Hypocalcaemia, 226
Hypocapnia, 29, 245
Hypochondriasis, 107
Hypogastric plexus, 116
Hypoglossal nerve (cranial nerve XII), 42, 68, 171–2
Hypoglossal nucleus, 171
Hypoglycaemia, 98, 215, 225–6
cerebral pathological changes, 61, 214
coma, 89, 213, 225
idiopathic leucine-induced, 216
Hyponatraemia, 89, 226
Hypoparathyroidism, 98, 226–7, 258
Hypophysis, see Pituitary gland
Hypopituitarism, 89, 226, 246
Hypotension
idiopathic orthostatic (Shy–Drager syndrome), 97, 122
postural, 97, 120
Hypothalamus, 35, 36
disease or dysfunction, 123, 124
functions of, 100–1, 114–16
Hypothermia, 226, 228, 245
Hypothyroidism (myxoedema), 89, 226
Hypotonia, 69, 176, 178
in lower motor neuron lesions, 181–2
in upper motor neuron lesions, 180–1

Hypoxia, 227, 245
Hypsarrhythmia in infantile spasms, 255
Hysterical symptoms, 107, 158
amnesia, 108
convulsions, 97–8
hyperventilation, 98
ocular convergence movements, 143
post-traumatic, 251
sensory, 205
trance, 89

Idazoxin, 14
Illusions, 105
Imipramine, 13, 17, 105–6
Immersion foot, 228
Impotence, 120
Impulsive disorders of conduct, 108
Incontinence, 121–2
Incoordination, 178–9
see also Ataxia
Indian spastic paraplegia, South, 230
Indoramin, 14
Infantile spasms, hypsarrhythmia in, 255
Infarction, anoxia caused by, 227
see also Cerebral infarction
Infections, neurological complications of, 236
Inflammation, pain in, 207
Inflammatory neurological disorders, 58
Infratentorial lesions, 247
Inherited neurological disorders, 61–2
Inhibitory postsynaptic potentials (IPSP), 10, 11, 37
Insomnia, 83, 85, 123
drug-induced, 84
Instinctive behaviour, control of, 100
Insulin, hypoglycaemia caused by excessive, 98, 215, 225–6
Intellect, 104–5
assessment of, 64, 107
defects of, 109–10, 227, 251
see also Dementia
Internal capsule, 35, 36, 159
Interneurons, 3
retinal, 128, 129
spinal (internuncial neurons), 49, 160–1, 164, 179, 194
Internuncial neurons, see Interneurons, spinal
Interoceptors, 5, 194
Interosseus nerve
anterior, 174, 176
posterior, 173, 176
Intervertebral discs, 21
prolapsed, 21, 242, 252, 261, 271
'Intracerebral steal syndrome', 29
Intracranial hypertension, benign, 248
Intracranial pressure (ICP)
effects of space-occupying lesions on, 244–7
raised, 241, 243–8
cerebral oedema and, 248, 249
lumbar puncture and, 240
papilloedema in, 135, 246
pneumoencephalography in, 247, 266
reduced, 208, 240, 241
Intracranial space-occupying lesions
diagnostic investigations, 256, 264, 266, 267
effects on intracranial pressure, 244–7
lumbar puncture and, 240
see also Cerebral tumours; Subarachnoid haemorrhage
Intrafusal muscle fibres, 167–9
Intraventricular haemorrhage, 260
Ionic membrane channels, 8, 11

drugs affecting, 12–15
techniques for investigating, 9–10
Iproniazid, 106
Iridocyclitis, 137
Ischaemic anoxia, 227
see also Cerebral ischaemia
Isoniazid, polyneuropathy due to, 230
Isoprenaline, 14
Isotope encephalography, 247, 256
Isotope ventriculography, 256
Isovaleric acidaemia, 219, 220

Jaeger's reading card, 66
Jaw jerk reflex, 69, 179
Jendrässik's manoeuvre, 70, 175–6
Joint receptors, 195, 199
Joint sense, impairment of, 197, 203

Kernicterus, 224
Kernig's sign, 65
Kernohan's sign, 246
Ketanserin, 14
3-Ketoacid CoA-transferase deficiency, 219
Klippel–Feil syndrome, 20
Knee jerk reflex, 69–70, 179
Korsakov (Wernicke–Korsakov) syndrome, 103, 107–8, 123, 229, 233
Krabbe's disease (globoid-cell leucodystrophy), 218, 221, 222
Krause end-bulbs, 195
Kufs' disease (late onset lipidosis), 220
Kyphosis, 21

Labyrinth, 152
assessment of function, 67, 153–5
structure of, 145, 146
see also Vestibular system
Labyrinthine disorders
ataxia in, 178
nystagmus, 144, 153
vertigo in, 155–6
Labyrinthitis, acute, 151, 155–6
Lactic acidaemia, 219, 220
Lactic acidosis, 225
Lafora body disease, 215
Language, disorders of, 75
Larynx, paralysis of, 171, 172
Lathyrism, 230
Lead poisoning, 235–6
Learning, 104
Leg, limitation in raising, 65
Leigh's disease, 215
Lemniscus (medial fillet), 46, 150, 198
Lenticular nucleus, 36, 183
Lentiform nucleus, 162
Leptomeninges, 22
Lesch–Nyhan syndrome, 217
Leucine-induced hypoglycaemia, idiopathic, 216
Leucodystrophies, 222
Levodopa, 163, 184
Lhermitte's sign, 202
Ligamenta denticulata, 22
Light
reflex of pupils, 136, 137
sensitivity of eyes to, 131, 132
Limbic system, 100
anatomy of, 102
functions of, 101–2, 103
Limbs
cutaneous areas of sensation, 201, 202
innervation of muscles, 172, 173–5, 176
pain in, 210–11
'phantom' sensations after amputation, 203, 211
weakness and paralysis of, 63, 174, 180–2
Lingual nerve, 126

Lipid metabolism, disorders of, 218–22, 223
Lipid storage diseases, 191, 192, 218, 220–1
Lipidosis, late onset (Kufs' disease), 220
Lipids, 222
Lipoproteins, disorders of, 221, 222
Locked-in syndrome, 86
Locus coeruleus, sleep and, 84
Longitudinal fasciculus, medial, 47, 142, 143, 152, 153
Lordosis, 21
Lower motor neurons, see Motor neurons, lower
LSD, see Lysergic acid diethylamide
Lumbar canal stenosis, 261
Lumbar discography 271
Lumbar puncture, 208, 240
Lumbosacral plexus, 164, 172
'Luxury perfusion syndrome', 29
Lysergic acid diethylamide (LSD), 14, 17, 105, 106, 234

McArdle's disease (muscle phosphorylase deficiency), 186, 216
Macroglia, 5
Magnesium ions, 15
Malabsorption, 232
Malingering, 251
Malnutrition, protein–calorie, 217, 229
Mamillary bodies (corpora mamillaria), 115, 123
Manganese poisoning, 236
Mania, 109
Mannosidosis, 216
Maple syrup urine disease, 219, 220
Marchiafava–Bignami disease, 233
Marijuana, 234
Masticatory muscles, 68, 169
Mechanoreceptors, 195
Medial longitudinal fasciculus, 47, 142, 143, 152, 153
Medial nucleus, 38
Median nerve, 174, 176
conduction velocity in, 189, 190
lesions, sensory loss in, 204
Median raphe, 105–6, 247
Medulla oblongata, 39, 41
development, 25
lesions, respiration in, 88
motor pathways, 159–60
sensory pathways, 197–8, 205
Medulloblastomas, 242
Megaloblastic anaemia, 232
Meige's syndrome, 184
Meissner's corpuscles, 195, 199
Melatonin, 16
Membranes
neuronal, 8, 223
postsynaptic, 5, 10, 12
see also Ionic membrane channels
Memory, 101, 102–3, 104
assessment of, 64, 107
disturbances of, 91, 107–8, 110, 123
short-term and long-term, 102–3
see also Amnesia
Ménière's disease, 151, 153, 154, 156
Meninges, 21–2
carcinomatosis of, 243
Meningiomas, 59
imaging techniques, 258, 259, 261, 268, 269
sphenoidal ridge, 141
Meningitis, 58
cerebrospinal fluid in, 240, 241–2, 243
clinical features, 88–9, 91, 208
deafness caused by, 151
pathological changes, 58, 59
signs of, 65
tuberculous, 59, 242, 243

278 Index

Meningoceles, 20
Menkes' kinky hair disease, 223
Mental disorders, 53, 64, 106–10
   in hepatic disease, 224
   post-traumatic, 251
   in Wernicke's encephalopathy, 229
Mental retardation (handicap), 106, 109–10
   in metabolic disorders, 215, 216, 220, 221
Mental state
   assessment, 64, 107
   influences on physical diseases, 53–4
Mepyramine, 14
Mercury poisoning, 183, 236
Merkel cells, 195
Mescaline, 234
Mesencephalon (midbrain vesicle), 24, 25, 26, 28
Mesenteric plexus, 116
Metabolic disorders
   inborn errors of metabolism, 110, 214, 215–24
   myopathies, 191
   pathological changes, 61, 214
   primary or endogenous encephalopathies, 213, 214–24
   secondary or exogenous encephalopathies, 213, 224–36
   see also Specific diseases
Metachromatic leucodystrophy, 218, 221, 222
Metal poisoning, 232, 235–6
Metastatic malignant tumours, 60, 155
Metergoline, 14
Methacholine, 14, 114
Methadone, 234
Methaemalbumin in cerebrospinal fluid, 241
Methoxamine, 114
Methyl alcohol poisoning, 134, 233
γ-Methyl-*p*-tyrosine, 13
Methyldopa, 14
Methylmalonic aciduria, 219
Methylphenidate, 17
Methysergide, 14
Microglia, 5, 6, 7, 57
Microphonics, cochlear, 148
Micturition syncope, 97
Midbrain, 41
   development and growth, 24–5, 26, 28
   lesions, 177, 205, 250–1
Migraine, 208–9
Migrainous neuralgia, periodic, 209
Mimetic paralysis, 170
Minamata disease, 236
Minnesota Personality Inventory (MPI), 107
Miosis, 121, 137
Mitochondrial myopathies, 191
Mongolism (Down's syndrome), 110
Monoamine oxidase (MAO), 16, 106
Monoamine oxidase (MAO) inhibitors, 14, 16–17, 105–6
Monoparesis, 63, 174
Monoplegia, 63, 174
Mood, disorders of, 107, 108–9
Moro reflex, 24
Morphine, 137, 206, 234
Morquio's disease, 216
Morvan's syndrome, 204
Mossy fibres, 39–40, 41
Motion sickness, 156
Motor cortex, 35, 159, 160, 161, 162, 164
Motor end-plate, *see* Neuromuscular junction
Motor nerve conduction velocity, 189, 190

Motor neuron disease (motor system disease), 58, 61, 172, 182, 184, 188
Motor neurons, 3
   development and growth, 24
   lower, 160
     lesions of, 77, 122–3, 181–2, 184
     see also Alpha motor neurons; Gamma motor neurons
   upper, 159
     lesions of, 180–1
Motor neuropathy, 184
Motor system, 158–92
   assessment of function, 67–70
   components of, 158–72
   disorders, 172–9, 180–92
   reflexes, 69–70, 179–80
   see also Movements; Muscles; Neuromuscular system; Paralysis; Weakness
Motor system disease, *see* Motor neuron disease
Motor units, 49, 164
   action potentials, 186, 187
Movements
   in delirium, 90
   incoordinated, *see* Ataxia
   involuntary, 68, 158, 163, 182–4
   see also Motor system; Muscles; Paralysis; Weakness
Mucolipidoses (sialidoses, types 1 and 2); 218, 221
Muller's muscle, 137
Multiple sclerosis
   cerebral imaging in, 263, 264
   cerebrospinal fluid (CSF) in, 242
   constitutional influences, 62
   euphoria in, 109
   nystagmus and vertigo in, 143, 144, 155, 156
   optic neuritis in, 135, 136
   pathological changes in, 58, 60
Multisystem degeneration, progressive, 122
Muscarinic receptors, 12, 15, 114
Muscimol, 14
Muscle fibres
   denervation hypersensitivity, 166
   fibrillation, 182, 186, 188
   intrafusal, 167–9
   types, 166
Muscle phosphorylase deficiency (McArdle's disease), 186, 216
Muscle spindles, 167–9, 195
Muscle tone, 174–8, 186
   abnormalities of, 158, 176–8
   see also Hypertonia; Hypotonia; Rigidity; Spasticity
   assessment of, 69, 175–6, 178
   postural, 175
Muscles
   assessment of function, 68–9
   atrophy, 63, 181, 182, 192
   biopsy, 191–2, 254
   contraction, 164–6
   contractures, 68, 185–6
   cramps, 185
   denervation of, *see* Denervation
   fasciculation, 182
   fatiguability, 68–9, 185
   hypertrophy, 63
   hypotrophy, 63
   influences on neuronal development and growth, 24
   pain, 185, 207
   power of individual, 68, 186
   sensory receptors, 161, 167–9, 195
   structure, 164, 165
   ultrastructure, 166, 167
   see also Motor system; Movements; Neuromuscular junction; Paralysis; Weakness

Muscular atrophy, progressive, 184
Muscular dystrophy
   Duchenne type, 61, 191, 192
   electromyogram (EMG) in, 186–7
   facioscapulohumeral, 61, 77
   limb-girdle, 61
   tendon reflexes, 186
Musculocutaneous nerve, 173, 176
Mutism, 77
   akinetic, 77, 86
Myasthenia gravis, 15, 167, 182, 185
   diagnostic tests, 191, 192
   muscular fatiguability, 68–9, 77
   ocular symptoms, 138, 141
   tendon reflexes, 186
Myasthenic–myopathic (Eaton–Lambert) syndrome, 185, 191
Myelin, 3, 217–18, 222
   disorders affecting, 222
   regeneration, 57
   sheath, lamination of, 6, 49, 50
   see also Demyelinating disorders
Myelinated neurons, 3, 4, 6, 49, 50
Myelography, 263, 269–71
Myelomatosis, 257
Myeloscintigraphy, 271
Myocardial pain, referral of, 207
Myoclonic epilepsy, 94–5, 97
Myoclonic jerks, 85, 95, 182
Myoclonus, 94–5, 182
   nocturnal, 85, 95
   palatal, 171, 184
Myoglobinuria, 191
Myoidema, 69
Myoneural junction, *see* Neuromuscular junction
Myopathy, 182, 184, 185
   alcoholic, 233
   clinical features, 182, 185
   diagnostic tests, 191–2
   electromyography (EMG) in, 186–7
Myopia, 127
Myotomes, 47
Myotonia, 69, 77, 185, 187
   congenita, 185
Myotonic dystrophy (dystrophia myotonica), 62, 185
Myxoedema, 89, 226

Narcolepsy, 17, 85
Neck reflexes, tonic, 177, 180
Neck stiffness, 65, 88, 246
Neocerebellum, 163–4, 178
Neocortex, 36–7
Neostigmine, 114, 137, 167
Nerve cells, *see* Neurons
Nerve conduction, 6–12
   across synapses, 10–12
   drugs affecting, 12–15
   measurement of velocity, 189, 190
   mechanisms of, 6–9
   new experimental techniques, 9–10
Nerve fibres, *see* Axon
Nerve growth factor, 24
Nerve-root compression, 211
Nervi erigentes, 119
Nervous system
   blood supply, 26–33
   degeneration and regeneration in, 55–7
   development and growth, 22–6
   morphology and organization, 19–50
   pathological reactions in, 57–61
   segmentation, 46, 47, 169, 200–1, 202
   structural units and their function, 1–19
Neural crest, 23, 24
Neural tube, 22–3, 24
   malformations, 23, 254

Neuralgia
   atypical facial, 210
   glossopharyngeal, 210
   periodic migrainous, 209
   postherpetic, 211
   suborbital, 210
   trigeminal, 209–10
Neurilemma, 6
Neurilemmal cells (Schwann cells), 3, 50
Neurilemmoma, 59
Neuroblasts, 23
Neuroeffector junctions, 4–5
   drugs affecting transmission across, 13–14
Neurofibrillary tangles, 55, 56, 217
Neurofibromas, 59
   spinal, 210, 261, 269
Neurofibromatosis, 136
Neurofilaments, 3, 217
Neuroglia, 5–6
Neurological disorders
   categories, 57–8
   constitution and heredity and, 61–2
   diagnosis, 54–5, 62–71
     aim of, 62
     approach to, 62
     clinical examination, 64–71
     eliciting symptoms (history taking), 63–4
     terminology, 63
   influences of mental state on, 53–4
   investigations, 253–72
   positive and negative symptoms, 55
Neuromodulators, 18–19
Neuromuscular disease, 184–92
   diagnostic principles, 185–6
   methods of differential diagnosis, 186–92
Neuromuscular junction (motor end-plate, myoneural junction), 5, 185
   cholinergic receptors, 12
   drugs acting at, 15, 166–7
   dysfunction, diagnosis of, 189–191
   transmission at, 11, 164–5
Neuromuscular system, 164–9
Neuromyelitis optica, 134, 135
Neuronal ceroid-lipofuscinosis, 220
Neurons
   cortical, 37
   degeneration and regeneration, 55–7
   development and growth, 23, 24
   epileptic, 92
   function, 6–12
   membranes, 8, 223
   morphological types, 2, 3
   orthograde and retrograde transport, 3
   sensitivity to lack of oxygen or glucose, 214
   soma (cell body), 1–3
   structure, 1–5
   see also Axons; Motor neurons; Myelin; Neuromuscular junction; Sensory neurons; Synapses; specific types of neurons
Neuropathies, 184
Neuropeptides, 18–19
Neurosis, 106
Neurotic symptoms, post-traumatic, 251
Neurotoxins, 236–7
Neurotransmitters, 4–5, 10, 11, 13, 15–19, 217
   agonists and antagonists, 13–14
   in autonomic nervous system, 113–14
   mechanism of action. 9
   in the retina, 129
   transport in neurons, 3

Index

Neurotubulin (neurotubular protein), 217
Nicotine, 14, 15
Nicotinic acid, 229, 231
Nicotinic receptors, 12, 15, 114
Niemann–Pick disease, 218, 220
Night blindness, 131
Night terrors, 85
Ninth cranial nerve, see Glossopharyngeal nerve
Nissl substance, 1
Nociceptors, 195, 206
Nodes of Ranvier, 3–4, 50
Nomifensine, 13
Noradrenaline (norepinephrine), 11, 13, 106, 113
  -containing neurons, 16, 84, 112, 113
  drugs influencing activity, 13–14, 16–17
  synthesis and breakdown, 15–16, 17
Notochord, 23
Nuclear magnetic resonance (NMR) scanning, 261, 262, 263, 268, 271
Nucleic acid metabolism, disorders of, 215–17
Nucleus accumbens, function of, 100
Numbness, 201
Nutritional amblyopia, 230
Nutritional deficiencies, 228–32
Nystagmoid jerks, 67
Nystagmus, 67, 143–4
  'ataxic', 143
  benign paroxysmal positional, 155, 156
  caloric tests, 144, 153, 154
  in cerebellar lesions, 144, 178
  optokinetic, 67, 142
  phasic, 144
  positional, 144, 154, 155
  post-traumatic, 251

Obesity, 123
Obsessive–compulsive neurosis, 107
Obturator nerve, 175, 176
Occipital lobe, 34, 142
Ocular movements, 125, 138–44
  in comatose patients, 88
  defects of, 139–41, 143–4
  examination of, 67, 139
  paresis, traumatic, 252
  pathways controlling, 138, 139, 142
  reflex, 133, 142–3
  saccadic and smooth-pursuit, 141–2
  types of, 138, 141–2
  vergence, 142
Ocular muscles
  extrinsic, 138–9, 140
  nuclei of, 138
  paralysis of, 139–41
Ocular myopathy, 141
Oculocephalic reflexes, 67, 88, 143
Oculogyric crises of postencephalic parkinsonism, 143
Oculomotor apraxia, 79, 143
Oculomotor nerve (cranial nerve III), 46, 125, 138
  palsy/lesions, 141, 246
  ptosis in, 137–8
  pupillary changes in, 121, 137
  parasympathetic outflow, 117, 118, 119, 136
Oculomotor nucleus, 117, 138, 139
Odontoid process, 21, 257
Olfactory nerves, 20, 125
  palsy, 252
Olfactory tract, 41, 126
Oligodendrocytes, 4, 5–6, 7
Olivary nuclei
  inferior, 41
  superior, 149, 150

Olivopontocerebellar degeneration, 122
Ondine's curse, 86
Ophthalmopathy, thyroid, 138, 226
Ophthalmoplegia, 137, 138, 141, 226
  anterior internuclear, 143
  posterior internuclear, 143
Ophthalmoplegic migraine, 209
Opiate intoxication and addiction, 89, 234–5
Opiate receptors, 15, 206
Opisthotonos, 177
Optic atrophy, 66, 135, 136, 230
Optic chiasm, 133, 134
Optic disc, examination of, 66–7, 135
Optic fundus, 66–7, 135–6
Optic nerve (cranial nerve II), 41, 66–7, 125, 133
  lesions, 134, 136
  neuritis or neuropathy, 135
Optic radiation, 133, 134–5
Optic tract, 46, 133, 134
Orbital cortex, 34–6
Orbital muscles, 137–8
Orbitofrontal cortex, functions of, 101–2
Organ of Corti, see Corti, organ of
Orotic aciduria, hereditary, 215–17
Orthograde axoplasmic transport, 3
Oscillopsia, 144
Ossicles, auditory, 145, 146
Osteomalacia, 227, 229
Otic ganglion, 117, 118
Otitic hydrocephalus, 248
Otitis media, headaches of, 208
Otoliths, 152
  tests of function, 155
Otosclerosis, 151
Ouabain, 92
Overactivity, 109
Oxotremorine, 15
Oxprenolol, 14
Oxygen
  hyperbaric, intracranial pressure and, 245
  supply to brain, 213, 214
  tension, cerebral blood flow (CBF) and, 29
  see also Cerebral anoxia
Oxytocin, 114

Pachymeninx, 22
Pacinian corpuscles, 195, 199
Paget's disease, 20, 257
Pain, 201, 205–11
  ascending pathways, 197–8, 199
  autonomic pathways of, 122, 123
  gate theory of, 206
  impaired appreciation of, 203
  individual differences in appreciation, 205
  mechanism of, 206
  nerve-root, 211
  neuropharmacology of, 206–7
  projected, 211
  referred, 122, 201, 207, 211
  skin receptors, 195
  testing perception of, 70, 197
  types of, 207–11
Pain asymbolia, 79
Palate
  myoclonus, 171, 184
  paralysis of, 171
Paleocerebellum, 163, 178
Palilalia, 77
Pallidum, see Globus pallidus
Pallium, see Cerebral cortex
Palsy, 174
Pan-dysautonomia with recovery, pure, 122
Panencephalitis, subacute sclerosing, 242, 255
Papilloedema, 66, 135–6, 246
  lumbar puncture and, 240
  pneumoencephalography in, 266

Pappenheimer's factor 'S', 84
Paraesthesiae, 202–3
  ischaemic, 189
  in migraine, 209
  in sensory jacksonian epilepsy, 205
Parageusia, 127
Parallel fibres, cerebellar, 39–40, 41
Paralysis, 158, 172–4
  in electrical injuries, 228
  in lower motor neuron lesions, 181–2
  mimetic, 170
  of muscles supped by cranial nerves, see under Specific nerves
  periodic, see Periodic paralysis
  postepileptic (Todd's), 95
  sleep, 84–5
  in spinal cord lesions, 181, 252–3
  in upper motor neuron lesions, 180–1
Paranasal sinuses, 20
Paranasal sinusitis, 208, 209
Paraparesis, spastic, 68, 122, 232
Paraphasia, 74
Paraplegia, 63, 174
  spastic, 181, 230, 252
Parasomnia, 86
Parasympathetic nervous system, 112–13, 118
  anatomy, 115, 117–19
  bladder and bowel function and, 119
  ganglia, 47, 115–16
  pupillary constriction, 136, 137
  sexual activity and, 113, 119–20
Parasympathomimetic drugs, 114
Paresis (muscle weakness), 158, 172–4, 181, 185
Pargyline, 14
Parietal lobe, 34
Parinaud's syndrome, 143
Parkinsonism, 163
  cerebrospinal fluid in, 243
  drug-induced, 16, 163, 236
  encephalitis lethargica causing, 108
  gait in, 68
  glabellar tap sign, 69
  postencephalitic, ocular movements in, 143
  tremor of, 183
Parosmia, 126
Past-pointing, 178
Patch-clamp technique, 9
Patellar clonus, 180
Pelizaeus–Merzbacher disease, 218, 221, 222
Pellagra, 231
Pelvic girdle weakness, gait in, 68
Penicillamine, polyneuropathy due to, 230
Perception
  control of, 36
  disorders of, 105–6
Perikaryon, 1
Periodic paralysis, 185, 191, 192, 226
Peripheral nerves, 49–50
  compound nerve action potentials, 49–50
  compression of, 189, 211
  disorders affecting, 184
  innervation of muscles of trunk and limbs, 172, 173–5, 176
  lesions, 122–3, 204
  nerve conduction velocity, 189, 190
  regeneration, 55, 57
  sensory fibres, cutaneous areas of distribution, 197, 201, 202, 204
  see also Polyneuropathy; Individual nerves
Peripheral nervous system, 19, 49–50

Peripheral neuropathy, 184
  in beri-beri, 229–30
  differential effects on sensory neurons, 197
  in lead poisoning, 235–6
  nerve conduction velocity in, 189
Pernicious anaemia, 231, 232
Peroneal nerve
  common, 175, 176
  deep, 175
  superficial, 175
Personality
  disorders, 106–7
  role of frontal lobes in, 104
Pethidine, 234
Petrosal nerve
  greater superficial, 117
  lesser, 117
Petrous apicitis, 141
pH of cerebrospinal fluid (CSF), 243
Phakomas, retinal, 136
Phalangeal (Dieters') cells, 145
Phantom limb sensations, 203, 211
Pharyngeal muscles, paralysis of, 171
Phasic sensory receptors, 12, 196
Phenelzine, 14
Phenothiazines, 14, 16, 245
  side-effects of long-term use, 163, 184, 236
Phenoxybenzamine, 14, 114
Phentolamine, 14, 114
Phenylephrine, 14
Phenylketonuria, 110
Phosphoinositides, 222
Phospholipids, 218, 222
Phototopic luminosity curve, 131, 132
Physostigmine, 14, 15, 167
Pia mater, 21–2
Pickwickian syndrome, 85
Picrotoxin, 17–18
Pigments, retinal, 128, 131
Pilocarpine, 114, 137
Pilomotor activity, autonomic control of, 120
Pineal gland, calcification of, 257
Pink disease (acrodynia), 236
Pinocytosis by neurons, 3
Pins and needles, feelings of, 202
Pirenzepine, 14
Pituitary gland, 20
  hypothalamic control of, 114
  tumours, 134, 257, 266
Plantar nerve
  lateral, 175
  medial, 175
Plantar response, 70, 177, 180, 246
Platybasia, 20
Pneumoencephalography, 247, 256, 261, 268
Poliomyelitis, cerebrospinal fluid (CSF) in, 242
Polyarteritis nodosa, 58–9
Polycythaemia vera, 135
Polymyositis, 186, 191, 192
Polyneuropathy, 61, 184, 185
  alcoholic, 233
  chemicals and toxins causing, 236
  sensory impairment in, 182, 204
Pons, 39, 41
  development and growth, 25
  lesions, 143, 205
  motor pathways in, 159, 161, 163
  see also Brain stem lesions
Pontine exotropia, paralytic, 143
Pontine myelinolysis, central, in alcoholics, 233
Popliteal nerve, lateral, conduction velocity in, 189
Porphyria, 223–4
Portosystemic encephalopathy, 224
Position sense
  ascending pathways, 197–8, 199
  impairment of, 203
  testing, 197

Index

Postanoxic encephalopathy, 227
Postcentral gyrus, sensory functions of, 200, 201, 205
Post-concussional (post-traumatic) syndrome, 250, 251
Posterior horn of spinal cord, 47, 49
Postsynaptic membranes, 5, 10, 12
Postural hypotension, 97, 120
Posture, abnormalities of, 68
Potassium (K^+)
 membrane channels, 8, 12–15
 serum levels, 92
Practolol, 14
Praxis, 36, 64, 72
Prazosin, 14
Precentral gyrus, 159
Prefrontal cortex, 34, 114
Prefrontal leucotomy/lobotomy, 104
Presbyacusis, 151
Presbyopia, 128
Presenile dementia (Alzheimer's disease), 55, 217, 260
Pressure
 receptors, 195
 testing perception of, 197
Presynaptic membranes, 5
Priapism, 120
Procaine, 12
Projection fibres, 39
Projector neurons, 3
Propionic acidaemia, 219
Propranolol, 14, 114
Proprioception, 161, 195
 ascending pathways, 197–8
 vertigo and, 155
Proprioceptors, 5, 194
Proptosis, 67, 138
α-Propyldopacetamide, 106
Propylphosphofluoridate, 14
Prosencephalon (forebrain vesicle), 24, 25, 26, 28
Prostaglandins, 18, 195, 209
Protein–calorie malnutrition, 217, 229
Proteins, 217–18
 in cerebrospinal fluid, 239, 242
 disorders of metabolism of, 217–18
 transport in neurons, 3, 217
Pseudoathetosis, 203
Pseudobulbar palsy, 76, 173
Pseudodementia, 110
Pseudopapilloedema, 136
Pseudotumour cerebri, 248
Psychiatric disorders, see Mental disorders
Psychogenic headache, 207
Psychogenic unresponsiveness, 89
Psychopathy, 107
Psychoses, 107
 post-traumatic, 251
 symptomatic, 90
Ptosis, 121, 137, 137–8, 141
Pulmonary insufficiency, chronic, 89, 227
'Punch-drunkenness' in boxers, 251
Punishment centres, 101
Pupils, 88, 136–7
 examination of, 67
 myotonic (Adie's/Holmes–Adie syndrome), 121, 137
 reflex pathways controlling, 133, 136–7
Purkinje cells, 2, 39, 40–1, 164, 214
Purkinje shift, 131, 132
Putamen, 35, 36, 162
Pyramidal cells, 2, 37
Pyramidal tract, see Corticospinal tract
Pyridostigmine, 14
Pyridoxine deficiency, 91, 229, 230–1
Pyruvic acidaemia, 220

Quadrigemina, superior corpora, 133, 134
Quadriplegia, 63, 174
Queckenstedt's test, 240

Radial jerk reflex, 69, 179
Radial nerve, 173, 176
Radiation injury, 228
Radiology, 256–72
Raeder's paratrigeminal syndrome, 121
Ramsay Hunt syndrome, 170
Ranitidine, 14
Receptors, 5, 12
Recovery potentials, 186
Red nucleus of midbrain, 41, 161, 162
Reflexes, 179–80
 autonomic, 120–1
 cutaneous or superficial, 70, 180
 H and F, 189
 in lower and upper motor neuron lesions, 181–2
 monosynaptic spinal, 168–9, 179
 multisynaptic, 179
 ocular movement, 67, 88, 133, 142–3
 primitive infantile, 69, 180
 pupillary, 133, 136–7
 stretch, 168–9, 179
 tendon, see Tendon reflexes
Refractory period, 9
Refsum's disease, 221, 222
Reissner's membrane, 145
Remak cells, 3
Renal failure, uraemic encephalopathy in, 89, 225
Reserpine, 13, 16, 84, 106, 163
Respiration
 apneustic, 88, 246
 ataxic, 88, 246
 autonomous, 88
 Cheyne–Stokes, 88, 246
 in chronic hypercapnia, 227
 pH of cerebrospinal fluid (CSF), 243
Respiratory centre, 41, 227
Respiratory insufficiency, chronic, 89, 227
Resting potential, 8
Reticular activating system, 82, 83, 249
Reticular formation, 39, 41, 82, 83
Reticulospinal tract, 161, 163, 176–7
Retina
 detachment of, 135
 function, 129–31
 structure, 128–9, 132
 vascular changes, 136
Retinal angiomas, 136
Retinal tubercles, 136
Retinitis pigmentosa, 128, 136
Retinol, see Vitamin A
Retinopathy, grades of, 136
Retrobulbar neuritis, 133–4, 135, 136
Retrograde axoplasmic transport, 3
Retro-orbital tumours, 134
Reward centres, 101
Rhesus group incompatibility, kernicterus in, 225
Rhinencephalon, 36
Rhodopsin, 128, 131
Rhombencephalon (hindbrain vesicle), 24, 25, 26
Right–left disorientation, 65
Rigidity, 69, 163, 176, 177
Riley–Day syndrome (familial dysautonomia), 122
Rinne's test, 150–1
RNA, role in memory storage, 103
Rods, retinal, 128, 129, 130
Romberg's sign, 203
Roof nuclei, 38
Rubrospinal tract, 161
Ruffini sensory endings, 195

Saccule, 145, 146, 152

Sacral nerves (nervi erigentes), 119
Salbutamol, 14
Salicylate intoxication, 89
Salivatory nuclei, 117, 118
Saltatory conduction, 4, 8
Sandhoff's disease, 220
Sanfilippo's disease, 216
Sarcoidosis, cerebrospinal fluid in, 242, 243
Sarcomere, 166, 167
Saxitoxin, 12–15, 236–7
Scarpa's ganglion, 152
Schizoid personality, 107
Schizophrenia, 106, 107, 243
Schonell's 'reading age', 107
Schwann cells, 3, 50
Sciatic nerve, 175, 176
Scoliosis, 21
Scopolamine, 15
Scotomas, 66, 133–4
Scotopic luminosity curve, 131, 132
Second cranial nerve, see Optic nerve
Sedative drugs, 234
Seizures, see Convulsions; Epilepsy
Selegiline, 14
Sella turcica, 20, 245–6, 257
Semicircular canals, 145, 146, 152
 caloric stimulation of, 144, 153
 paresis, 153, 154
Senile argyrophilic plaques, 55, 56
Senile dementia, 55
Senile tremor, 183
Sensation
 affective responses to, 196, 199–200
 conscious awareness, 194
 parameters of, 195–6
 types of, 197
 see also Pain; Position sense; Proprioception; Tactile discrimination, Thermal sensation; Touch; Vibration sense
Sensation–stimulus intensity, relationship between (Weber–Fechner law), 125, 196
Senses, special, see Specific senses e.g. Hearing; Smell; Vision
Sensory ataxia, 68, 178, 203
Sensory cortex, 199, 200
 lesions, 203, 205
Sensory disorders
 pathophysiology and clinical significance of, 182, 203–5
 types of, 201–3
 see also Dysaesthesiae; Pain; Paraesthesiae
Sensory evoked potentials, 37, 189
Sensory fibres, types of, 197
Sensory inattention, 70, 79, 203
Sensory nerves
 conduction velocity, 189, 190
 lesions, 123, 204, 211
 studies of function, 189
Sensory neurons, 3, 197
Sensory neuropathy, 184, 204, 232
Sensory receptors, 5, 12, 194–5
 in muscles, 167–9, 195
 phasic, 12, 196
 tonic, 12, 167
Sensory system, 194–211
 anatomical pathways, 49, 197–200
 assessment of function, 70, 120, 196–7
 cutaneous segmentation, 200–1
 sensory parameters, 195–6
Serotonin, see 5-Hydroxytryptamine
Seventh nerve, see Facial nerve
Sexual activity, autonomic control of, 113, 119–20
Sexual development
 impaired, 123
 precocious, 120
Sexuality, excessive, 120

Shoulder–hand syndrome, 123
Shy–Drager syndrome, 97, 122
Sialidoses, types 1 and 2, 218, 221
Sinus thrombosis, see Venous sinus thrombosis
Sixth cranial nerve, see Abducens nerve
Skeleton, examination of, 65
Skin
 changes in coma, 88
 pain sensation in, 207
 sensory receptors in, 5, 194–5
 sensory segmental areas, 200–1, 202
Skull
 basilar impression of, 20, 257
 'crack-pot' sound, 246
 development and morphology, 20
 examination, 65
 fractures, 248, 250, 252
 hyperostosis of, 20, 257
 radiography, 256–8
Sleep, 83–6
 apnoea, 85–6
 disorders, 84–6, 123
 paralysis, 84–5
 rapid eye movement (REM) or paradoxical, 83
Sleep-promoting substance (SPS), 84
Sleep-walking, 85
Smell, sense of, 65–6, 125–6
Snake venoms, 237
Snellen's test types, 66
Snout reflex, 69
Sodium (Na^+)
 extracellular levels, 214
 membrane channels, 8, 12–15, 131
Somnambulism, 85
Sound, 145
 conduction in the ear, 148
 intensity of, 144, 145
 localization by ears, 150
Space-occupying lesions, intracranial, see Intracranial space-occupying lesions
Spasmodic torticollis, 184
Spastic paraparesis, 68, 122, 232
Spastic paraplegia, 181, 252
 West Indian and South Indian, 230
Spasticity, 69, 176, 177, 181, 232
Speech
 assessment, 65
 control of, 36, 72–3
 disorders, 73–8
 in childhood, 77–8
 see also Specific disorders e.g. Aphasia; Dysarthria
Sphenopalatine ganglion, 117, 118
Sphingolipids, 218
Sphingomyelin, 218, 222
Spina bifida, 20–1, 23, 254
Spinal accessory nerve (cranial nerve XI), 42, 47, 68, 171, 176
Spinal canal, 21, 261
Spinal column
 development and morphology, 20–1
 fracture–dislocation, 252, 253
 pain in, 210–11
 radiography of, 261, 264
Spinal cord
 blood supply, 32–3
 central canal, 25–6
 compression, 253
 cerebrospinal fluid in, 242
 imaging techniques, 264–6, 269–71
 contusion, 252
 development and growth, 23–4, 25
 general morphology 46–7, 48
 hemisection (Brown–Séquard syndrome), 204, 253

Index

injury, 252–3
 aetiology, 252
 clinical features, 252–3
 pathology, 252
 ischaemia and/or infarction, 32
 meninges around, 22
 motor pathways, 49, 160–1, 164, 172
 segmental organization, 46, 47, 169, 172, 200–1
 sensory pathways, 49, 197–8, 199
 subacute combined degeneration, 204, 231–2
 see also Syringomyelia
Spinal cord angiography, 271
Spinal cord lesions, 181, 184, 252–3
 autonomic effects, 119, 121–2
 Horner's syndrome, 121
 pain in, 210
 reflexes in, 180
 sensory impairment in, 202, 204–5
 sexual function in, 120
Spinal ganglia, 47, 116
Spinal interneurons, see Interneurons, spinal
Spinal muscular atrophy, 182, 184
Spinal nerves, 47, 48, 169, 172, 200–1
Spinal reflexes, monosynaptic, 168–9, 179
Spinocerebellar tracts, 163
Spinothalamic tracts, 198, 199, 202
Splanchnic nerves, 116, 118
Spondylosis, 261, 270, 271
Spongioblasts, 23
Squint (strabismus), 139–40, 141
 concomitant, 139
 latent concomitant, 139–40
 paralytic, 139
Stammering, 78
Stapedius muscle, 145
Status lacunosus, 61
Steele–Richardson–Olszewski syndrome, 141
Stellate cells, 2, 37
 cerebellar, 40, 41
Stellate ganglion, 116
Stereoanaesthesia, 203
Sternomastoid muscle, paralysis of, 171
Steroids in cerebral oedema, 248
Strabismus, see Squint
Streptomycin, deafness caused by, 151
Striate (visual) cortex, 34, 35, 37, 133
Striatonigral degeneration, 122
Strychnine, 18
Stupor, 86
 catatonic, 89
 common causes, 87
 diagnosis, 88–9
 in head injured patients, 250
 postepileptic, 87, 95
Sturge–Weber syndrome, 258
Subacute combined degeneration of the cord, 204, 231–2
Subacute necrotizing encephalomyelopathy (Leigh's disease), 215
Subacute sclerosing panencephalitis, 242, 255
Subarachnoid haemorrhage, 60, 123, 250, 264
 cerebrospinal fluid in, 241, 242
 coma in, 88
 lumbar puncture in, 240
 retinal changes, 136
Subarachnoid space, 22
'Subclavian steal', 27
Subdural haematoma, 88, 250, 260, 267
Subdural haemorrhage, 250, 264
Subdural hygroma, 249
Subdural space, 22

Subfalcial herniation of cingulate gyrus, 87, 244, 245, 246
Subhyaloid haemorrhage, 136
Submandibular ganglion, 118
Submaxillary ganglion, 117
Substance P, 17, 195, 207
Substantia gelatinosa, 49, 194, 195, 197, 206
Substantia nigra, 41, 162, 163
Subthalamic nucleus, 162
Sucking reflex, 69
Sudeck's atrophy, 123
Sulci, 34
Sulcus limitans, 23, 25
Sulphatide lipidosis (metachromatic leucodystrophy), 218, 221, 222
Sulpiride, 14
Superior corpora quadrigemina, 133, 134
Sural nerve biopsy, 254
Suxamethonium, 15, 167
Sweating
 excessive, 122, 123
 gustatory, 121, 170
 loss of, 120, 121, 137
Sydenham's chorea, 183
Sympathetic chain, 115, 116, 117
Sympathetic nervous system, 112, 113
 anatomy, 116–17
 bladder and bowel function and, 119
 control of pupillary dilatation, 136, 137
 eyelid innervation, 137–8
 ganglia, 47, 115, 116–17
Sympathomimetic drugs, 13, 14, 114
Synapses, 1, 4–5
 chemical transmission, 4–5, 15–19
 electrical, 5, 10
 formation and development, 24
 neuronal degeneration across (transneuronal), 57
 transmission across, 4–5, 10–12
 see also Neurotransmitters
Syncope, 96–7, 98
Syphilis, 58
 cerebrospinal fluid (CSF), 242, 243
 optic atrophy, 135, 136
 pupillary reflexes in, 137
 see also General paresis; Tabes dorsalis
Syringobulbia, sensory impairment of, 205
Syringomyelia, 26, 247, 253, 261
 myelography in, 270, 271
 sensory impairment in, 204–5
 traumatic ascending, 252
Systemic lupus erythematosus, 58–9, 192

Tabes dorsalis, 58, 60
 Argyll Robertson pupil, 137
 cerebrospinal fluid (CSF) in, 242
 sensory impairment in, 204
Tactile agnosia (astereognosis), 79, 203
Tactile discrimination, 70, 196, 197, 198, 203
 ascending pathways, 197–8, 199
Tactile inattention, 70, 79, 203
Tangier disease, 221, 222
Tarichotoxin, 12
Taste, sense of, 66, 125, 126–7
Tay–Sachs disease, 136, 220
Tegmental tract, central, 46
Telencephalon, 24, 25
Telodendria, 3, 4
Temperature sensation, see Thermal sensation
Temporal cortex, medial 36
Temporal lobe, 34

lesions, 103, 105, 151, 153
 tentorial herniation, 244, 245, 246–7, 251
Temporal lobe epilepsy (complex partial), 93, 94, 96, 105, 254, 255
Tendon organs, Golgi, 167–9, 195
Tendon reflexes, 168–9
 in disease, 175–6, 177, 179–80, 181, 186
 examination of, 69–70, 179
Tensilon, 191
Tensor tympani muscle, 145
Tenth nerve, see Vagus nerve
Tentorial herniation, 244, 245, 246–7, 251
Tentorium cerebelli, 21, 38
Tetanus toxin, 18, 236
Tetany, 98, 226
Tetrabenazine, 106
Tetraethylammonium ions, 15
Tetraplegia, 63, 174
Tetrodotoxin, 9, 12, 14
Thalamic pain, 201–2, 211
Thalamus, 35, 36
 behavioural functions, 100, 101, 104
 connecting pathways, 99–100, 198–200
 lesions, sensory impairment in, 205
 motor functions, 161, 162, 163
 reticular activating system, 41, 82, 83
 sensory pathways, 198–200
Thallium poisoning, 236
Thermal sensation
 ascending pathways, 198, 199
 testing, 70, 197
Thermoreceptors, 195
Thermoregulation, 123
Thiamine deficiency, see Vitamin B₁ deficiency
Thioxanthenes, 14, 16
Third nerve, see Oculomotor nerve
Thomsen's disease, 185
Thoracic sympathetic ganglia, 116, 118
Thought, processes of, 72–3
Thrombosis
 cerebral, coma in, 88
 intracranial venous sinus, 32, 242, 248
Thyrotoxicosis (Graves' disease), 138, 183, 226
 myopathy, 192, 226
 ophthalmic, 138, 226
Tibial nerve, 175, 176
Tic (habit spasm), 182
Tic douloureux (trigeminal neuralgia), 209–10
Tinel's sign, 203
Tinnitus, 151–2
Tobacco amblyopia, 134, 230
Todd's paralysis, 95
Tolosa–Hunt syndrome, 141
Tongue, lesions affecting, 171–2
Tonic neck reflexes, 69, 180
Tonic seizures, 94
Tonic sensory receptors, 12, 167
Tonsillar herniation, see Cerebellar tonsillar herniation
Torsion spasm, 183–4
Torticollis, spasmodic, 184
Touch
 ascending pathways, 197–8, 199
 impaired appreciation of, 203
 receptors, 195
 testing perception of, 70, 197
Toxic disorders, 236–7
Toxic encephalopathy, 236
Toxic hydrocephalus, 248
Toxoplasmosis, 258
Trauma
 craniocerebral, see Head injury
 pathological responses to, 58
Traumatic cerebral compression, acute, 251

Traumatic encephalopathy, 250–1
 chronic ('punch-drunkenness'), 251
Tremor, 182–3
 benign familial or essential, 183
 in hepatic disease, 183, 224
 intention, 178–9, 183
 in parkinsonism, 183
 senile, 183
Triceps jerk reflex, 68, 179
Trichopoliodystrophy (Menkes' kinky hair disease), 223
Tricyclic antidepressants, 17, 105–6
Trigeminal nerve (cranial nerve V), 41–2, 252
 lesions, facial pain in, 209
 motor function, 68, 169
 sensory pathways, 198, 201
Trigeminal neuralgia (tic douloureux), 209–10
Trochlear nerve (cranial nerve IV), 125, 138, 139
 palsy, 141
Tropical ataxic neuropathy, 230
Trunk muscles, innervation of, 172, 176
Tryptophan, 105, 106
Tuberculosis, retinal tubercles, 136
Tuberculous meningitis, 59, 242, 243
Tuberous sclerosis, 136
Tubocurarine, 15, 167
Tumours of the nervous system, 59–60
 see also Specific types of tumours
Twelfth cranial nerve, see Hypoglossal nerve
Two-point discrimination, see Tactile discrimination
Tyramine, 13
Tyrosinaemia, hereditary, 220

U-fibres, 37
Ulnar nerve, 174, 176
 conduction velocity, 189
 evoked motor action potentials, 189–91
 lesions, sensory loss in, 204
Ultrasonic imaging, 31, 256
Uncal herniation, 87
Uncus, lesions of, 127
Unmyelinated neurons, 3, 4
Uraemic encephalopathy, 89, 225
Urine, retention of, 121, 122
Utricle, 145, 146, 152

Vagus nerve (cranial nerve X), 42, 170–1
 autonomic function, 117–19, 121
 motor function, 68, 170–1
Vallecula, 38
Valsalva's manoeuvre, 120–1
Vascular lesions, 60–1
 granulomatous, 58–9
 headache in, 209
 imaging techniques, 31, 256, 264, 267–8, 271
 local tissue anoxia in, 227
 retinal, 136
 in spinal cord, 32, 271
 see also Cerebral infarction; Cerebrovascular disease
Vasoconstriction reflex, 120
Vasodilatation reflexes, 120
Vasovagal attacks, 97
Vegetative state, persistent, 249, 251
Veins
 cerebral, 32, 33
 spinal cord, 32–3
Venography, extradural, 271
Venous sinus thrombosis, 32, 242, 248
Venous sinuses, cerebral, 32, 33
Ventricular puncture, 241

Ventricular system, 25–6, 28
  pneumoencephalography, 265, 266
Ventriculography, 247, 256, 261, 264, 265, 266, 268
Vermis, 38, 39
Vertebrae, development and morphology, 20–1
Vertebral angiography, 261, 264, 266, 267, 268
Vertebral arteries, 26–7
Vertigo, 67, 153, 155–6
  acute labryinthine, 144, 155–6
  in benign positional nystagmus, 155, 156
  post-traumatic, 156, 251
  recurrent aural (Ménière's disease), 151, 153, 154, 156
Vestibular nerve, 67, 152
  lesions, 155, 178
Vestibular neuronitis, 153
  'acute', 155–6
Vestibular nuclei, 152, 161, 163
Vestibular system, 142, 152–6
  assessment of function, 67, 153–5
  disorders, 155–6
  see also Vertigo
  function, 125, 142, 153
  structure, 152–3
Vestibular tracts, 163

Vestibule, 145, 146
Vestibulospinal tracts, 152, 161
Vibration sense, 196
  ascending pathways, 197–8
  testing, 70, 197
Vincristine, 217
Violent behaviour, 108
Virchow–Robin spaces, 22
Virus infections, cerebrospinal fluid (CSF) in, 242, 243
Viruses, neurotropic, 58
Visceral sensation, 117, 122, 194, 196
  referral of, 122, 207
Vision, 125, 127–44
  assessment, 66–7, 131–2
  colour, 66, 132–3
  critical fusion frequency, 132
  nervous pathways, 133, 134
  optical defects of, 127–8
  tubular, 135
  see also Eyes; Ocular movements; Optic nerve; Retina
Visual acuity, 66, 131–2, 133
Visual agnosia, 79
Visual aphasia, 75
Visual asymbolia, 75
Visual cortex, see Striate cortex
Visual fields, 133–5
  defects in migraine, 209

  erroneous projection of, 140–1
  testing, 66
Visual inattention, 79–80
Vitamin A (retinol), 129–31
  deficiency, 131, 229
  excess, 229
Vitamin B$_1$ (thiamine) deficiency, 107–8, 215, 228–9
Vitamin B$_6$ deficiency, see Pyridoxine deficiency
Vitamin B$_{12}$ deficiency, 61, 134, 230, 231, 232
  neuropathy (subacute combined degeneration of the cord), 204, 231–2
Vitamin D
  deficiency, 229
  excess, 229
Vitamin deficiencies, 228–32
Vitamin E deficiency, 232
Vocal cords, paralysis of, 171, 172
Voltage–clamp technique, 9–10
Vomiting centre, 41
Vomiting in raised intracranial pressure, 246
von Frey hairs, 197
von Hippel–Lindau disease, 136

Wallerian degeneration, 56
Water intoxication, 89, 225, 226

Weakness, muscular, 158, 172–4, 181, 185
Weber–Fechner law, 125, 196
Weber's test, 150
Wechsler intelligence scales (WISC and WAIS), 107
Wernicke–Korsakov syndrome, see Korsakov syndrome
Wernicke's area, 73, 74, 75
Wernicke's encephalopathy, 229, 233
West Indian spastic paraplegia, 230
Willis, circle of, 26, 27
Wilson's disease (hepatolenticular degeneration), 61, 183, 223
Wolman's disease, 221
Word blindness, 74
  cortical, 75
  pure subcortical, 75
Word deafness, 74
  congenital, 78

X-linked disorders, 61
Xanthochromia of cerebrospinal fluid, 241
Xanthomatoses, 221

Young–Helmholtz theory of colour vision, 132–3

Zimelidine, 13